AF678979

Color Atlas of
LENS IMPLANTATION

Editor

S.P.B. Percival
MA, MB, B Chir, FRCS, FCOphth, DO
Department of Ophthalmology
Scarborough District Hospital
Yorkshire
United Kingdom

Mosby Year Book

St. Louis Baltimore Boston Chicago London Philadelphia Sydney Toronto

Mosby
Year Book
Dedicated to Publishing Excellence

Mosby–Year Book, Inc.
11830 Westline Drive
St. Louis, MO 63146

Copyright © S.P.B. Percival, 1991
All rights reserved.
Published with rights in the USA, Canada and Puerto Rico by Mosby–Year Book, Inc.
A Year Book Medical Publishers imprint of Mosby–Year Book, Inc.
ISBN 0-8151-6664-8

English edition first published by Wolfe Publishing Ltd,
2–16 Torrington Place, London WC1E 7LT, UK.

All rights reserved. No part of this publication may be reproduced, stored in a retrieval system, or transmitted, in any form or by any means, electronic, mechanical, photocopying, recording, or otherwise, without written permission from the publisher.

Permission to photocopy or reproduce solely for internal or personal use is permitted for libraries or other users registered with the Copyright Clearance Center, provided that the base fee of $4.00 per chapter plus $.10 per page is paid directly to the Copyright Clearance Center, 21 Congress Street, Salem, MA 01970. This consent does not extend to other kinds of copying, such as copying for general distribution, for advertising or promotional purposes, for creating new collected works, or for resale.

Contents

Foreword

As the population of the world grows and social conditions improve, many more people reach advanced age and so may become victims of degenerative disorders, of which senile cataract is probably the most common and certainly the most disabling. Fortunately, its effects are now almost completely remediable.

In the past 40 years it has proved possible, after a cataract extraction, to restore the optical system within the eye by implanting an artificial lens, which in some respects is actually superior to a natural lens because it provides better light transmission and colour vision. We no longer tell the patient that the cataract needs removal, but instead that the eye requires a new lens, which will provide a second 'lease' of almost natural sight.

Half-a-century ago cataract surgery was a difficult and hazardous procedure requiring a high degree of skill and, for the patient, two weeks in hospital lying perfectly still. Now, with improved anesthesia, pharmaceutical control of inflammation and infection and a new generation of surgical instruments with, not least, efficient operating microscopes, excellent results have been brought within the reach of every well-equipped ophthalmic surgeon. Furthermore, modern cataract surgery now requires only a day in hospital or can sometimes be undertaken as an out-patient procedure.

Now that, it is said, over 10 million lens implants have been inserted, many patients with developing cataract have learned of this revolution in surgery, which now produces such quick and vastly improved results. The almost instant restoration of natural sight has produced it's own problems for it has led to a demand for cataract surgery which, throughout the world, is insatiable.

This book sets out to describe just how far ophthalmic surgery has now progressed in its efforts to restore, safely and consistently, sight of the highest quality to millions throughout the world. It also discusses the complications and problems that pose a challenge, for nothing stands still, especially in ophthalmology. What better teachers can we have than the active surgeons at work each day in many different countries, who are themselves deeply committed to the better relief of the most common and crippling penalty of advancing age?

HAROLD RIDLEY

Preface

In 1972 approximately 1000 lens implantation operations were performed worldwide. By 1982 the annual rate had reached 1,000,000, half of which were in North America. The annual rate is now over three million, and by 1992 should have trebled again, such is the explosion in this fascinating field of medicine. Cataract extraction has always been the most common major surgical operation and, with 30 million sufferers in the Indian sub-continent alone, there is clearly much to be done in the expansion of surgical training. However, lens implantation has brought a need for changes in technique. The patients' expectations and the visual prognosis can now be so much better when advanced methods are used that everywhere on Earth should be expected to benefit from these changes. Eye surgeons the world over are now anxious to appraise their work and learn the techniques that can ensure safety for their patients, whether by using the more traditional methods or the new intercapsular methods, whereby virtually all the surgery is carried out inside the membrane that encapsulates the cataract, so affording greater protection to the delicate tissues inside the eye and greater stability for the lens implanted. Perfection may be heightened by the new method of circular capsulorhexis.

The purpose of this book is to explain in pictorial form the options now available, the reasoning behind change and the management of problems and complications. Simple maneuvers are preferred to the complicated, thereby encouraging the trainee and facilitating an easy transition for those experienced surgeons now changing from the intracapsular to intercapsular approach or phacoemulsification.

It is a book for experts wishing to enhance their skills with the very latest information, for example in histopathology, endophacoemulsification, implant design and scleral fixation, as well as a guide for those just beginning in this new and exciting field.

Finally, any success of this Atlas will be due to the dedication of the contributors, leading exponents of lens implantation from all over the world, who, with their associates, secretaries and photographers, have combined to provide a comprehensive account of one of the most fascinating subjects in modern medicine. I most sincerely thank each and every one. For the readers, I can do no better than to wish them a 'lift' towards new horizons in their approach to help those who cannot see.

PIERS PERCIVAL

Acknowledgements

I am very deeply grateful to Mrs. Verne Wright for her immense help in ensuring that communications with the contributors were successfully completed and for retyping many of the manuscripts before presentation to the publishers. I also thank R. Bijster, L.I. Los and A.M. Worst van Dam (Chapter 13), and Emily Hindman (Chapter 36) for their help in preparing manuscripts for individual chapters. Much of the information concerning the blindness problem in Kenya was supplied by Dr Randy Whitfield (Chapter 47), for which I am grateful.

For illustrations I am indebted to numerous colleagues, photographers and artists, who have helped to supply the contributing authors with up-to-date material, and must acknowledge, in particular, Krystina Strodulski of The Center for Intraocular Lens Research, Charleston, South Carolina (Front cover, **36.32**), T. Mole of Southampton Eye Hospital (Chapters 3 and 12), W. Velt for the drawings in Chapter 13, Sue Ford of the Western Ophthalmic Hospital (**16.30, 16.31, 23.21**), Calver Townsend of the Western Ophthalmic Hospital (**16.30, 16.31**), Zvi Friedman of the Goldschleger Eye Institute (Chapter 19), Sandra Brown, RN, and Catherine Barry of The Medical University of South Carolina (Chapter 36), Rayner Intraocular Lenses Ltd (**12.1, 12.3, 17.2, 32.7, 32.8, 32.10**), Allergan Medical Optics (**19.6**), Alcon Ltd. (**19.9, 19.10, 20.1**), Pharmacia Ophthalmics (**21.2**), Iolab Corporation (**21.1, 32.5**), Rodenstock Ltd (**44.2**), Sigmacon Ltd (**44.3**), as well as the authors and publishers of various books and journals in giving ideas or permission for reproduction, including *The American Journal of Ophthalmology* (**10.4, 10.5, 15.1, 41.9, 41.10, 41.19**), *Archives of Ophthalmology* (**15.22**), *Highlights of Ophthalmology* (**44.4**), *Implants in Ophthalmology* (**19.1–19.5, 27.2, 27.4, 46.1–46.8, 46.10, 46.11**) and *Intraocular Lenses; Evolution, Designs, Complications and Pathology* Williams and Wilkins (**25.1, 36.1, 36.3, 36.4, 36.9, 36.11, 36.14, 36.17, 36.28–36.31**), and *Ocular Surgery News* (**27.8, 27.9**).

The line illustrations not listed above were drawn by Joanna Cameron and Gill Ellsbury.

PIERS PERCIVAL

Contributors

Mr Michael Absolon, FRCS, FCOphth,
Southampton Eye Hospital,
Wilton Avenue,
Southampton SO9 4XW,
England

Dr Peter J. Agapitos, MD, FRCS(C),
Assistant Professor of Ophthalmology,
University of Minnesota,
Department of Ophthalmology,
Ramsey Clinic and St Paul-Ramsey Medical Center,
St Paul, Minnesota,
United States of America

Prof. John Alpar, MD,
St Luke Eye Institute,
5311 West 9th Avenue,
Amarillo, Texas,
United States of America

Dr Aziz Y Anis, MD FACS,
The Anis Eye Institute,
1919 South 40th Street, Suite 206,
Lincoln, Nebraska 65806,
United States of America

Prof. David Apple, MD,
Department of Ophthalmology,
Medical University of South Carolina,
171 Ashley Avenue,
Charleston, South Carolina 29425,
United States of America

Mr Eric J. Arnott, FRCS,
11 Milford House,
7 Queen Anne Street,
London W1N 9FD,
England

Prof. Danièle Aron Rosa, MD,
The Rothschild Eye Institute,
25 Rue Manin,
75019 Paris,
France

Prof. Georges Baikoff, MD,
Centre d'Ophthalmologie,
Clairval-Saugeaie,
36 Boulevard du Redon,
13009 Marseille,
France

Dr Graham Barrett, MD,
Lions Eye Institute,
2 Verdun Street,
Perth 6009,
Australia

Prof. Michael Blumenthal, MD,
Goldschleger Eye Institute,
Sackler School of Medicine,
Tel Aviv University,
Tel Aviv,
Israel

Mr Tom Casey, FRCS,
Queen Victoria Hospital,
East Grinstead,
Sussex,
England

Dr Varda Chen, MD,
Goldschleger Eye Institute,
Sackler School of Medicine,
Tel Aviv University,
Tel Aviv.
Israel

Mr D. Peter Choyce, MS, FRCS, FCOphth,
9 Drake Road,
Westcliff-on-Sea,
Essex SS0 8LR,
England

Dr Patrick I. Condon, FRCS,
Regional Eye Department,
Ardkeen Hospital,
Waterford,
Ireland

Prof. Ulrich Demeler, MD,
Eye Department,
Augenklinik Zentralkrankenhaus,
St-Juergen-Strasse,
D-2800 Bremen 1,
Federal Republic of Germany

Prof. Robert C. Drews, MD,
Washington University School of Medicine,
211 North Merame Avenue,
Clayton, Missouri 63105,
United States of America

Dr Richard J. Duffey, MD,
The Mobile Eye, Ear, Nose and Throat Center,
2880 Dauphin Street,
Mobile, Alabama,
United States of America

Dr John Dunphy, FFARCS,
Regional Eye Department,
Ardkeen Hospital,
Waterford,
Ireland

Dr Henry F. Edelhauser, PhD,
Emory University Eye Center,
1327 Clifton Road NE,
Atlanta, Georgia 30322,
United States of America

Dr Richard Erdey, MD,
Rochester Eye Institute,
Rochester,
New York,
United States of America

Dr Albert Galand, MD,
Centre Hospitalier Universitaire et Clinique Sainte Rosalie,
Rue des Wallons 72,
B-4000 Liège,
Belgium

Mr Michael Hayward, FRCS,
Leeds General Infirmary,
Great George Street,
Leeds LS1 3EX,
England

Prof. David A. Hiles, MD,
3518 Fifth Avenue,
Pittsburgh, Pennsylvania 15213,
United States of America

Prof. Richard H. Keates, MD,
Professor and Chair,
Department of Ophthalmology,
University of California,
Irvine, California 92717,
United States of America

Dr Manus C. Kraff, MD,
Northwestern University,
JFK Eye Institute,
5600 W. Addison St, 4th Fl,
Illinois 60634,
United States of America

Dr Marvin L. Kwitko, MD,
Assistant Professor of Ophthalmology,
McGill University,
5591 Cote des Neiges Road,
Montreal, Quebec H3T 1Y8,
Canada

Mr Arthur Lim, FRCS,
Chief, Dept of Ophthalmology,
National University Hospital,
Lower Kent Ridge Road,
Singapore 0511

Dr Richard L. Lindstrom, MD,
Clinical Professor of Ophthalmology,
University of Minnesota,
Attending Surgeon, Philips Eye Institute and Veteran's Administration Medical Center,
Minneapolis, Minnesota,
United States of America

Dr Ole J. Lorenzetti, PhD,
University Texas South Western,
1945 Berkley Place,
Fort Worth, Texas 76110,
United States of America

Dr Kensaku Miyake, MD,
Shohzankai Medical Foundation,
Miyake Eye Hospital,
1070 Kami 5,
Higashiozone-Cho Kita-Ku,
J-462 Nagoya,
Japan

Dr Robin Morgan, MD,
Department of Ophthalmology,
Medical University of South Carolina,
171 Ashley Avenue,
Charleston, South Carolina 29425,
United States of America

Dr Cosme I.N. Naval, MD,
61 Buchanan Street,
North Greenhills,
San Juan,
Metro Manila,
Philippines

Mr Bruce A. Noble, FRCS,
Consultant Ophthalmic Surgeon,
Leeds General Infirmary
Great George Street,
Leeds LS1 3EX
England

Dr Terry O'Brien, MD,
The Wilmer Ophthalmological Institute,
The Johns Hopkins University School of Medicine,
The Johns Hopkins Hospital,
601 N. Broadway,
Baltimore, Maryland 21205,
United States of America

Dr Stephen Obstbaum, MD,
Department of Ophthalmology,
Lenox Hill Hospital,
100 East 77th Street,
New York, New York 10021,
United States of America

Dr Robert Osher, MD,
Cincinnati Eye Institute,
10494 Montgomery Road,
Cincinnati, Ohio 45242,
United States of America

Mr John Pearce, ChM, DO, FCOphth,
2 Windsor Street,
Bromsgrove,
Worcestershire B60 2BG,
England

Mr Clive Peckar, MSc, FRCS, FCOphth,
Warrington District Hospital,
Lovely Lane,
Warrington,
Cheshire WA5Y 1QG,
England

Mr Piers Percival, FRCS
Scarborough Hospital,
Scarborough,
North Yorkshire YO12 6QL,
England

Dr John Retzlaff, MD
91 Black Oak Drive,
Medford,
Oregon 97504,
United States of America

Mr Emanuel Rosen, MD, FRCS(E),
10 St John Street,
Manchester M3 4DY,
England

Dr Donald R. Sanders, MD, PhD,
University of Illinois at Chicago,
Center for Clinical Research,
815 W. Van Buren St, Suite 300,
Chicago, Illinois 60607,
United States of America

Dr C. William Simcoe, MD, PC,
Utica Square Medical Building,
Suite 110,
Tulsa, Oklahoma 74114,
United States of America

Dr William Smiddy, MD,
Boscom Palmer Eye Institute,
University of Miami School of Medicine,
P.O. Box 016880,
Miami, Florida 33101,
United States of America

Dr Leon D. Solomon, MD, FRCS(C),
Assitant Professor
McGill University, Montreal,
5775 Cote des Neiges Road 107,
Montreal, Quebec H3S 2S9,
Canada

Prof. Walter Stark, MD,
John Hopkins Hospital,
No 100 Baltimore,
Maryland 21205,
United States of America

Prof. Ahti Tarkkanen, MD,
Helsinki University Eye Hospital,
Haarthaninkatu 4,
SF-00290 Helsinki,
Finland

Dr Spencer P. Thornton, MD, FACS,
Department of Ophthalmology,
Baptist Hospital,
2010 Church Street, Suite 207,
Nashville, Tennessee 37203,
United States of America

Dr Julie Tsai, MD,
Department of Ophthalmology,
Medical University of South Carolina,
171 Ashley Avenue,
Charleston, South Carolina 29425,
United States of America

Dr Daniel Vörösmarthy, MD,
Head of Department of Ophthalmology,
Semmel Weiss Hospital,
1085 Budapest,
Gyulai Pal u 2,
Hungary

Mr Hugh Williams, FRCS,
5 Harmont House,
20 Harley Street,
London W1N 1AL,
England

Dr Mark Wood, DO, FRCS(C),
Consultant Ophthalmologist,
Presbyterian Church of East Africa
Kikuyu Hospital Eye Department,
P.O. Box 45,
Kikuyu,
Kenya

Dr Jan G.F. Worst, MD,
Refaja Hospital Stadskanaal,
Julianalaan 11,
97510 BM Haren,
The Netherlands

Dr Akio Yamanaka, MD,
Kobe Kaisei Hospital,
11–15 Shinihara-Kitamachi,
3 Chome,
Nada-Ku,
Kobe 657,
Japan

Dr Ralph Zabel, MD,
Department of Ophthalmology,
9-240 Health Sciences Unit C,
Box 493 UMHC,
516 Delaware Street SE,
Minneapolis, Minnesota 55455,
United States of America

Dedication

To my family,
and to the International Friendship
of Ophthalmic Surgeons

Section 1:
EXTRACTION OF CATARACT

1: Basic concepts and evolution

Aziz Anis

Our concept of any object of matter or mind depends on the diligence of our research, our background information, our faculties of deduction and our personal convictions and philosophies. All these factors are variable and thus concepts of the same object of interest can be differently perceived by different individuals.

It is not unusual, however, for a large number of individuals working in the same field to come up with similar concepts of the same object, thus establishing a basic concept but sometimes erroneously considering it to be a fact.

The point is that our so-called basic concepts are directly related to our times and the intellectual plane in which we function. We should always, therefore, be sufficiently open-minded when new evidence is convincing enough to challenge established ideas, not to hang on to them stubbornly, hiding behind a facade of false conservatism.

An exaggerated illustration of this point is the comparison between our concept of a cataract and that of the ancient Egyptians. They perceived it to be a miniature watershed, the frothy white foam of which cascaded behind the pupil, turning it white and obstructing vision. We still keep the literal name of the waterfall phenomenon 'Cataract' to indicate the state of clouding of the crystalline lens.

Evolution, which is a state of perpetual change when applied to disciplines and techniques, is also necessary for progress. We should always seek to evolve our methods in the direction of eliminating shortcomings and enhancing benefits. If we ever reached a stage where we considered our methods to need no further evolution, however elaborate and sophisticated, we would deny our patients all hope of progress. Imagine where we would be if couching had been accepted as the ultimate method of surgical treatment!

Now the basic concepts concerning cataract are as follows:

- Cataract is a structural, physical, biochemical, and optical change in the crystalline lens of the eye that interferes with the normal transmission and refraction of light rays. This interference affects the overall sharpness of definition of the retinal image.
- Long before substantial decrease in the visual acuity is detected, functional visual acuity may be reduced under certain levels of light. This is due to the drop in contrast of the retinal image induced by abnormal light distribution resulting from aberrant light scattering within the vitreous cavity.
- In order to restore normal visual acuity the visual axis must be cleared.
- So far the only means known to clear the visual axis is the surgical removal of the defective lens. The refractive power should be replaced and so far the intraocular lens (IOL) has proved to be the best option.
- Prior to contemplating the surgical removal of a cataract, the potential for improvement in functional visual acuity should be tested and proven to be significant enough to justify the surgical risk.
- Whatever method the surgeon elects to achieve this objective, it should be with the minimum of damage to or interference with the neighboring structures in the eye.

Until the late 1950s, extracapsular cataract extraction (ECCE) of relatively mature cataracts was the preferred method. The anterior capsule was grasped with a toothed capsule forceps to tear off the central portion and the nucleus expressed. The anterior and posterior chamber were then copiously irrigated to wash out the degenerated cortex. The 10 mm limbal incision, usually made with a Graefe knife, was then closed with a single silk suture.

Intracapsular extraction flourished and saw its golden age during the 1960s and early 1970s. The lens was grasped by smooth capsule forceps or the erysiphake. Later, the cryoprobe became fashionable and removal of the lens was facilitated by the use of the enzyme α-chymotrypsin to dissolve the zonular fibers.

About 20 years ago, Kelman introduced phacoemulsification. Using an ultrasonic vibrating cannula he was able to emulsify the nucleus in the inflowing irrigating fluid in the anterior chamber and aspirate the emulsion. The instrument was introduced through a 3 mm limbal incision. This was the first return to ECCE. However, because of the intricacies of the machine and the technique, it was practiced by only a limited number of surgeons.

The resurrection of IOLs during the 1960s by Binkhorst, Choyce and others further reduced interest in phacoemulsification, since the incision had to be enlarged to introduce the implant and thus negated the main advantage, which was the small incision.

Nevertheless, evidence was accumulating in favor of ECCE as a safer operation that leaves the eye in a more normal physiologic state with its anatomic compartmentalization intact. Moreover, the posterior chamber and the capsular bag in particular proved to be a reliable and more stable location for IOL fixation.

This led to the development of several manual techniques for ECCE. Lately there has been a resurgence of interest in phacoemulsification due to the development of new concepts for IOL implants that can be introduced through small incisions. It is also conceivable that the future will provide an injectable lens implant that would fill the emptied and cleaned intact capsular bag. In anticipation of these new approaches and techniques, phacoemulsification and its alternatives that can be performed through a small incision are in an active stage of development. Also, the instrumentation for standard phacoemulsification has been greatly improved to reduce the damage from excessive fluid turbulence in the anterior chamber.

Initially, removal of a large part of the anterior capsule was recommended, but the realization that the adhesions of the anterior capsule to the posterior capsule, sandwiching the implant haptics between them, provided strong fixation and reliable stability led to alternative methods.

Kelman advocated a triangular or 'Christmas tree' shape but the majority of extracapsular surgeons preferred a circular anterior capsulectomy.

In 1980, intercapsular cataract extraction was introduced by Baikoff and Sourdille. The same year Galand and I adopted the technique and taught it widely. The technique has flourished and presently claims a very substantial following.

In this technique a linear anterior capsulotomy is performed from 10 to 2 o'clock through which the contents of the capsular bag are removed and the lens implant is inserted. A small central semicircular portion of the inferior anterior capsular flap is then removed after insertion of the IOL.

This technique, even though it requires some training and practice, has proved to be superior to any other technique in protecting the corneal endothelium and the rest of the anterior segment structures, since all the surgical manipulations are performed within the cavity of the capsular bag. It also provides the best conditions for foolproof placement of the implant totally within the capsular bag.

In its standard form, continuous flow irrigation to maintain the anterior chamber is used, just like all other standard manual or machine extracapsular techniques.

The Dry Intercapsular Cataract Extraction (DICE) technique, in which the anterior chamber is maintained with a viscoelastic compound so avoiding turbulence of the irrigating fluid, is one modification (see Chapter 6).

In all these techniques, the initial anterior capsulectomy or capsulotomy may be performed with a cystitome or bent needle of 25 to 30 gauge. Small punctures are made very close to each other; each one is connected to the previous one in what has come to be known as the 'can-opener' technique. This leaves a scalloped edge with tears or cracks running from the edge of the capsulotomy between adjacent tags and ending blindly in the anterior capsular flap. Any slight pull or stretch of the capsule is liable to extend one or more of these cracks radially towards the capsular fornix.

We now know that a smooth edge to the anterior capsulotomy has an extraordinary strength which preserves the integrity of the flaps and enhances the strength of the capsular bag as a whole. The fashioning of a smooth break in the anterior capsule has come to be termed capsulorhexis. Modern capsulorhexis is an evolutionary concept which may be tailored to different circumstances. The following illustrates some methods now in use.

Round capsulorhexis suitable for ECCE or phacoemulsification

1.1

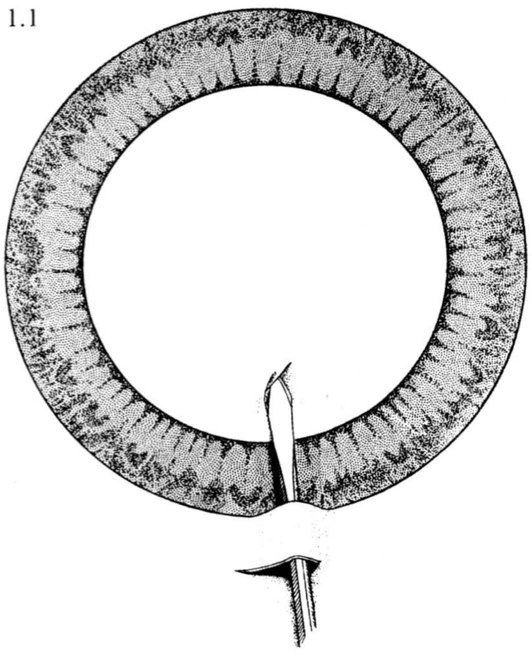

1.2

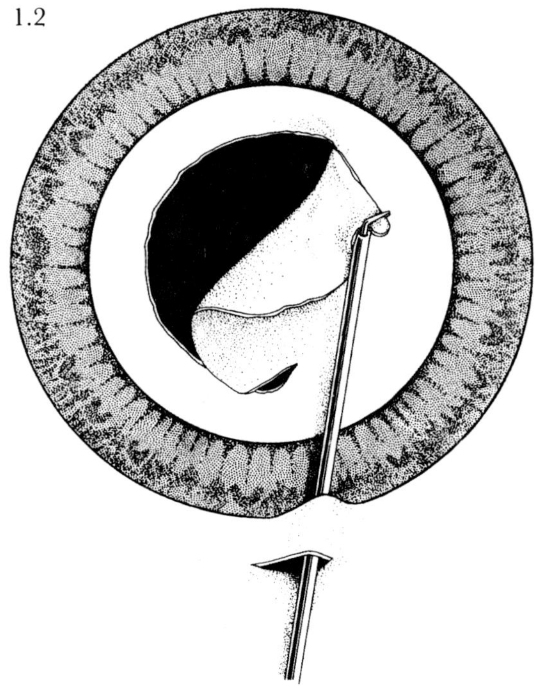

1.3

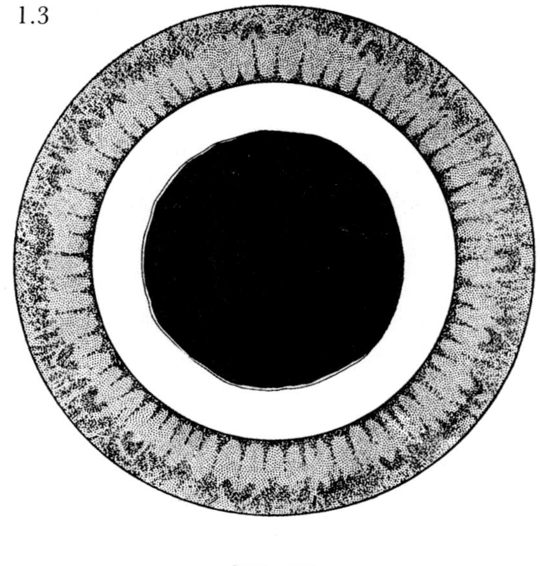

1.1 A small incision is made in the anterior capsule diagonal to the vertical meridian of the pupil. This is done using a double-edged, very sharp lance. While the tip of the blade is underneath the peripheral end of the incision, it is lifted slightly anteriorly to extend the tear circumferentially for a small distance, thus fashioning a small triangular flap. The position of this flap determines the eventual diameter of the final round capsulectomy.

1.2 Using the Anis® microforceps, the capsular flap is held and the tear extended circumferentially slowly and deliberately. It is released and repositioned several times to grasp the central flap closer to the end of the extending tear in order to have better control, until it joins the start of the tear at the junction between the diagonal and circumferential components.

1.3 The completed round capsulectomy with smooth edge. For phacoemulsification the diameter may be up to 1 mm smaller than the diameter of the implant's optic. The capsule is resistant to extension by tearing, provided its edges remains smooth. If the overall diameter of the compressed or folded implant is larger than the diameter of the opening, the implant will stretch the capsulotomy during insertion, producing an oval rather than a round shape. Care must be taken as this may put a substantial stress on the zonular fibers positioned 90° to the long axis of the oval.

For nucleus extraction, the nucleus, provided it is not too hard, may be made smaller by hydrodissection to separate the core from its outer shell. The diameter of the capsulotomy should be large enough to permit exit of the nucleus or an obstructed delivery may result in rupture of the zonules.

Linear and arcuate capsulorhexis suitable for large incision intercapsular cataract extraction

1.4

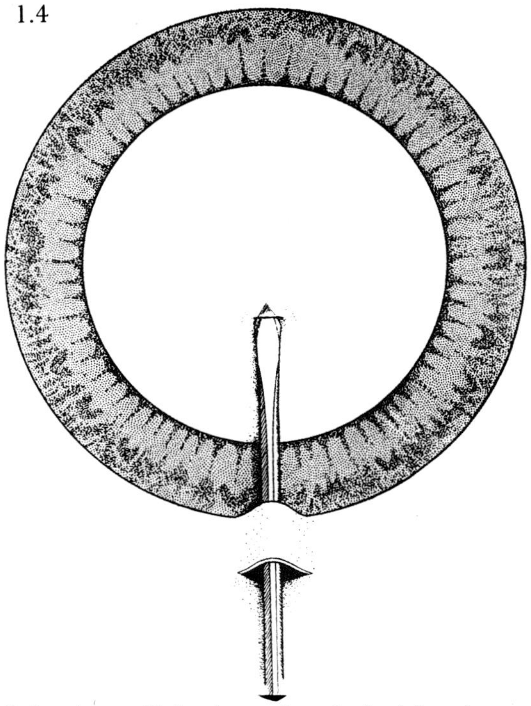

1.5

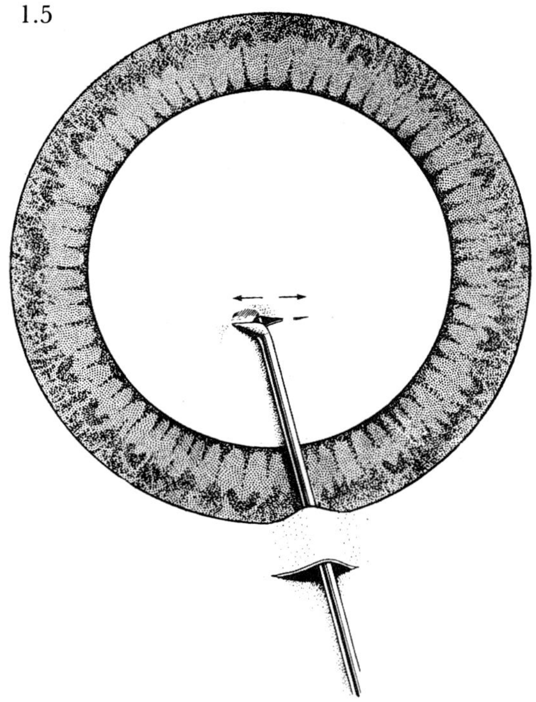

1.6

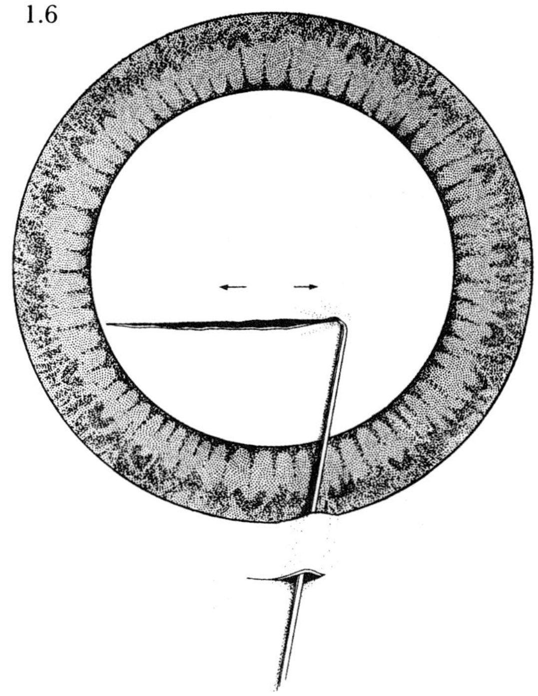

1.4 A small horizontal stab incision is made using a very sharp, double-edged narrow lance at the junction of the superior third and inferior two-thirds of the vertical diameter of the pupil.

1.5 The Anis® microscissors are used to make a horizontal extension of the incision to either side.

1.6 The bent tip of the Sinskey hook or capsulotomy needle is inserted in the capsular incision and controlled extension of the linear tear is made to either side. This fashions a clean linear capsulotomy extending from 10 to 2 o'clock free of capsular tags. Through this capsulotomy the nucleus is extracted, the cortex is aspirated and the intraocular lens implant is introduced.

1.7 After the IOL has been positioned, a vertical cut is made in the inferior flap with fine long-bladed scissors.

1.8 Using microforceps the central flap is held near the end of the vertical cut and the tear is extended in an arcuate fashion by changing the vectors of pull until the tear joins the horizontal capsulotomy.

1.9 The final, U-shaped capsulectomy opposite the center of the IOL optic.

1.7

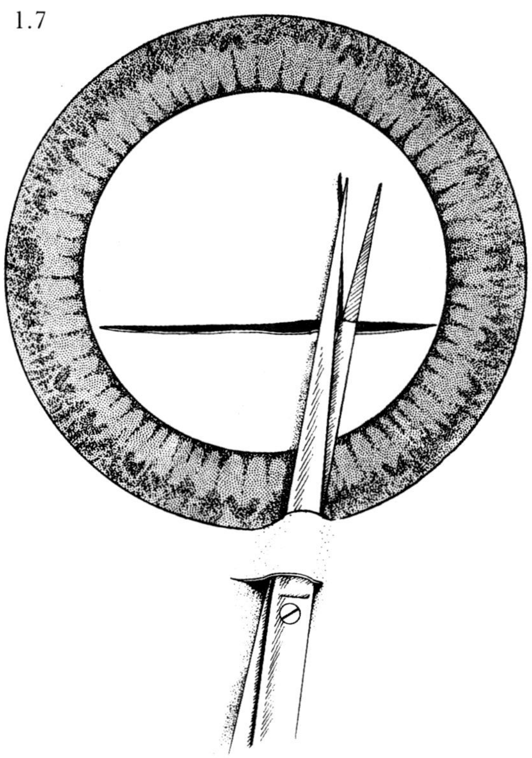

1.8

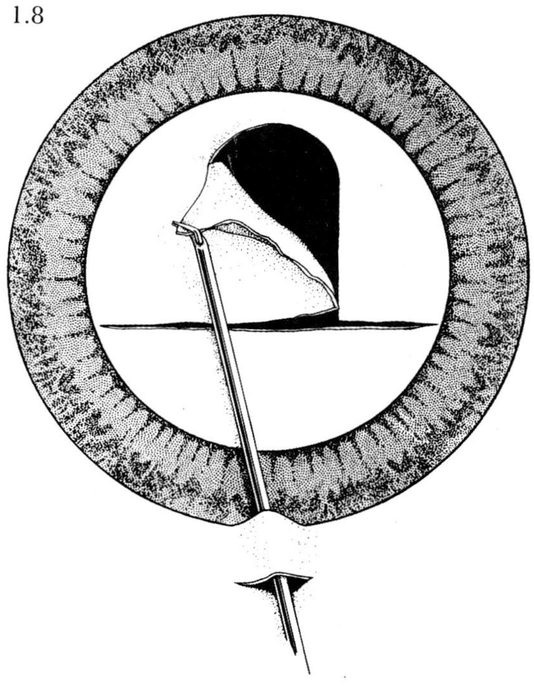

1.9

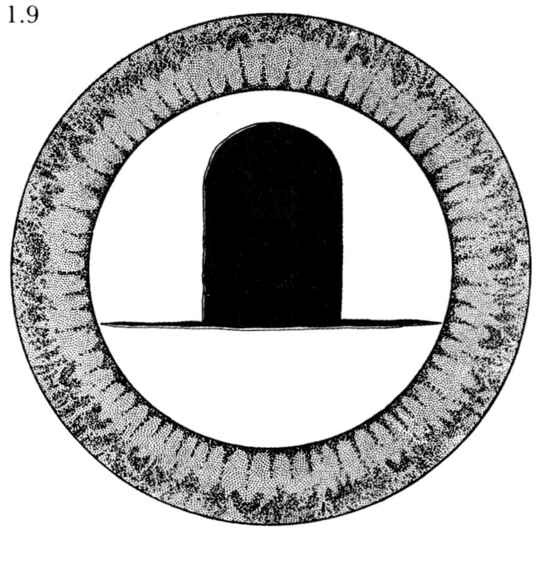

Capsulorhexis suitable for small incision intercapsular cataract extraction including intercapsular phacoemulsification or DICE

1.10

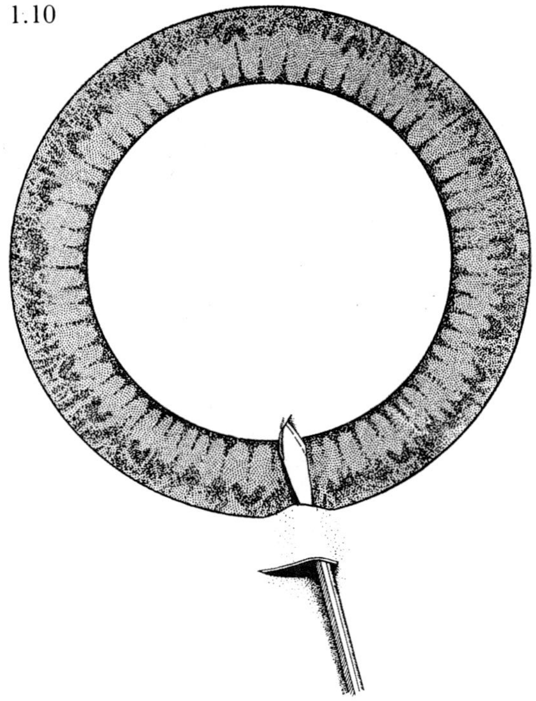

1.11

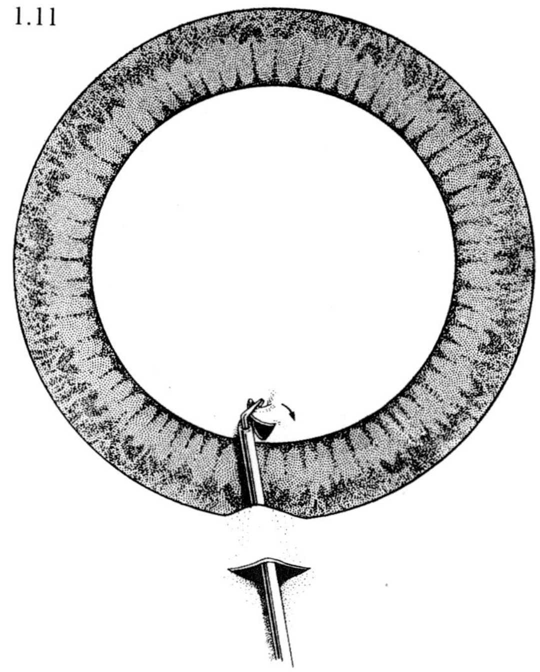

1.10 A small diagonal stab incision in the anterior capsule is performed with a fine lance at 12 o'clock, close to the border of the fully dilated pupil. The point of the knife is placed underneath the upper end of the incision and lifted slightly anteriorly to extend the tear circumferentially, thus fashioning a small, tongue-like flap.

1.11 With the Anis® microforceps the capsular flap is extended in a circular fashion to form a small round capsulectomy 1–2 mm in diameter.

1.12

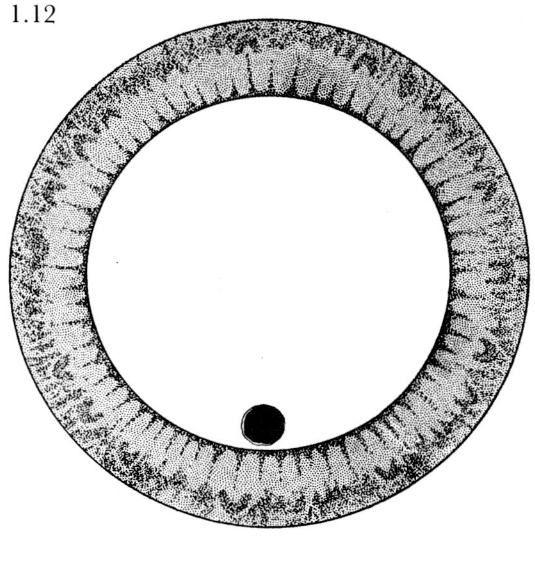

1.13

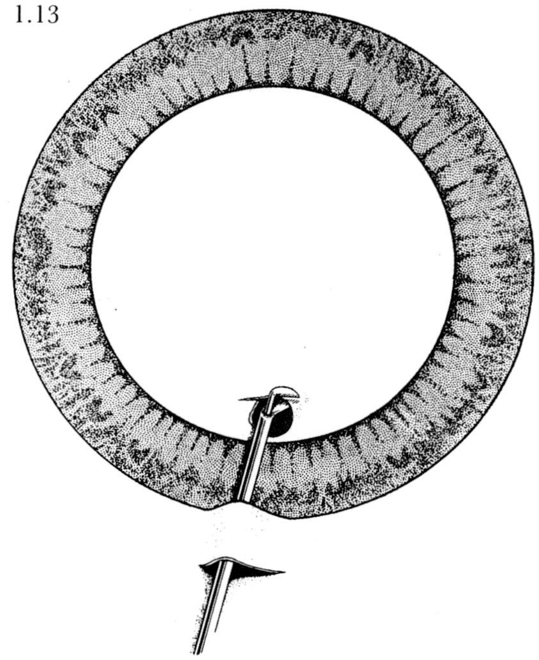

1.12 Small round capsulectomy at 12 o'clock with smooth edge without breaks. Through this the lens content is removed, and the capsular bag cleaned. Sometimes a radial extension occurs at 12 o'clock towards the fornix of the capsular bag. This is not critical and should not extend further during the intercapsular manipulations.

1.13 To implant a small incision IOL, a small cut with microscissors is performed to either side tangential to the central edge of the small round capsulectomy.

1.14

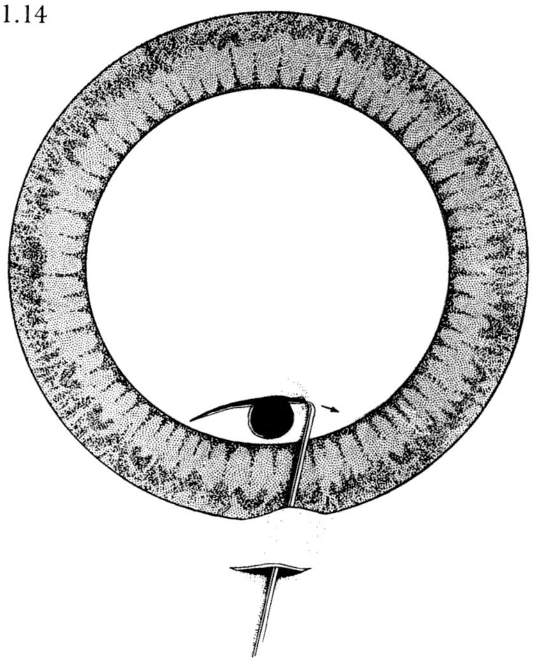

1.15

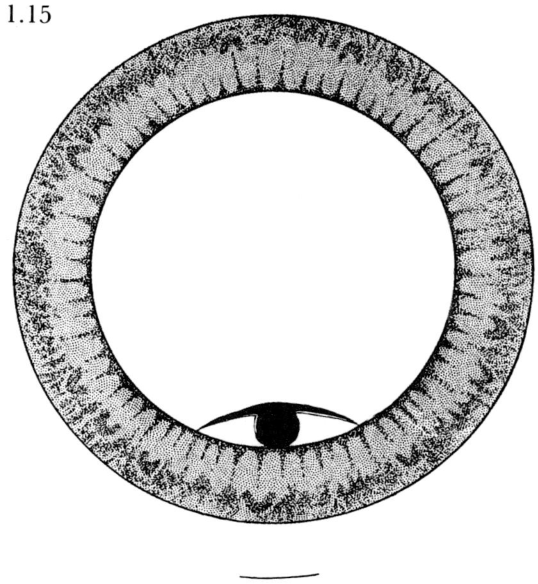

1.14 A Sinskey hook is inserted and the capsulorhexis extended to either side to form an entry large enough for the lens implant.

1.15 Opening for small incision IOL.

1.16

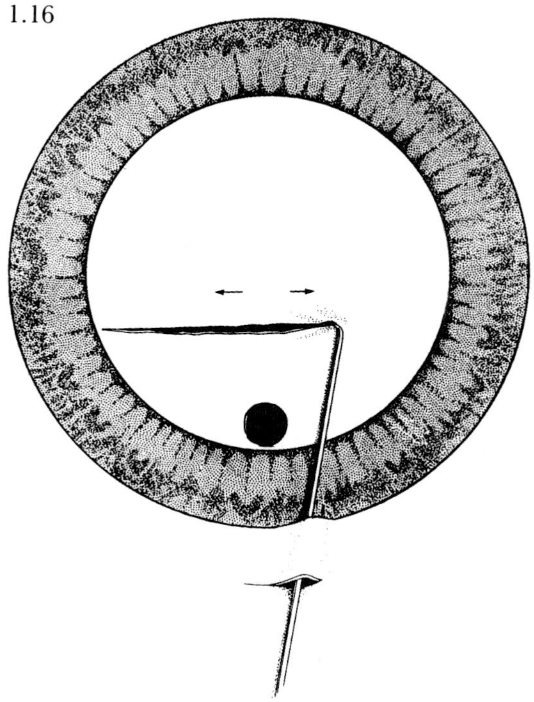

1.17

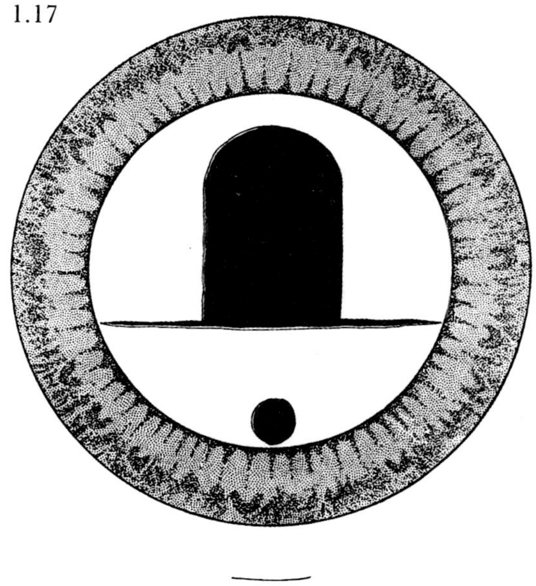

1.16 To implant a standard size IOL, repeat **1.10–1.12** above then introduce a viscoelastic compound through the small round capsulectomy to create a wide separation between the anterior and posterior capsules. A stab incision is made and extended as in **1.4–1.6**.

1.17 After insertion of the IOL, capsulorhexis is completed as in **1.7–1.9**.

2: Incisions and sutures

Emanuel Rosen

Decisions on incisions for cataract surgery depend on:

- What is to be removed through the incision.
- What is to be inserted through the incision.

Basic concepts of cataract incisions

- The keratometric effect of corneal, limbal or scleral incisions is an eventual flattening of the surgical meridian.
- Transverse or arcuate incisions placed close to the corneal apex induce greater meridional flattening than do more peripheral incisions.
- The longer the incision, the greater the keratometric flattening in the surgical meridian. For longer incisions, an additional steepening of the opposite meridian is observed, the so-called 'coupling effect'.

Astigmatic effects of suturing incisions

In the case of a superior cataract incision, suture closure induces a temporary keratometric steepening or 'with the rule' astigmatism which is the initial phase of a two-stage keratometric swing from 'with' to 'against the rule'.

The effects of suture closure of an incision depend upon suture orientation, suture tension and suture material.

Wound compression results in central steepening (**2.1**). Thus a tight suture at 12 o'clock will induce plus astigmatism at 90° (with the rule). The tighter the suture the steeper the change.

The variables of an incision are:

- **Location.**
- **Extent.**
- **Form.**
- **Closure.**
- **Instrumentation.**

2.1

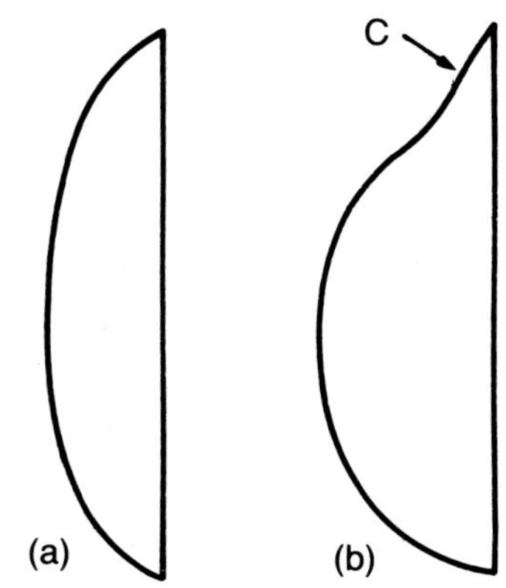

2.1 Corneal curve (a) before and (b) after wound compression due to an overtight suture at C. Peripheral flattening is associated with central steepening.

Location

Meridian

Cataract surgery is usually performed through an incision centered on the 12 o'clock meridian. It is thus concealed and protected maximally under the upper eyelid. This approach is obviously the most convenient for the microsurgeon. Occasionally a lateral or inferior approach is required in complicated cases especially, where the upper cornea has been compromised by previous intervention.

Small incision surgery based on the phacoemulsification technique, or lens aspiration in younger patients, utilizes an incision based on the 11 o'clock meridian (for a right eye) with a view to extension later for IOL implantation, across the 12 o'clock and towards the 1 o'clock position.

Anteroposterior location

The options for access to the anterior chamber are corneal, limbal or scleral.

In each case further variation is possible with an anteroposterior band of tissue in each area being utilized for the incision by individual surgeon preference. Criteria for choice may depend on: tissue vascularity, potential astigmatic effects, suture access, conjunctival surgery, chord length versus length of arc, iris management, closed chamber surgery, or suture material.

Tissue vascularity: The cornea is avascular, the limbus and sclera moderately vascular. This aspect of these tissues influences surgical control of bleeding and wound healing rates. The more vascular the tissue, the more rapid the healing process, but the need for hemostasis is increased. There are occasions when absence of bleeding is a necessity in cataract surgery, for example when patients are on anticoagulant therapy or have blood dyscrasias.

Astigmatism (see also Chapter 26): Preoperative astigmatism that is corneal in origin may be usefully adjusted as a planned part of the surgical process. The principal involved is to either relax the steeper meridian or tighten the flatter meridian, whichever is the easier of the two options, remembering that in the case of a superior cataract incision, suture closure induces 'with the rule' astigmatism which is the initial phase of a two-stage keratometric swing from 'with' to 'against the rule'. Also, tighter sutures produce steeper changes in the vertical meridian. Induced astigmatism is avoided primarily by understanding the natural history of the healing process in relation to the individual incision. This is achieved by studying the keratometric regression pattern of an incision for a six month postoperative period wherein most incisions will heal to a stable position (**2.2**).

Thus, a surgically induced 'with the rule' astigmatism (plus cylinder at 90°) will regress as a wound heals, a process accelerated when necessary by release of over-tight sutures at least two months after surgery, but depending on the incision site, remembering that corneal wounds are slower to heal than more posterior incisions.

Astigmatic effects may be induced by poor alignment of wound edges (e.g. overlap of wound edges, lateral shift of anterior and posterior wound lips or poor suturing technique with over-tight or loose interrupted sutures), by poor tensioning of a continuous suture, or by a suture too superficial or too long (**2.3–2.5**).

2.2

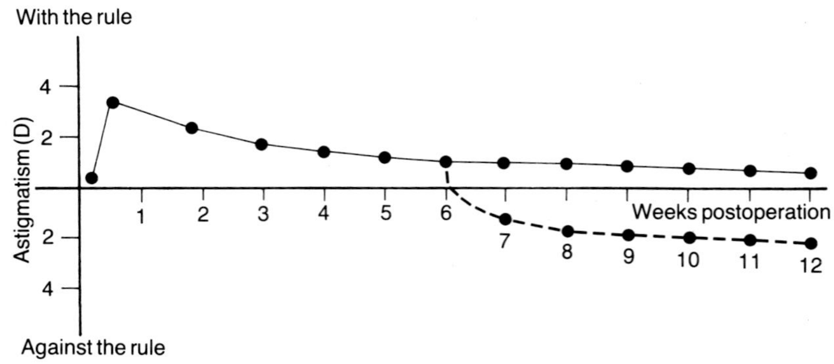

2.2 Schematic postoperation astigmatic decay curve indicating a sharp rise in astigmatism in the first postoperative week as suture compression of the wound is allied to tissue swelling. The subsequent decay (solid line) is due to resolution with wound healing and flattening of the central cornea. Enhanced decay (dotted line) may be caused by removal of sutures at six weeks.

2.3

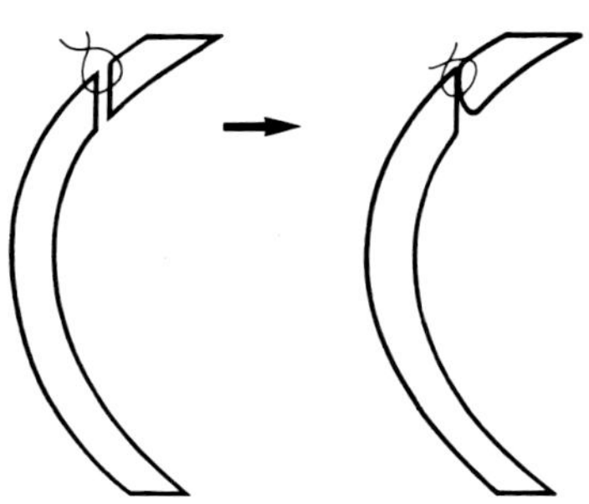

2.3 Bevelled corneal incision: a suture too superficial causes internal gape.

2.4

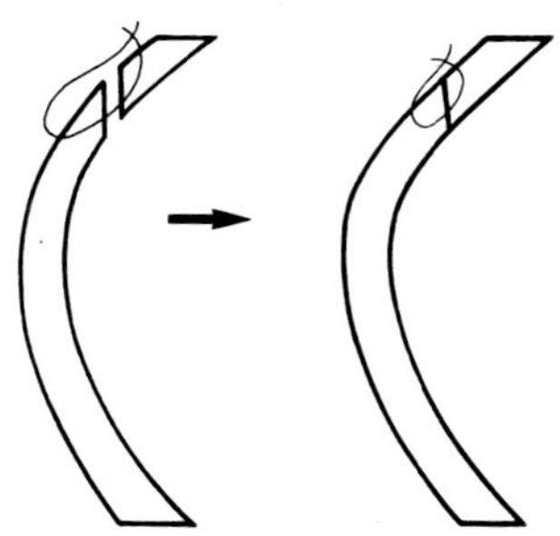

2.4 Bevelled corneal incision: a suture too long causes unnecessary steepening.

2.5

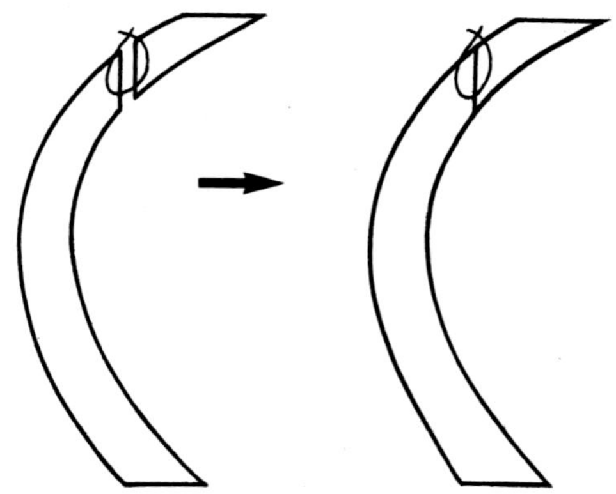

2.5 The correct suturing method for a bevelled corneal incision.

Suture access: Postoperative suture management is a factor in deciding where to place an incision. If the sutures are placed in the cornea, then access to them for division or removal in the postoperative period is easy either by laser, knife or needle. In contrast, a posterior suture location with consequent conjunctival overlay makes such access more difficult and therefore more invasive.

Conjunctival surgery: An incision posterior to the limbus must involve surgery to the conjunctiva whether a fornix-based conjunctival flap, a limbal-based conjunctival flap, or involving bipolar cautery debridement of the anterior conjunctiva for an anterior scleral incision.

A fornix-based conjunctival flap with limbal peritomy should extend beyond the anticipated scleral incision site with full access provided thereby. Retraction of the conjunctival flap and bipolar cautery hemostasis are usual. Anterior insertion of Tenon's capsule, more obvious in the younger patient, must also be retracted using a knife edge. The combined operation of trabeculectomy and cataract may utilize this approach for creation of either a triangular or a rectangular scleral flap.

The limbal-based conjunctival flap is a traditional approach involving a decision on flap size. This incision is created by scissors and Tooke's knife or an equivalent device and is 'inelegant' when compared with more anterior incisions in cataract surgery. Bipolar cautery is necessary to provide hemostasis. The approach is time consuming and offers no advantage over a fornix-based flap.

Bipolar debridement of anterior conjunctiva combines conjunctival removal and hemostasis in one simple and rapid process. The bipolar power setting should be just adequate to achieve its visible end, thereby avoiding the potential complication of tissue shrinkage. Adequate irrigation with balanced salt solution is essential. This approach is followed by rapid re-epithelialization of the debrided area in the first few hours of the postoperative period and will automatically bury monofilament nylon sutures.

Iris management: An incision into the anterior chamber at the iris plane risks iris tissue prolapse; therefore a corneal or limbal incision which leaves a lip of limbal tissue anterior to the iris plane is often preferred for planned ECCE.

Closed chamber surgery: Phacoemulsification is specifically planned as a closed chamber procedure. Therefore, it utilizes a small incision capable of extension for IOL implantation. Planned ECCE may be performed as a partial closed chamber technique involving suture control of the incision during surgery as well as at completion.

Incision extent

The relationship between the transverse length of an incision or chord length (the operational factor), and the arcuate incision length necessary to achieve the desired opening into the anterior chamber, is shown in **Table 2.1.**

Table 2.1. The relationship between an arcuate wound length and its chord length at various distances from the center of the cornea

Distance from center of cornea (mm)	*Transverse incision (chord) length (mm)* 7	8	9	10
	Arcuate wound length (mm) if circumferential:			
4	8.5	12.6		
4.5	8.0	9.9	14.1	
5	7.8	9.3	11.2	15.7
5.5	7.6	9.0	10.5	12.6
6	7.5	8.8	10.2	11.8
6.7	7.4	8.6	9.9	11.4
7	7.3	8.5	9.8	11.1

Form

The wound profile may be bevelled, reversed, perpendicular, two plane or pocket.

'Bevelled' implies a corneal or limbal incision which is cut at any angle to the surface other than a right angle (**2.6**). It is simple to perform with one sweep of a sharp blade, but requires more meticulous closure than a two-plane incision, which 'locks' the two surfaces of an incision more effectively and with a simpler suturing technique.

A reversed corneal incision is made solely with a knife, with its point angled towards the upper anterior chamber angle (**2.6**). The rationale is to utilize intraocular pressure to force closure of the incision and maintain a watertight junction. If intraocular pressure rises post-operatively, the wound is less likely to gape than with a bevelled or perpendicular incision.

A perpendicular incision (**2.7**) is simple but prone to leakage and lateral shift.

A two plane incision (**2.7**) is the most popular corneo-limbal incision form. This incision is watertight and encourages exact apposition of wound edges, especially when correctly sutured through the angle of the two planes in the wound. The two plane incision may be reversed (**2.8**) to combine the advantages of the reverse incision and obviate the need for cautery. A further variant is the step incision (**2.8**), useful when combined with trabeculectomy.

Pocket incision (**2.7**) refers to a scleral incision where a tunnel or pocket from this posteriorly oriented incision is made to gain access to the anterior chamber. It is the incision of choice for phacoemulsification as it is suited to the small incision (see **2.9**).

2.6

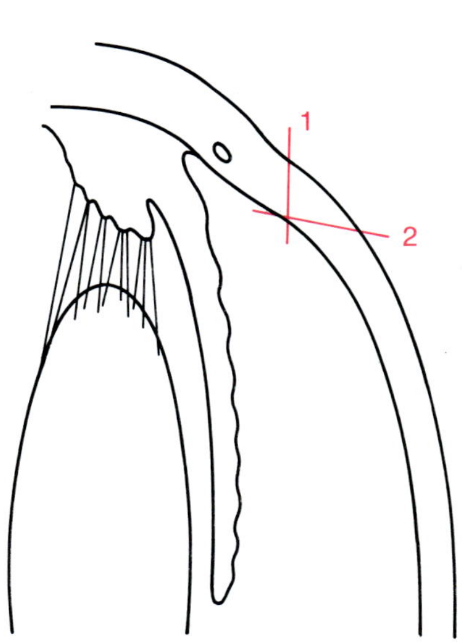

2.6 Diagrammatic representation of bevelled (1) and reversed (2) corneal incisions.

2.7

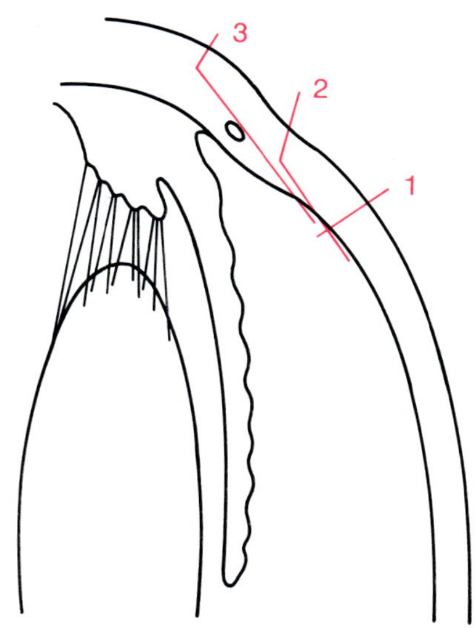

2.7 Diagrammatic representation of perpendicular corneal incision (1), two-plane limbal incision (2) and a scleral pocket incision (3).

2.8

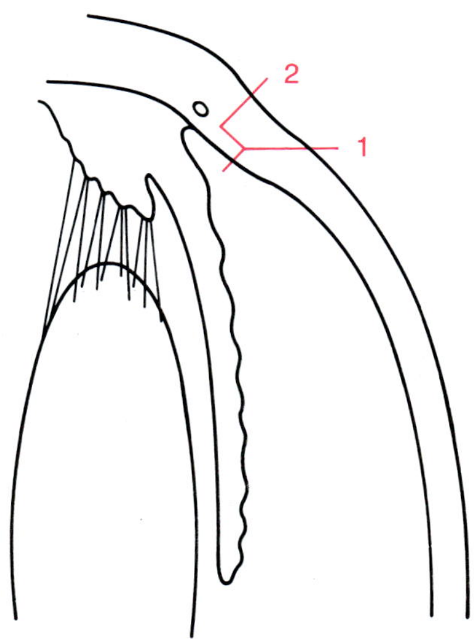

2.8 Diagrammatic representation of reversed two plane (1) and step (2) limbal incisions.

Closure

It is necessary to consider the suture material, suture orientation, number of bites and suture needles.

Suture material

Monofilament nylon of 10-0 gauge is overwhelmingly the material of choice for cataract wound closure. Its qualities of integrity, tensile strength, uniformity, moderate elasticity and ultimate biodegradability, combined with the excellent range of fine needles to which it is swaged, make alternative materials less satisfactory (**Table 2.2**). Finer and coarser gauge monofilament nylon, polypropylene, synthetics such as mersilene and absorbable materials such as vicryl, as well as virgin silk, are used by a tiny minority of surgeons who see a particular virtue in a material in relation to their own technique. In general, tougher suture materials extend the period of wound compression and therefore induced astigmatic effects will persist. This can be used to advantage. On the other hand, material such as virgin silk induces tissue resorption around it, with wound weakening and unpredictable astigmatic effects.

Table 2.2 Suture material characteristics

Material	*Biodegradability*	*Tissue reaction*	*Other features*
A) *Nonabsorbable*			
1. Nylon (Polyamide)	Loses 15% per year	Minimal	Monofilament High tensile strength Relatively elastic Stiff suture ends
2. Silk			
a) Virgin silk	3–6 months	Moderate	Ties easily Soft suture ends Inelastic
b) Braided silk			More drag Nidus of infection? Frays easily
3. Polypropylene	Semi-permanent	Minimal	Monofilament High tensile strength Most elastic suture Stiff suture ends
4. Polyester a) Mersilene b) Dacron	Permanent	Minimal	Braided or monofilament High tensile strength Not elastic
5. Stainless steel	Permanent	Minimal	High tensile strength Staples?
B) *Absorbable*			
1. Polygalactin 910 e.g. Vicryl	2–3 weeks	Mild	High tensile strength Hydrolytic degradation Monofilament or braided
2. Polyglycolic acid e.g. Dexon	2–3 weeks	Mild	High tensile strength Braided Hydrolytic degradation

Suture orientation and number of bites

Figures 2.9–2.13 show the alternatives for both interrupted and continuous suture patterns. All bites should be radial (at right angles to the incision), except for the continuous style shown in **2.12**, and spaced little more than 1 mm apart. Spacing wider than 2 mm may lead to wound leak and poor control of astigmatism.

Interrupted sutures may be single or X-shaped. Knots are usually buried to avoid irritation. Individual sutures can have variable induced tension to adjust for the astigmatic effects of the incision or to overcome preexisting astigmatism. Use of a surgical keratometer may be helpful in positioning and tensioning interrupted sutures, though precautions in simulating postoperative intraocular pressure are required for improved accuracy. Interrupted sutures also have the virtue of individual removal or tension release to control postoperative astigmatism.

Continuous sutures have the theoretical virtue of evenly spreading the tension load across an incision, though the longer the incision the more variable the astigmatic result. Release or removal of a continuous suture has an 'all or none' effect compared with the interrupted variety. Continuous sutures, accordingly, are best suited to small posterior (scleral pocket) incisions unless divided into two (**2.11**).

2.9

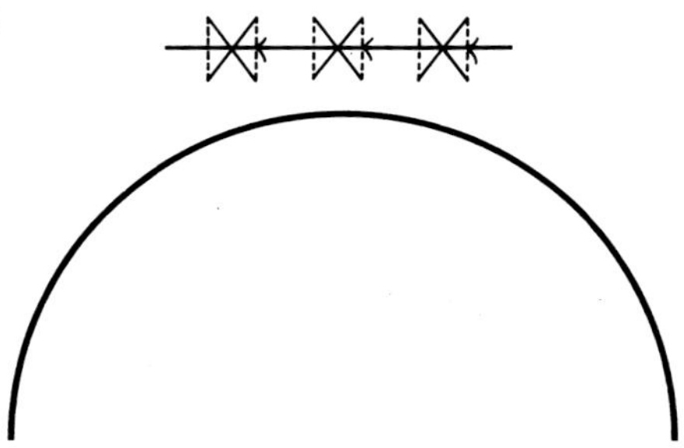

2.9 Interrupted monofilament nylon X suture closure of a scleral pocket incision. X sutures may also be used for closure of a limbal section.

2.10

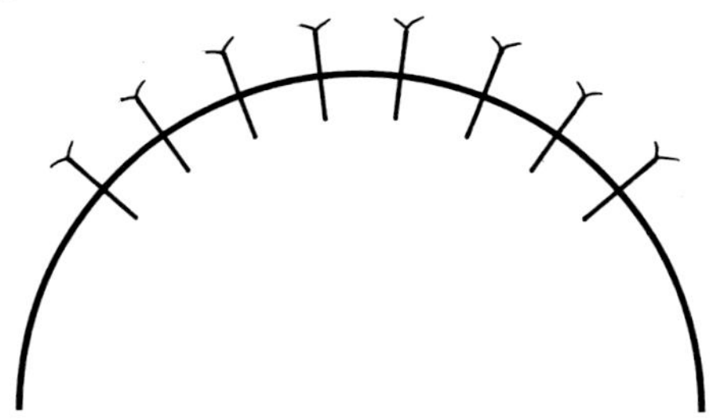

2.10 Interrupted monofilament nylon suture closure of a limbal incision.

2.11

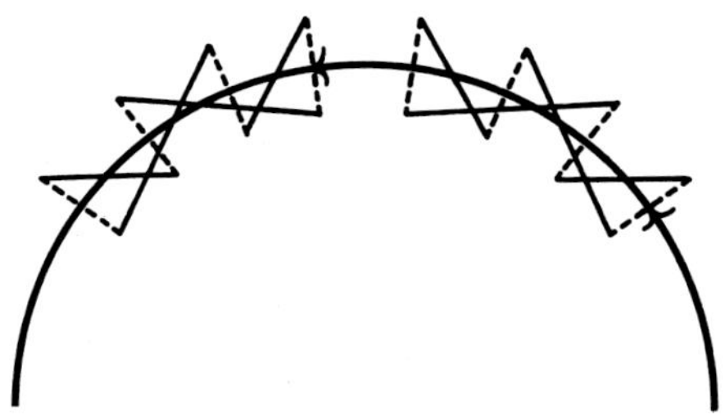

2.11 Two double-X continuous sutures, each with a single knot. After limbal section, this enables half the wound to be closed prior to lens implantation.

2.12

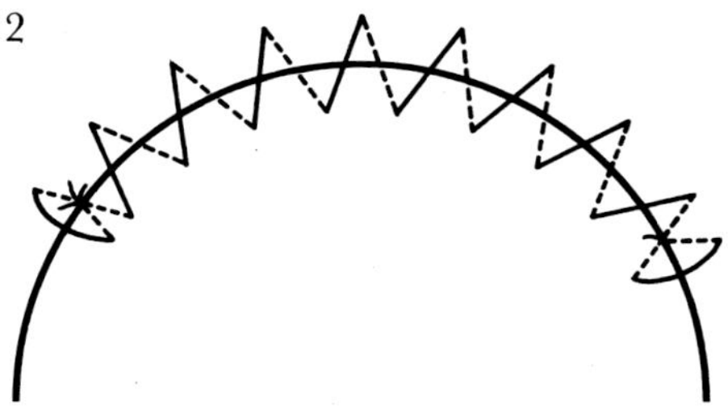

2.12 Continuous monofilament nylon suture closure of a limbal incision with buried knot at each end. Suture bites should be at about 35° to the radial to avoid lateral shift of wound edges. The disadvantage is poor control of astigmatism.

2.13

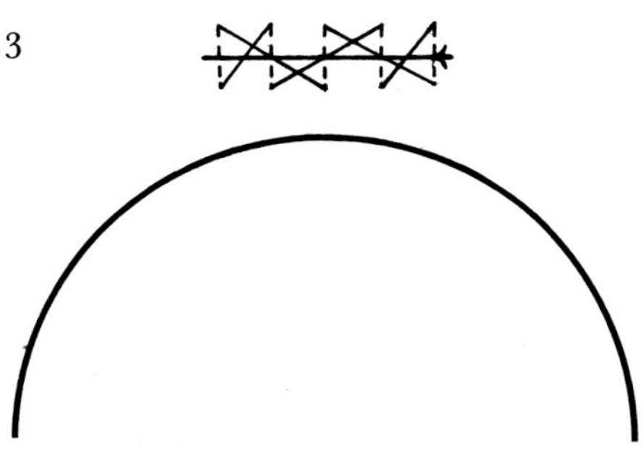

2.13 Continuous monofilament (5 bite) 'bootlace' suture (single knot) for a scleral pocket cataract incision extended to admit an intraocular implant.

Suture needles

Needle dimensions (**2.14**) include wire diameter, radius of curvature and length. *Compound curvature* needles have a progressively shorter radius of curvature towards the tip and are favored by some surgeons for short bites with deep suture placement.

Tip designs include cutting, reversed cutting, spatula and round taper point. *Cutting designs* have a triangular profile, cutting at the tip and three edges. As there is a cutting edge superiorly, the effect is to create a suture canal superficial to the path of the needle, which may therefore cut out of the tissue.

A *reverse cutting* needle is triangular with the cutting edge below. Its effect is to create a suture path beneath the path of the needle and therefore it penetrates tissue more easily. It is used for full thickness suturing of tissue. Special care with scleral suturing is required to avoid penetration.

A *spatula needle* is four- or six-sided with cutting edges on the sides. It cuts at the tip and sides parallel to the tissue plane. It displaces tissue above and below its plane of travel and therefore avoids tissue penetration. This is the most commonly used style for suturing of cataract incisions.

A *round taper point* only cuts at the tip and therefore tissue penetration is more difficult. It provides a wide suture canal for easy knot burial by suture rotation.

2.14

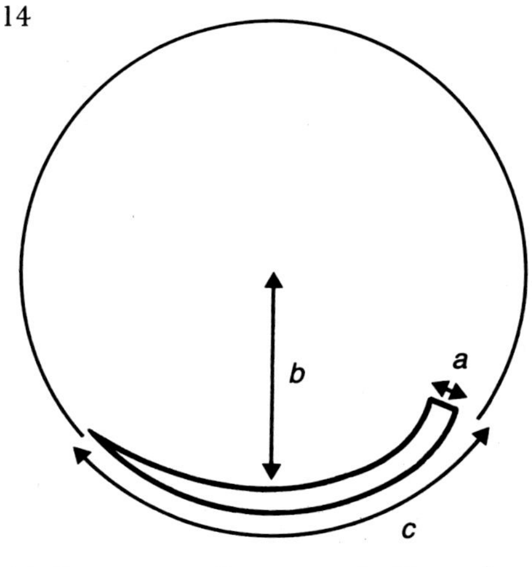

2.14 Suture needle general dimensions: *a*, diameter; *b*, radius of curvature; *c*, length.

Instrumentation

The choice of instruments for cataract incisions is simple. The incision has to be made initially by a sharp knife, steel, ceramic or diamond whose form is a matter of individual preference. Control is aided by a pair of atraumatic micromanipulating forceps held in the other hand and applied to the eye near the incision site. A partial thickness incision through cornea or limbus may be completed by knife or angled corneal scissors whose effect is to create the two plane incision favored by many surgeons. The extent of an incision may be gauged precisely by use of a rule or caliper, utilizing the data in **Table 2.1**. Posterior incisions associated with bleeding require hemostasis by bipolar cautery of which the hemeraser (a concentric bipolar tool) is the most effective and the least likely to induce tissue shrinkage, a phenomenon with potentially serious wound effects.

Incision closure requires a fine needle holder used in conjunction with the micromanipulating forceps. The needle holder, if well designed, may double as suture-tying forceps, though an additional pair of dedicated suture-tying forceps is necessary with interrupted sutures for suture rotation to bury the knot.

Future developments

- Biochemical and pharmacological control of wound healing, (acceleration or deceleration), will give further control and precision to the cataract surgeon. Developments of such agents are being keenly researched and animal experimental data will before long be transformed into a practical surgical and postoperation tool.
- Fine stainless steel staples may soon be used to close cataract incisions. The material is of proven value even inside the eye, but engineering development is required to provide a simple and consistent method of stapling a cataract wound, i.e. miniaturization of a well-established if gross surgical principle.
- Cyanoacrylate adhesives have had a role in ophthalmic trauma and corneal techniques for some years. Their development for closure of cataract incisions would seem to be logical, but present results are unreliable.

Further reading

Jolson A.S. The etiology and control of iatrogenic astigmatism in cataract incision closure. In: Ginsburg S.P. (Ed.), *Cataract and intraocular lens surgery; a compendium of modern theories and techniques*. Birmingham, Alabama, Aeselapius Publishing Co., Vol 2, pp 537–569, 1984.

Lindstrom R.L., Destro M.A. Effects of incision size and Terry keratometer usage on post operative astigmatism, *Am. Intraocular Implant Soc. J.*, **11,** 469–473, 1985.

Rowsey J.J. Ten caveats in keratorefractive surgery. *Ophthalmology*, **90,** 148–155, 1983.

Swinger C.A. Post operative astigmatism. *Surv. Ophthalmol.*, **31,** 219–248, 1987.

Thrasher B.H., Boerner C.F. Control of astigmatism by wound placement. *Am. Intraocular Implant Soc. J.*, **10,** 176–179, 1984.

3: Intracapsular techniques

Michael Absolon

By *intracapsular cataract extraction* (ICCE) is meant the removal of the whole cataractous crystalline lens intact, including its capsule (**3.1**). The term should not be confused with intercapsular or endocapsular extraction, a method of extracapsular cataract extraction (ECCE) in which the nucleus and cortex of the lens are removed through an opening in the anterior capsule.

3.1

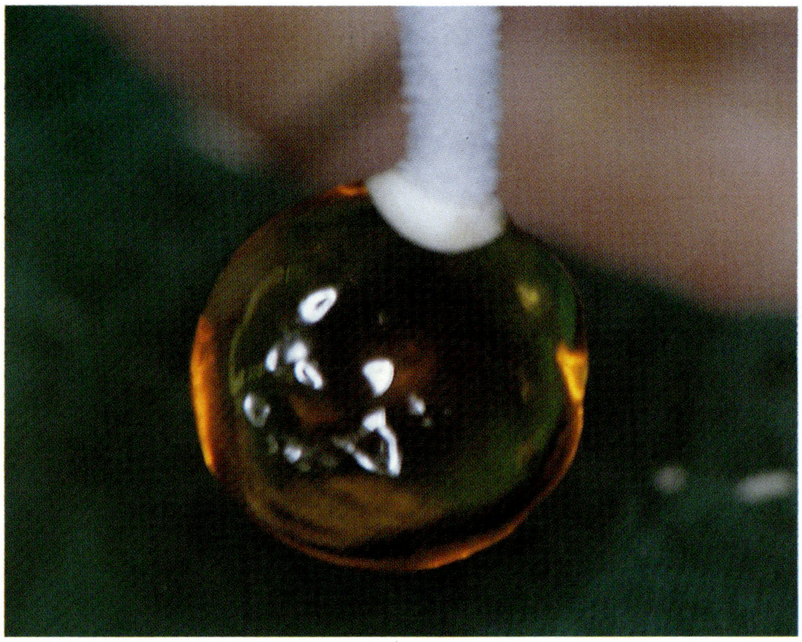

3.1 Intact cataractous lens.

Advantages and indications

- An immediate and permanent clear visual axis, with no capsulotomy required.
- Excellent postoperative visualization of the fundus.
- Capability (when implantation is not contemplated) of being easily performed in basic conditions in developing countries using a simplified technique without an operating microscope.
- Hypermature cataracts and small pupils (a sector iridectomy may be helpful) are added reasons for ICCE when operating under basic conditions (**3.2**).
- Cataract removal when the cornea is cloudy but a graft is not comtemplated or when the anterior chamber is flat. Such a situation arises with acute glaucoma secondary to an intumescent cataract. Expression or cryoextraction after sector iridectomy and chymotrypsin may be the procedure of choice.
- Lens dislocation or rupture of the zonule for more than 40% of its circumference (as may be found with traumatic cataract) generally merits ICCE followed, if indicated, by an anterior chamber lens.

3.2

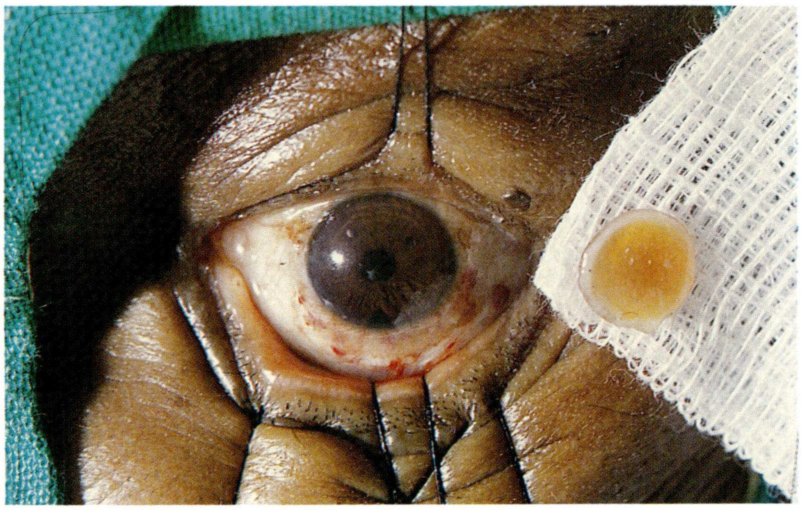

3.2 ICCE in rural Kenya.

Disadvantages

These are mainly related to the removal of the barrier effect of the posterior capsule, the consequences of which may be:

- Aphakic retinal detachment (ARD) in 1–2% of cases (less than this in eyes of normal axial length and in which no complication occurred, and greater than this in myopic eyes and those in which vitreous loss occurred).
- Clinical cystoid macular edema (CME) in up to 1% of cases. This incidence is higher when the vitreous is disturbed or when there is a brisk postoperative uveitis.

In addition, ICCE commits the surgeon to using an anterior chamber lens implant (ACL) or an iris fixated implant.

Contraindications

- Patients under 35 (because of the adherence of the anterior hyloid to the posterior capsule).
- High myopia.
- Occurrence of permanent CME following ICCE for the first eye.
- Occurrence of ARD following ICCE for the first eye, unless 360° prophylactic cryotherapy is carried out.
- Patients with proliferative diabetic retinopathy.

Myopia and ICCE: Practical guidelines

Myopia of <7D: ICCE permissible provided careful pre- and post-operative examination of the retinal periphery is carried out, and prophylactic cryotherapy is performed if necessary.

Myopia of 7–10D: ECCE is preferable. If ICCE is performed, 360° prophylactic cryotherapy should be carried out.

Myopia >10D: ECCE is advisable.

Minimization of Late Complications

ARD is minimized by no traction on the zonules, no disruption or forwards movement of the vitreous face, no vitreous loss and adherence to guidelines in the presence of myopia.

CME is minimized by minimal intraocular manipulation, elimination of operative complications and appropriate pre- and post-operative medication (when ICCE is accompanied by an ACL, a nonsteroidal anti-inflammatory drug such as diclofenac is given the day before surgery and for two weeks postoperatively, and topical steroids are given in a tapered dosage for three months).

Corneal decompensation, which is extremely rare following properly performed ICCE, is minimized by minimal corneal manipulation, no endothelial touch and care in irrigation of the anterior chamber.

Technique

Either general or local *anesthesia* may be employed. The author's preference is for general anesthesia because it provides satisfactory operating conditions, it is pleasant for the patient, and the anesthetist controls the vital functions.

Adequate exposure with minimal pressure on the globe is obtained with a suitable speculum or lid sutures, together with a superior rectus suture.

Mydriasis is achieved by cyclopentolate 1% and phenylephrine 10% instilled three times during the hour before surgery.

The incision should be in two planes, and should extend for 150°. A limbal incision with a diamond knife produces a small limbus-based conjunctival frill, and combines the advantages of a corneal and corneoscleral incision, while having the disadvantages of neither. A deep vertical groove is cut (**3.3**) and bleeding vessels are cauterized (**3.4**). The anterior chamber is entered at one side of the section, and some viscoelastic substance injected. The section is completed by cutting an oblique shelf, with the knife angled forwards (**3.5**).

3.3

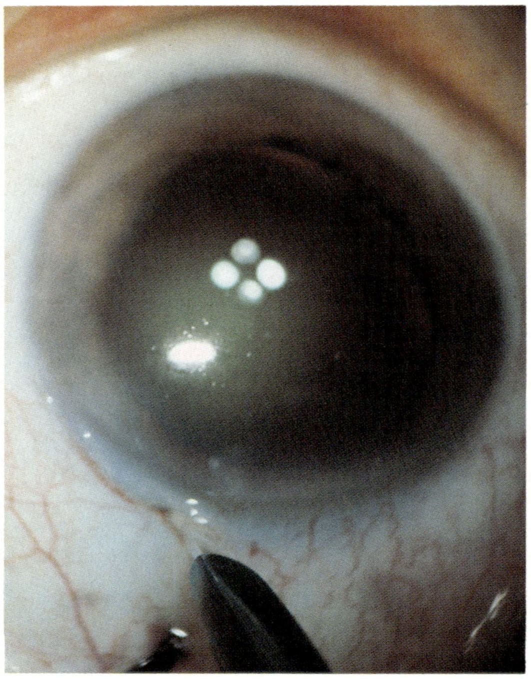

3.3 Deep vertical groove with diamond knife.

3.4

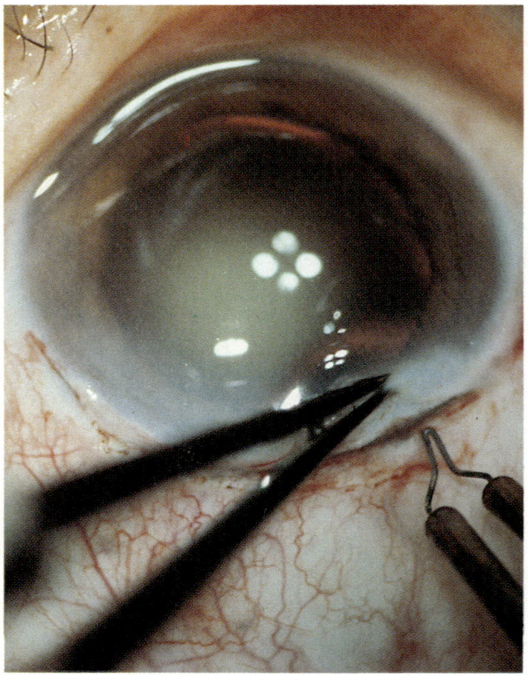

3.4 Cautery to bleeding vessels.

3.5

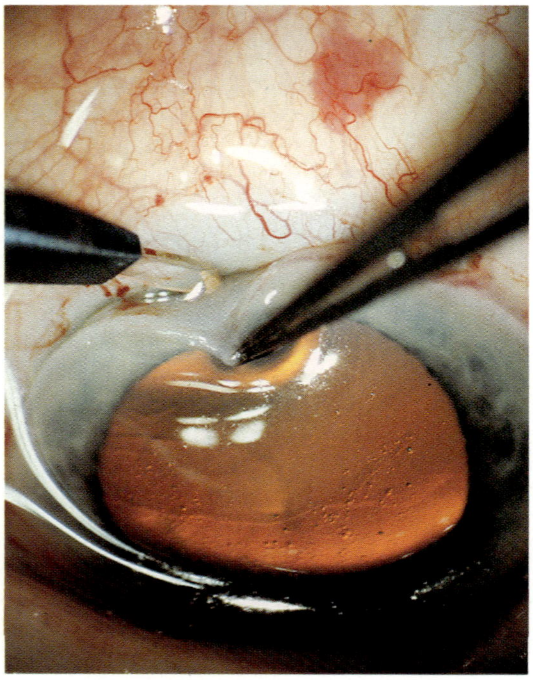

3.5 Cutting the oblique shelf.

A peripheral iridectomy is performed (**3.6**) (two if an ACL is to be implanted) and chymotrypsin is injected through the 12 o'clock iridectomy to each side, using a lacrimal cannula (**3.7**) and then beneath the pupil margin from 3 o'clock to 9 o'clock. Three 10-0 nylon sutures are now placed (**3.8**) making sure that the 11 o'clock and 1 o'clock sutures are a minimum of 6 mm apart if an ACL is to be implanted. The anterior chamber is irrigated with balanced salt solution to remove zonular fragments (**3.9**), and the lens is then removed either with Arrugas' capsule forceps or with the cryoprobe.

3.6

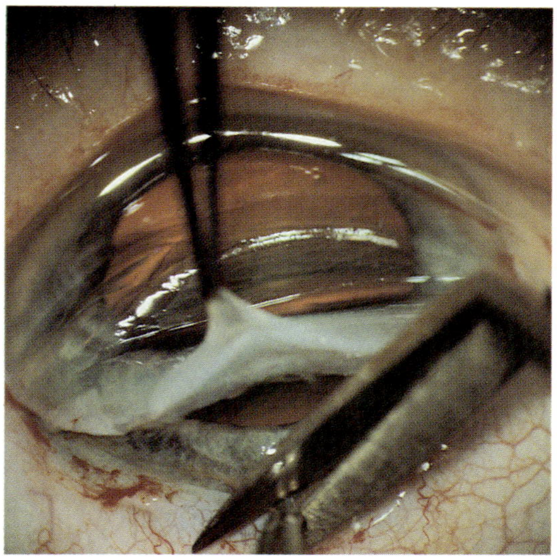

3.6 Peripheral iridectomy.

3.7

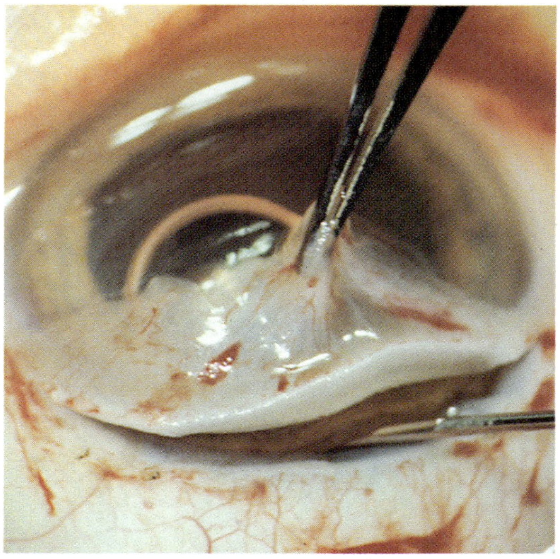

3.7 Chymotrypsin injected through iridectomy.

3.8

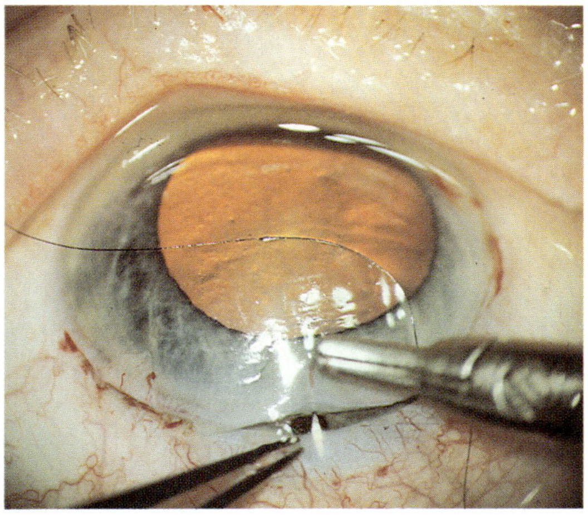

3.8 Placing a 10-0 nylon suture.

3.9

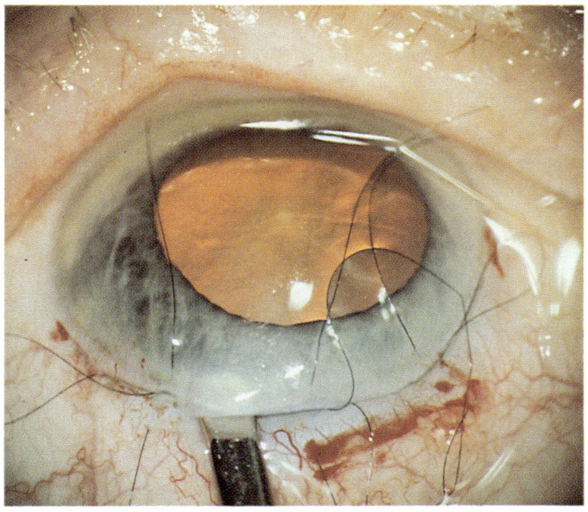

3.9 Irrigation with balanced salt solution.

Forceps delivery: Gentle pressure with a squint hook just below the inferior limbus causes the upper pole of the lens to tilt forwards. The iris is brushed off the lens with a Marten hair brush (**3.10**) or microsponge and the capsule is grasped with Arrugas' forceps (**3.11**). The lens is removed by gentle side-to-side movements, aided initially by gentle expression, though all pressure should be removed from the eye by the time the lens is half way out (**3.12**).

Alternatively, the iris may be retracted and the lens capsule grasped with forceps, but the risk of capsule rupture is greater.

3.10

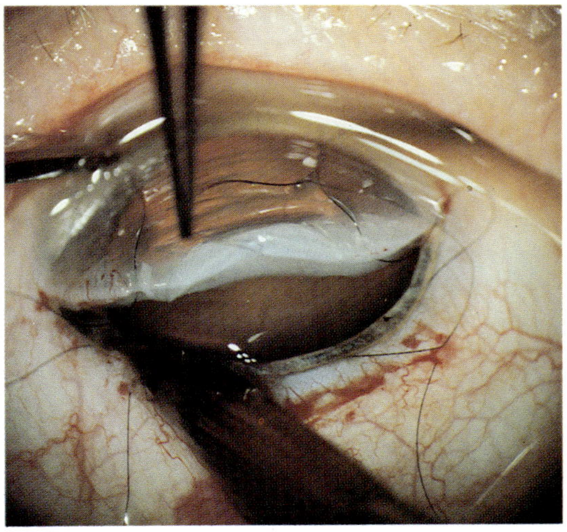

3.10 Iris retraction with brush.

3.11

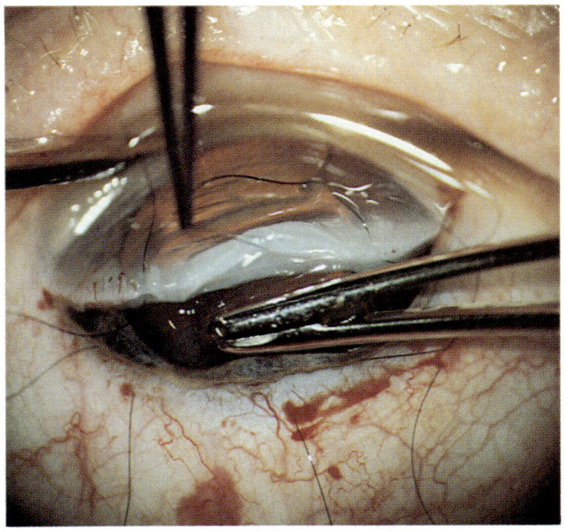

3.11 Capsule grasped with Arrugas' forceps.

3.12

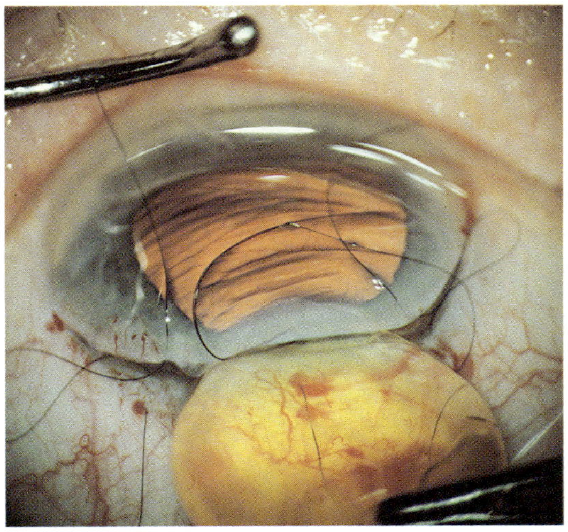

3.12 Removal of lens with forceps.

3.13

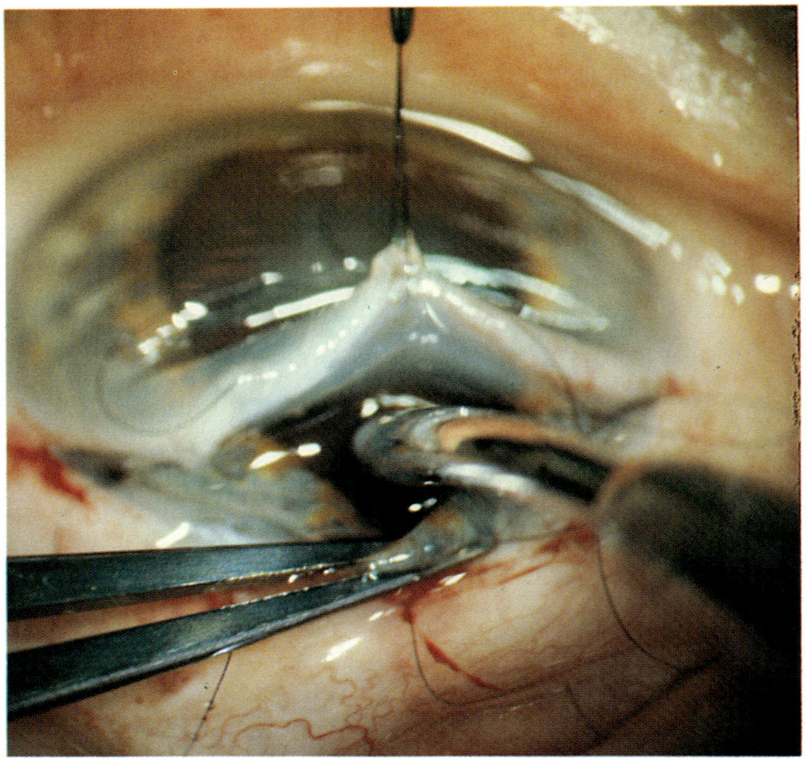

3.13 Cryoprobe applied to lens after iris retraction using forceps.

3.14

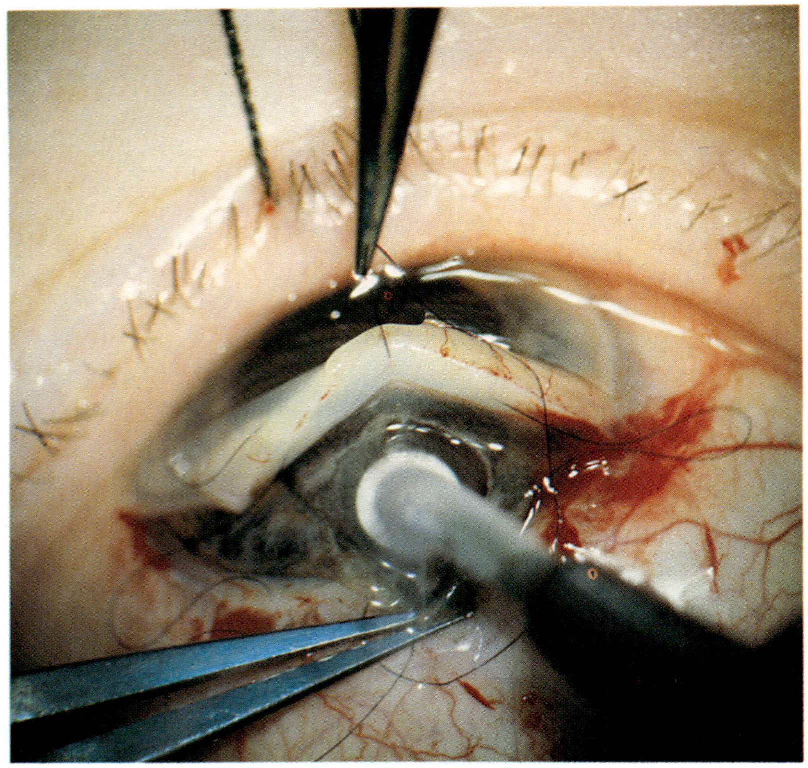

3.14 Cryoprobe activated.

3.15

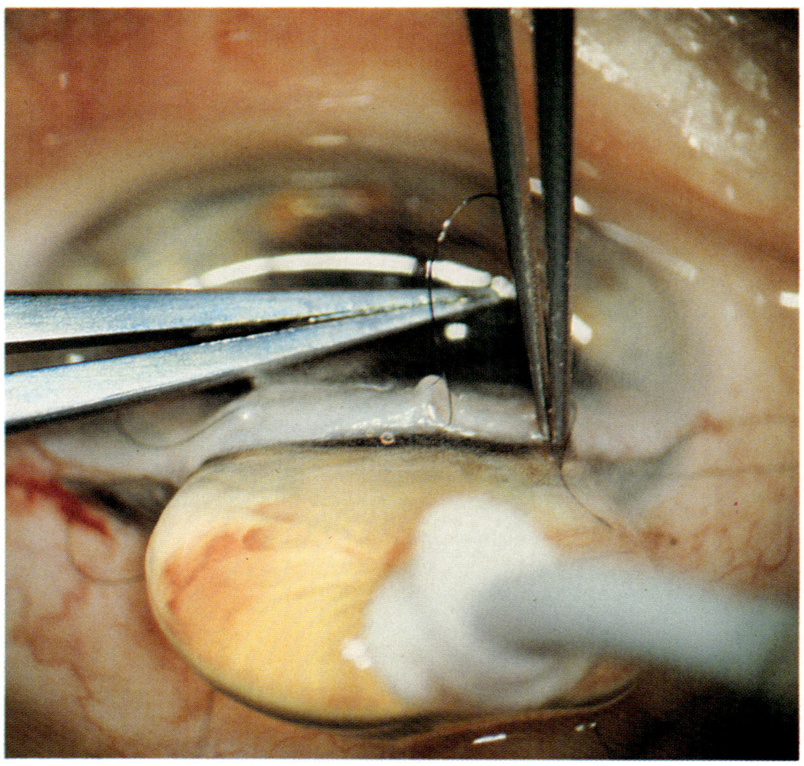

3.15 Lens delivered with cryoprobe.

Cryoextraction: The iris is retracted by a brush, microsponge, or fine curved forceps (**3.13**), and the nonactivated cryoprobe is applied to the lens capsule. The probe is then activated (**3.14**), and delivery of the lens is achieved by side-to-side rocking movements (**3.15**), taking care to avoid touching the cornea or iris with the ice-ball. This is most likely to happen immediately the ice-ball forms, and there should therefore be an initial rapid lifting movement to avoid touch.

Conclusion of the operation: The iris is reposited with a brush or repositor if necessary. The anterior chamber is reformed if necessary with balanced salt solution *via* a Ryecroft cannula. The sutures are tied, and additional sutures inserted as necessary. The knots are cut short and are buried beneath the conjunctival flap. Antibiotic drops and ointment are instilled, and the eye is padded for 24 hours.

Postoperative care: A mydriatic is instilled twice daily and guttae prednisolone with neomycin four times daily for two weeks: thereafter the steroid is tapered off over the next month.

4: Extracapsular techniques

Clive Peckar

During the 1960s and early 1970s the majority of cataract operations were carried out using the intracapsular technique. However, with the advent of second generation posterior chamber lenses, which required capsular support, it soon became apparent that extracapsular cataract extraction (ECCE) associated with posterior chamber lens implantation offered better visual results with greater lens stability than intracapsular extraction. The continued use of implants after intracapsular surgery was associated with an unacceptable risk of subluxation, retinal detachment, corneal decompensation, cystoid macular edema and uveitis (pupil supported lenses whether anterior or posterior chamber); and macular edema, uveitis, glaucoma and corneal decompensation (anterior chamber lenses). These lenses have now fallen into disfavor and ECCE has become established as the procedure of choice for primary lens implantation.

Surgical technique

Technique may be varied according to the planned method for lens implantation and length of incision. The following steps offer simplicity and guidance for those surgeons new to the technique of ECCE.

Capsulotomy

Following the first stage of a two-plane limbal section (chord length 10 mm), a 1 mm incision is made into the eye. A viscoelastic agent is injected into the eye prior to capsulotomy. This produces a controlled operation with greater safety and is invaluable, particularly for surgeons in training. Its effect is fourfold:

- Protection of the corneal endothelium, particularly from direct contact with a hard lens nucleus or polymethylmethacrylate (PMMA) intraocular lens.
- Creates space and prevents collapse of the anterior chamber.
- Helps prevent trauma to the superior iris.
- Provides tamponade to prevent the anterior capsule lifting off the lens nucleus prematurely during anterior capsulotomy.

In the presence of a mature cataract a slightly larger volume of viscoelastic agent is used to prevent lens milk escaping into the anterior chamber and obscuring the view of the capsulotomy. If the view of the capsulotomy is obscured by an excess of fluid cortex, this should be aspirated before the capsulotomy is continued.

The traditional capsulotomy is a round or 'D'-shaped 'can-opener' incision (**4.1**), but many surgeons have now switched to a linear capsulotomy (**4.2**) in association with an 'in the bag' (intercapsular, endocapsular or envelope) technique. Linear capsulotomy has the advantages of:

- Simplicity.
- Additional protection of the endothelium during infusion or aspiration and other anterior chamber manipulations, particularly during expression of the lens nucleus.
- Accurate placement of the intraocular lens within the capsular bag, prior to capsulorhexis.
- Maintenance of an intact anterior capsule which, in the event of posterior capsule rupture, can be placed posterior to a sulcus fixated posterior chamber intraocular lens in order to support it.

4.1

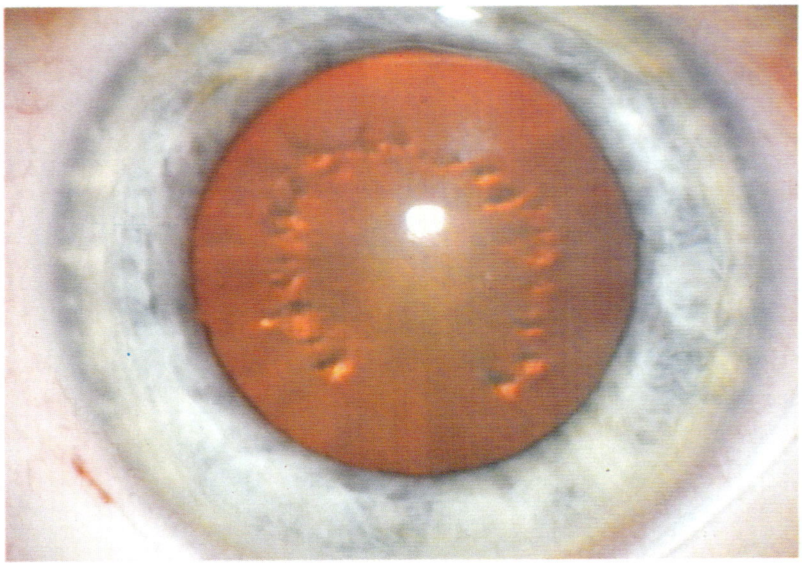

4.1 The can-opener capsulotomy made by multiple pricks on the anterior capsule with a capsulotomy needle attached to a syringe of viscoelastic material, four fifths completed.

4.2

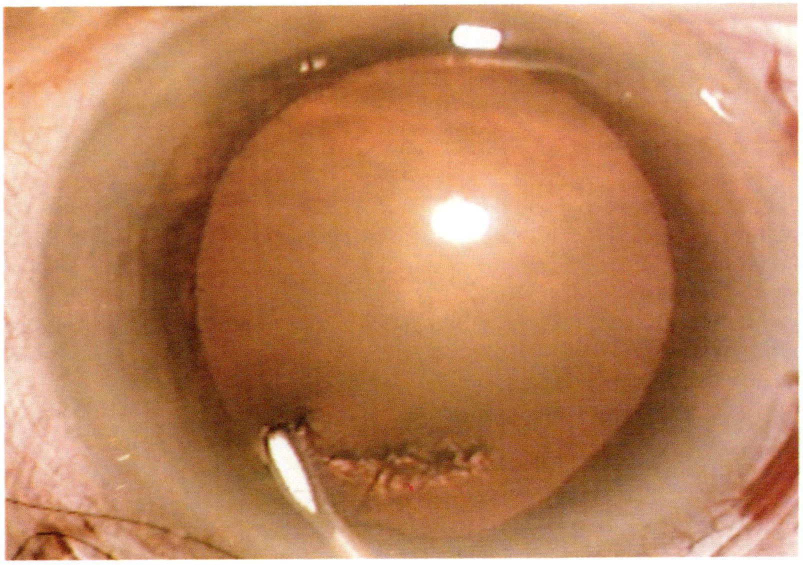

4.2 Linear capsulotomy two thirds completed.

The can-opener method has the advantage of good visibility and may be chosen by surgeons new to ECCE before progressing to other methods. The disadvantages are disturbance to the integrity of the zonule and peripheral lens capsule and uncertainty in placement of IOL haptics, particularly if the pupil constricts.

Where a linear capsulotomy has been carried out, the anterior capsule may be dissected off the lens nucleus using balanced salt solution 'hydrodissection', and the lens nucleus then mobilized with the same irrigating Rycroft cannula.

The incision is then opened to its full extent.

Removal of lens nucleus

The nucleus may be expressed by gentle pressure involving depression of the inferior pole of the nucleus at 6 o'clock, depression of the superior section at 12 o'clock, or depression of the superior section in association with the use of a vectis, or irrigating vectis at 12 o'clock to help float out the nucleus.

When the nucleus is small and freely mobile any of these procedures is satisfactory. However, in a number of cases there may be difficulty in expressing the nucleus without undue folding of the cornea. For this reason a combination of all three methods can be used. The inferior pole of the nucleus is depressed, just posterior to the 6 o'clock limbus, with a squint hook, and an irrigating vectis is used to depress the section at 12 o'clock. While the inferior pole of the nucleus is depressed the superior nucleus enters the anterior chamber (**4.3**) and is then floated out over the depressed superior section (**4.4**). In most cases it is not necessary to enter the eye with the vectis, but this can be easily carried out if the nucleus proves resistant to expression. Extreme care must be taken to prevent undue pressure being exerted on the lens zonule. For those nuclei most resistant to expression, a viscoelastic agent may be injected underneath the anterior capsule superiorly and behind the nucleus to lift it forwards.

4.3

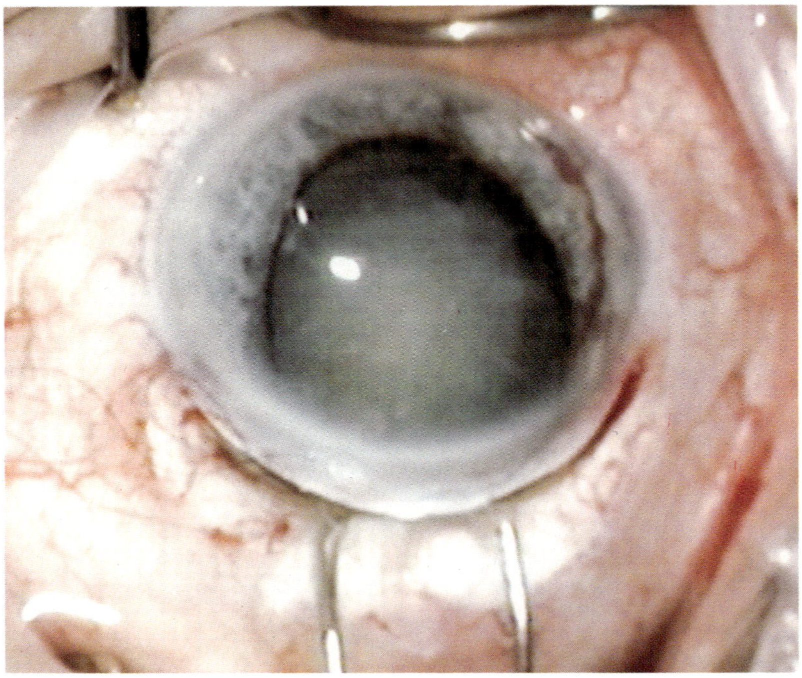

4.3 Depression of posterior lip of section with counter pressure at 6 o'clock.

4.4

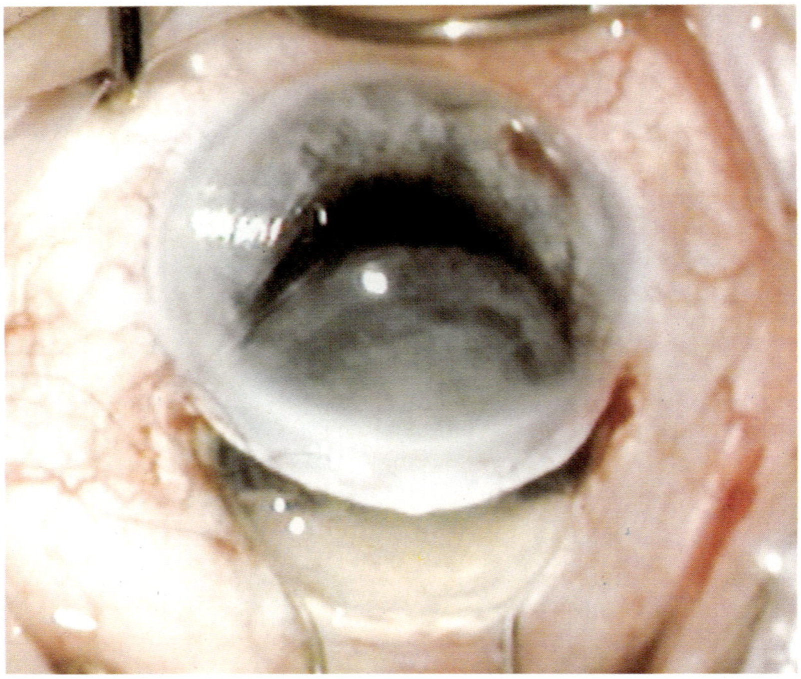

4.4 The nucleus is floated onto an irrigating vectis.

Irrigation/aspiration

Following removal of the lens nucleus the residual lens cortex must be aspirated in total from the capsular bag, using either a manual or automated system of irrigation/aspiration (I/A). It is vital that all the cortex is removed from the equatorial region of the capsular bag to reduce the incidence of postoperative capsular fibrosis. Surgeons vary in their preference as to whether to use a manual or automated system. A spring syringe (**4.5**) connected directly to an infusion aspiration cannula and via a drip set to a bottle of irrigating fluid (ideally BSS® or BSSPLUS®) provides a simple, cheap and efficient method for I/A. The system can be completely disposable (**4.5**) or, where financial constraints

4.5

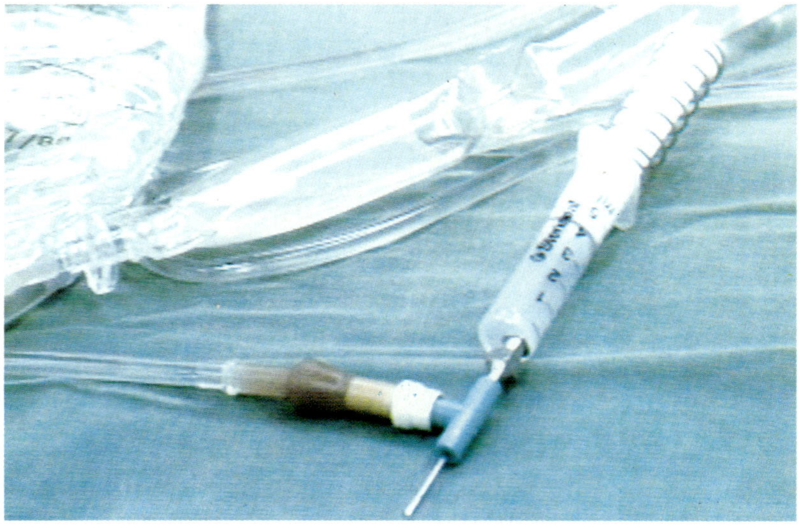

4.5 Inexpensive hand-held I/A system.

or availability prevent this, the cannulas can be reused. The spring on the syringe is optional and can offer controlled suction for a one-handed technique, although a two-handed technique generally should be preferred.

Three methods of providing mechanical vacuum for automated aspiration exist:

- Peristaltic pumps.
- Diaphragm pumps.
- Venturi systems.

By measuring the 'pre-port vacuum' in front of a 0.3 mm I/A cannula, it is possible to make comparisons between these three systems and the

4.6

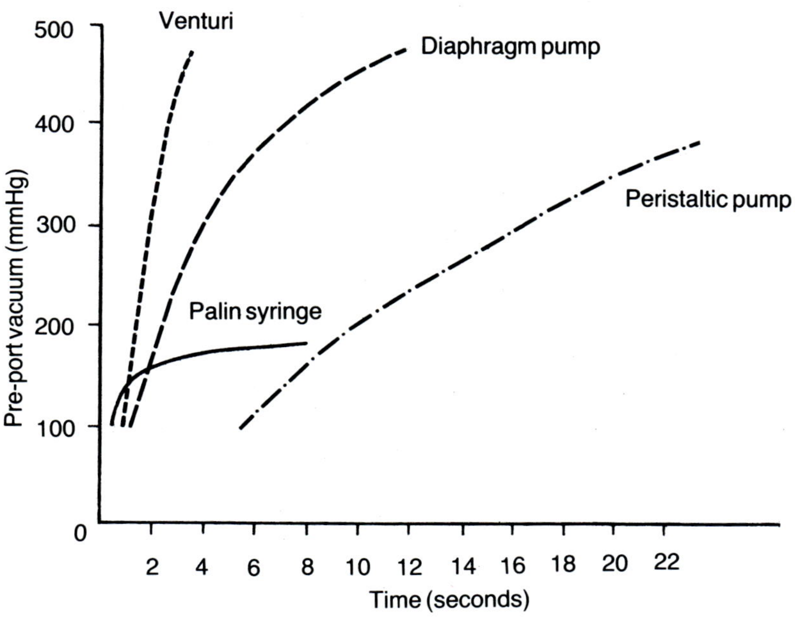

4.6 Graph showing vacuum achieved by different systems against time.

simple spring Palin syringe in the laboratory. Owing to the dead space that exists in the aspiration tubing, all the automated systems produce a delay between activation and achieving vacuum at the infusion cannula. The pre-port vacuum measurement can therefore be plotted against time (**4.6**). It can be seen that although the spring syringe has a limited effective volume (2 ml for a 5 ml syringe), its speed of onset is very fast due to the lack of dead space. This, combined with the fact that it is hand controlled rather than foot controlled, is an advantage over the automated systems. It must be remembered, however, that with the spring syringe it is either necessary to keep removing the I/A cannula from the eye, or to use a disposable one-way valve that can be fitted between the syringe and the hub of the cannula. Excessive delay in achieving reasonable vacuum levels with a peristaltic pump is clearly demonstrated, as is the relative speed of the newer venturi systems, which utilize the operating room piped-air supply. To achieve aspiration of 'soft cortex' and adequate grasping of 'thick sticky cortex' within the port for 'stripping' requires a pre-port vacuum of between 100–160 mmHg, while aspiration of 'sticky cortex' requires a pre-port vacuum of at least 250 mmHg. Where a spring syringe is used, therefore, it is necessary to strip sticky cortex from the capsular bag, having engaged it in the cannula port first, and remove it piecemeal from the eye (**4.7, 4.8**). Soft cortical matter can be purely aspirated. When using an automated I/A system, pre-port vacuum measurements of 400 mmHg may be required in order to aspirate 'sticky cortex'.

Problems exist with the removal of residual cortex from the 12 o'clock position, particularly when the pupil is not fully dilated. Maximum mydriasis should have been obtained preoperatively by the use of cyclopentolate and phenylephrine drops, and is maintained by using 1/1000000 adrenaline in the irrigation solution. Aspiration of the cortex from 12 o'clock may be aided using a micro-iris retractor in the other hand. Most surgeons, however, prefer not to have two instruments in the eye at any one time and cannulas with curved ends help to retract the iris and superior capsular flap to gain access to the '12 o'clock cortex'. Where access to the 12 o'clock cortex is still difficult, an irrigating–aspirating iris retractor has been designed, which deepens the anterior chamber and forces the 12 o'clock cortex into the aspiration port, while retracting

4.7

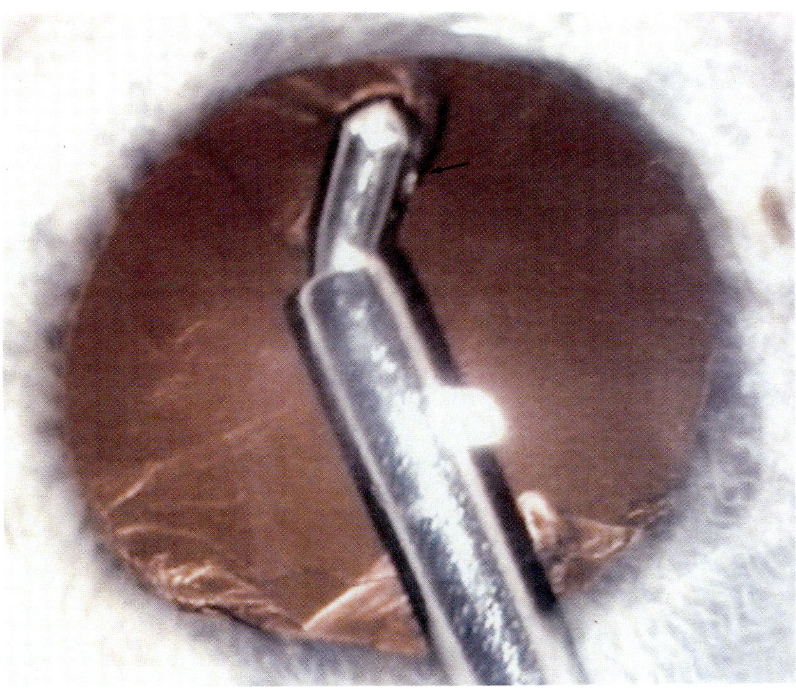

4.7 Grasping of cortex inside the capsular bag by engagement into aspiration port (arrow) of coaxial cannula. Intercapsular (envelope) extraction.

4.8

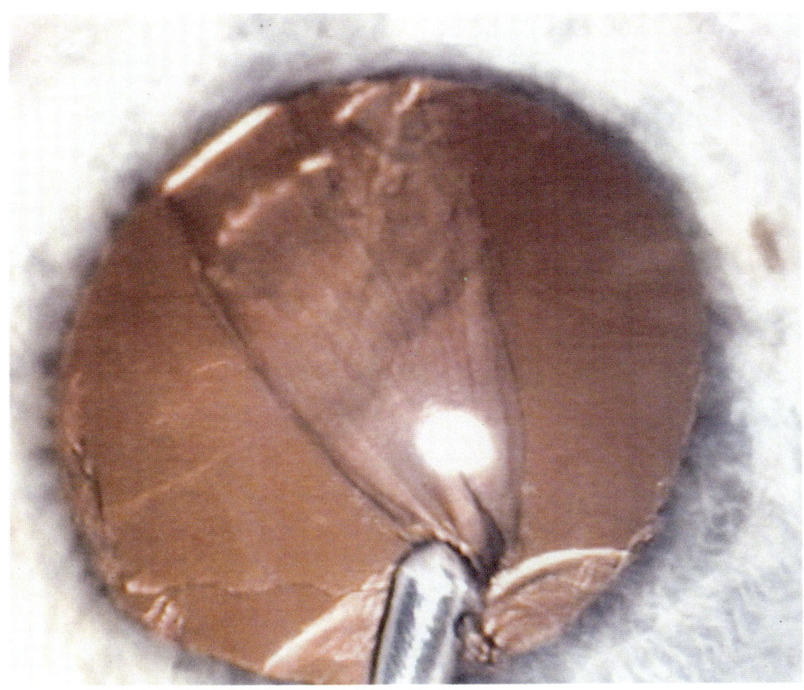

4.8 Same piece of cortex as in **4.7** being stripped from the eye. When the cortex is sticky it does not readily aspirate into a hand-held syringe and the cannula may have to be removed from the eye for each piece.

the iris and superior capsular flap (**4.9, 4.10**). Alternative methods for aspiration at 12 o'clock using a straight aspirating cannula with the port directed upwards or a J-shaped aspirating cannula with the port directed underneath the capsular flap are shown on p. 308. A set of 'reusable' cannulas is shown on p. 307.

4.9

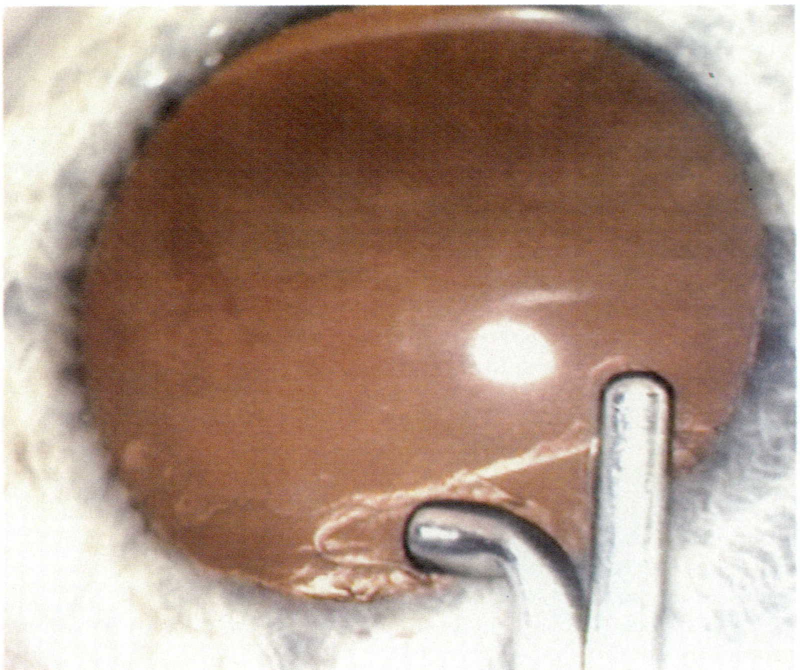

4.9 Peckar double cannula: the curved irrigating limb retracts the iris and superior capsular flap while the 0.3 mm port, which faces posteriorily on the straight, round-ended limb, aspirates the cortex. The irrigation, by blowing the cortex backwards, makes for easier retraction of the capsule.

4.10

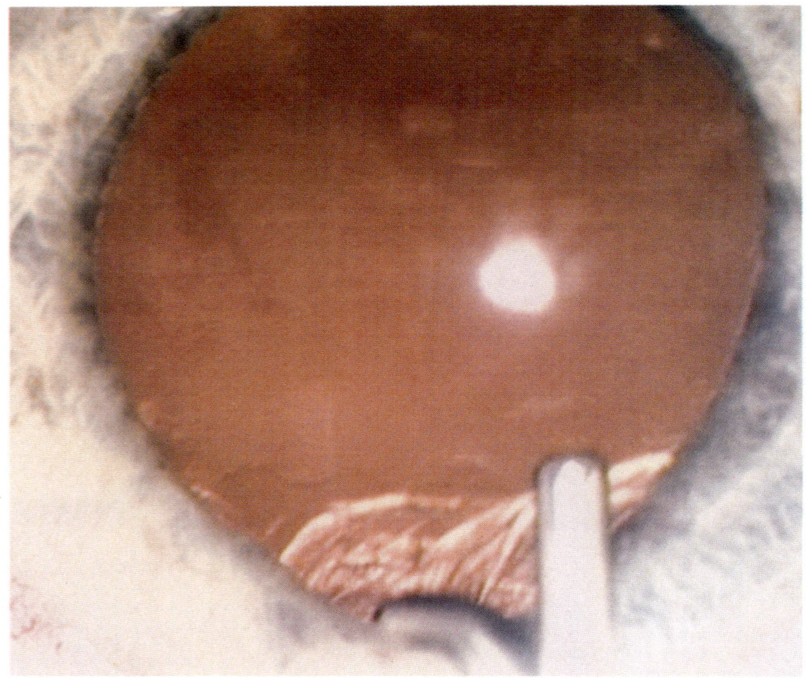

4.10 Same eye as in **4.8** and **4.9** showing aspiration of the 12 o'clock cortex.

Insertion of IOL

For capsule fixation the intercapsular (endocapsular or envelope) technique should be used and it may be desirable to inflate the capsular bag with viscoelastic agent prior to inserting the intraocular lens.

The intraocular lens is grasped by its optic and inserted directly into the capsular bag (**4.11**). The superior haptic is grasped at its tip (**4.12**) and by rotating and pronating is placed horizontally within the capsular bag (**4.13**). By this maneuver, dialling becomes unnecessary in the majority of cases. Certain types of lenses that require perfect centration in a vertical plane (eg. bifocal IOLs) may be better placed in the bag with the haptics vertical.

4.11

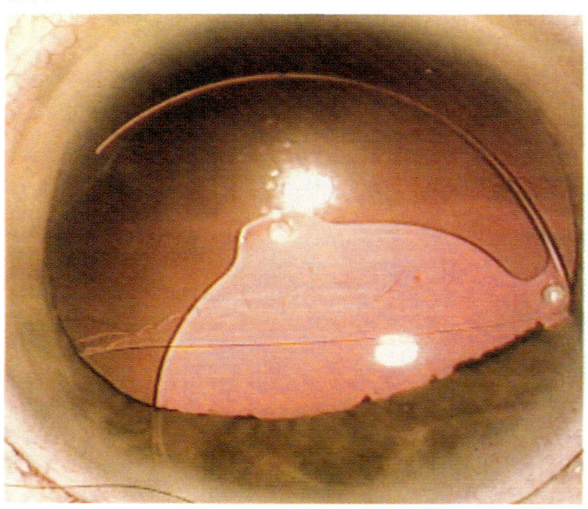

4.11 Insertion of the inferior loop and haptic into the 'envelope' of capsule.

4.12

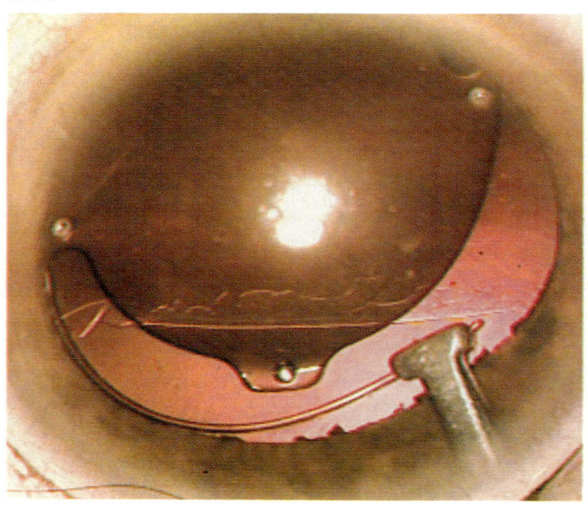

4.12 The tip of the superior loop is grasped with forceps.

4.13

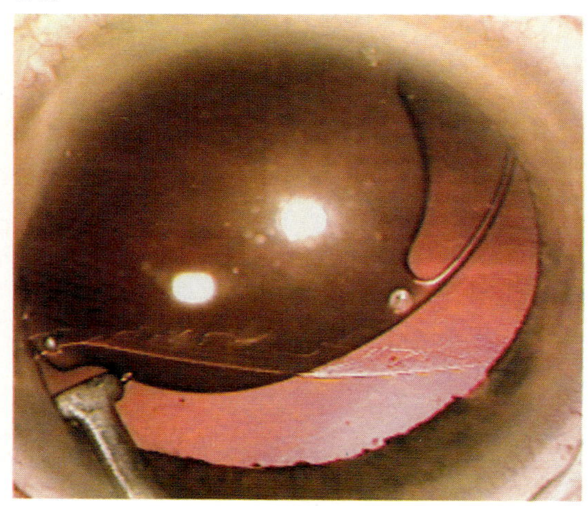

4.13 Rotation and pronation of the upper loop into the superior capsular fornix.

Where the intercapsular technique has been used, an anterior capsulotomy is now carried out. One or two vertical incisions are made using scissors (**4.14, 4.15**) and these are joined together by a capsulorhexis, having grasped the end of one of the vertical incisions with angled forceps (**4.16**).

For sulcus fixation the above capsulorhexis may be completed before lens implantation, alternatively the can-opener method (which is more suited for sulcus fixation) may be used. For this it is important to inject a viscoelastic agent behind the iris border to compress the remnant of anterior capsule against the posterior capsule and to offer free access to the sulcus prior to lens implantation. Extracapsular techniques for sulcus fixation are described on p. 301.

4.14

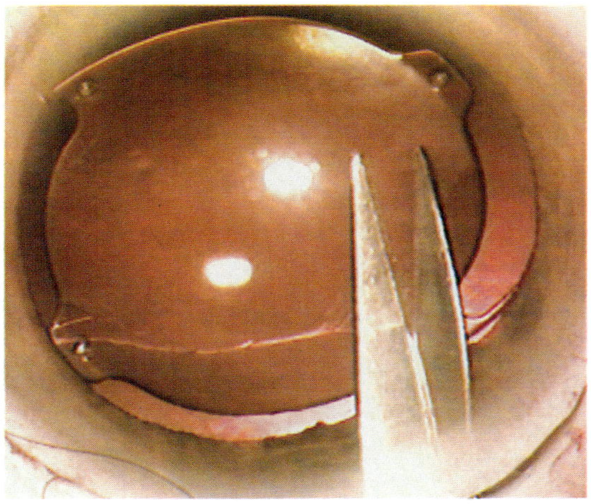

4.14 Vertical incision with fine capsulotomy scissors.

4.15

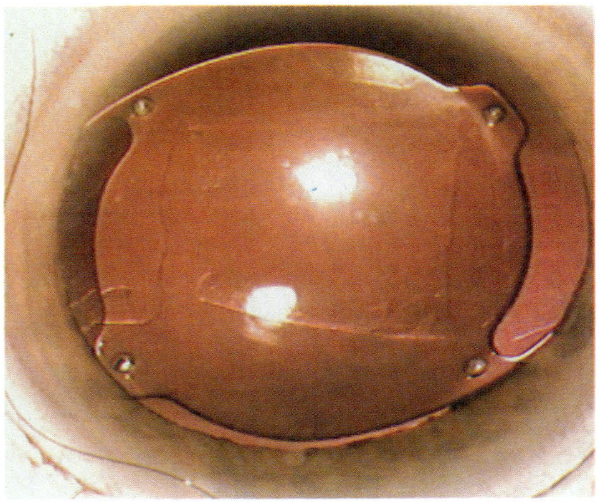

4.15 Completion of two vertical incisions into the anterior capsule.

4.16

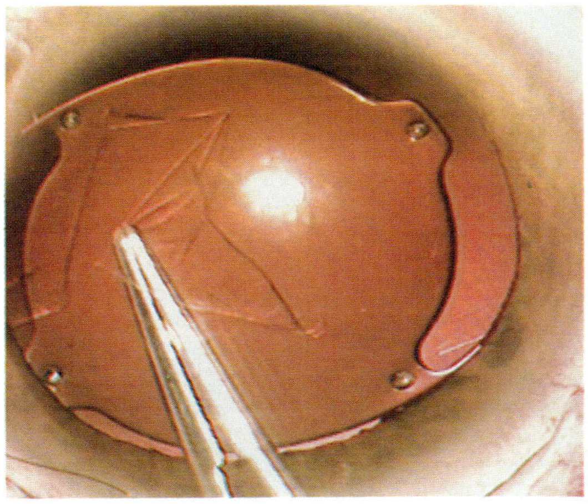

4.16 The anterior capsule is torn between the incisions with Kelman–McPherson forceps.

Technical information

All the illustrations in this chapter were produced electronically from routine surgical U-matic video recordings using a Sony Mavigraph 5000 Colour Video Printer®.

5: Development of the intercapsular technique

Georges Baikoff

Intercapsular surgery means surgery performed *between* the anterior and posterior leaves of the lens capsule. The inherent advantages are protection of adjacent intraocular structures and improved certainty of IOL placement. Further, if a break should occur in the posterior capsule, a posterior chamber lens can be safely implanted in front of the anterior capsule without primary capsulectomy, assuming the facility of a YAG laser if this capsule later opacifies.

In the late 1970s, 2-loop Binkhorst implants were implanted by the author with large horizontal flaps of the capsule in place (**5.1**) to aid positioning of the loops. This allowed an early fixation of the lens in the sac which, in turn, permitted excellent mydriasis. Unfortunately, the healing of the capsular sheets rapidly led to the development of a white opacity in all but the most central part. With the advent of posterior chamber flexible loop lenses it again seemed advisable to place the lens in the capsular sac in order to prevent contact with the ciliary body (**5.2**). In 1980, we were able to publish a technique for intercapsular insertion. This was modified later by Albert Galand into what is now known as the envelope technique.

Purely capsular fixation (**5.3**) maintains the implant at a distance from the fragile structures of the eye, avoids chronic uveal irritation, or vascular lesions at the level of the major arterial circle of the iris and, theoretically, permits long-term tolerance in totally isolating the implant.

The guiding principle for ensuring capsular fixation by the intercapsular method was to conserve the anterior lens capsule so that the IOL

5.1

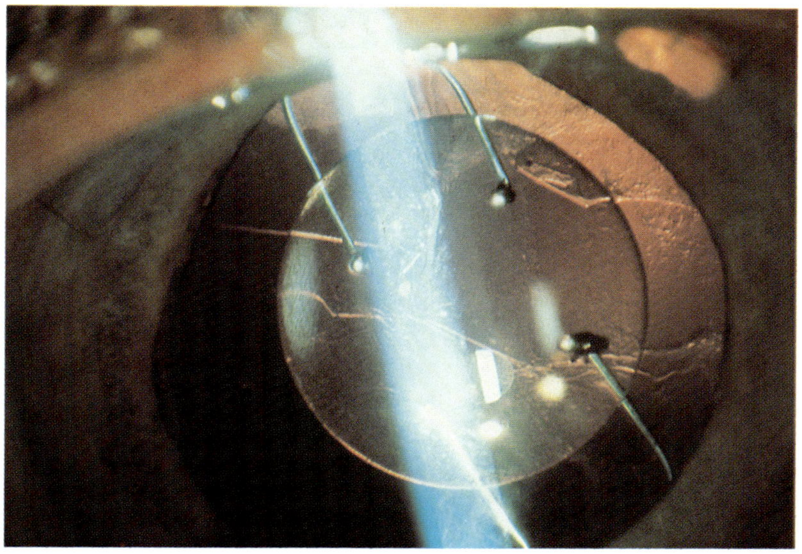

5.1 Early intercapsular technique to fixate a 2-loop Binkhorst lens. Shown postoperatively with pupil dilated.

5.2

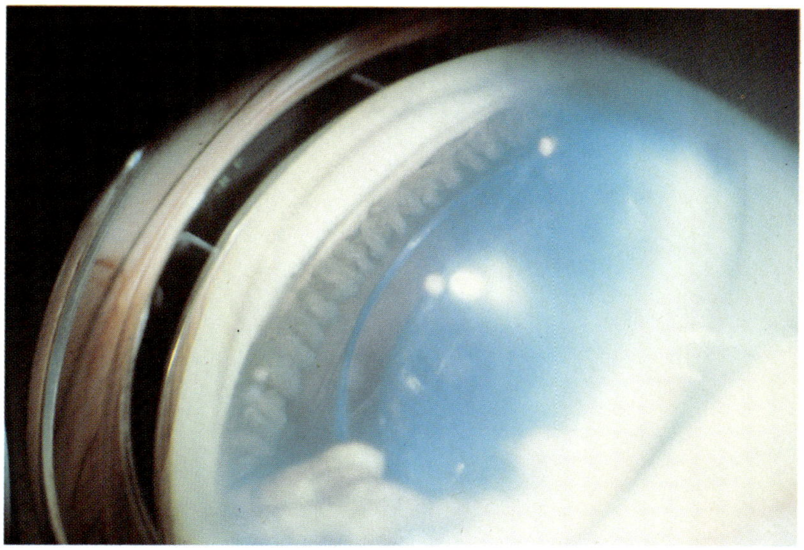

5.2 Gonioscopy of traumatic iris coloboma showing suspension of lens loop in capsular sac and no contact with the ciliary body.

5.3

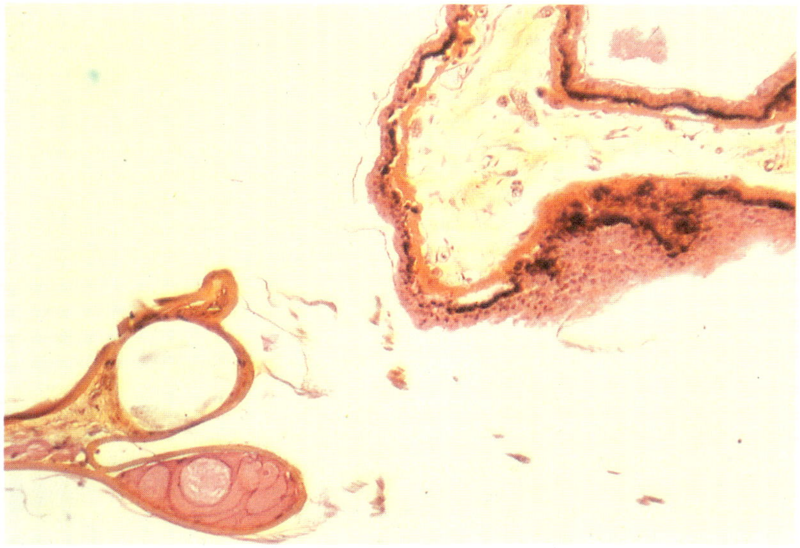

5.3 Histology showing encapsulated loop devoid of inflammatory reaction.

could glide into the capsular sac (**5.4, 5.5**).

The initial capsulotomy was performed in the shape of a semicircle (**5.6**). After guiding the lens into the sac (**5.7**), the IOL was dialled 90° in order for the upper loop to lodge in the capsular fornix (**5.8**). Once the lens had been centered, the anterior capsule was torn or cut so as to conserve the peripheral border (**5.9**). However, this method sometimes led to decentering of the IOL because of uncertainty of the size or shape of the retained anterior capsule. If it was too small, the loop could slide forward and come to lie in the iridociliary sulcus. The envelope technique of Galand reduced this possibility by making a larger upper flap: the initial capsulotomy was made horizontal between the upper third and lower two thirds of the anterior capsule. Intercapsular extraction was performed with expression of the nucleus and irrigation of the cortex *in situ*. After insertion of the IOL two cuts were made in the anterior capsule and a 'U'-shaped piece torn between the cuts with Kelman–McPherson forceps.

5.4

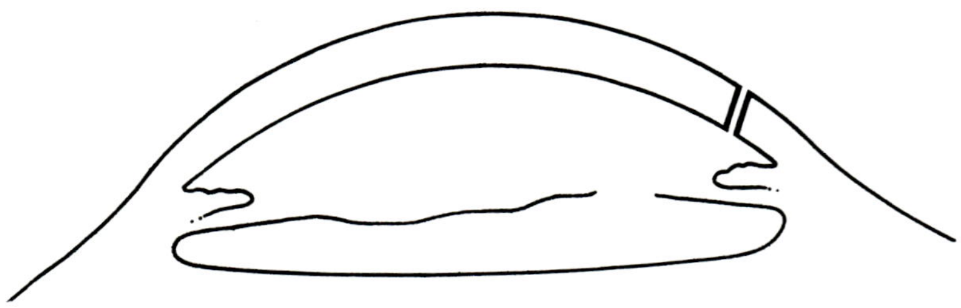

5.4 Conservation of anterior capsule after removal of cataract.

5.5

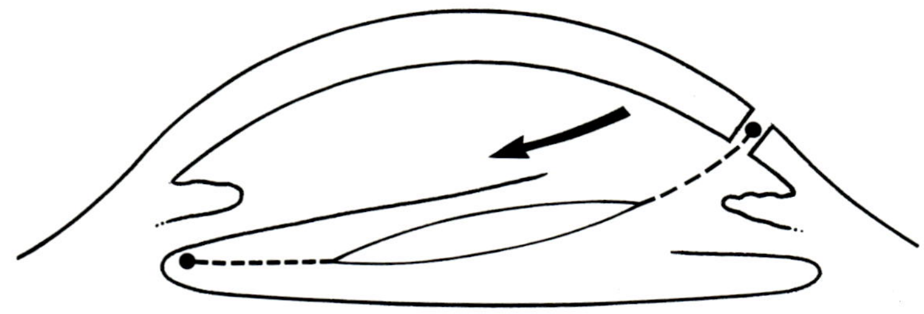

5.5 Capsular glide.

5.6

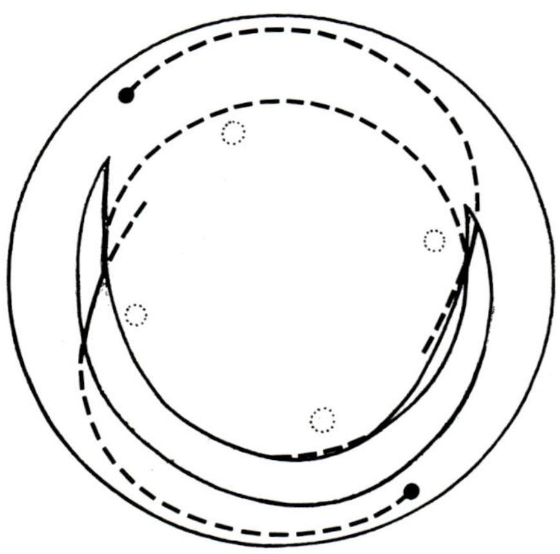

5.6 Semicircular capsulotomy convex upwards.

5.7

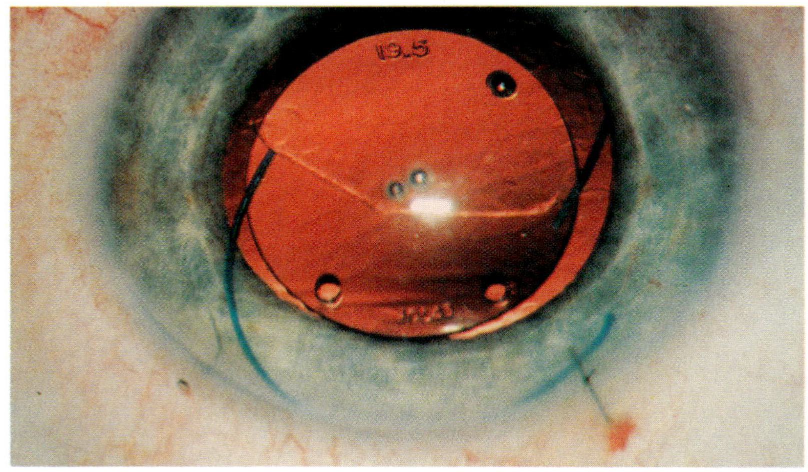

5.7 The IOL has been guided into the capsular sac.

5.8

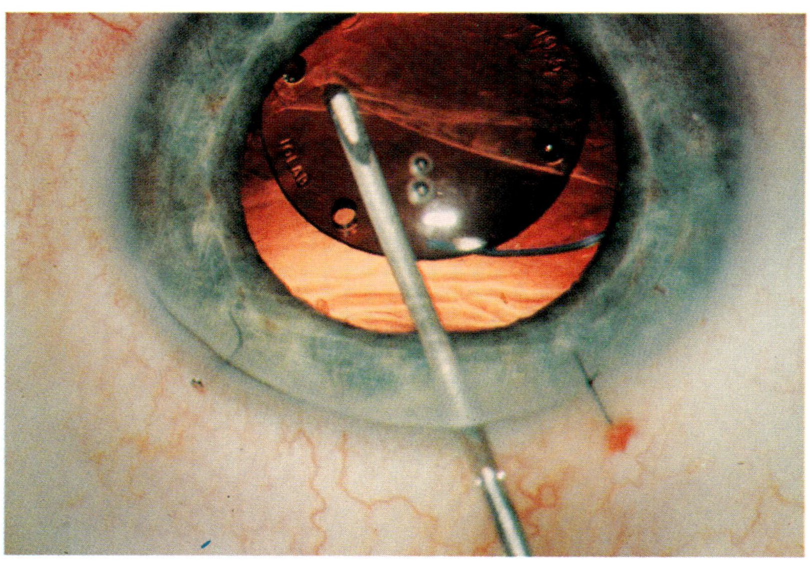

5.8 Dialling to achieve total encapsulation.

5.9

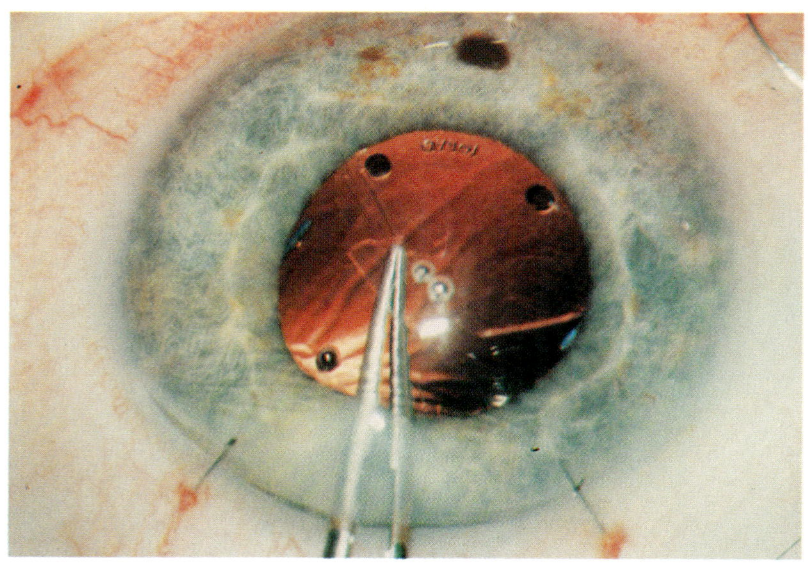

5.9 A semicircular tear completes the removal of a disc of anterior capsule. Note well centered IOL within the sac.

All these techniques of capsulotomy are based on the introduction of dotted perforations on the anterior surface of the capsule. A useful analogy may be to compare the anterior capsule to a sheet of stretched cellophane. It has the possibility of tearing in any direction. The unintentional appearance of such a tear (**5.10, 5.11**) can lead to asymmetric placement and later decentration of implants, whether of the opened or closed loop type. However, if there is a smooth rim to the anterior capsulotomy the integrity of the zonule and capsular fornix is preserved (**5.12**) and decentration will be prevented because there is an even contracture of the capsule throughout its circumference and because it is impossible for loops to slide through a tear or in front of a leaf of capsule. Continuous circular capsulotomy or capsulorhexis was first described by Thomas Neuhann. The capsule is torn in a controlled circular fashion, without any dotted perforations. The cellophane-like sheet can tear circularly by simple traction and if a circular opening is made with a smooth rim it can be deformed during lens implantation like a buttonhole (**5.13**) with no risk of ripping. Associated with this evolution of capsulorhexis, the routine use of viscoelastic substances has rendered obsolete the need to conserve the anterior lens capsule.

5.10

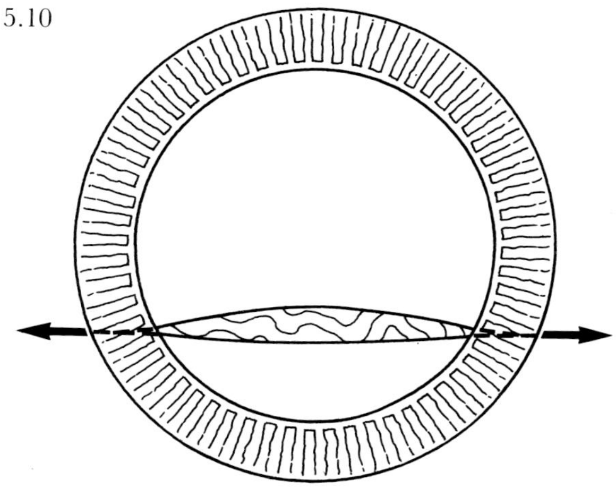

5.10 Diagram showing the direction of unwanted tears after linear capsulotomy used for the envelope method.

5.11

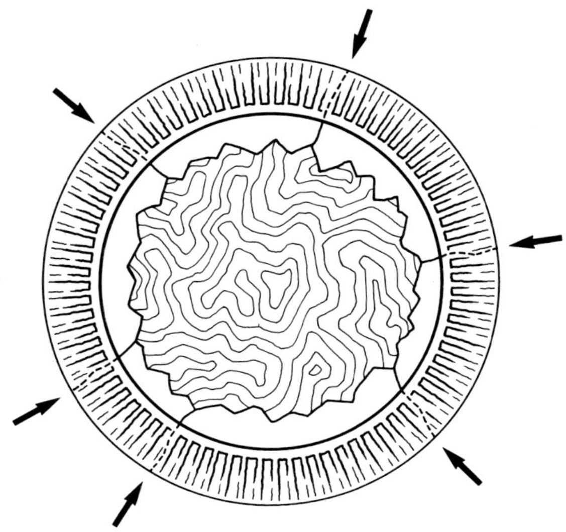

5.11 If a can-opener capsulotomy is used with dotted perforations, multiple radial tears (arrows) may develop, often hidden by the iris.

5.12

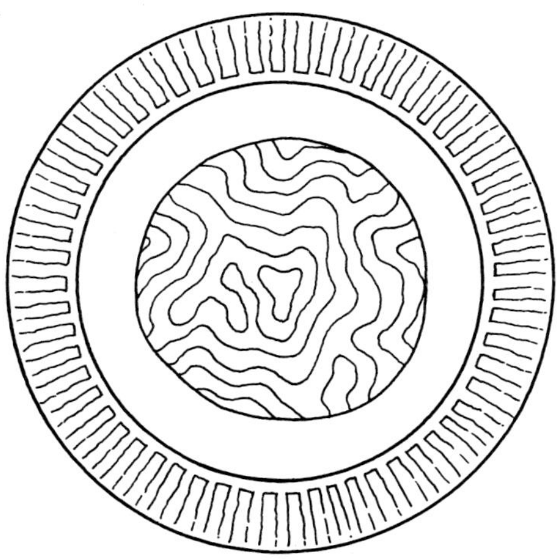

5.12 Smooth circular capsulorhexis preserves the integrity of the zonule and capsular fornices.

5.13

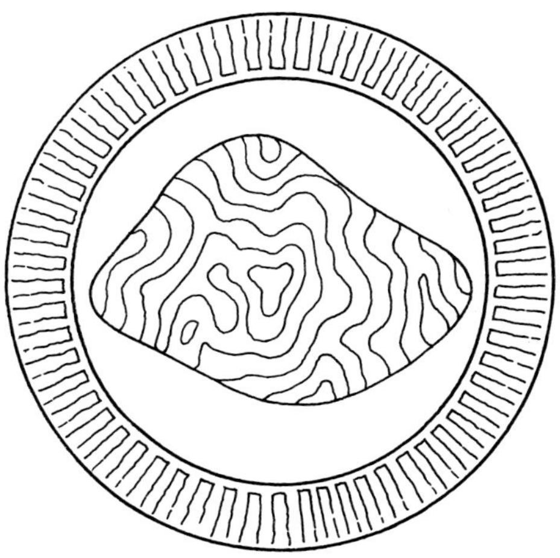

5.13 Deformation of circular opening without risk of developing a radial tear.

Technique for capsulorhexis

The chamber is sealed by either air or a viscoelastic substance. It is important to increase the pressure in the anterior chamber in order to relax the tension of the anterior capsule. Using a 25- or 30-gauge needle with a bent tip, the opening is commenced with a radial puncture at one o'clock (**5.14, 5.15**). A fragment of the anterior capsule detaches and using the needle point, is made to fold back on itself (**5.16, 5.17**). A circular movement is continued in the direction indicated (**5.18–5.23**) until an arc of 360° is completed (**5.24, 5.25**). The edge remains smooth

5.14

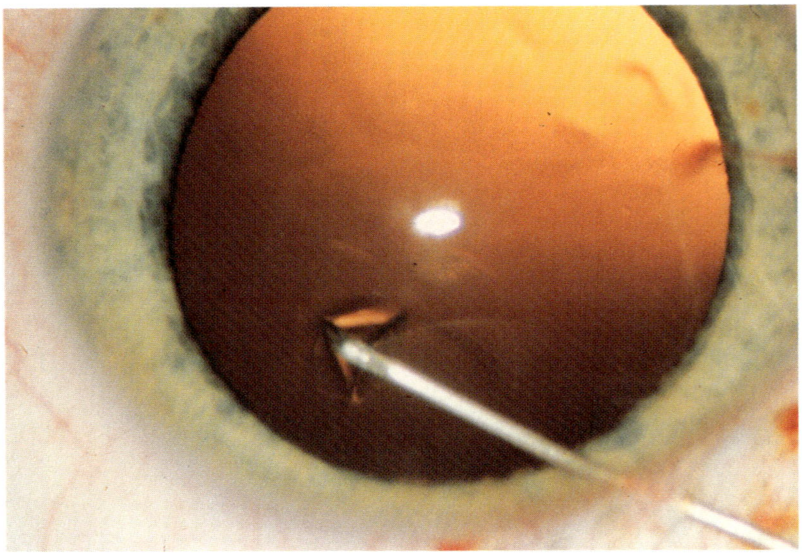

5.15

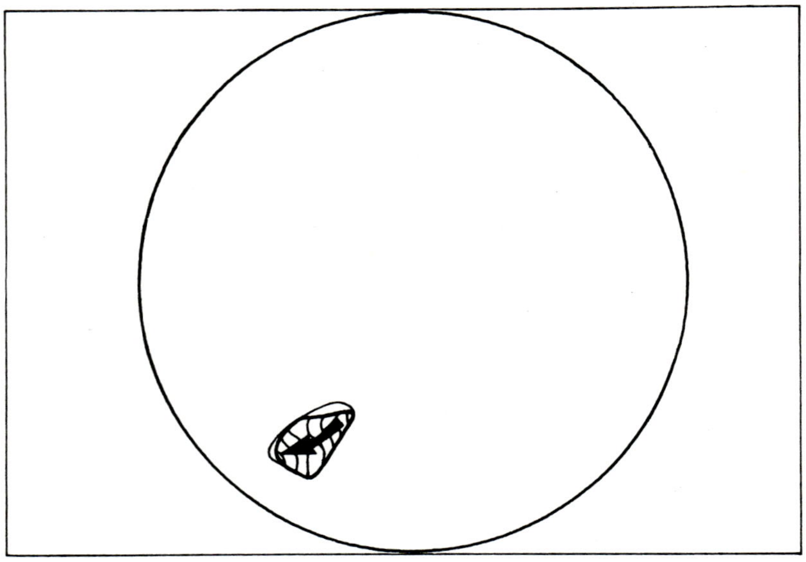

5.16

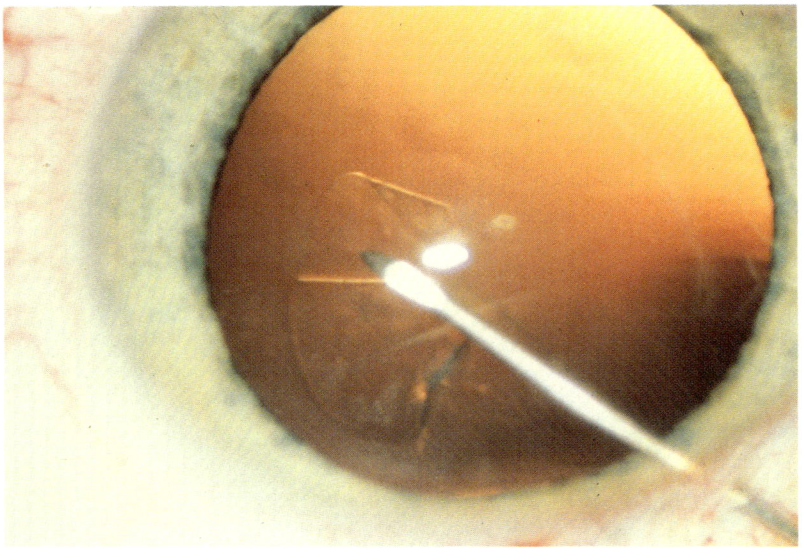

5.17

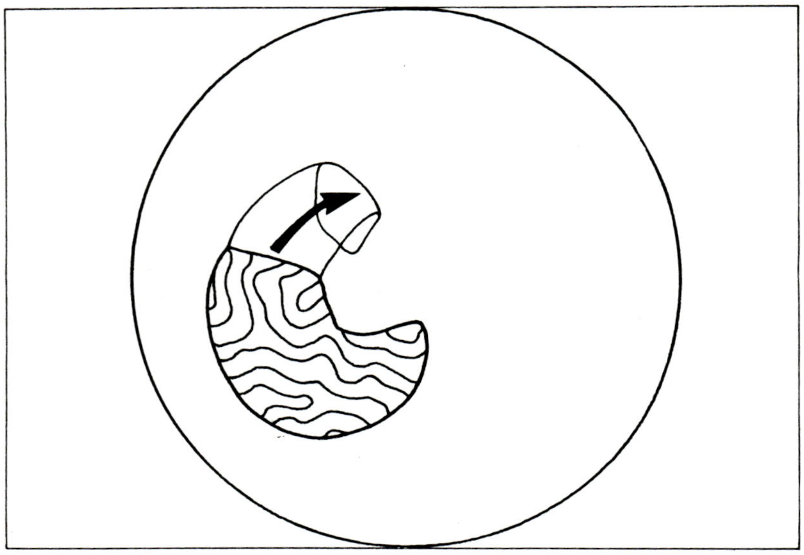

5.18

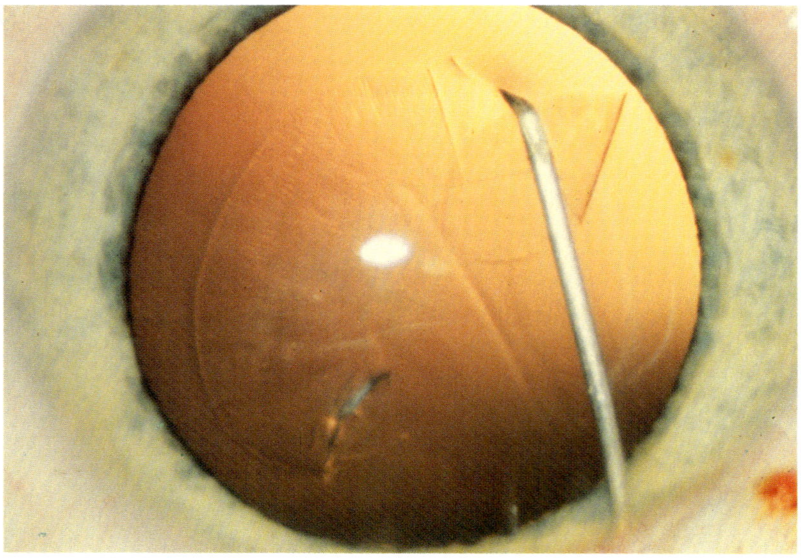

5.19

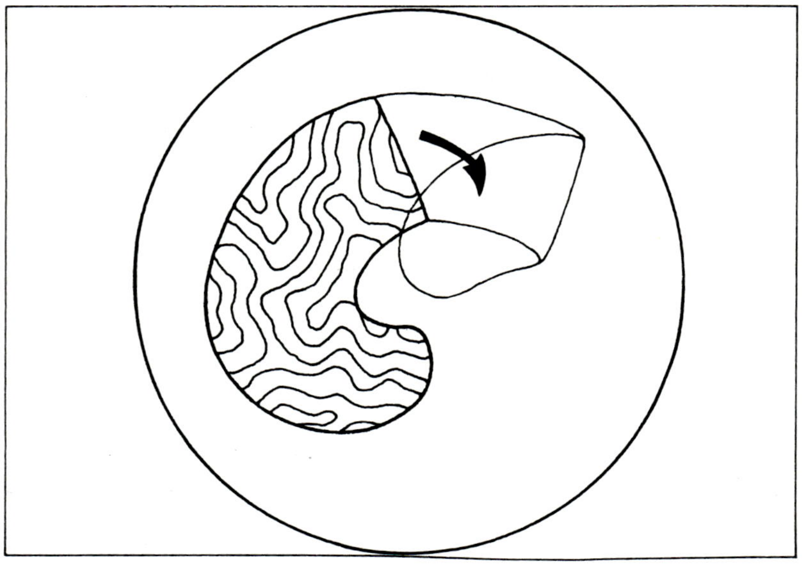

and ideally has a diameter of 6.5 mm. Small indentations (**5.25**) do not matter because they are not associated with radial tearing. The separated disc of capsule can be extracted with the nucleus or aspirated with the cortex. The nucleus is then extracted by phacoemulsification or planned ECCE. For the latter, hydrodissection of the nucleus core may be necessary before lifting the nucleus through the relatively small opening. For hydrodelineation of nuclear layers, see p. 40. If the nucleus is hard or large, a purpose-made relaxing incision is made at the edge of

5.20

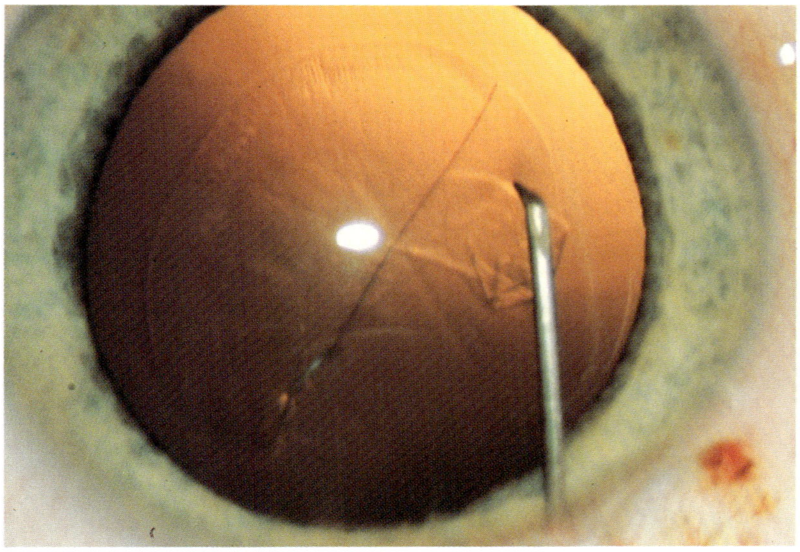

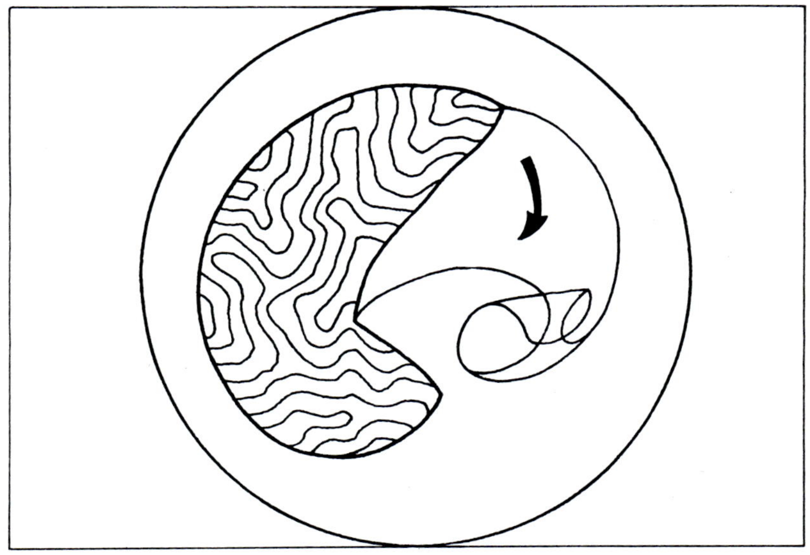

5.21

5.22

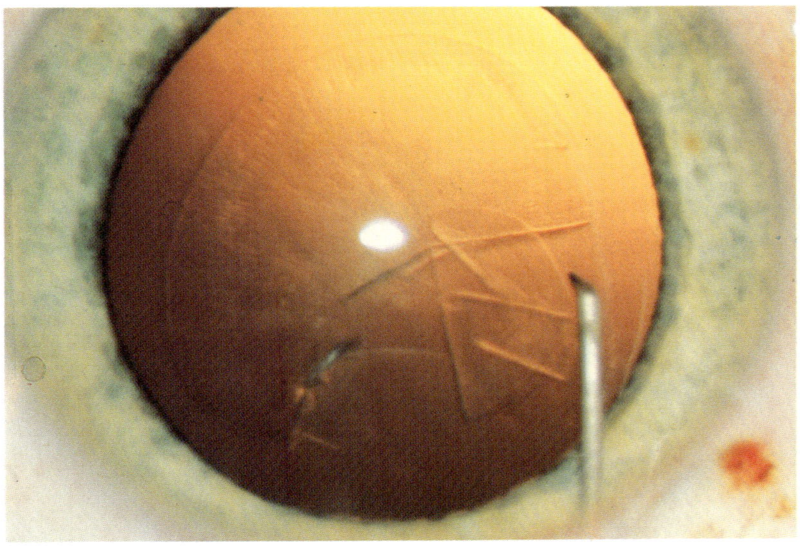

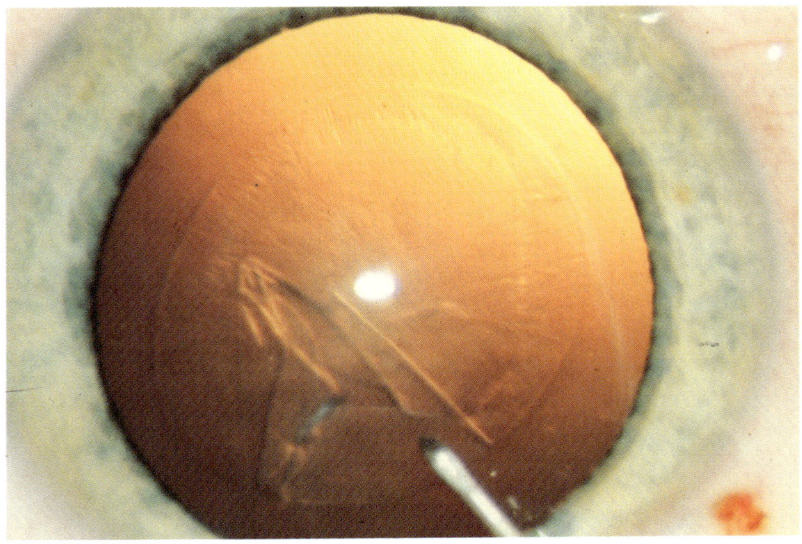

5.23

5.24

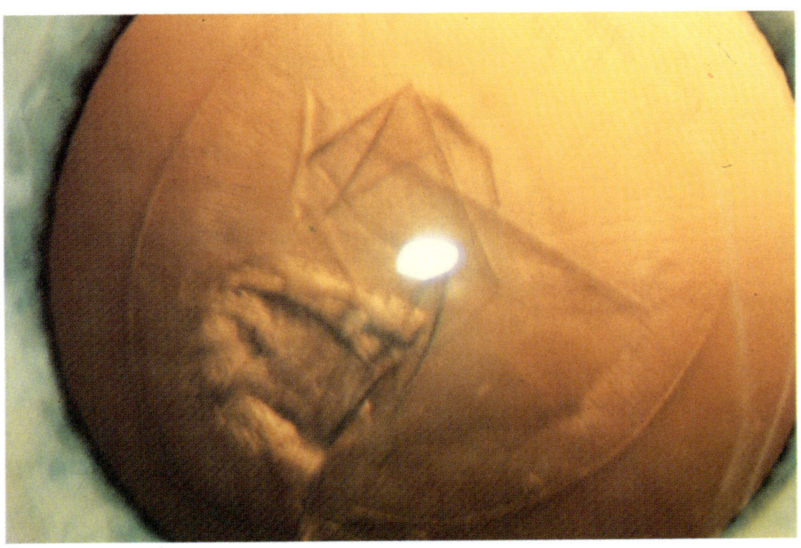

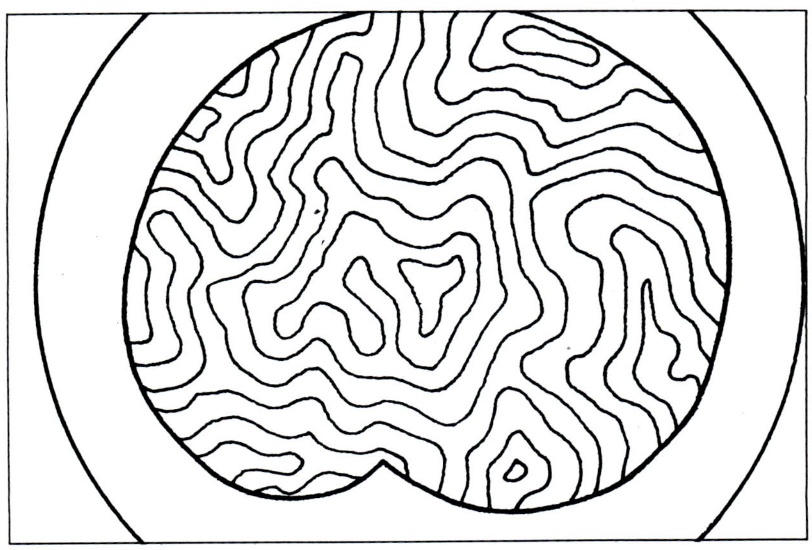

5.25

5.14–5.25 Technique for capsulorhexis. The arrows indicate the direction of movement of the needle tip.

the capsulotomy (see p. 96). If the pupil is not well dilated, the envelope method may be preferred.

After aspiration of the cortex, the capsule is carefully cleaned (**5.26**), and finally, a circular ring (**5.27**) remains that is stable and amenable to deformation during the passage of implants even of large size (**5.28, 5.29**).

5.26

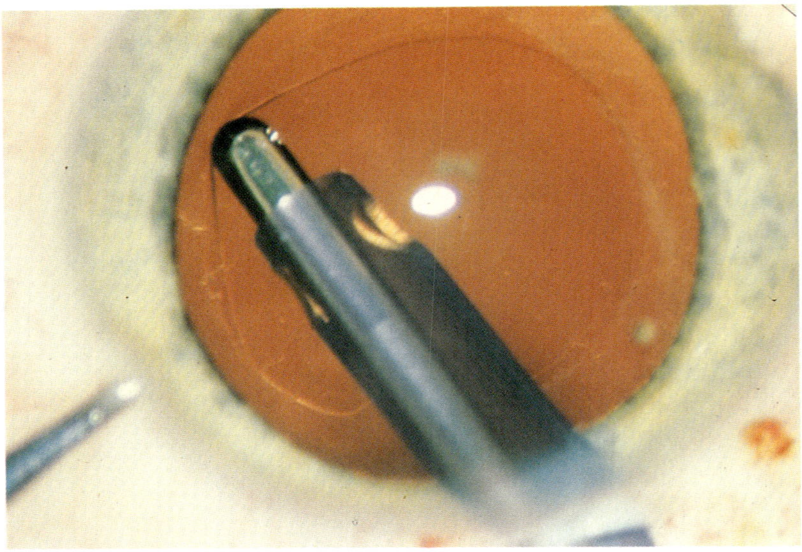

5.26 Cortical cleanup with aspiration/irrigation probe.

5.27

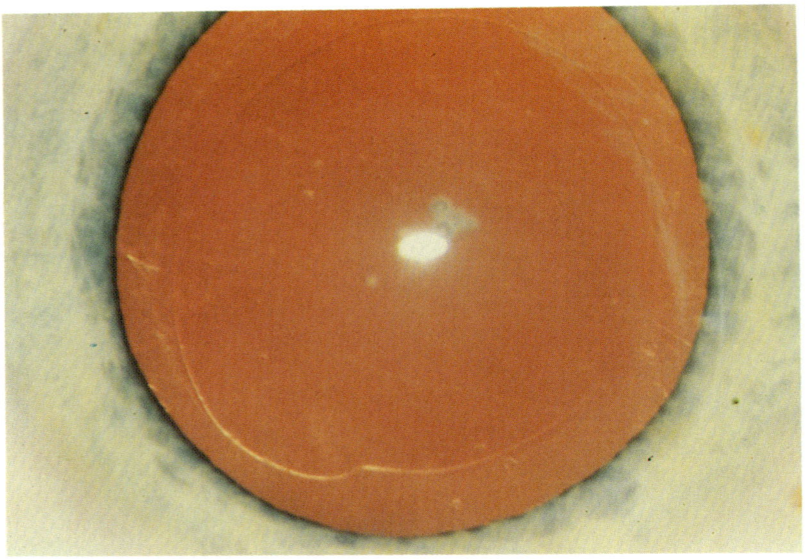

5.27 6.5 mm circular opening with one small indentation.

5.28

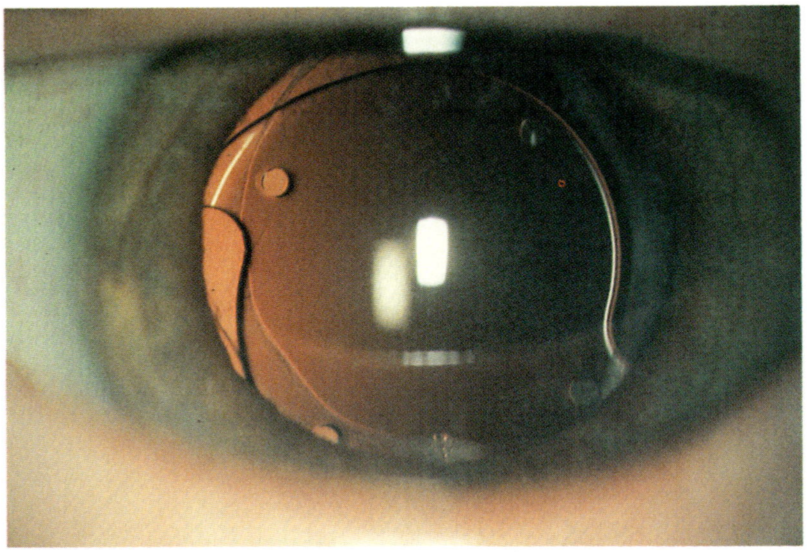

5.28 Implantation of an IOL with C loops and a 7 mm optic.

5.29

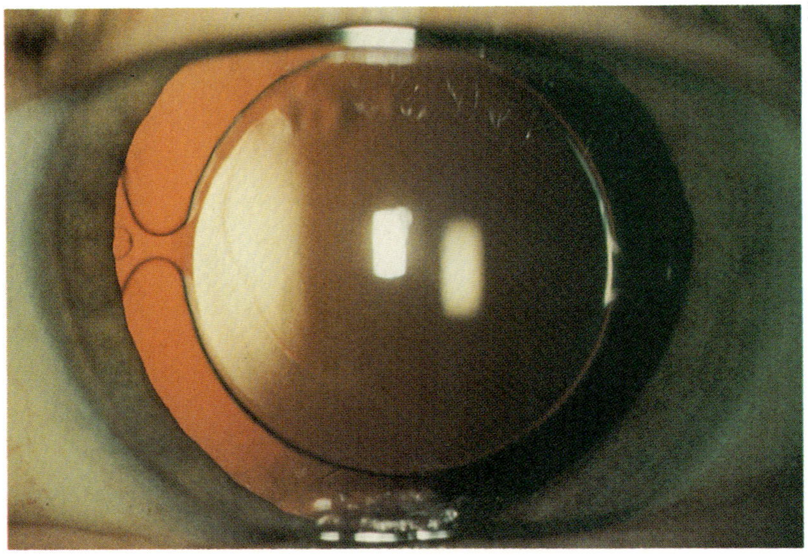

5.29 Implantation of a 9 mm compressible disc lens.

6: Small incision dry intercapsular cataract extraction and hydrosonic emulsification

Aziz Anis

The science and art of cataract extraction surgery has gone through a revolution of progress and innovation within the past two decades.

Starting with Kelman's introduction of his revolutionary phacoemulsification method of cataract extraction and stimulated by the development and evolution of lens implants from their conception to their current status, many refinements and creative concepts in cataract surgery, specifically in the different techniques for extracapsular cataract extraction (ECCE), have since followed. The following is a new method for small incision ECCE.

Objections to phacoemulsification concern the relatively large volume (up to 500 ml) of irrigating solution flowing in and out of the eye, which creates excessive turbulence in the anterior and posterior chambers. This may damage corneal endothelial cells and iris pigment epithelium, and disturb the natural integrity of the zonular membrane. This last damage can be demonstrated by the observation of lenticular fragments swirling behind the posterior capsule during surgery in the absence of any capsular tear.

Moreover, phacoemulsification fragments the compacted nuclear matter into minute particles which may then bombard the corneal endothelium. Studies conducted by Apple have shown a significant correlation between the amount of endothelial cell loss and the volume of irrigating fluid and duration of ultrasound. He has also shown that the preservation of the anterior capsule reduces the endothelial damage.

However, there are merits in small incision surgery provided the main objectives of the operation are not compromised.

The method for disposal of the nucleus in the small incision dry intercapsular cataract extraction (DICE) technique is a novel approach based on anatomical structure. The nucleus is no more than compacted layers of cortex, layered from the periphery within the limited space of the capsular bag. The most central layers are subjected to the most pressure for the longest duration and are therefore the most compact. This inner core constitutes the hardest part and, excepting brunescent cataracts, has a diameter of 2 to 5 mm.

The mechanism of nucleus removal is dependant on separation of the nuclear layers by injecting minute amounts of fluid at consecutively deeper levels. This may be achieved with the Anis HydroSonic™ machine which utilizes special cannulas attached to a hydrosonic injection handpiece. The 29-gauge cannula separates or decompacts the layers and the 20-gauge cannula, which has an end port with a sharp edge, is used to shave off each layer consecutively. Both the 29-gauge decompacting cannula and the 20-gauge shaving cannula can be propelled through the nuclear layers manually, provided the nucleus is relatively soft, or they can be propelled mechanically using a mini-motor in a self-contained handpiece or hydrosonically using the HydroSonic™ handpiece of the machine to produce linear oscillation.

The ultrasound energy is used not to fragment and emulsify the compact nuclear matter, but to propel first the 29-gauge cannula through the harder central layers of the nucleus and then the sharp edge of the 20-gauge cannula. The amount of ultrasound energy used is less than 10% of the energy used in standard phacoemulsification and is delivered in pulses only when needed.

Illustrations **6.1–6.18** show a step by step description.

6.1

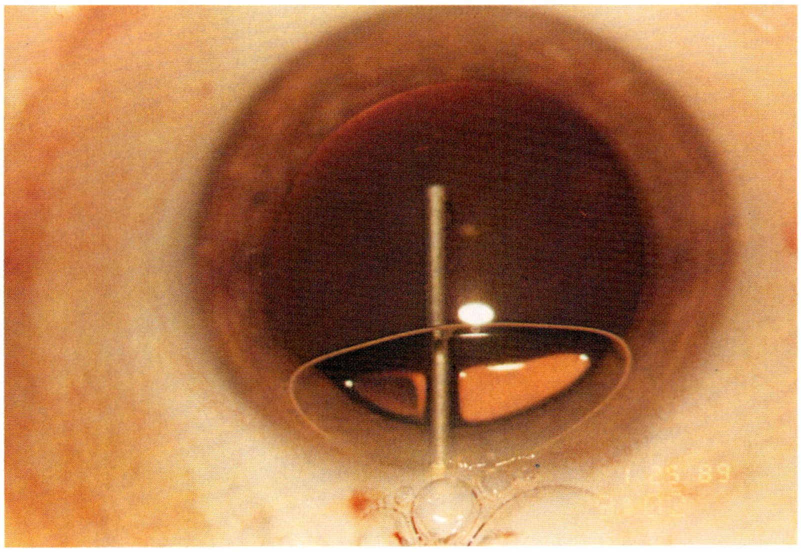

6.1 After wet field cautery to the limbal area at 12 o'clock along a 6 mm arc, a 2 mm vertical groove 0.5 mm posterior to the cornea at 12 o'clock has been made with the diamond blade. The scleral flap has been undermined and the anterior chamber entered to complete the incision. Air is injected into the anterior chamber to evacuate the aqueous and is replaced with a viscoelastic compound.

6.2

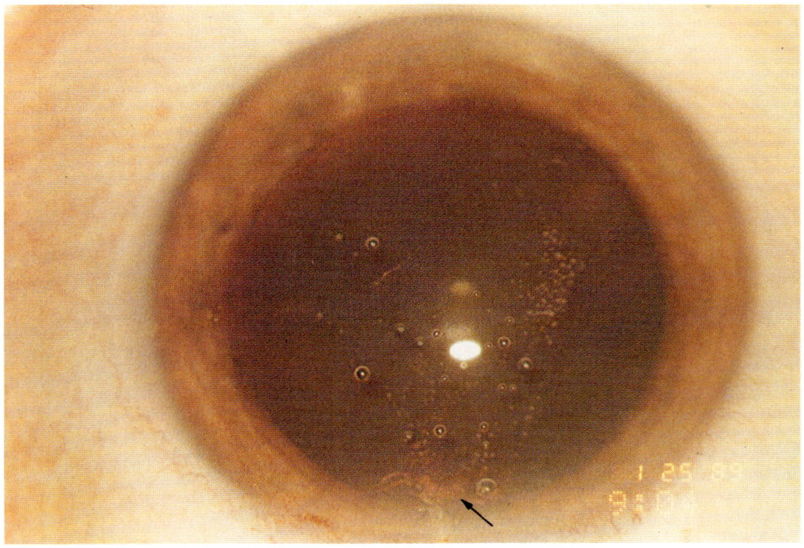

6.2 A small diagonal stab incision (arrow) in the anterior capsule is performed with a fine double-edged blade very close to the border of the fully dilated pupil to make a small round capsulectomy 1–2 mm in diameter (see **1.10–1.12**).

6.3

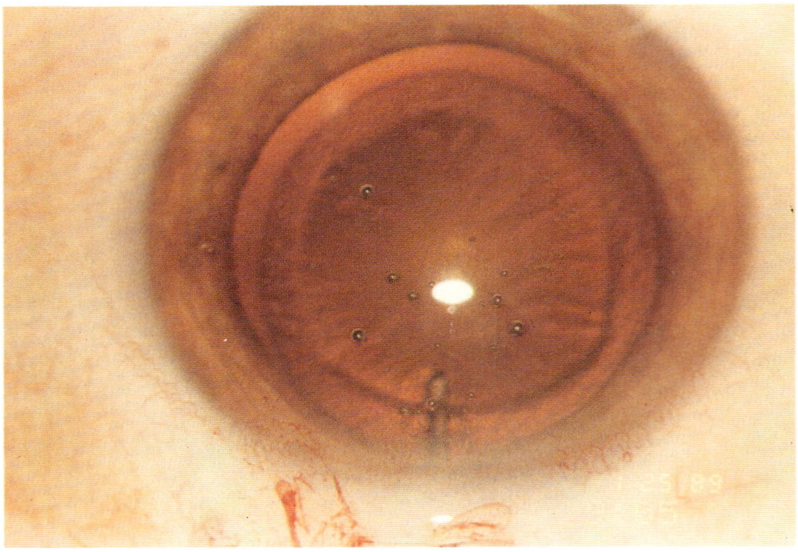

6.3 The 29-gauge cannula of the hydrosonic handpiece is introduced through the small round capsulectomy for a short distance and a small amount of irrigating solution is injected to create a cleavage plane between the superficial and underlying layers of cortex.

6.4

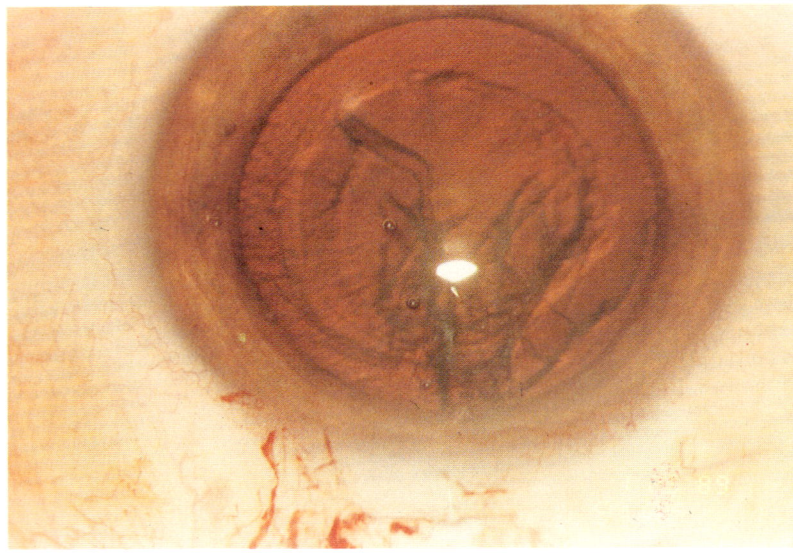

6.4 The cannula is now advanced for a short distance towards the center of the nuclear core and another small amount of irrigating solution is injected. This process is repeated until the center of the nucleus is reached. As each cleavage plane is made, its circular outline is delineated in the red reflex and a series of concentric circles appear. (This process is called hydrodecompaction and the visual appearance of the concentric circles is hydrodelineation.)

6.5

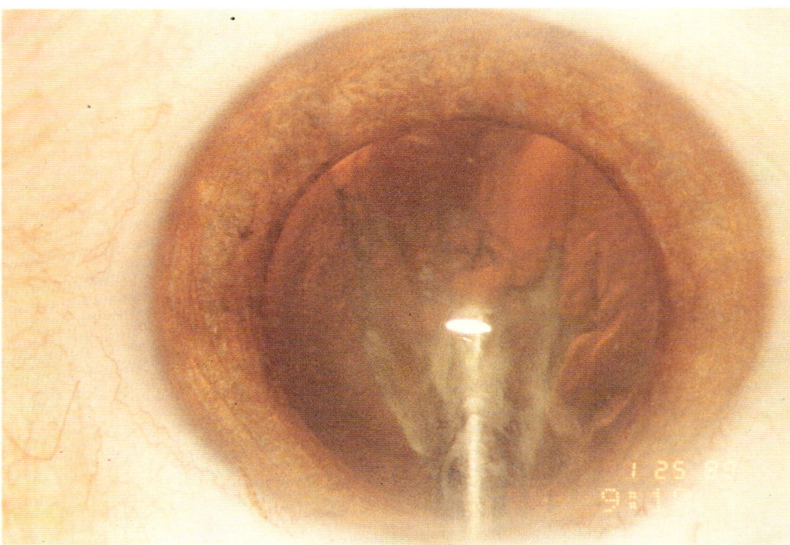

6.5 The 20-gauge cannula of the hydrosonic handpiece is now introduced and advanced underneath the anterior capsule through the most anterior decompacted layer and, with gentle aspiration, a gutter is shaved. The cannula is withdrawn to the capsular opening and advanced again to shave an adjacent gutter. This process is repeated, forming a pattern of diverging gutters from the capsular opening.

6.6

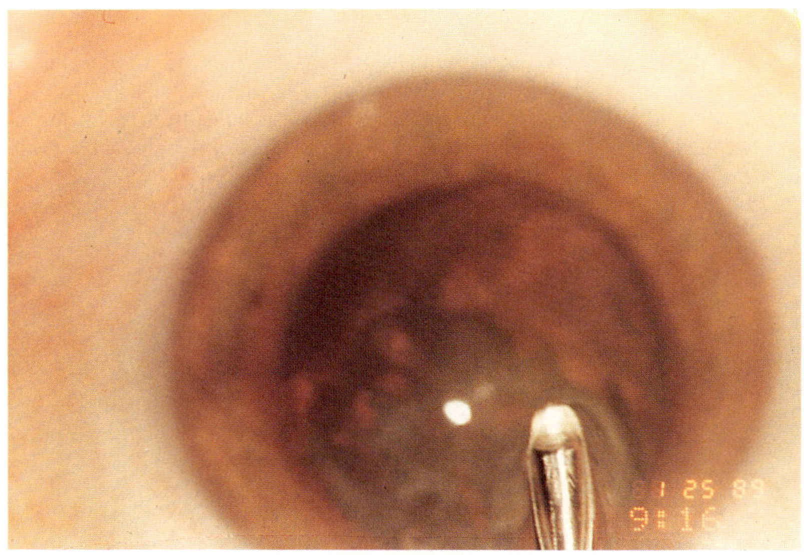

6.6 The irrigating protective sleeve is now advanced over the aspirating cannula beyond the posterior sharp edge of the cannula.

6.7

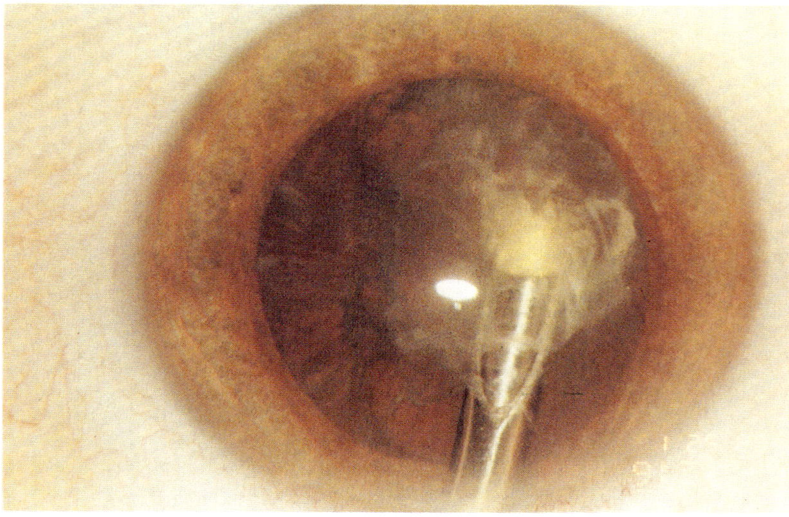

6.7 This lip is now gently inserted between the posterior capsule and the remaining thin nuclear plate, which is shaved off.

6.8

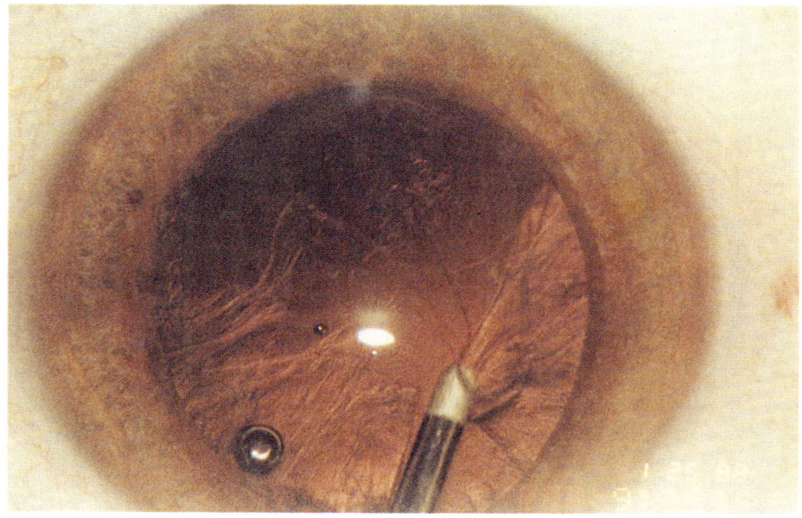

6.8 Manual aspiration of the cortex from within the capsular bag is now completed using a 23-gauge cannula on a plastic 6 ml syringe. The anterior chamber is maintained with viscoelastic agent.

6.9

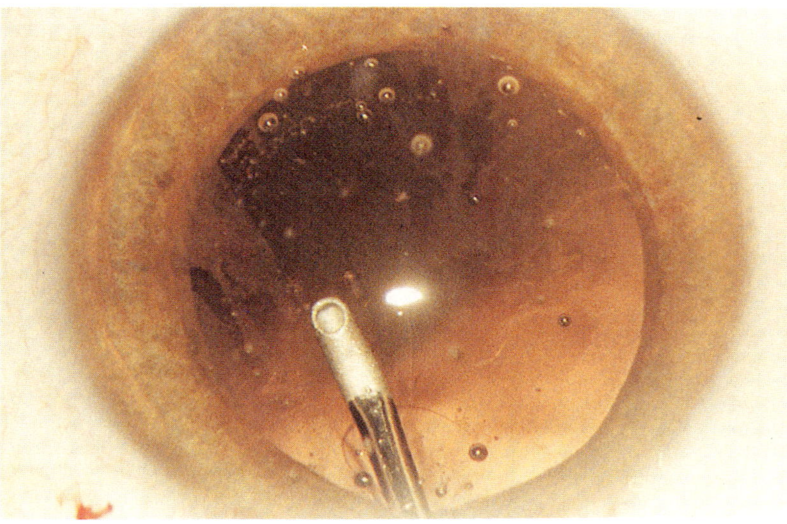

6.9 The epithelium is vacuumed off the anterior and posterior capsules using the 23-gauge cannula.

6.10

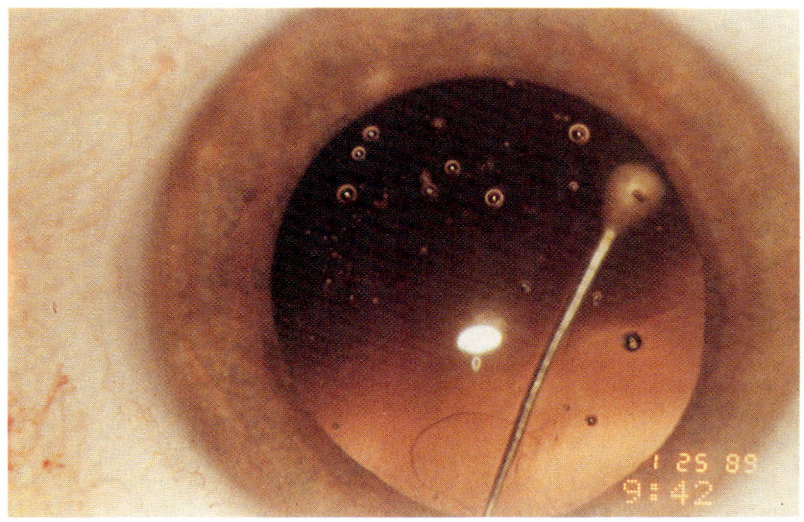

6.10 The capsular fornix is scrubbed using the Anis® capsular scrubber.

6.11

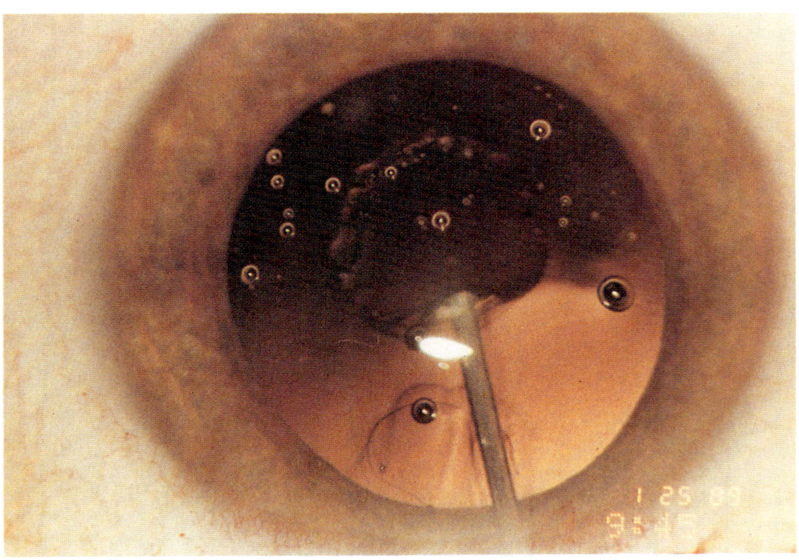

6.11 A small amount of viscoelastic agent is injected between the anterior and posterior capsules.

6.12

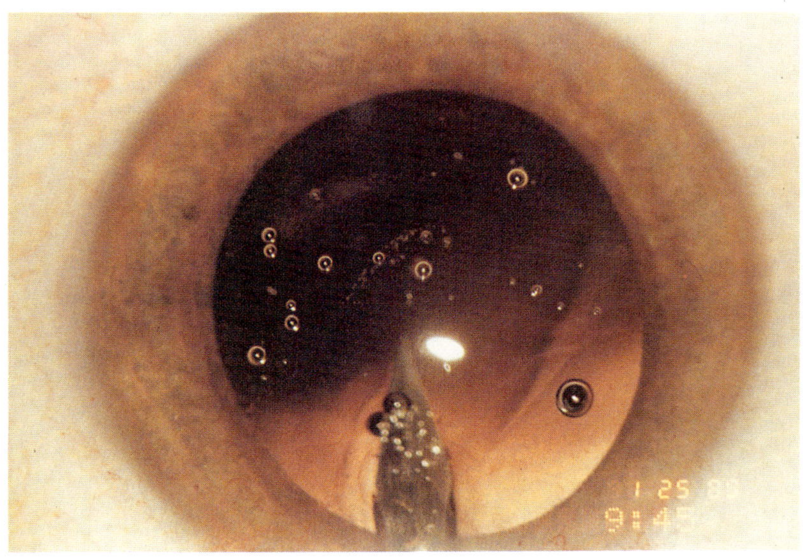

6.12 A small horizontal stab incision is made with a sharp microlance in the anterior capsule (see **1.16**).

6.13

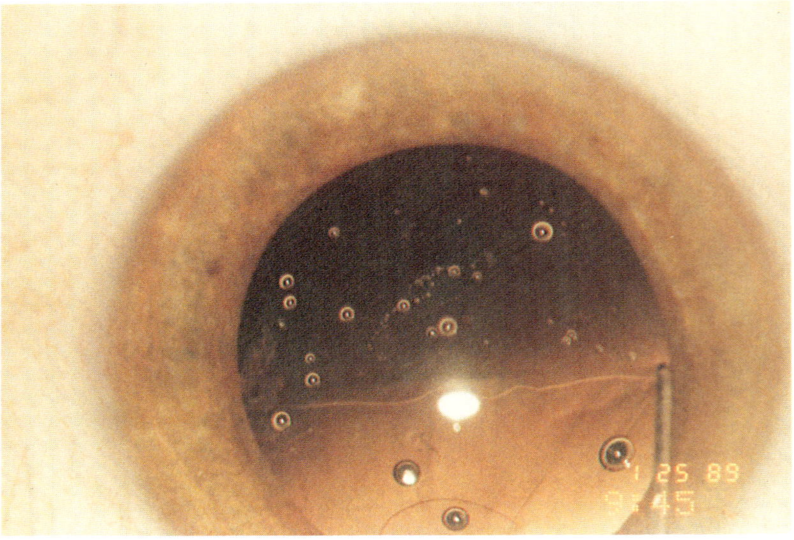

6.13 The bent tip of the Sinskey hook is inserted into the anterior capsular incision and moved horizontally to extend the incision from 10 to 2 o'clock.

6.14

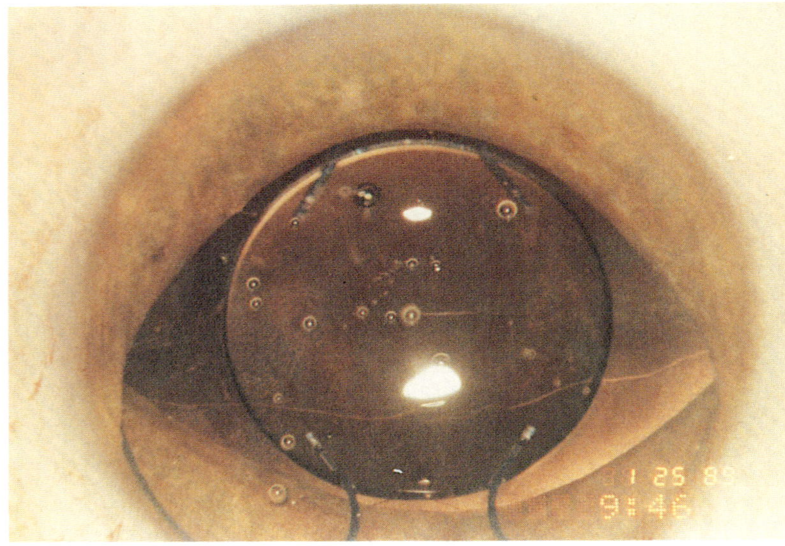

6.14 The scleral incision is enlarged to between 6.5 and 7 mm and the Anis® lens implant is introduced into the inferior capsular bag through the linear capsulorhexis.

6.15

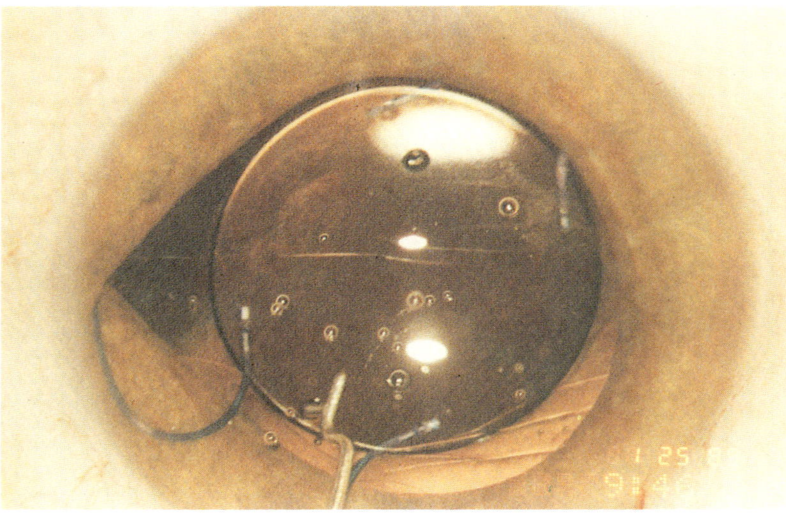

6.15 The lens is rotated to position its upper part within the upper capsular bag.

6.16

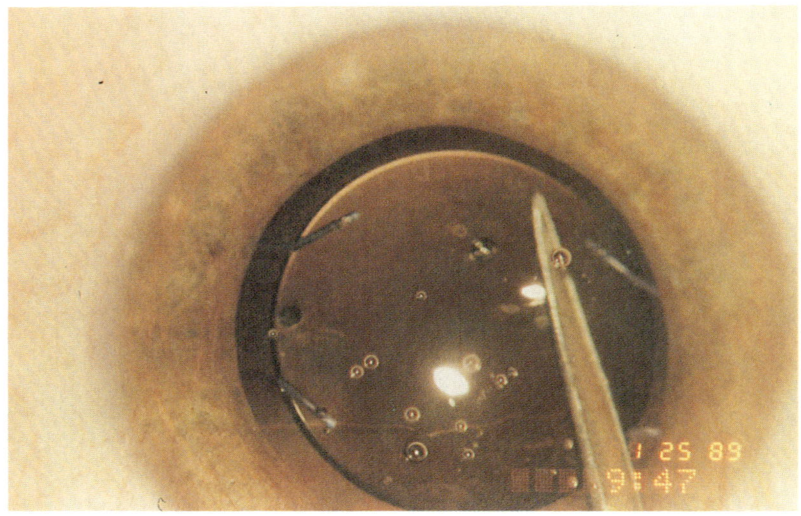

6.16 A vertical cut in the inferior capsular flap is made 1 mm inside the edge of the optic.

6.17

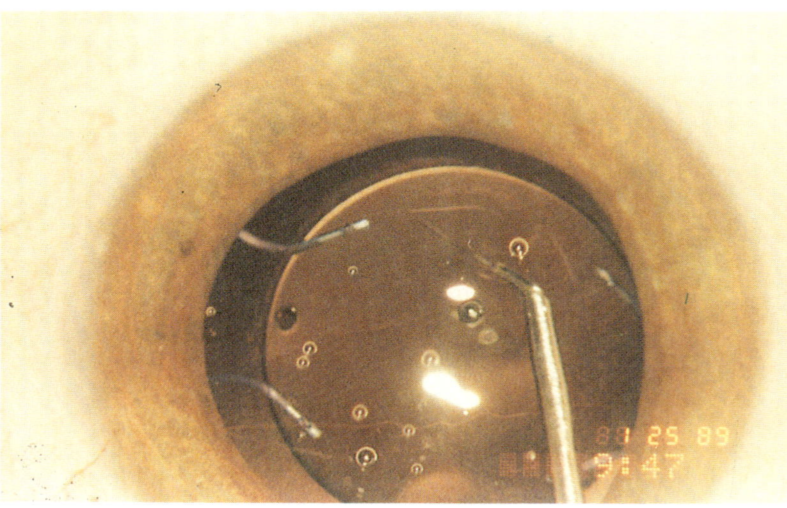

6.17 Microforceps are used to tear the central part of the flap in an arcuate fashion to leave a 4 mm gap in front of the optic.

6.18

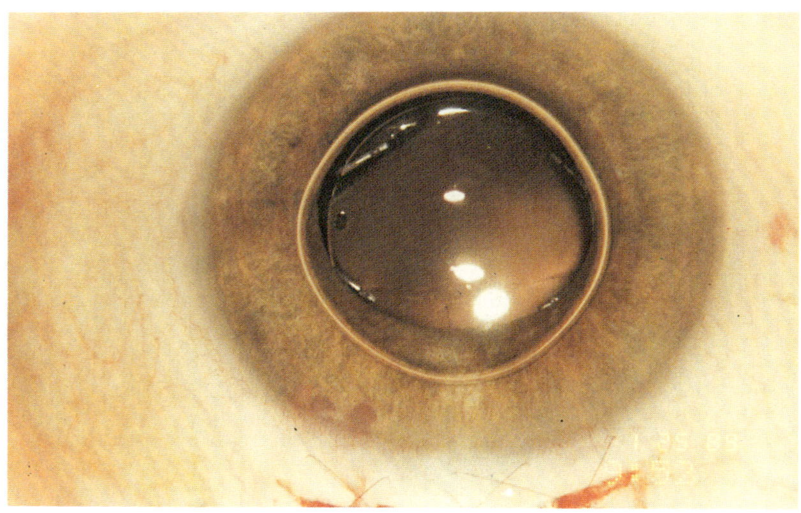

6.18 The viscoelastic agent is removed from the anterior chamber and replaced with air. The scleral incision is then sutured and the air is replaced with balanced salt solution.

7: Phacoemulsification

Eric Arnott

Phacoemulsification was introduced in the late 1960s by Dr Charles Kelman as a means for removing the adult cataractous lens through a small incision.

The lens is emulsified with ultrasonic agitation of a needle at 55,000 cycles per second, the needle making an excursion of 3/1000 of an inch with an acceleration of 80,000 G. With each thrust the point of the needle will pass into the nucleus of the lens before its inertia is overcome. It is the high acceleration of the needle by ultrasonic energy that makes this system more effective than other cutting devices.

Phacoemulsification offers several advantages over simple extracapsular cataract extraction. The smaller incision can be closed more effectively than the larger incision necessary for manual removal of the nucleus. An eye with a smaller incision is less likely to be damaged by minor trauma and allows patients total immediate postoperative ambulatory freedom. The chances for suturing to cause postoperative astigmatism are reduced. Complications, such as wound rupture, iris incarceration through the wound, cystoid macular edema and exposure to endophthalmitis pathology, are also less likely.

Despite the advantages with the small incision, the popularity of phacoemulsification over the last 20 years has waxed and waned owing to several factors. Phacoemulsification is a difficult procedure to learn, the average surgeon requiring at least 50 cases before becoming at all skilled in its use. The high cost of acquiring the equipment for this type of surgery has deterred many surgeons from using this procedure. Moreover, with the increased incidence of intraocular lenses being used, the 3 mm phacoemulsification wound had to be enlarged to 6 or 7 mm in length, to some extent nullifying the advantage of the small incision – although, in fact, the astigmatism and other problems associated with surgical incision are markedly reduced with an incision of this size compared with that of 10–12 mm required for manual removal of the nucleus.

Over the last few years the introduction of lenses that could be inserted through the small 3 mm incision has again revived further interest in phacoemulsification. The greatest factor in the increased use of phacoemulsification at the present time is the refinement of the instruments. While the irrigating/aspirating (I/A) part of the instrument has remained standard over the years, with the side port 0.3 mm in diameter used in conjunction with an aspirating pressure of up to 400 mmHg, the ultrasonic tip itself has been modified greatly and the ultrasonic energy refined. The present generation of phacoemulsifiers provide functions such as linear control of fragmentation and aspiration (**7.1**). The fragmentation can be carried out with a needle which is activated by continuous ultrasonic energy or it can be pulsed and the power levels used for fragmentation modified (**7.2**). The power level available is now sufficient for even the hardest nucleus to be phacoemulsified. Also available is an immediate response reflux infusion to maintain the anterior chamber when entering the globe and to eject ocular material trapped in the mechanical orifice. Some emulsifiers can be programed to computer function, tailored to the individual surgeon's needs. Several forms of ultrasonic tip are now available. In all the tips the diameter is approximately 1 mm. The needle is surrounded by a sleeve leaving the final 1–2 mm of tip free (**7.3**). The angulation of the tip may be varied from 15° to 70° and another option is a turbo tip with variable angulation.

7.1

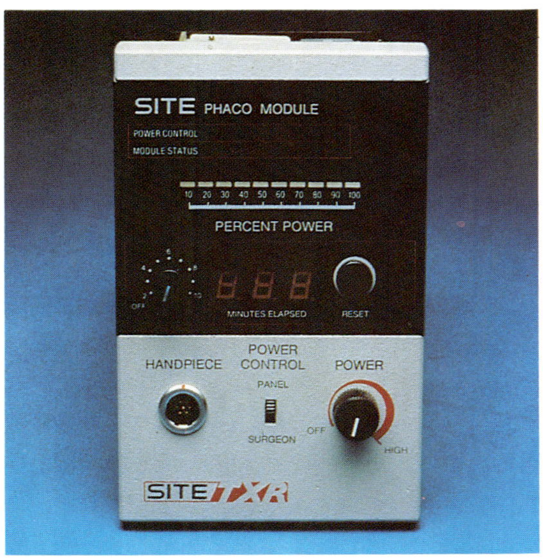

7.1 The Site® system for irrigation, aspiration and phacoemulsification.

7.2

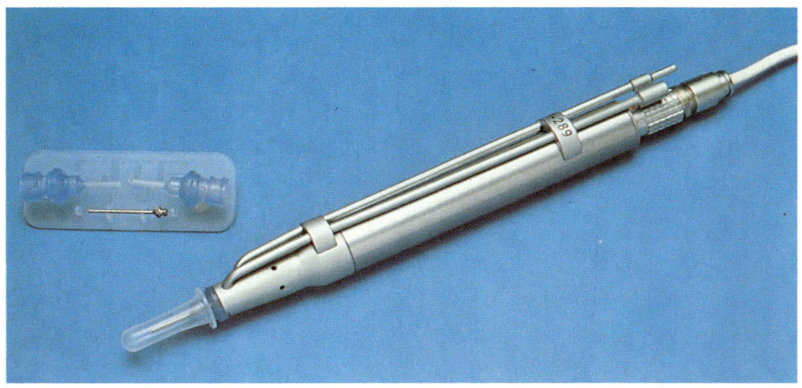

7.2 Handpiece for phacoemulsification.

7.3

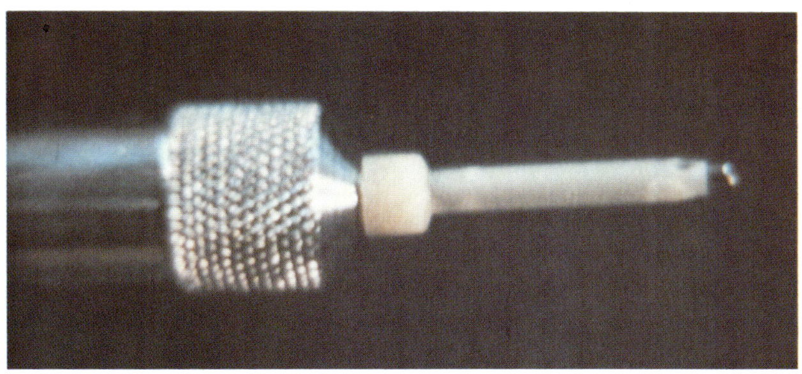

7.3 Ultrasonic probe for phacoemulsification showing the sleeve that covers the probe, apart from the tip.

In all operations involving phacoemulsification, certain standard calibrations need to be determined. The phacoemulsification instrument should be on a trolley of such a height that the pump is at the same level as the patient's eye. The infusion bottle is normally raised 65 cm above the head of the patient. Under differing circumstances the bottle may be raised or lowered. During the capsulotomy the infusion bottle may be levelled to 80 cm. The aspirating pressure available is modified depending on the stage of the operative procedure. During phacoemulsification the flow of fluid averages 25 cm^3/min, whereas with cortical aspiration it averages 40 cm^3/min. The setting of the aspirating pressure is invariably proportional to the diameter of the aspirating port. The ultrasonic tip has a diameter of 1 mm, with which the maximum aspirating pressure is 70 mmHg. The I/A tip for cortical removal usually has a diameter of 0.3 mm; with this the aspirating pressure may be increased to 400 mmHg. When 'hoovering' the posterior capsule for cortical cleanup the aspirating pressure is reduced to 65 mmHg.

Technique of phacoemulsification

Phacoemulsification entails four stages:

- Entry into the eye.
- Capsulotomy and entry into the lens.
- Removal of the nucleus
- Removal of the remaining contents of the lens, leaving the posterior capsule intact or purposely open.

Entry into the eye

The simplest form of phacoemulsification may be performed with a 3.2 mm opening at the corneoscleral junction, this opening being enlarged to any desired degree before the insertion of the intraocular lens.

At the other extreme is the scleral tunnel approach with the incision being made 2–3 mm from the corneoscleral junction. In between these two forms of incision are all the variables associated with either a corneal, limbal or scleral section.

Capsulotomy

The can-opener form of anterior capsulotomy (**7.4**) replaced the original 'Christmas tree' approach. In this technique, using a cystitome, small nicks are made in the anterior capsule at a variable distance from the equator of the lens. With 360° cuts the appearance was similar to an open can, hence the name. As an alternative to using the cystitome to make nicks in the capsule, it can be used to engage the capsule and tear it (capsulorhexis).

The opening should be made near to the equator so as to remove as many of the anterior subcapsular cells as possible, but most surgeons advocate leaving at least 2–3 mm of peripheral anterior capsule intact so as to avoid any damage to the zonular fibers which can encroach up to 3 mm from the equator over the anterior capsule. This form of capsulotomy has remained popular because of good exposure on the nucleus. It is ideal when used in conjunction with the insertion of an implant which has haptics for ciliary sulcus fixation.

7.4

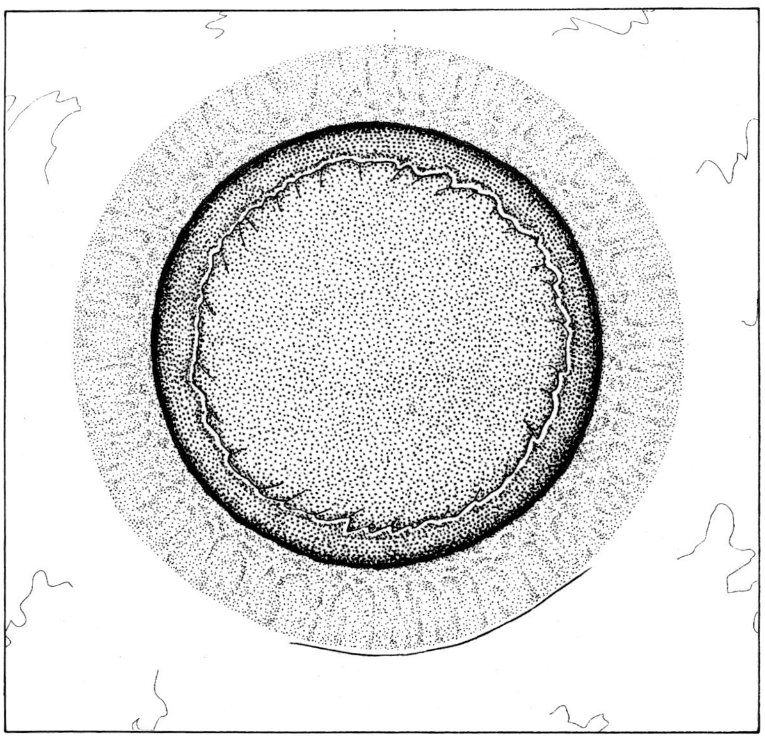

7.4 Illustration of corneoscleral section and can-opener capsulotomy.

However, the main emphasis with posterior chamber implants is to achieve fixation of the haptics within the capsular bag. This has necessitated the need for further modifications in the shape and size of the anterior capsulotomy, with the opening being of a variable diameter and either circular, elliptical or semilunar (**7.5**).

The method of actually cutting the anterior capsule also has some variations. Kelman introduced the cystitome for tearing the capsule. More recently, an ultrasonically agitated cystitome has been produced to tailor cut the capsule.

Continuous circular capsulorhexis (pp 36–38) is preferred by many. In this technique a cut is made into the anterior capsule and then the remainder of the capsule is torn in the appropriate direction, leaving a smooth edge to maintain the integrity of the peripheral capsule and zonule.

The envelope opening is performed by making an incision into the anterior capsule, usually some 3.5 mm from the equator of the lens at 12 o'clock. This incision is made of variable length and, although Galand (who pioneered the technique) recommended a linear incision, a more physiological type is one that follows the line of the equator, producing a 'happy smile' appearance in the capsule (**7.6**).

The totally endocapsular approach is to make a small circular hole in the capsule near to the section, through which the ultrasonic tip is placed (see Chapter 8).

7.5

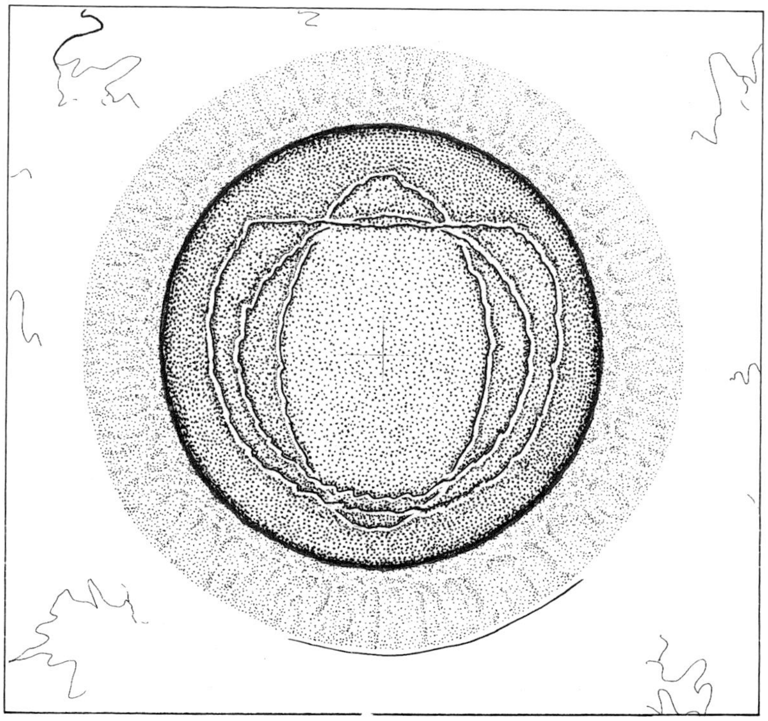

7.5 Illustration of various configurations for anterior capsulotomy suitable for phacoemulsification.

7.6

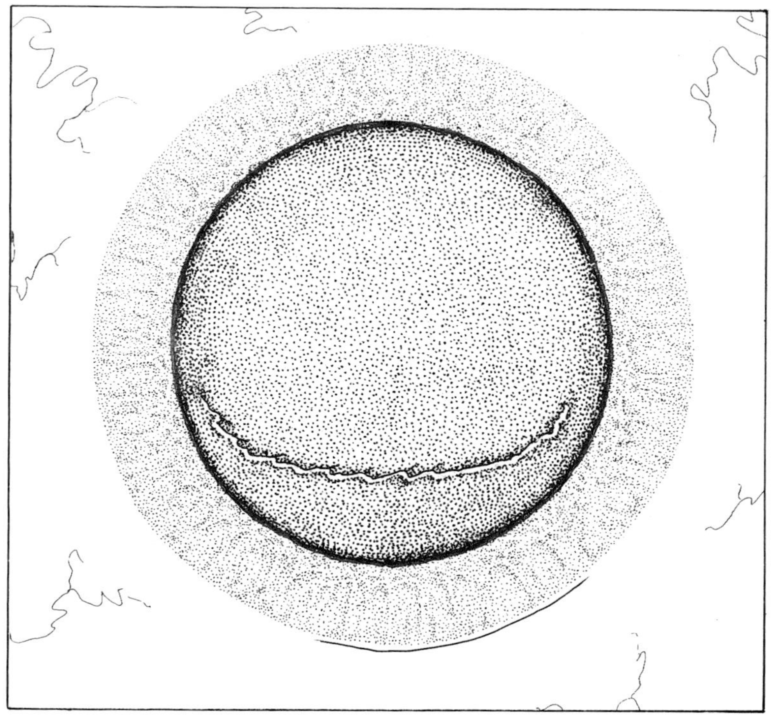

7.6 Illustration of an 'envelope' incision producing a 'happy smile' appearance in the capsule.

Removal of lens nucleus and cortex

To some extent, the technique of phacoemulsification will vary depending on the form of anterior capsulotomy that has been performed. The method of phacoemulsification is similar in the can-opener capsulotomy and with the circular or semilunar smaller opening into the anterior capsule. In the envelope technique, however, a modified approach must be made.

For can-opener, semilunar or circular capsular openings there are four basic approaches to emulsification of the cataract:

- Emulsification of the nucleus after it has been dislocated into the anterior chamber (Kelman).
- A single-handed technique with initial removal of the nucleus in the posterior chamber and final removal of nucleus fragments in the anterior chamber (Sinskey).
- The single-handed endocapsular technique (see also p. 95).
- A bimanual technique with the surgeon holding the phacoemulsifier in one hand and a fine spatula in the other to control the position of the nucleus in the posterior chamber, to steady the nucleus onto the tip of the emulsifier and to aid rotation (Maloney).

7.7

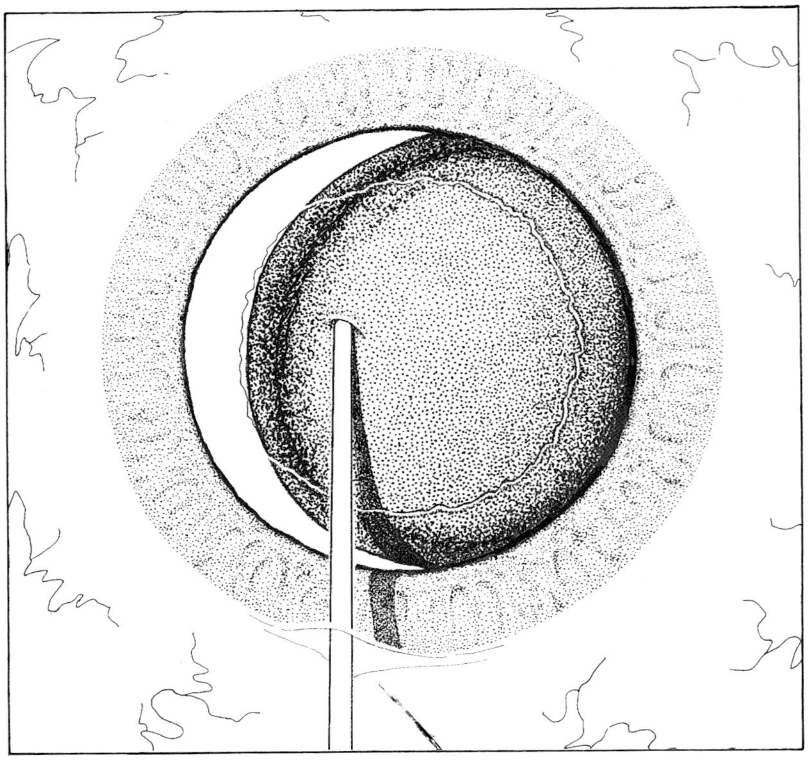

7.7 Illustration showing dislocation of nucleus into the anterior chamber with a cystitome.

7.8

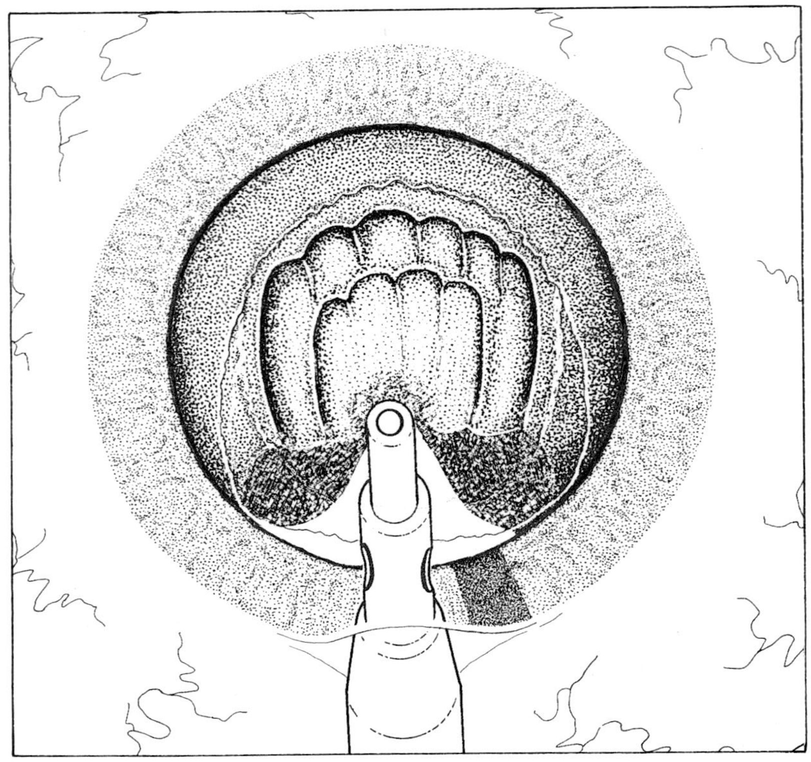

7.8 Illustration of the croissant technique, in which the central part of the nucleus is removed first.

Removal of the nucleus after its dislocation into the anterior chamber is the method advised by Kelman.

After the anterior capsulotomy has been completed, the nucleus of the lens is engaged with the cystitome in the 3 o'clock meridian near to the equator. The cystitome is drawn over to the right, which disengages the left lateral pole of the nucleus from the fornix (**7.7**). It is important that the cystitome be brought beyond the midline of the cornea to effect disengagement of the equator of the lens from the fornix of the capsular bag. The cystitome engages the lens in a similar position in the 9 o'clock meridian and in a reverse movement the other pole of the lens is disengaged into the anterior chamber.

Once the nucleus is in the anterior chamber several methods can be employed for its emulsification. The tip of the ultrasonic handpiece can be engaged in the lens at 12 o'clock and, with gentle to and fro movements, the center part of the nucleus can be removed; this is the croissant technique. Once the harder central part of the nucleus has been removed (**7.8**), the peripheral softer part of the nucleus can be removed, usually with reduced ultrasonic power.

An alternative technique is to sculpt first the peripheral part of the nucleus. With this carousel technique the lens gently rotates as the outer portion of it is emulsified. The lens will slowly cartwheel around in the anterior chamber (**7.9**) until the central harder part of the lens is reached, which is also emulsified. These techniques of removing the lens in the anterior chamber are undoubtedly the easiest and certainly, for the beginner, the safest as, if the posterior capsule should be inadvertently ruptured, there is less likelihood of the lens nucleus falling into the vitreous cavity. These techniques do more damage to the corneal endothelium than does the alternative of removal in the posterior chamber.

7.9

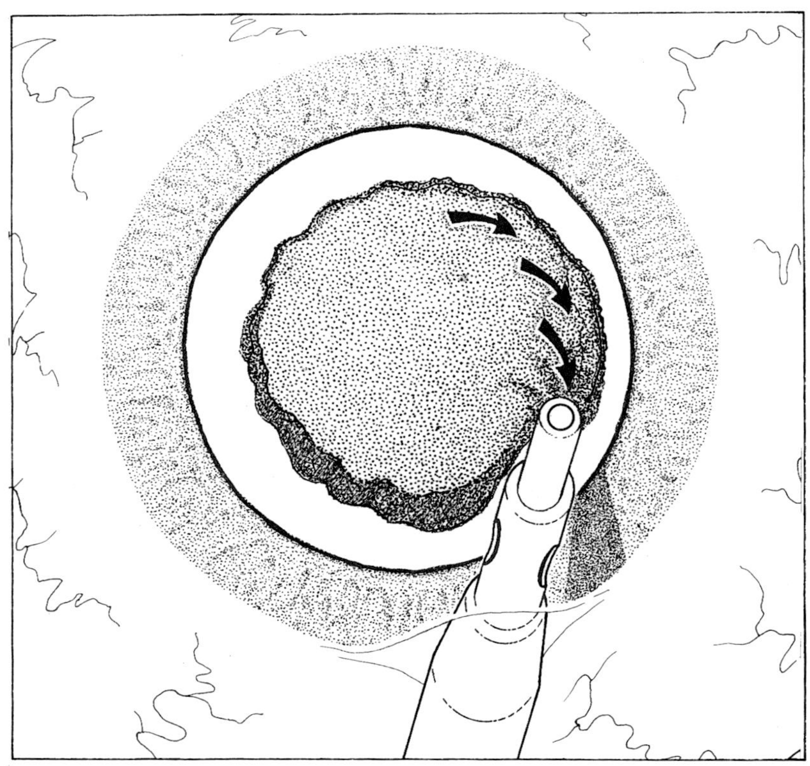

7.9 Illustration of the carousel technique of removing the central nucleus after the peripheral nucleus has already been sculpted.

Removal of the lens using a single-handed technique – first in the posterior chamber and the final fragments in the anterior chamber is the method taught by Sinskey. After completing the anterior capsulotomy the ultrasonic handpiece is held in the surgeon's dominant hand. The tip of the emulsifier is inserted into the anterior chamber and the superficial surface of the lens is gently scalloped. Not more than half the diameter of the phaco tip is buried in the surface of the nucleus (**7.10**). Once approximately one-third of the nucleus has been removed, the ultrasonic tip is withdrawn to lie over the pupil at 12 o'clock. With a hard nucleus, more is removed at this stage than with a softer nucleus.

With cessation of inflow and aspiration, the anterior chamber naturally shallows. With the anterior chamber shallowed, the tip of the needle is passed over the iris to engage the nucleus of the lens, which is then rotated a small amount and the process of scalloping the surface of the lens is continued using I/A ultrasound. These two stages of the emulsification are repeated several times with progressive shallowing of the width of the lens.

Finally, when a very flat biscuit of lens is left, the anterior chamber is again shallowed with cessation of inflow and outflow. The nucleus is pushed down and the upper pole of the nucleus at 12 o'clock is again engaged with the tip and the final part of the nucleus is aspirated and emulsified (**7.11**).

7.10

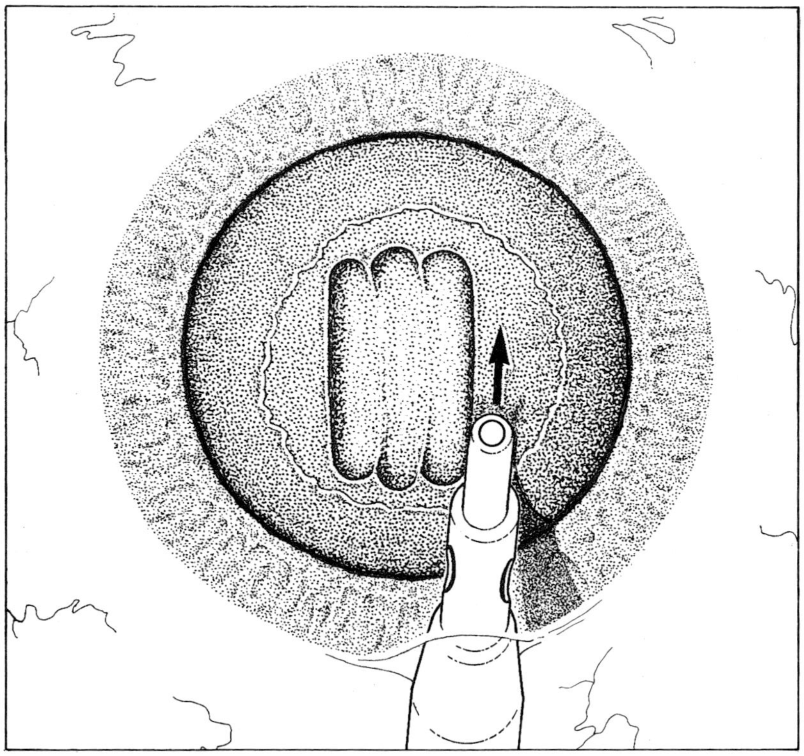

7.10 Illustration of superficial scalloping as advised by Sinskey.

7.11

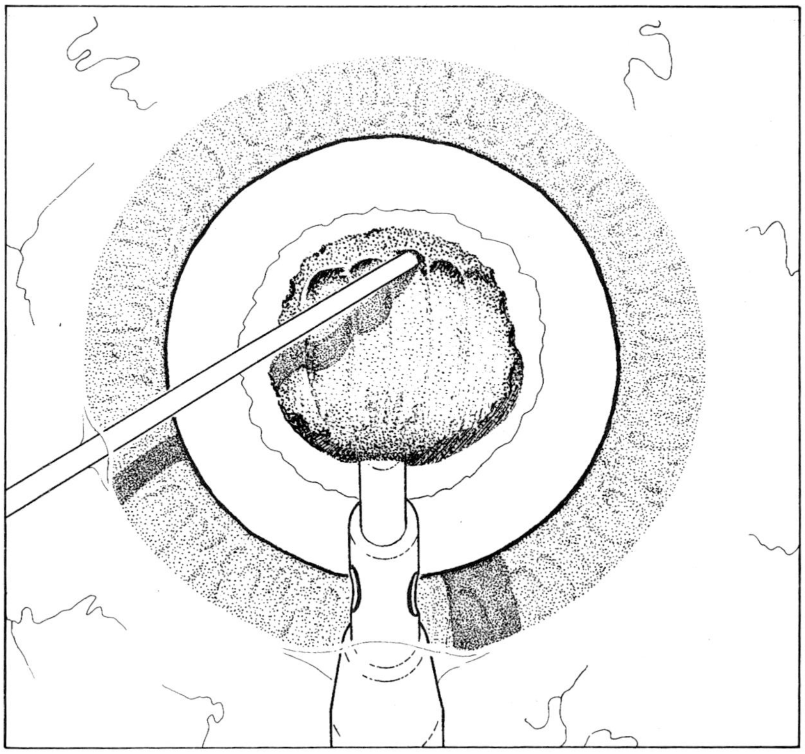

7.11 Illustration of nibbling the final part of the nucleus at 12 o'clock, while the inferior pole is depressed with a spatula.

The single-handed endocapsular technique for removing the nucleus within the capsular bag is most suitable after a relatively small opening has been made in the anterior capsule, either circular (about 5.5 mm in diameter) or semilunar (with a width of 5.5 mm in the vertical plane and 6 mm in the horizontal). An advantage of continuous tear capsulorhexis is that the zonules and the rim of the anterior capsule are maintained intact. Once the capsulotomy has been completed, a Rycroft cannula is placed under the rim of the anterior capsule and buffered salt solution is gently injected to hydrodissect the nucleus from the surrounding cortex. This technique differs from some of the alternative methods of phacoemulsification in that the nucleus is freed from the surrounding cortex before phacoemulsification commences. The nucleus is, however, contained within the limits of the capsular bag, which allows for its controlled movement during removal. First, the superficial surface of the nucleus is scalloped. At intervals the anterior chamber is shallowed by cessation of inflow and the nucleus, mobile within the capsular bag, is rotated so that the sculpturing process can be continued at a different plane. During its removal the nucleus is repeatedly rotated to the emulsification tip, which remains stationary. The diameter of the nuclear remnant is reduced as the rotations continue. After the lens has been rotated through half a revolution with intermittent sculpturing, a thin posterior equatorial portion of mobile nucleus will remain. In the removal of this final plaque, a cyclodialysis spatula may be used to support the disc so that the ultrasonic tip is kept at a safe distance from the posterior capsule. A modification introduced by Fine is the flip technique whereby the spatula pushes the nuclear remnant towards 6 o'clock, which is then flipped back-to-front for easier emulsification.

Using the endocapsular technique, the superior tip of the anterior capsule limits access to the superior pole of the lens nucleus. To overcome this difficulty and to remove the periphery of the nucleus, an inferior approach with the ultrasonic tip may be adopted, as described by Davison, whereby the ultrasonic tip is used to nibble small wedges of peripheral nucleus in the 5–6 o'clock meridian. Very low ultrasonic power is used at this stage. Once the inferior wedge of peripheral nucleus has been removed, the nuclear remnant is rotated and a fresh area attacked. Once the remnant has been drawn centrally, the remainder of the small plaque will be readily emulsified. It is imperative that during this stage the nucleus is freely mobile, thus ensuring that the upper polar remnant of nucleus does not remain incarcerated in the upper capsular fornix.

Gimbal, who pioneered the continuous tear form of capsulotomy, suggested that the nucleus, after superficial scalloping, should be cracked into four pieces; first, by a vertical split and then by horizontal splits. This would obviate problems with the upper pole underneath the anterior capsule, but it may be dangerous, for if the posterior capsule were to rupture, large chunks of nucleus would fall into the vitreous.

7.12

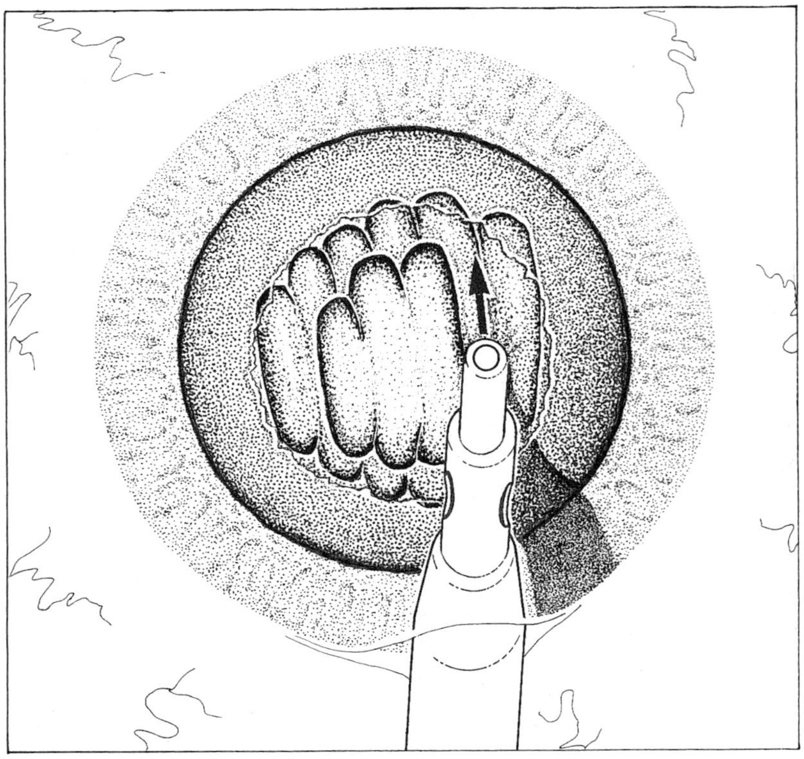

7.12 Illustration of the first stage of the Maloney technique.

7.13

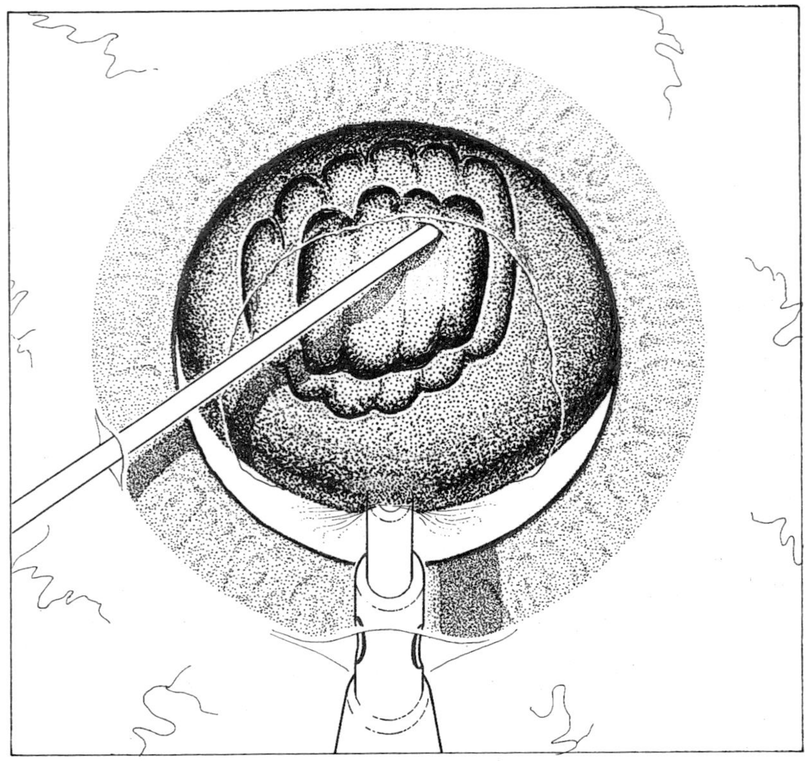

7.13 Illustration of the second stage of the Maloney technique.

The bimanual technique of emulsifying the nucleus in the posterior and anterior chambers involves a second incision at either the 3 or 9 o'clock meridian 1 mm long and large enough to allow a fine spatula to be inserted into the anterior chamber. As stressed by Maloney there are three stages.

Firstly, the superficial surface of the nucleus is scalloped. Less than half the diameter of the needle engages the nucleus with a power setting of 50%. A rim of peripheral nucleus is left intact. The softer the nucleus the wider the rim that is left intact. Since the tip is 1 mm in diameter and the thickness of the average lens is 3.5 mm, the depth of the scalloped cortex can be gauged by noting its extent relative to the diameter of the needle. As the crater in the nucleus becomes deeper, the red reflex from the fundus will increase (**7.12**).

Secondly, when a sufficient portion of the nucleus has been sculpted, the nucleus is freed from the surrounding cortex. With the anterior chamber shallowed by stopping the inflow of fluid, the spatula held in the surgeon's other hand is used to push the nucleus towards the 6 o'clock meridian, thus exposing the upper rim of nucleus within the pupil margin where it is engaged with the tip of the phaco needle (**7.13**). With inflow of fluid the nucleus will be freed from the surrounding cortex. Once the nucleus has been freed it is allowed to drop back into the posterior chamber.

Thirdly, with the thinned nuclear bowl now lying free within the posterior capsule, the spatula is used to control the position of the nucleus while the phaco tip progressively removes peripheral segments of the remaining nucleus in the 11 o'clock meridian. The spatula engages the rim of the remaining nucleus, which is rotated so that fresh areas of peripheral nucleus are presented to the phaco tip. The phaco tip should be held just over the pupil margin at 12 o'clock, with the allowance of fine movement towards the 11 o'clock meridian. In this way, segment by segment of the peripheral nucleus is emulsified (**7.14**). Finally, the small central plate of nucleus is steadied with the spatula and emulsified.

With all the above methods, once the nucleus has been emulsified the automated I/A cannula is used to remove the residual cortex. This is simply performed, since with the small section the anterior chamber remains well formed. Following the removal of the cortex the posterior capsule and fornix area are cleaned using either a Kratz Scratcher or the I/A tip with an aspirating pressure of 65 mmHg.

7.14

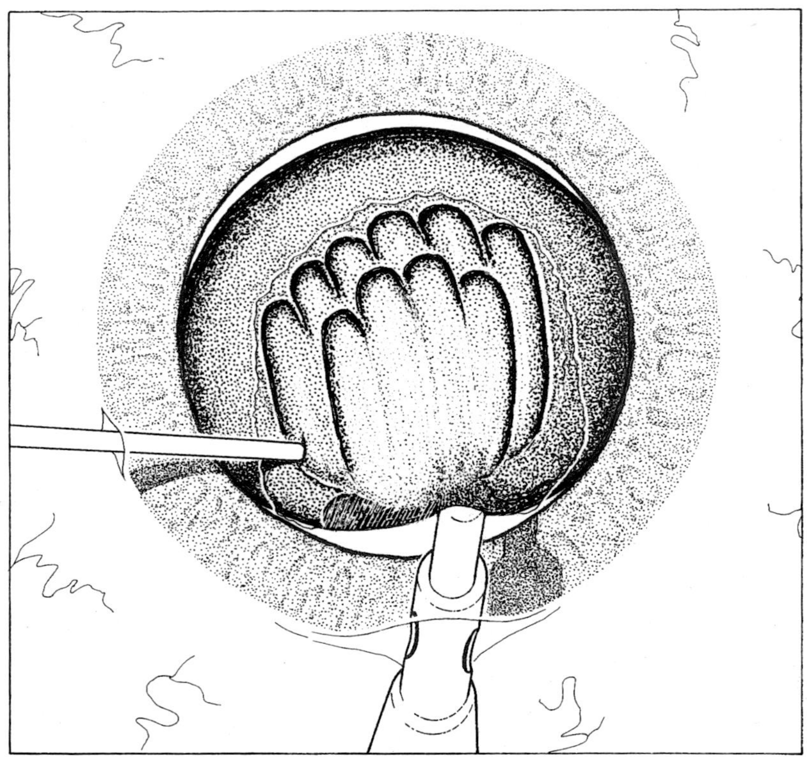

7.14 Illustration of the third stage of the Maloney technique.

Technique of phacoemulsification for the envelope (intercapsular) method

With this technique the contents of the lens are removed within the confines of the capsular bag. An opening is made into the anterior capsule from 10.30 around to 1.30, being slightly curvilinear and parallel to the equator of the lens (**7.6**). Vanna's scissors may be used to make this incision and employed to disengage the upper pole of the nucleus from the upper fornix. A viscoelastic solution is injected under the anterior capsule.

With the injection of viscoelastic solution, one can see it spreading beneath the anterior capsule and then around the side of the nucleus towards the posterior capsule. The whole procedure is performed with the nucleus freed from the surrounding cortex. The nucleus, however, is well fixed for phacoemulsification since it is within the almost intact confines of the capsular bag. If the nucleus is hard, it is probably best emulsified without the preliminary hydrodissection to free it from the surrounding cortex.

Initially, a small amount of the nucleus is emulsified within the lips of the anterior capsule. This allows enough opening to be made within the capsular bag so that the tip of the needle can pass between the nucleus and the anterior capsule. The nucleus is scalloped away with horizontal thrusts of the tip over the superficial surface of the nucleus. It is protected from the anterior capsule by viscoelastic solution. As in the other forms of phacoemulsification approximately one-third to one-half of the nucleus is removed in this manner. Care is taken to see that the tip does not extend too far inferiorly so as to perforate the periphery of the anterior capsule. The second stage is to emulsify the periphery of the nucleus that is presenting in the 12 o'clock meridian (**7.15**). A small amount of nucleus is emulsified and then, using either the tip of the needle or a separate spatula, the nucleus is rotated a little and the adjacent segment of nucleus emulsified. This process continues until all the peripheral nucleus has been emulsified (**7.16**).

The cortex is removed, again keeping the anterior surface of the capsule intact. The posterior capsule is polished, and the capsular bag is now ready for the insertion of the implant.

The difference between this and the other forms of phacoemulsification is essentially that the surgeon is working within a more confined space. Instead of having the anterior chamber superficial to the working needle, one has the intact anterior capsule. Moreover, the lens lying within the capsular bag is placed more posteriorly than it is with the more conventional form of phacoemulsification. Less power is used for the nucleus emulsification, hence the procedure is more delicate and time consuming and should be recommended only for the softer forms of cataract. An envelope phaco tip is available which has a reduced diameter of 0.53 mm.

7.15

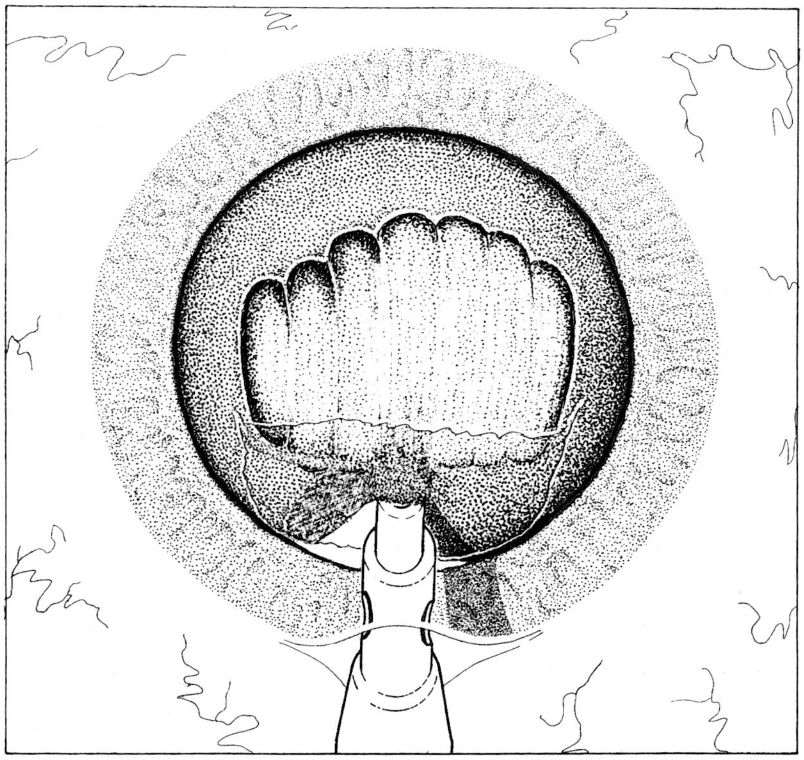

7.15 Illustration of intercapsular phacoemulsification.

7.16

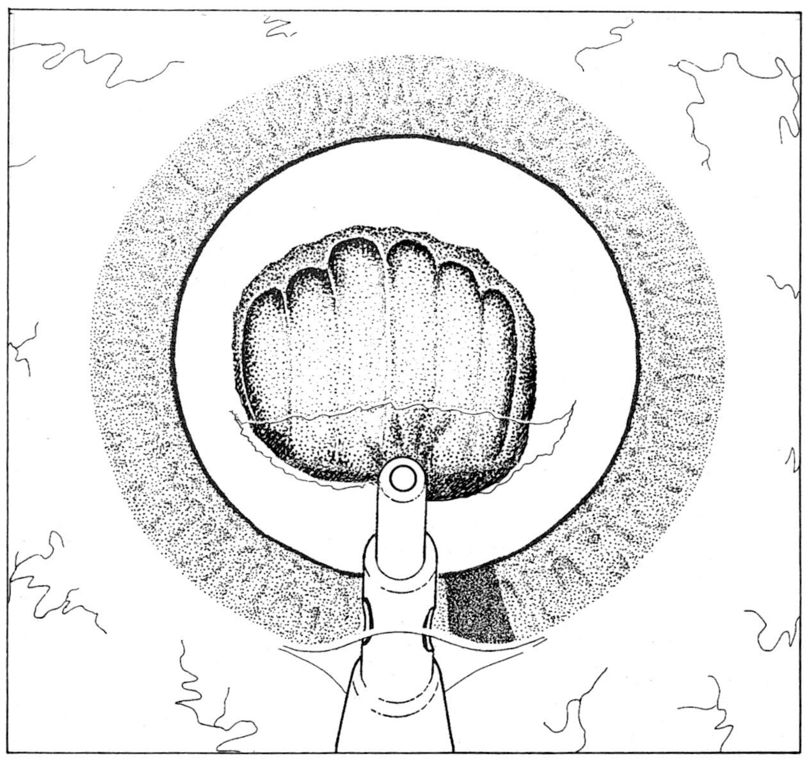

7.16 Illustration of the flat plate of residual nucleus after emulsification of the central and peripheral nucleus.

Insertion of implant after phacoemulsification

The incision into the eye is enlarged to 6.5 mm and viscoelastic solution is injected into the capsular bag and anterior chamber. A one-piece polymethylmethacrylate (PMMA) lens with totally encircling loops is recommended for capsule fixation. The insertion technique will depend on the form of anterior capsulotomy.

Using the semilunar incision (**7.17**), the lens is inserted into the eye and, using a Hirschman probe, the inferior loop is gently guided into the capsular bag in the 6 o'clock meridian, as is the gusset of the upper loop in the same movement.

A Lester hook is then used to nudge and improve the positioning of the lens. This hook is inserted into the upper gusset of the lens, which is dialled slowly in a clockwise direction. With a quarter revolution, the gussets will lie in the 3 and 9 o'clock meridians and the superior loop should, with the dial, have progressively been fed into the capsular bag single-handedly (**7.18**).

An alternative two-handed technique may be preferred for insertion of the upper loop. With the upper gusset lying in the 2 o'clock meridian, a hook held in the surgeon's other hand may be used to bend and push the end of the upper loop into the capsular bag (**7.19**).

7.17

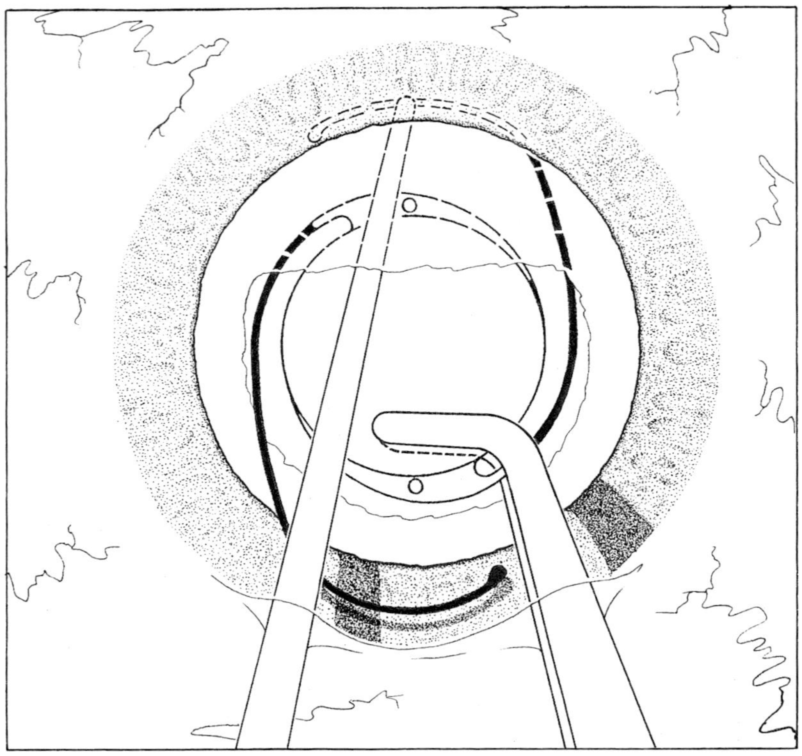

7.17 Illustration of implantation through a semilunar capsulotomy.

7.18

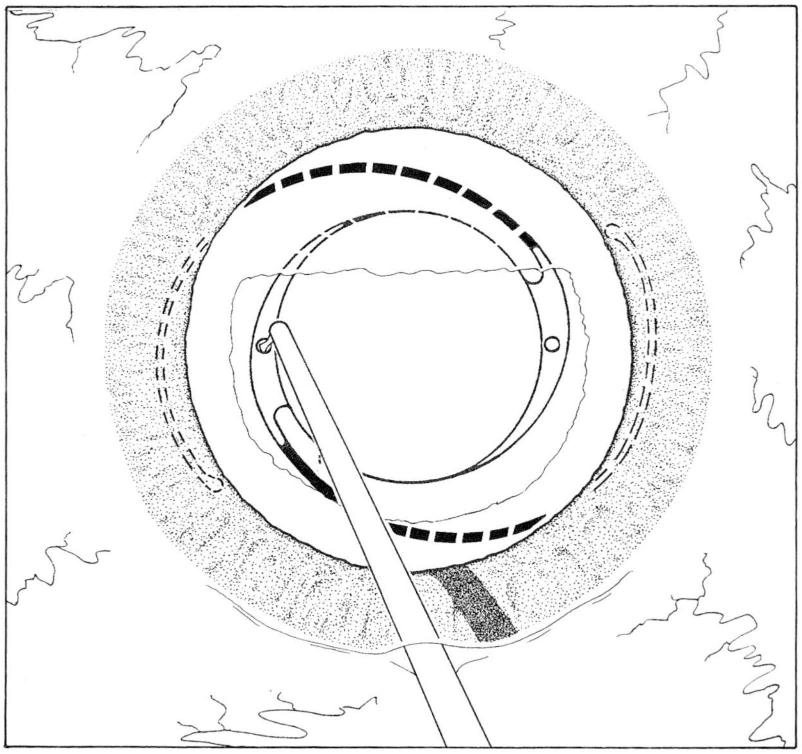

7.18 Illustration of dialling hook in hole at upper gusset of the lens.

7.19

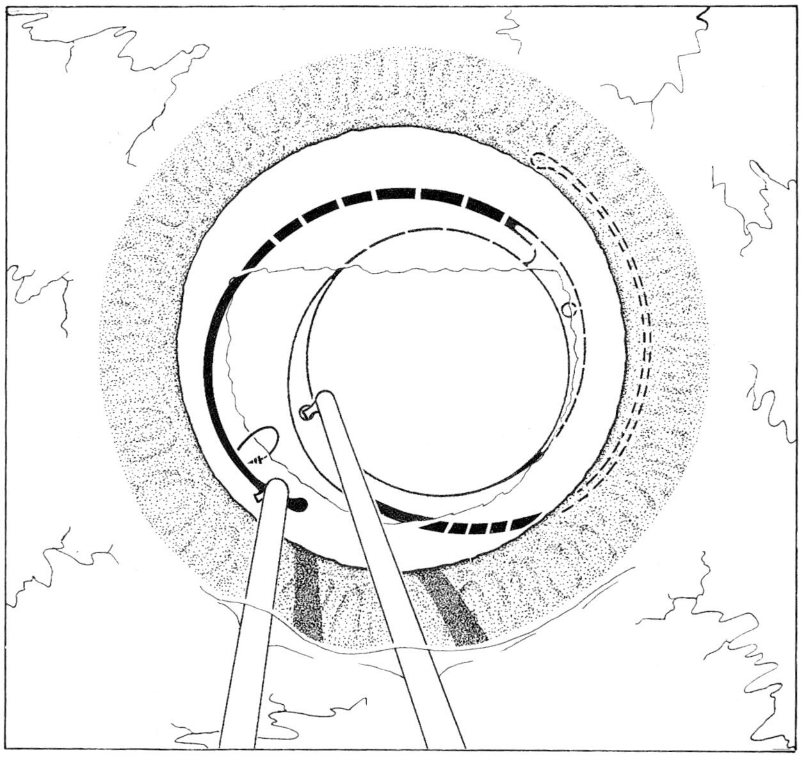

7.19 Illustration of the use of a Kuglen hook to flex the upper loop into the capsular fornix.

Considerations for the surgeon commencing phacoemulsification

Selection of cases

A surgeon skilled in the use of phacoemulsification may use this procedure in any form of cataract extraction. A surgeon new to phacoemulsification may be more cautious. The cataractous nucleus has stages of density. In a young patient with an inherited or developmental cataract, the nucleus will invariably be soft and easily emulsified. In some eyes the cataract may even be aspirated without phacoemulsification. In the adult the density of the nucleus can be determined by its color. A pale gray nucleus in a middle-aged patient will be soft and is the easiest to emulsify. With increasing density the nucleus will develop a yellowish tinge which with time will darken to brown and finally become black in appearance. These color changes are caused by an increase of lipofuscin in the nucleus and are associated with increased hardness. While modern ultrasonic machines can cope with any density of nucleus, it must be realized that the harder nucleus will require more ultrasonic time for its removal, not only on account of its composition but also because these nuclei are usually relatively larger. The beginner should not choose patients over the age of 75.

The ideal eye has a blue iris and a pupil dilated to at least 6.5 mm. Contraindications for the beginner include pupils stuck down due to posterior synechiae, pupils that have been constricted for a long period of time with miotics, those in the elderly patient that have hyaline degeneration of the sphincter, pupils in diabetic eyes which dilate poorly and those in eyes with pseudoexfoliation of the lens capsule.

Opacities in the cornea will markedly reduce the exposure and make the operation more difficult. Arcus senilis and marginal opacities will restrict the view of the periphery of the anterior segment. With trachomatous scarring of the cornea, frequently the cornea will become progressively more opaque as surgery proceeds. The beginner should also avoid an eye that is small or sunken or patients with heavy overhanging brows.

Instrumentation and surgical procedure

Before starting the surgical procedure the surgeon should carry out a checklist to verify that the equipment is in perfect running order. The fluid level of the inflow solution should be some 65 cm above the level of the eye. The aspirating pressure should be set between 65–85 mmHg. The ultrasonic power level should be set at the required setting. For most procedures the initial power level will be 70%, being adjusted as required according to nuclear density. The ultrasonic tip should be aligned with a 2 mm clearance of the surrounding sleeve. The ultrasonic handpiece should be held comfortably. Most surgeons hold it in the same way as a fountain pen, between the index and second finger and gripped by the thumb. An alternative method, as adopted by Kratz, is to hold the handpiece like a snooker cue with the hand pronated.

All instruments working within the eye are working around a fulcrum centered at the incision and so have limited mobility. For this reason it is important that the surgeon is seated at the patient's head in a position that leaves the surgeon's hands relaxed and mobile: the incision into the eye should then be in the 10.30 or 1.30 meridians. When at the 12 o'clock meridian, the surgeon's hand will be hyper-extended at the wrist and relatively immobilized.

The ultrasonic tip should be inserted through the incision into the eye with the bevel facing posteriorly, ensuring that the sharp tip does not damage the iris during its insertion. Once within the anterior chamber the angle of the tip is reversed before being engaged into the nucleus.

The tip should be moved as little as possible within the confines of the chamber and kept well clear of the corneal endothelium, iris and capsule, as it has the potential for aspirating tissue 2 mm distal to its end. The instrument should be kept in the plane of the iris and not dipped posteriorly.

Further reading

Maloney W.F. Tutorial in phacoemulsification. *European J. Implant Refractive Surgery*, **2,** 125–133, 1990.

8: Phacoemulsification within the capsular bag

Leon Solomon

The most suitable cases for beginning intercapsular (endocapsular) phacoemulsification (endophaco), are those with wide pupillary dilatation (>7 mm), good exposure of the globe, and mild to moderate nuclear density. The harder the nucleus, the more difficult the procedure will be, as the surgeon may not be able to plunge the ultrasonic (U/S) tip directly into the paracentral nuclear core, but will have to start at the midperiphery. However, since the anterior capsule is maintained in place, endophaco has the advantage over standard phacoemulsification of better endothelial cell protection, particularly when the duration of surgery is prolonged. It is also preferred in the presence of soft nuclei with posterior subcapsular cataract because it is a one-handed technique and there is no need for a second instrument, which can be dangerous in the presence of soft nuclei.

A posterior scleral incision approximately 7 mm in length, 1.5 mm posterior to the limbus, is created and continued forward to the cornea. The anterior chamber is entered using a 3.0 mm keratome which results in a snug fit around the phacoemulsification handpiece. Sodium hyaluronate is injected to fill the anterior chamber. A 5–6 mm crescentic anterior capsulorhexis is performed with a cystitome (**8.1**). Alternatively, a small circular capsulorhexis can be made as shown on p. 14.

The handpiece should be tested for operating defects and proper fluid flow, prior to its insertion into the eye. Depending on the density of the nucleus, using the Site® or Phacotron® linear machine, a power setting of 50–60% is chosen, a pulse mode of 5 or 6, and a vacuum level of 1. With the Storz Daisy® machine, using the linear pulse mode of 5 or 6, the power is set between 30 and 60% and the vacuum between 30 and 40 mmHg. The pulse mode is particularly useful for less dense nuclei. The non-pulsed, continuous mode can be selected for any type of case if the surgeon prefers and is particularly useful for the more dense nuclei.

The handpiece is passed into the eye in the 'bevel down' position (to prevent stripping Descemet's membrane) and is then rotated to the 'bevel up' position. The operation is started by plunging the tip through the anterior capsulorhexis and emulsifying into the paracentral nuclear material (**8.2**). Hydrodissection under the anterior capsule is not

8.1

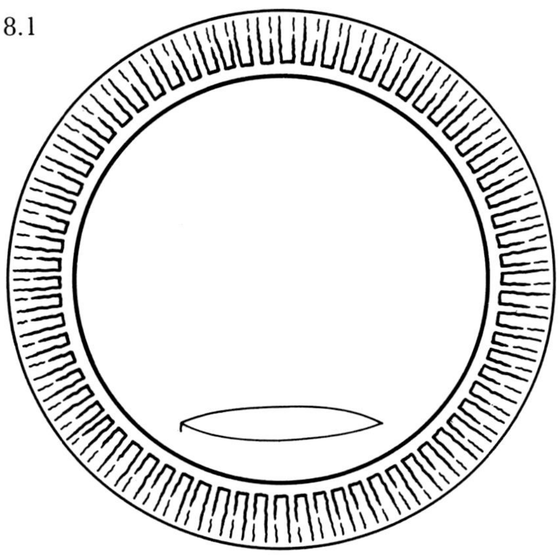

8.1 Crescentic capsulorhexis. The right-handed surgeon first makes a 1 mm vertical cystitome puncture to the left-hand end. From this the capsule is pulled to the right with the cystitome point and the sweep will be found to make a smooth crescentic opening.

8.2

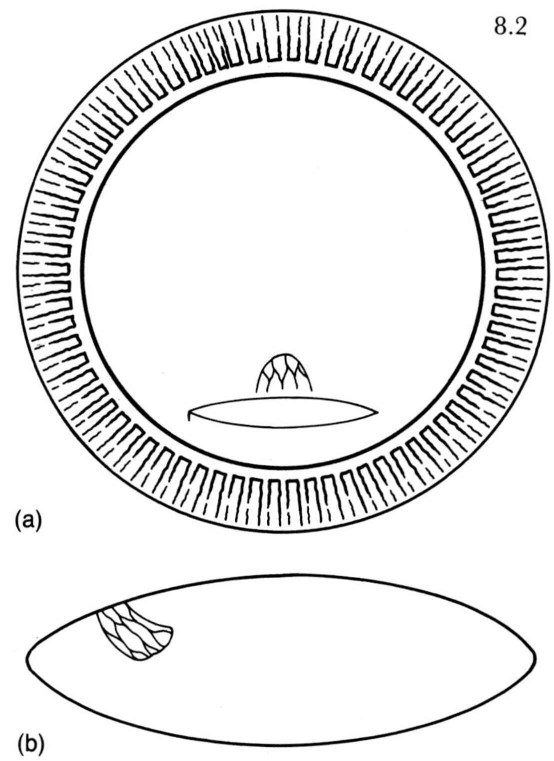

8.2 Excavation of entrance and commencement of paracentral core penetration: (a) front view; (b) side view.

8.3

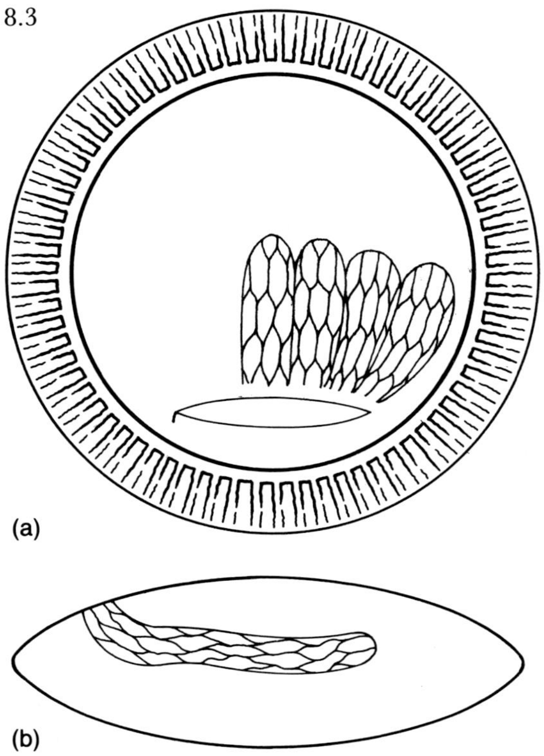

8.3 Emulsifying the central core: (a) front view; (b) side view.

8.4

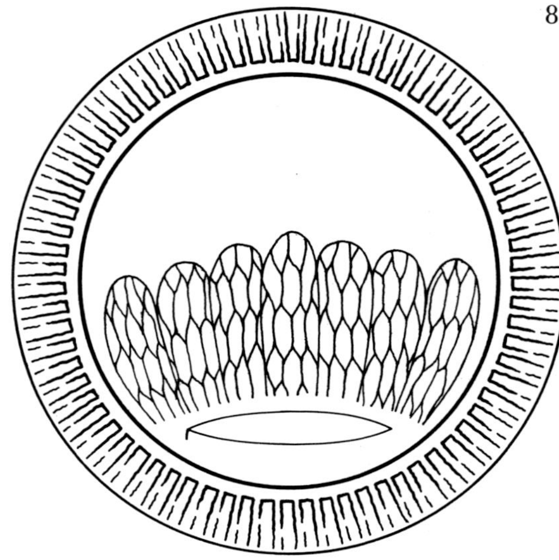

8.4 Completion of the central core. Do not rotate the nucleus.

8.5

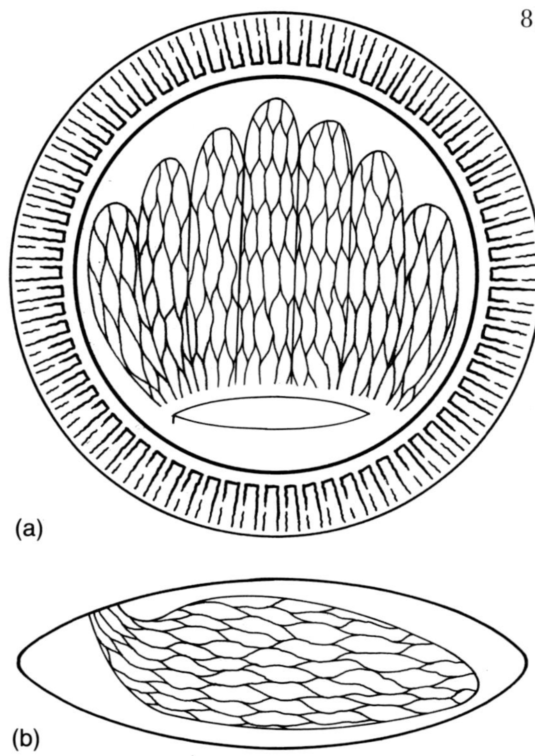

8.5 Extension into inferior and side peripheries of the nuclear core: (a) front view; (b) side view.

performed as it is most important to maintain the nucleus in its fixed position until the final stages. The density of the nuclear material will determine how rapidly one can continue to emulsify through the nucleus. A tunnel is created near the center of the nucleus; this tunnel is expanded first to one side (**8.3**), then back towards the center and the other side (**8.4**), and is then deepened (**8.5**). Duration will depend on the density of the nuclear material. If the tip does not cut sufficiently through the nuclear material, then the U/S power setting should be increased by 10. In some cases, increasing the vacuum level slightly may be more useful than a power increase. If the power is increased, it must be reduced after the central nucleus has been emulsified.

Tunnelling through the nuclear core is continued by extending the sculpting medially, laterally, inferiorly (**8.5**, side view), and finally to the peripheral shell. Medial and lateral sculpting is best accomplished by positioning the U/S tip bevel sideways, while inferior and peripheral sculpting is best served by the bevel up position. The peripheral nucleus will be seen to split away from the surrounding cortical material as it is drawn towards the aspirating port. This is a tricky maneuver which should be carefully observed before it is undertaken.

It is important to note that all of the above is accomplished **without rotating the nucleus.** When the nucleus loses its adhesion to the surrounding cortical material and becomes loose within the bag, the one-handed sculpting maneuver is difficult to perform and rupture of the posterior capsule is possible. Very hard nuclei tend to rotate early and easily. Care must be taken to prevent or control excessive rotation. It is important not to 'push excessively' as the U/S tip sculpts its way through the core. Pushing can cause the nucleus to rotate or even tear the posterior capsule and is unnecessary since the U/S tip will move on its own with minimal guidance from the surgeon's hand.

Once the peripheral sculpting is finished, the depth of the remaining nuclear core should be assessed; its remaining thickness should measure approximately 25% of the fully intact nucleus. When this is achieved, and the nucleus is still in position, the surgeon can elevate the superior nuclear pole (12 o'clock) by releasing the foot pedal on the machine to position 0, which will cause the anterior chamber to shallow and the nucleus to rise. The phaco tip (bevel up) is now passed just under the superior nuclear pole to entrap it and then the foot pedal is depressed to position 1 (infusion). This will permit infusion flow, which will help to separate the superior pole of the nucleus (by hydration) from its posterior cortical adhesions. A 45° angulation on the phaco tip is best for superior pole elevation and entrapment, and it also provides a more efficient cutting action.

8.6

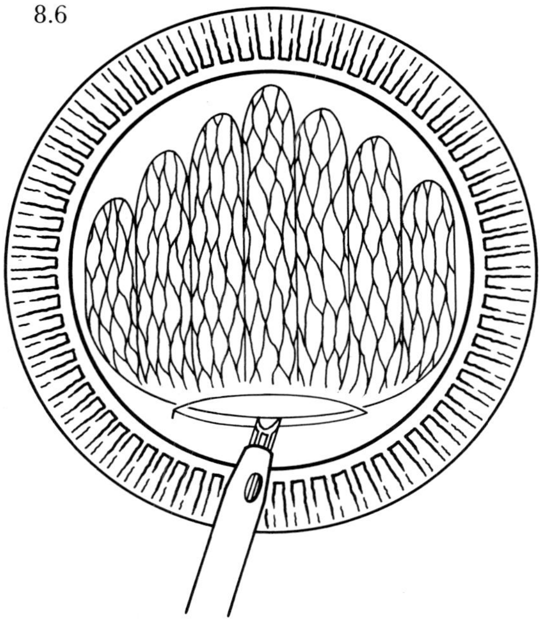

8.6 Elevation of superior pole at 12 o'clock. A 45° U/S tip is preferred for posterior hydrodissection.

The medial and lateral peripheral cortical adhesions are almost completely separated by the previous U/S sculpting in those areas. The remaining nucleus can now be emulsified by sculpting the entrapped superior pole at 12 o'clock and at its adjacent medial and lateral positions (**8.6**). The U/S tip can now be used to peel the remainder of the peripheral nucleus towards a more centrally medial or lateral position for better surgical exposure. What remains is the nuclear plate, a flat plate of nuclear core of about 25% thickness of the intact nucleus, thinning out towards the periphery. It is approached first at the 12 o'clock position, holding the U/S tip below the plate, bevel up. The central area is sculpted to split the plate in half (**8.7**). This will create a 'croissant', which can be drawn towards the superior pole by placing the phaco tip at the inside entry of the bag and slowly increasing the aspiration power (vacuum) from 1 to 2 (Site® and Phacotron® machines) or 30 to 40 mmHg (Daisy®) and collapsing the material towards the port of the U/S tip. Several bursts of U/S energy will then remove the material upon contact. Chasing this loose material around inside the bag can result in errors. It is best to emulsify any remaining fragments by holding the U/S tip in the 12 o'clock position in the bag just inside the anterior capsulorhexis (**8.8**).

Once all the nuclear material has been removed, the U/S tip can be taken out of the eye. The surgeon can then proceed with the infusion and aspiration (I/A), keeping in mind that the anterior capsule is still in place. After the cortical material has been completely emptied from the capsular bag and the posterior capsule polished, the bag should be expanded with Healon. The sclerocorneal penetration (which was originally 3 mm) has to be extended to 7.5 mm (7 mm PMMA optic), or 6.5 mm (6 mm PMMA optic). The appropriate incision for foldable intraocular lenses (IOLs) is 4.5 mm. The IOL is now inserted into the capsular bag and the loops are rotated to the horizontal position. The remaining flap of anterior capsule is removed with curved capsulotomy scissors and Kelman–McPherson forceps. The surgeon may choose to remove the anterior capsule flap prior to IOL insertion. This maneuver requires a small scissor snip at the edge of the crescentic anterior capsulorhexis and then a circular tear capsulorhexis (using Kelman–McPherson forceps), encompassing approximately a 5.0–5.5 mm diameter. Viscoelastic material should not be placed into the capsular bag

8.7

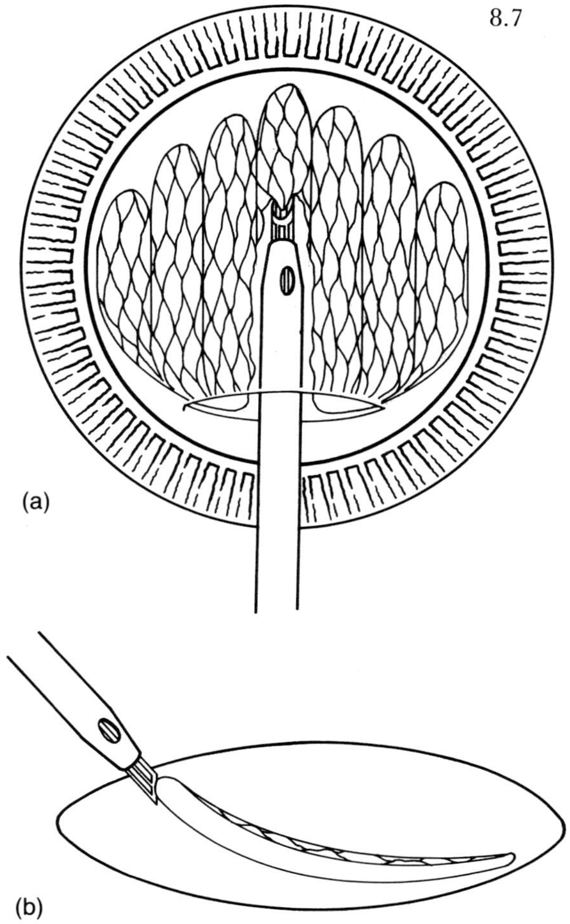

8.7 Splitting and collapse of the nuclear plate: (a) front view; (b) side view.

8.8

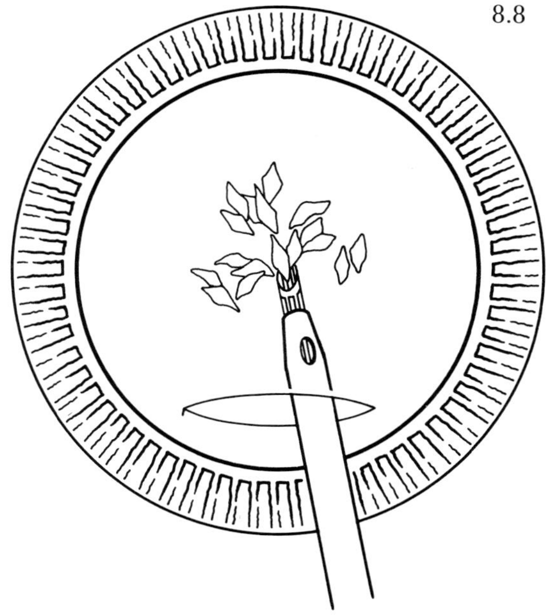

8.8 Fragment cleanup; aspiration near the superior pole causes nucleus fragments to present at the U/S tip.

prior to this maneuver, but should be used to expand the bag once the anterior flap has been torn away. The IOL is then placed into the circular opening and rotated into a horizontal position. The wound is sutured and the sodium hyaluronate aspirated.

The problems associated with this procedure are the same as with general phacoemulsification, with the additional importance of preserving the integrity of the anterior capsule. Manipulation of the phaco tip will sometimes cause the anterior capsule to split down the middle. If this happens, the bag is no longer complete, but has two flaps. The IOL can still be placed underneath the flaps and the latter can then be removed with capsulotomy scissors in two sections, instead of one. A tear in the posterior capsule can seriously alter the safety of this operation. Fragments of the nucleus can fall through the rent into the vitreous body. The surgeon must be alert to this possibility and the remaining nucleus must be kept in position until a vitrectomy machine can be brought to cut away the vitreous. Then a Sheets Glide is inserted into the bag, covering the rent in the posterior capsule, after which the nucleus fragments can be expressed, aspirated, or emulsified. The vitrectomy can be completed to guarantee that there are no vitreous remnants anterior to the capsule or in contact with the wound. Following the vitrectomy, a posterior chamber IOL may still be inserted in front of the anterior capsule and the haptics glided into the sulcus. The use of the intact anterior capsule for central support is one advantage of this endocapsular technique. In the event of sulcus placement, an IOL should be chosen with a loop span of 14 mm.

Once mastered, endophaco is an extremely beneficial procedure for both patient and surgeon. The surgery, which can usually be completed within 20–30 minutes, may well become the standard method for cataract surgery. Experience with the manual technique of intercapsular (endocapsular) cataract extraction is considered to be of benefit prior to starting intercapsular (endocapsular) phacoemulsification.

9: Excimer laser phakoablation

Danièle Aron Rosa

It has been demonstrated since 1978 that intraocular surgery is possible using short-pulsed lasers such as the neodymium: yttrium aluminium garnet (YAG) laser, and there is an increasing interest in the ophthalmological surgical applications of short pulsed lasers of various wavelengths (**9.1**). Attempts had been made already to apply YAG photodisruption to cataract surgery, however this, although possible, provides less precision than pure photoablation with an excimer laser (exited dimer).

The excimer lasers were first used in industry to etch metal and plastics. The first application of the excimer laser to ophthalmic corneal surgery was carried out by Srinivasan and Trokel who ablated the cornea using an argon fluoride 193 nm excimer laser. The laser–tissue interaction of the argon fluoride 193 nm excimer laser allows removal of corneal tissue with submicron precision and nearly no thermal effects.

Excimer lasers at wavelengths of 193, 248 and 308 nm have been evaluated for use in other human structures, such as in eyelids, in angioplasty and in dermatology. However, attempts at ablation of the lens are still experimental; non-human primates and rabbits have been the only live experimental models; human cadaver eyes have also been used.

The recent development of ultraviolet (u.v.) grade fused silica fibers with a greater transmission of u.v. light has made it possible to use short wavelength lasers, such as the xenon chloride (XeCl) excimer 308 nm laser or the fifth harmonic of a crystal YAG laser (210 nm) for intraocular procedures.

The excimer lasers are magnetically switched lasers. (The laser currently used at the Rothschild Eye Institute laboratory is a SOPRA® French XeCl excimer laser.) The pulses so generated are of 50–60 ns duration. The repetition rate can be varied from 1 to 500 Hz. The energy delivery system includes: a system of quartz, spherical, diverging and converging, lenses (20 mm diameter), a u.v. grade fused silica fiber optic, of 600 µm core diameter, which includes cladding and coating. The central part of the fiber is at the output of the laser, its distal part is included at the center of a 1 mm diameter irrigation aspiration (I/A) system, specially made for the purpose by FCI (France Chirurgie Instruments) (**9.1**). The total length of the fiber optic is 50 cm. The optical system of lenses allows the laser beam to be focused at 200 µm from the distal part of the fiber optic, thus avoiding damage to the fiber optic.

9.1

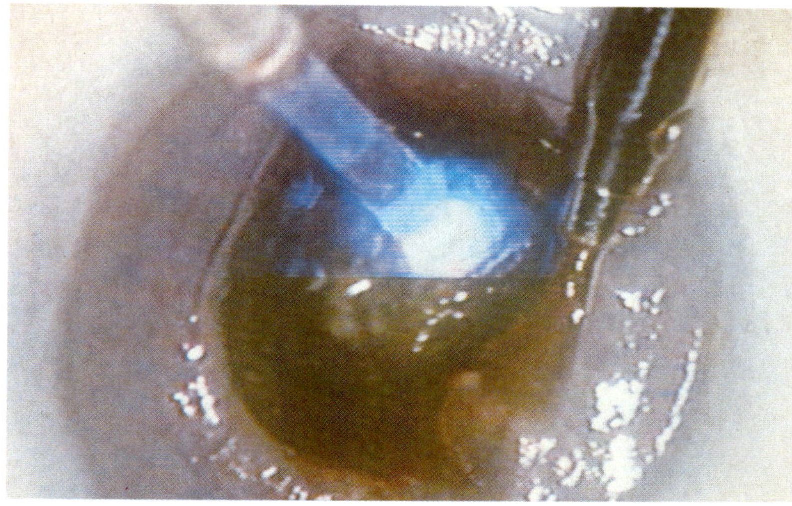

9.1 Laser phakofragmentation using the XeCl excimer laser on a cadaver eye from which the cornea has been removed. The u.v. grade fused silica fiber optic has a diameter of 600 µm, and the emission of the pulse light is clearly visible.

After the fiber optic has been introduced into the I/A cannula, the cannula is normally connected to the I/A FCI automatic system. From our experience the best flux is from 2.7 to 3.5 J cm^{-2}. The repetition rates were varied from 2 to 20 Hz, the lower repetition rates being used to ablate the cortex and nucleus in the vicinity of the two capsules.

Surgery is performed under an independent operating microscope (Wild Leitz) whose eyepieces are specially treated to avoid u.v. irradiation of the eyes of the surgeon.

Sequences of the operation

A limbal-based conjunctival flap is made 4 mm from the limbus to expose the pars plicata zone of the sclera. A supporting transparent plastic mask, 2 mm x 75 µm, is then placed so that it faces the sclera parallel to the limbus and the laser is focused. The sclera and the choroid are opened 1.5 mm posterior to the limbus. A laser hole is then made in the capsule and the I/A tip containing the fiber optic is introduced into the cortex. While the laser is working, the system is progressively pushed forward to the center of the nucleus, which is progressively photoablated and photodisrupted from the center towards the periphery (**9.2**). The cortex is then aspirated without further opening the lens capsule. This technique could, in the future,

9.2

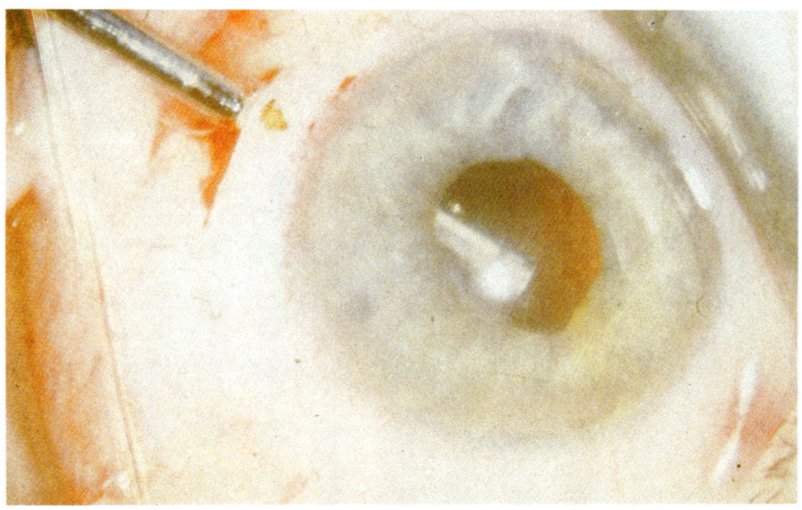

9.2 XeCl excimer laser phakoablation using the pars plana approach. At the end of phakoablation, the light of the laser pulse is visible at the tip of the fiber optic.

enable a total in-the-bag lens removal, *whatever the hardness of the cataract*, and the introduction of a liquid or semiliquid intraocular lens. A transcorneal approach and laser phakoablation in the anterior chamber is also possible but not recommended (**9.3**).

The ideal XeCl excimer 308 nm laser setting is regularly 2.7 to 3 J cm^{-2} ± 15% with a pulse rate of 5 Hz. The average number of pulses required to ablate cadaver nuclei (in the eye) of humans aged 70 to 85 years, maintained at a normal pressure of 15 mmHg, is 5000 pulses, which represents 1000 seconds. For non-human primates and rabbits whose lenses are clear and soft, the number of pulses required for ablation averages 1000: the density of the nucleus seems to affect the number of pulses required, but the I/A system working at the same time may play a major role when the lens is soft.

However, during the sequences other events occur. There is always gas bubble formation around the site of laser impact (**9.4**), which seems to prove that the XeCl excimer laser at this flux does not generate pure photoablation, but that there is also a plasma surface formation. Supporting this hypothesis, there is also a strong shock-wave formation with ejection of the liquified lens material from the target area.

A wavelength of 308 nm is more penetrating than one of 193 nm. It could be considered that a partial distant irradiation of the lens capsules may destroy the epithelial cells; however, one should also consider that there is, at this wavelength when used in air, a possible mutagenicity and retinotoxicity: it still has to be proven whether phakoablation in a fluid medium will reduce these risks. Furthermore, cornea endothelial cell toxicity of the XeCl excimer laser has to be seriously studied.

Ezra Maguen *et al.*, whose experimental work corroborates our experience, have measured the decrease in flux from the fiber optic tip as the distance increases in saline: for an output flux of 2.8 J cm^{-2} at the tip, the flux at 3 mm distance is 0.2 J cm^{-2}. However, new fiber optics are coming onto the market that are transparent to shorter wavelengths and in the near future lasers producing 193, 200 or 210 nm, which are less toxic and so safer, may be in use.

9.3

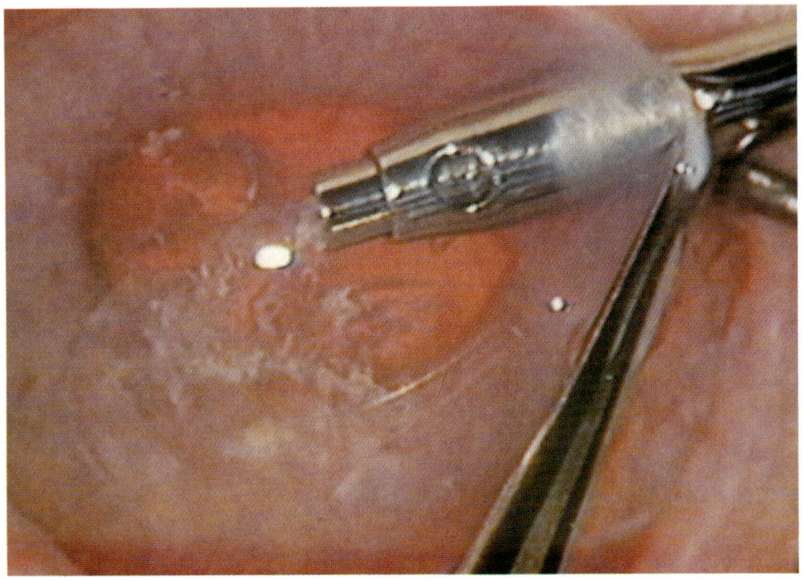

9.3 XeCl excimer laser phakoablation is the anterior chamber of a rabbit eye, showing a partially fragmented lens and cavitation bubbles.

9.4

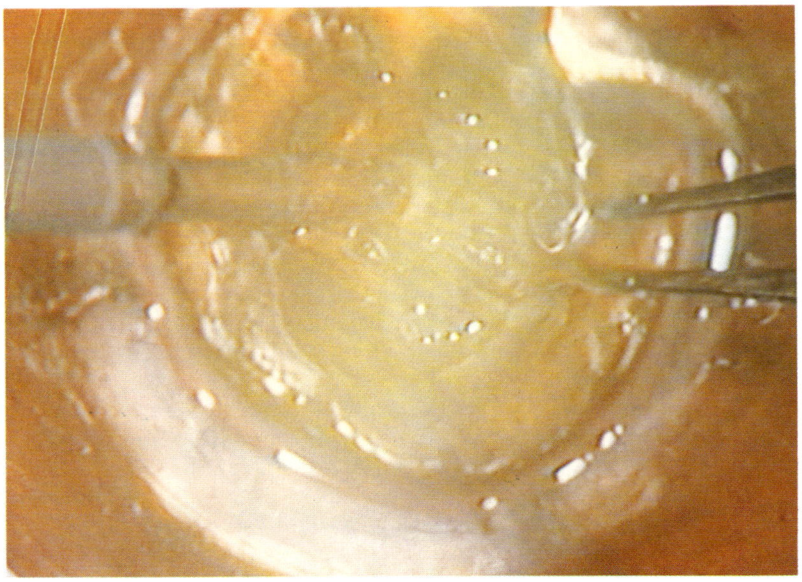

9.4 XeCl excimer laser phakoablation of a cadaver eye with the cornea removed. The fiber optic has been introduced deeply into the lens and ejected particles and bubbles that surround the tip are visible, suggesting that XeCl ablation is a combination of photoablation coupled with surface plasma and shock wave effects.

Further reading

Aron-Rosa D. Use of a pulsed Neodymium YAG laser for anterior capsulotomy before extracapsular cataract extraction. *Am Intraocul. Impl. Soc. J.*, **7,** 332–333, 1981.

Aron-Rosa D., Carre F., *et al.* Keratorefractive surgery with the excimer laser. *Am. J. Ophthalmol.*, **100,** 741–742, 1985.

Haefliger E., Parel J.M., *et al.* Accommodation of an endocapsular silicone lens (phacoersatz) in the nonhuman primates. *Ophthalmology*, **94,** 471–477, 1987.

Maguen E., Martinez M., *et al.* Excimer laser ablation of the human lens at 308 nm with a fiber delivery system. *J. Cat. Refract. Surg.*, **15,** 409–414, 1989.

Trokel J.L., Srinivasan R. and Braren B. Excimer laser surgery of the cornea. *Am. J. Ophthalmol.*, **96,** 710–715, 1983.

10: Ophthalmic irrigating solutions

Ole Lorenzetti and Henry Edelhauser

Irrigating solutions have undergone a considerable improvement since the early 1960s. Many of the advances have progressed with our increased knowledge of corneal physiology, anterior segment dynamics, improved methods for evaluating irrigating solutions, and the requirements of improved surgical procedures with the demands of microsurgical techniques offered by operating microscopes.

The evolution of ocular irrigating solutions has been from sterile distilled water in the 19th century, to normal saline in the early part of the 20th century, to various modifications of lactated Ringer's solution, Tyrode's solution, tissue and organ media, tissue irrigants (Plasma-Lyte^{TM}), to balanced salt solution (BSS®) and finally to glutathione bicarbonate Ringer's (GBR), which evolved commercially into balanced salt solution Plus (BSS PLUS®) (**Table 10.1**).

Table 10.1 Composition of intraocular irrigating solutions (all concentrations expressed in mmol l^{-1} of solution)

Ingredient	*Normal Saline* (0.9% NaCl)*	*Lactated Ringer's**	*Hartmann's Solution**	*Plasma-Lyte 148™**	*BSS®**	*BSS PLUS®**	*GBR†*
Sodium chloride	154	102	102.6	86	110	122.2	111.6
Potassium chloride		4	4	5	10	5.08	4.8
Calcium chloride		3	2.4	–	3	1.05	1.1
Magnesium chloride		–	–	1.5	1.5	0.98	0.78
Magnesium sulfate		–	–	–	–	–	–
Sodium lactate		28	27	–	–	–	–
Sodium acetate			–	27	29	–	–
Sodium gluconate			–	23	–	–	–
Sodium citrate			–		6	–	–
Sodium acid phosphate			–			–	0.86
Disodium phosphate			–			3.0	–
Sodium bicarbonate			–			25.0	29.2
HEPES			–			–	–
Glucose			–			5.11	5.01
Glutathione (reduced)			–			–	0.30
Glutathione (oxidized)			–			0.30	–
Adenosine			–			–	0.50
Ascorbic acid							
Potassium phosphate							
Dextran 40							
pH	4.5–7.2	6.0–7.2	6.2–7.0	7.4	7.4	7.4	7.4
Osmolality (mosmol)	290	277	256	299	305	305	274

Ingredient	*Modified AME*	*SMA®**	*Opeguard-MAr®**	*Cardiff Solution*	*Schachar‡*	*PHS*
Sodium chloride	120	112.9	112.9	120.46	111.6	107
Potassium chloride	3.1	4.8	4.8	4	4.82	5.2
Calcium chloride	1.15	1.2	1.2	2.54	1.04	1.45
Magnesium chloride	–	–	–	–	0.78	1.18
Magnesium sulfate	1.2	1.2	1.2	1.0	–	–
Sodium lactate	–	–	–	–	–	–
Sodium acetate	–	4.4	–	–	–	–
Sodium gluconate	–	–	–	–	–	–
Sodium citrate	–	3.4	–	–	–	–
Sodium acid phosphate	–	–	–	1.0	0.86	–
Disoidum phosphate	–	–	–	–	–	–
Sodium bicarbonate	23.0	25.0	25	–	25.0	25.8
HEPES	–	–	–	20.0	–	–
Glucose	10	8.3	8.3	4.45	5.01	5.1
Glutathione (reduced)	–	–	–		–	
Glutathione (oxidized)	–	–	–		0.30	–
Adenosine	–	–	–			
Ascorbic acid						6.8
Potassium phosphate	0.5				20.0	
Dextran 40						0.49
pH	8.2		7.2	7.2		
Osmolality (mosmol)	292	290	284			283

* *Commercially available.* † *pH adjusted by bubbling with 5% CO_2/95% air.* ‡ *US Patent 4620979.*

Today, lactated Ringer's, BSS® and BSS PLUS® form the basis for many variations, including Hartmann's, Peyman, Schachar, SMA_1, SMA_2®, SMA_3, Freeman's, and Cardiff solution.

Studies in the early 1970s showed that a bicarbonate Ringer's solution containing glucose, adenosine, and glutathione, prevented the cornea from swelling and maintained the cellular endothelial integrity, and that the best irrigating solution should contain concentrations of inorganic and organic constituents similar to aqueous humor. A GBR solution was formulated, containing in addition to the basic salts, sodium bicarbonate, glucose, glutathione, and adenosine. It was maintained at a pH of 7.4 and had an osmolality of 274, slightly hypotonic to human endothelial tissues but isotonic to rabbit tissue.

Plasma-Lyte 148™ was the first solution used for phacoemulsification because it had a stable pH of 7.4. However, it lacked glucose and the critical ion calcium, and it has been shown that with infusion to the anterior chamber, the junctions between the endothelial cells become broken (**10.1, 10.2**) with marked corneal edema.

The major problems with Ringer's solution and lactated Ringer's, which contain calcium, were a variable pH and the lack of a buffer and energy source. With the addition of bicarbonate ion to a solution of variable pH, precipitation of the calcium could occur and the medium occasionally turned cloudy. During the late 1970s BSS® 500 ml became available for large volume intraocular surgery. Later a GBR type of solution became commercially available as BSS PLUS®, which is similar to GBR except that oxidized glutathione is used in place of reduced glutathione, and adenosine is lacking. Such a formula is necessary in order to develop a solution that is stable with a long shelf life.

10.1

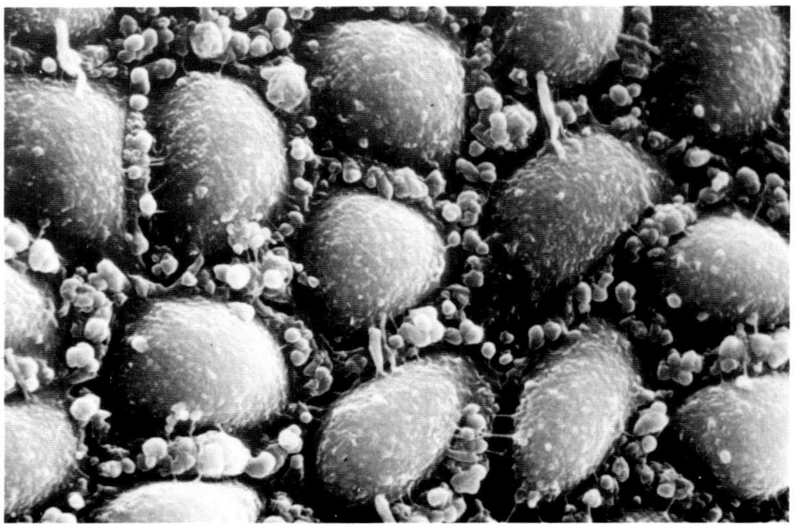

10.1 Influence of Plasma-Lyte 148™ on corneal endothelium. SEM of rabbit corneal endothelium perfused with Plasma-Lyte 148 for 2 h. The endothelial cells are swollen and the junctions between cells have become disruptive. Magnification x 2000.

10.2

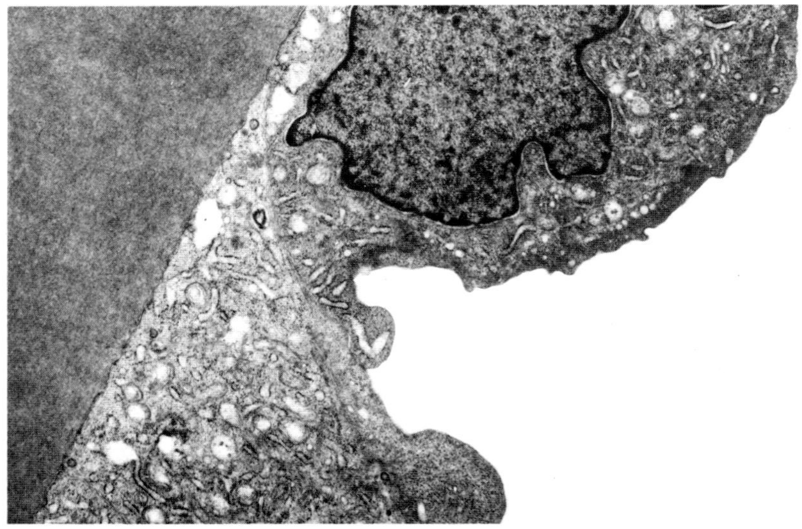

10.2 TEM of the same cornea as in **10.1**. The junction between cells is broken, cytoplasmic vacuoles are present, and mitochondria are condensed. Magnification x 9700.

Aqueous and vitreous humor

Ophthalmic irrigating solutions should mimic aqueous and vitreous humor in ingredients, pH and osmolality (**Table 10.2**). Extensive studies have shown that a proper irrigant should have a pH of 7.4 ± 0.6, osmolality of 310 ± 30 mosmol and a physiological bicarbonate–phosphate buffer system. In addition, the importance of glucose, glutathione and electrolytes (sodium, potassium, calcium and magnesium) in concentrations that mimic human aqueous and vitreous has been demonstrated in several publications.

Table 10.2 Chemical composition of human aqueous humor, vitreous humor, BSS PLUS®, and BSS® (all concentrations expressed in mmol l^{-1} or meq l^{-1} solution)

Ingredient	*Human aqueous humor*	*Human vitreous humor*	*BSS PLUS®*	*BSS®*	*Ingredient*	*Human aqueous humor*	*Human vitreous humor*	*BSS PLUS®*	*BSS®*
Sodium	162.9	144	160.0	155.7	Glucose	2.7–3.7	3.4	5.0	–
Potassium	2.2–3.9	5.5	5.0	10.1	Ascorbate	1.06	2.0	–	–
Calcium	1.8	1.6	1.0	3.3	Glutathione	0.0019	–	0.3	–
Magnesium	1.1	1.3	1.0	1.5	Citrate	–	–	–	5.8
Chloride	131.6	177.0	130.0	128.9	Acetate	–	–	–	28.6
Bicarbonate	20.15	15.0	25.0	–	pH	7.38	–	7.4	7.6
Phosphate	0.62	0.4	3.0	–	Osmolality				
Lactate	2.5	7.8	–	–	(mosmol)	304		305	298

Aqueous flow plays an important part with the use of irrigating solution. Factors such as volume differences, buffering capacity, and flow rates, are of relative importance in tissue injury. Whereas intravascular drugs, which often contain potentially toxic additives, are rapidly diluted and buffered by the intravascular volume, this is not the case intraocularly, because no such dilution or buffering potential exists. There may be prolonged contact of irrigants with intraocular structures postoperatively. While the duration of surgical irrigation is important, it, nevertheless, represents only a small fraction of the overall time the solution is in direct contact with the corneal endothelium and other intraocular structures. **Table 10.3** demonstrates mathematically that 4 h 23 min is required for aqueous secretions to fill the fluid capacity of the normal nongeriatric eye (in which the crystalline lens has been replaced by a posterior chamber IOL). Since surgery, as well as other factors, often reduces aqueous inflow and outflow by as much as 50%, a reforming solution frequently remains in the postoperative eye for over eight hours.

Table 10.3 Aqueous replacement of irrigation solution vs. time

Fluid capacity	
Anterior chamber	0.250 ml
Posterior chamber	0.060 ml
Space left by extracted crystalline lens	0.250 ml
Subtotal fluid capacity	0.560 ml
Aqueous flow rate	
Normal eye (average)	0.002 ml min^{-1}
Aqueous replacement	
Minimum time $\dfrac{0.025\text{ ml}}{0.002\text{ ml min}^{-1}}$	= 262.5min (4h, 23min)
Flow rate following surgery	
Aqueous flow may be reduced by surgery by 50%. Thus irrigating solution may remain for up to 8.75 hours	

Blood aqueous barrier effects of anterior chamber irrigation have been evaluated by Miyake and Asakura (1985) on rabbits using physiological saline, lactated Ringer's solution, BSS® and SMA_2® with the irrigation aspiration tip of a phacoemulsifier.

Fluorophotometry showed that physiological saline yielded the most damage, lactated Ringer's solution and BSS® yielded moderate damage, while SMA_2® showed only slight damage to barrier function. These results suggest that glucose, as well as Ca^{2+}, Mg^{2+} and the bicarbonate (HCO_3) buffer system, are essential constituents for maintaining function in the blood–aqueous barrier.

Corneal endothelium barrier function has been studied by Araie *et al.*, (1988), in the rabbit *in vitro*, comparing the effect of GBR, BSS PLUS® and SMA_2® on the endothelial permeability (P_{ac}) to carboxyfluorescein. The major chemical differences between SMA_2® and GBR or BSS PLUS® are that SMA_2® does not contain glutathione and phosphate but does contain acetate and citrate. All are buffered with bicarbonate. Results showed a significant increase in permeability for SMA_2®, confirming the importance of glutathione in improving the safety of intraocular irrigating solutions.

Additive drugs in the irrigating solution may cause a variable *uveal response* and may be potentially toxic to the corneal endothelium. Intraoperative mydriasis and miosis can be rapidly effected by the addition of pharmacological agents directly to irrigating solutions. It is important that agents introduced intracamerally be in a physiologically buffered vehicle which complements the irrigating solution that should mimic the natural intraocular fluids. The safety of a properly formulated solution may be seriously compromised by the deliberate introduction of adjunctive solutions. Several surgeons have advocated routine addition of mydriatics, miotics and antibiotics to irrigants in cataract surgery. Epinephrine, acetylcholine, thrombin and carbachol are frequently used. In these instances, drugs that have been formulated for intravenous, intracardiac, or intratracheal use are being introduced into a compartment for which they have not been designed. Additive drugs also contain various chemicals (preservatives, solubilizers, antioxidants) that may not be safe. The potential exists for direct endothelial toxicity or for a weak inflammatory response from the drug itself, the vehicle, its preservative, or any number of interactions with the irrigant, which may result in an altered electrolyte balance, pH or osmolality.

Examples of toxicity to endothelium include *thrombin* (McDermott *et al.* 1988), the sodium bisulphite buffer in 1:1000 epinephrine (Edelhauser *et al.* 1982) and 1% acetyl choline (Yee and Edelhauser 1986), which is formulated in water for injection containing no buffers or essential electrolytes. Carbachol is contained in a balanced salt solution and has demonstrated no ultrastructural or functional abnormalities.

Comparative effects of formulations currently used

Lactated Ringer's (LR) solution contains the essential ions to maintain intraocular tissues. However, it contains 28 mmol l^{-1} of lactate, which is a much higher concentration than is found in the intraocular fluids (**Tables 10.1** and **10.2**). LR was formulated as an intravenous solution, and the high concentration of lactate was to supply the heart with a substrate that would serve as an energy source while it was under metabolic stress. Intraocular tissues do not use lactate as a major substrate for metabolism. Another difficulty with LR is the variability in pH (6.0 to 7.2) from one sample to another. Several studies have shown the harmful effects of LR as compared with BSS PLUS® on the corneal endothelium when perfusion is prolonged (**10.3**). Neither LR nor *Hartmann's solution*, which has the same deficiencies, should be used for phacoemulsification or pars plana vitrectomy.

Balanced Salt Solution (BSS®) became available for large volume intraocular irrigation (500 ml) in the 1970s. Although adequate for intraocular use, it is not similar to human aqueous (**Table 10.2**), and Glasser *et al.* (1985) have shown a significant effect on corneal endothelium when compared with BSS PLUS® (**10.4, 10.5**).

SMA$_2$® is similar in formulation to BSS® and GBR. The essential ingredients of SMA$_2$® and GBR are the bicarbonate ion and glucose; the difference between the two solutions is that SMA$_2$® lacks glutathione but contains sodium acetate and sodium citrate as buffers to maintain the pH. Since acetate and citrate buffers are not normally found in the eye, SMA$_2$® may not support cell metabolism as well as

10.3(a)

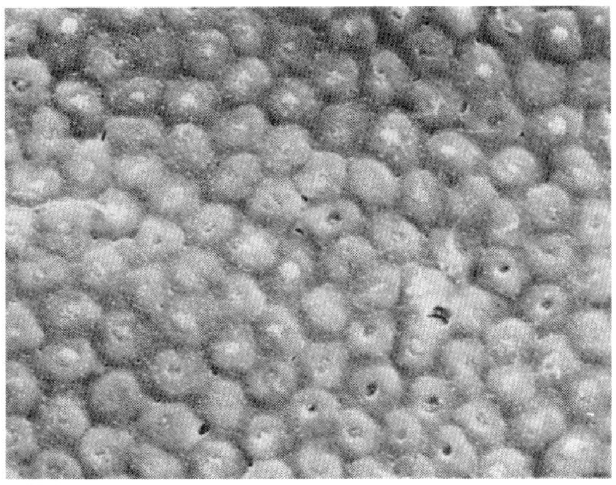

10.3(b)

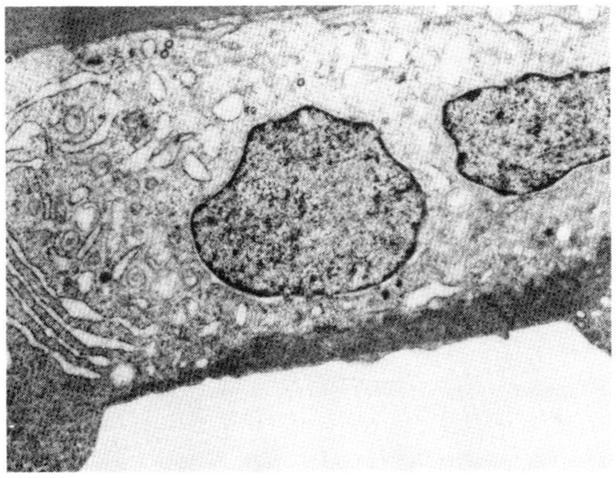

10.3(c)

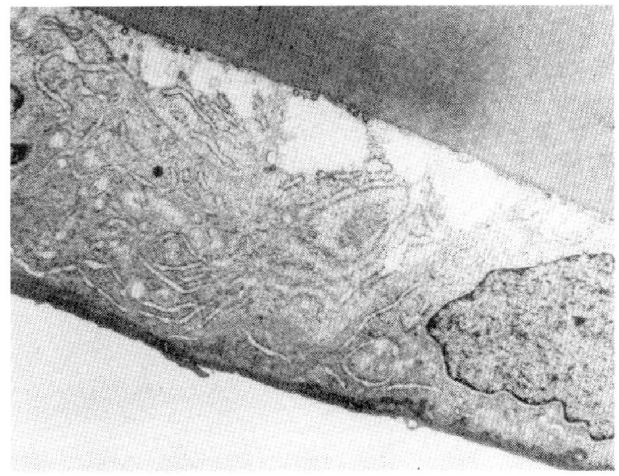

10.3 Influence of lactated Ringer's on the corneal endothelium. (a) SEM of rabbit corneal endothelium perfused with lactated Ringer's for 3 h. The endothelial cells are swollen, cytoplasmic blebbing has occurred, and there are areas of junctional breakdown and cell loss. Original magnification x 1000. (b) TEM of the same cornea perfused with lactated Ringer's for 3 h. Note the cytoplasmic blebbing, dilation of the endoplasmic reticulum, and area of clarified cytoplasm. Original magnification x 12000. (c) TEM of the same cornea illustrating the area of clarified cytoplasm adjacent to Descemet's membrane. Magnification x 9600.

10.4

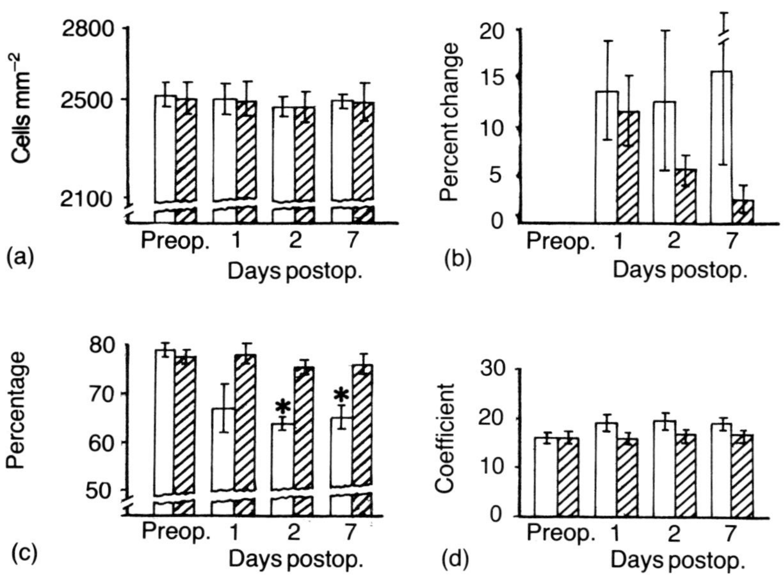

10.4 (a) Endothelial cell density, (b) corneal swelling, (c) percentage of hexagons, and (d) coefficient of variation (standard mean cell area/mean cell area) after anterior chamber irrigation for 15 min. Open histogram, BSS®; lined histogram, BSS PLUS®. Bar gauge, mean ± SEM. Asterisk denotes $p < 0.05$. $N = 5$ for each measurement (Glasser *et al.* 1985).

10.5

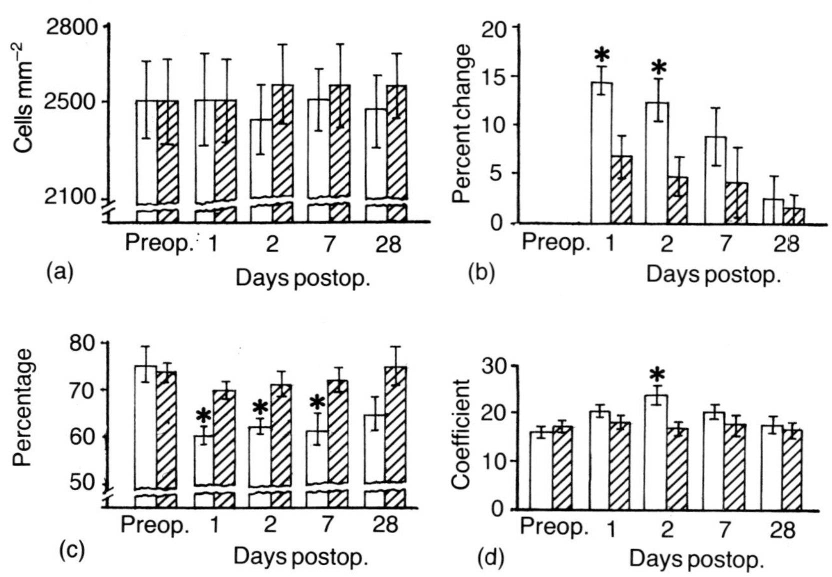

10.5 Comparison of ocular damage in the cat following 60 min irrigation of anterior chamber with BSS® (open histogram) or BSS PLUS® (lined histogram): (a) changes in corneal endothelial cell density, (b) corneal swelling, (c) percentage of hexagonal cells, and (d) variability of cell area (coefficient of variation = standard deviation/mean). Bar gauge, mean ± SEM. Asterisk denotes $p < 0.05$. $N = 5$ for each measurement (Glasser *et al.* 1985).

does a solution without acetate and citrate. Recent studies (**10.6, 10.7**) have compared BSS® (acetate–citrate–phosphate buffer), SMA_2® (acetate–citrate and bicarbonate buffer), and BSS PLUS® (bicarbonate buffer) for their ability to protect the human corneal endothelium following *in vitro* perfusion. BSS® maintained the corneal thickness without swelling; SMA_2® caused the corneas to swell at 7 μm h^{-1}; BSS PLUS® promoted temperature reversal, and the human corneas deswelled at 13 μm h^{-1}. One possibility is that the citrate chelates the calcium. By comparison, BSS PLUS® protected the corneal endothelial integrity throughout the perfusion period.

10.8 shows that SMA_2®, like BSS®, may cause significant morphologic alterations of the endothelium.

10.6

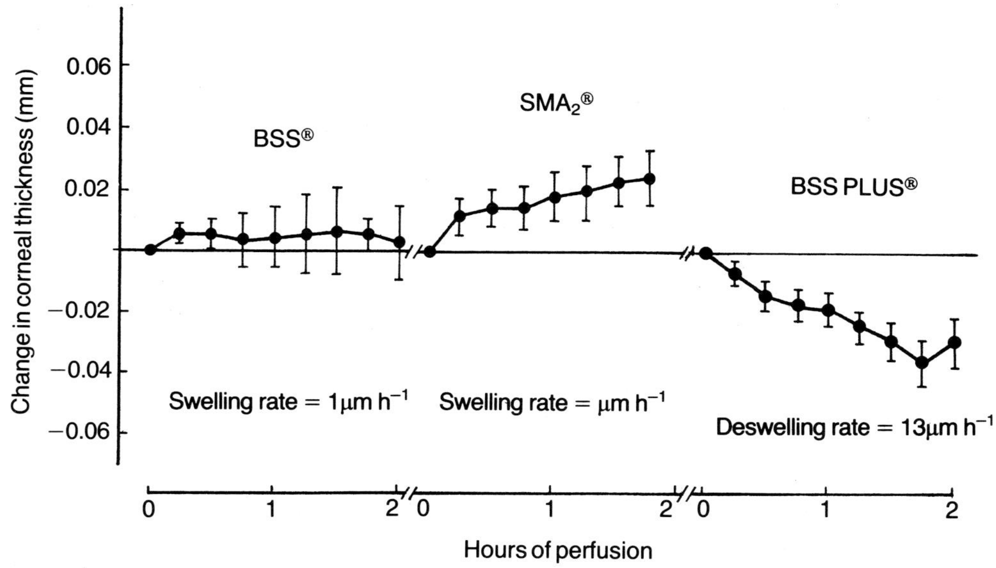

10.6 Corneal swelling following *in vitro* corneal endothelial perfusion with BSS® ($N = 6$), SMA_2® ($N = 8$), and BSS PLUS® ($N = 14$).

10.7(a)

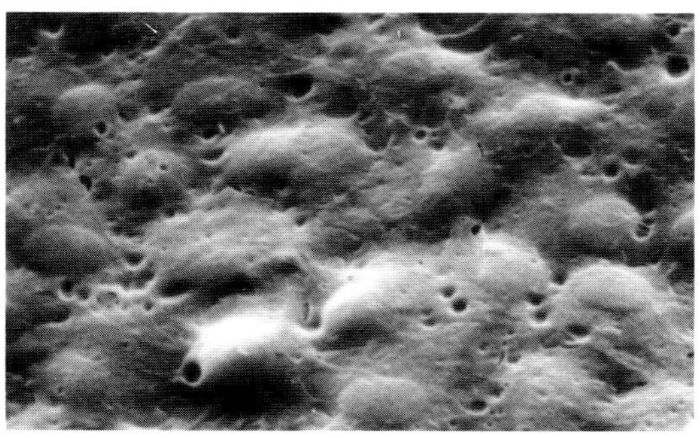

10.7(b)

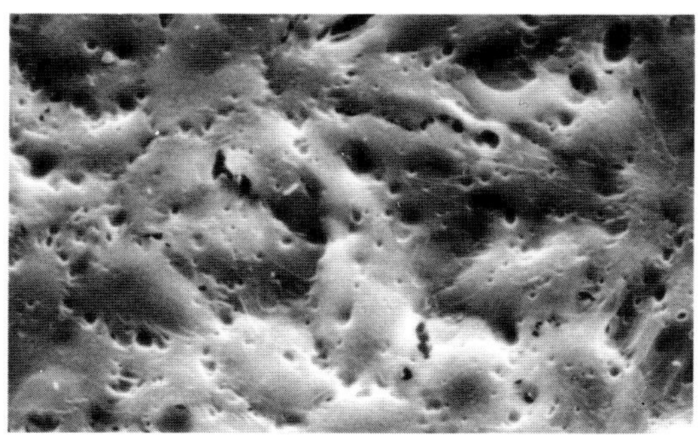

10.7(c)

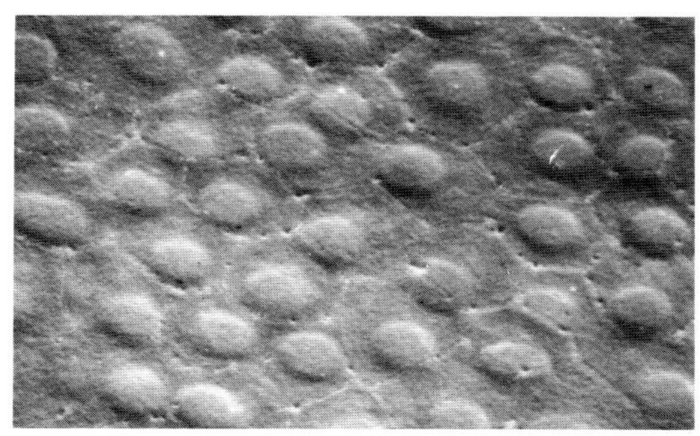

10.7 Scanning electron micrographs (magnification x 1000) of human corneas following 2 h of endothelial perfusion with (a) BSS®, (b) SMA_2® and (c) BSS PLUS®.

10.8

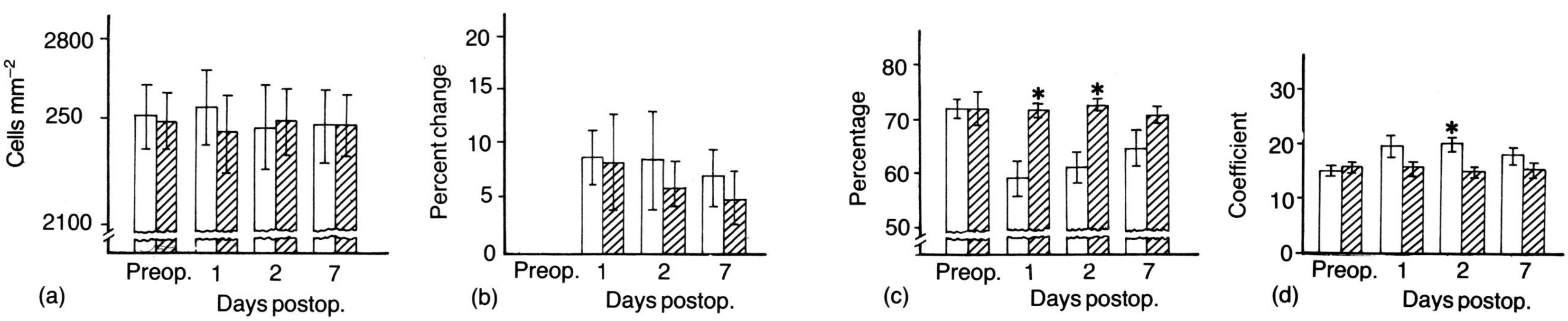

10.8 Morphologic changes in (a) corneal endothelial cell density, (b) corneal swelling, (c) percentage of hexagonal cells and (d) coefficient of variation, in the cat after anterior chamber irrigation for 60 min with SMA_2® (open bars) and BSS PLUS® (hatched bars). Bar gauge, mean ± SEM. Asterisk denotes $p < 0.05$. N = 5 for each measurement.

A forerunner of SMA_2® was SMA_1, but this was found to form precipitates. SMA_3 does not form precipitates, but was discontinued because of an excess of bicarbonate, which formed bubbles during surgery. A recently developed modification of the Japanese SMA formulas is *Opeguard-MA*®, which more nearly approaches BSS PLUS® in composition.

BSS PLUS® is chemically similar to human aqueous and vitreous (**Table 10.2**). It is stable for 6 h after parts I and II have been mixed. The presence of the proper bicarbonate buffer, of glucose to provide energy for intracellular metabolic pathways, and of glutathione to prevent oxidative damage, all represent improvements over BSS® and SMA_2®.

The Cardiff irrigating solution has the addition of *N*-2-hydroxyethyl-piperazine-N^1-2-ethanesulphonic acid (HEPES) in a basic salt solution with glucose. The effect of HEPES was to stabilize the formulation and improve the buffering capacity, but more recently it has been found to be toxic to the corneal endothelium.

Formulations have also been described containing other additives but are unproven. Dextran has been proposed as an ingredient by Textorius *et al.* (1986) and Peyman (PHS, **Table 10.1**). Schachar discussed a formulation with ascorbate and provided illustrations with the use of reduced glutathione and adenosine, but which have known instability and cannot be commercialized on a large scale.

Functional use of intraocular irrigating solutions

Ocular surgery involving irrigation requires solutions that can maintain normal cellular metabolism, function, structure and integrity of the corneal endothelium, iris, ciliary body, lens and retina. When moderate to high volumes of irrigation are required the solutions used must contain the necessary components to protect the delicate balance existing within the endothelial cell structure.

The morphologic characteristics of corneal endothelial cells are markedly changed by aging with an increase in cell size and an increasing variation in cell shape indicating a loss of the regularly sized hexagonal-shaped cells normally found in youth. These changes are more pronounced in the eyes of diabetics. The act of surgery, especially if tissues are traumatized, will compound this problem since mitotic proliferation is rare and large cells appear as a consequence of cell loss when neighboring cells expand to cover denuded areas. Clinical trials conducted by Kline (1983) showed the superiority of BSS PLUS® compared to BSS® in 100 cases of planned extracapsular extraction with automated irrigation/aspiration and insertion of a posterior chamber IOL.

The extremely sensitive *in vitro* models have also demonstrated the superiority of BSS PLUS® over other irrigating solutions, and although *in vivo* studies are of necessity much less sensitive, BSS PLUS® should be considered the solution of choice for high risk cases and during phacoemulsification and vitrectomy operations. The essence of this superiority is the combination of: calcium, which is essential for maintaining endothelial cell junctions; glucose, which is necessary for aerobic metabolism; glutathione, which aids in membrane protection; and a bicarbonate buffer, which is the normal buffer in human aqueous.

Further reading

Araie M., Shirasawa E., and Hikita A. Effect of oxidized glutathione on the barrier function of the corneal endothelium. *Invest. Ophthalmol. Vis. Sci.*, **29,** 1884–1887, 1988.

Edelhauser H.F. and MacRae S.M. Irrigating and viscous solution. In Sears M. and Takkonen A. (Eds), *Surgical Pharmacology of the Eye*. Raven Press, NY, 363–388, 1985.

Edelhauser H.F., Hyndiuk R.A., Zeeb A., and Schultz R.O. Corneal edema and the intraocular use of epinephrine. *Am. J. Ophthal.*, **93**, 327–333, 1982.

Glasser D.B. *et al.* Effects of intraocular irrigating solutions on the corneal endothelium after anterior chamber irrigation. *Am. J. Ophthal.* **99,** 321, 1985.

Kline O.R., Jr., Symes D.J., Lorenzetti O.J., and deFaller J. Effect of BSS PLUS® on the corneal endothelium with intraocular lens implantation. *J. Cutaneous and Ocular Toxicology,* **2,** 243–247, 1983.

McDermott M.L., Edelhauser H.F. and Mannic M.T. Intracorneal thrombin and the corneal endothelium. *Am. J. Ophthal.,* **106,** 414–422, 1988.

Miyake K. and Asakura M. Effect of anterior chamber irrigation and irrigating solutions on the blood aqueous barrier. *Graefe's Archive Ophthalmology,* **222,** 254–255, 1985.

Peyman G.U., Sanders D.R., and Ligara T.H. Dextran-40-containing infusion fluids and corneal swelling. *Arch. Ophthal.,* **97,** 152–155, 1979.

Textorius O., Nilsson S.E.G., and Anderson B.E. Effects of intraocular perfusion with two alternating irrigation solutions on the simultaneously recorded ERG of albino rabbits. *Documenta Ophthalmol.,* **63,** 349–358, 1986.

11: Management of intraoperative complications

Ulrich Demeler

Prolapse of the iris

The prolapse of the iris, depending on its extent, can be a disastrous complication during intra- and extra-capsular cataract extraction and can be difficult to manipulate. To avoid this complication, both in local and in general anesthesia, the intravenous injection of 250 mg acetazolamide is recommended, 20–30 min prior to the opening of the eye as well as oculopression for about 10–15 min. After the eye is opened, care should be taken not to fill the anterior chamber with too much viscoelastic substance or to have the irrigating solution flowing at too high a pressure. The management of an iris prolapse depends on the time of its occurrence. If it happens immediately after the opening of the anterior chamber prior to any surgical manipulation in the eye, in most cases it can be easily replaced with a spatula. The anterior chamber should be deepened by the injection of a viscoelastic substance or, in the case of phacoemulsification, by the outflow of the irrigating solution. If the prolapse of the iris occurs while enlarging the incision, when nucleus delivery is planned, the iris should be pressed down with a spatula and the nucleus expression performed over the spatula. The iris can then be replaced easily in most cases. If the eye becomes hard because of an increasing *vis a tergo*, and the iris prolapses recurrently, the eye should be closed immediately with preplaced sutures.

After deepening of the anterior chamber with a viscoelastic substance, the implantation of a posterior chamber lens is still possible, but an anterior chamber lens may be preferred if other intraoperative complications have occurred. After successful implantation of the intraocular lens, the prolapsed iris is often flabby and necrotic. If the pupil is not round, anterior synechiae can be expected, and it is advisable to perform a small peripheral iridectomy or even a sector iridectomy with restoration of the pupil by a 10-0 nylon suture.

If, during wound closure, iris prolapse is found to complicate proper wound suturing, it may be helpful to inject a small amount of viscoelastic agent just inside the wound.

Small pupil

Successful extracapsular surgery depends on adequate mydriasis, which will facilitate the anterior capsulotomy and provide a full field of view throughout the operation when performing the nucleus delivery, the removal of all cortex, the polishing of the posterior capsule and the implantation of the posterior chamber lens.

Aids to mydriasis may be the subconjunctival injection of 0.5 ml of a mixture of 100 mg cocaine HCl and 20 mg atropine sulfate in 10 ml solution of balanced salt solution (e.g., BSS®) or the injection of 0.3 ml of a mixture of 1 ml of adrenaline 1:1000 in 10 ml balanced salt solution in the anterior chamber. Normally, 0.3–0.5 ml of adrenaline 1:1000 should be added to the irrigating solution of 500 ml balanced salt solution. Passing the irrigating solution through a thermostatically controlled blood warmer may additionally help to preserve pupil dilatation.

If, in spite of all these mydriatics, the pupil diameter is too small to do an adequate capsulotomy, two inferior sphincterotomies at the 5 and 7 o'clock position will usually ensure a large enough pupillary dilatation. If the sphincterotomies are insufficient, the creation of a sector iridectomy will allow safe continuation of the surgery (**11.1**).

If an anterior capsulotomy is attempted through a small pupil followed by delivery of the nucleus, there is considerable risk of sphincter tears, iridodialysis, iris hemorrhage and rupture of the zonule or posterior capsule. The pupil may constrict after nucleus delivery, and dislocation of the nucleus prior to expression is an additional irritation to the iris, also making removal of the cortex difficult.

If the pupil is rigid with posterior synechias from previous surgery, iritis or miotic therapy, then, under the protection of a viscoelastic substance, a peripheral iridectomy should be performed and converted with scissors into a sector iridectomy. This may or may not be performed in conjunction with inferior sphincterotomies. The posterior synechias are divided with a spatula or the blunt edge of the cystitome, as well as with the help of a viscoelastic substance.

In some cases it is recommended to resuture the sector iridectomy with 10-0 nylon in order to have a protecting iris diaphragm, e.g. if capsular or sulcus fixation is intended, or to enable an easy and safe haptic fixation in the anterior chamber.

11.1

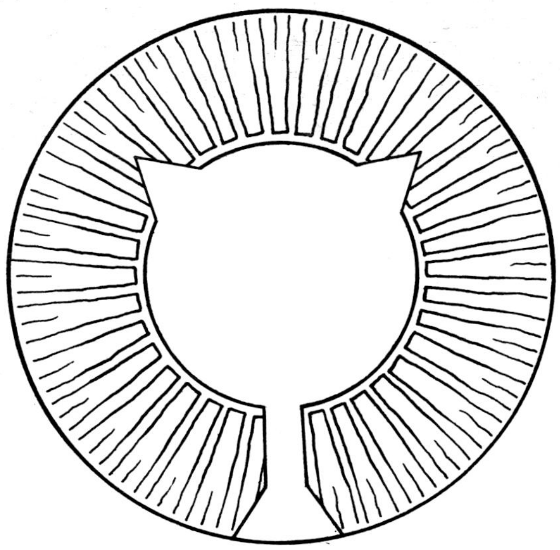

11.1 Posterior synechias or small pupil during surgery. If two sphincterotomies at 5 and 7 o'clock positions are insufficient, a peripheral iridectomy is converted into a sector iridectomy at the 12 o'clock position.

Detachment of Descemet's membrane

Minor detachments of Descemet's membrane during extracapsular cataract extraction are not associated with serious complications. Extensive detachments, however, will be followed by corneal edema, bullous keratopathy and reduced vision, often requiring the patient to be given a penetrating graft. Descemet's detachment can occur when any surgical instrument enters the anterior chamber. It can also happen during insertion of the lens, when the lens haptics become entangled with Descemet's membrane at the wound edge. To avoid this complication an air bubble or viscoelastic substance should be injected into the anterior chamber before entering it. When performing phacoemulsification or automated irrigation/aspiration, the same effect can be achieved by a relatively high pressure inflow passing the corneal wound edge at a steep angle.

Small and circumscribed detachments of Descemet's membrane do not require treatment. Large and extensive detachments should be detected at least before the eye is closed, because they require special surgical intervention. Depending on the extent of the detachment, the injection of an air bubble or, better, a viscoelastic substance in the anterior chamber after lens implantation is necessary (**11.2**). Only thus can the replacement of the detached Descemet's membrane be achieved. In very large detachments of more than half of Descemet's membrane (**11.3**), it is necessary to resuture the detached membrane with 10-0 nylon in addition to the injection of a viscoelastic substance.

11.2

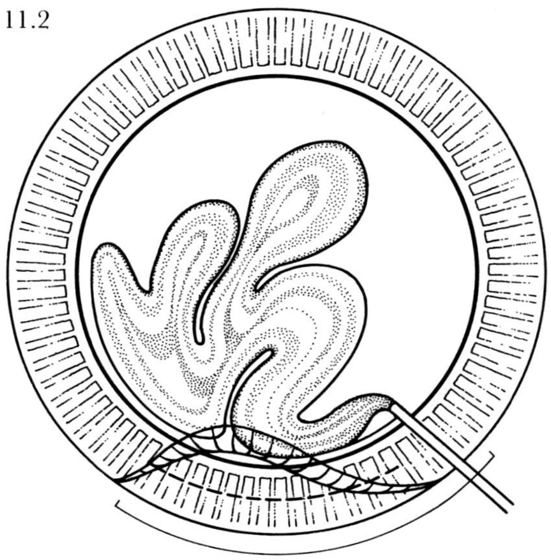

11.2 A significant detachment of Descemet's membrane, but viscoelastic substance in the anterior chamber is sufficient for reattachment.

11.3

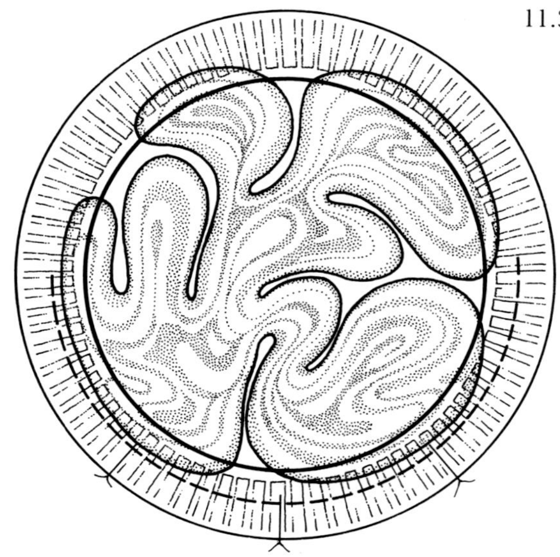

11.3 In a very large detachment of Descemet's membrane, the membrane should be sutured with 10-0 nylon additionally to the viscoelastic substance in the anterior chamber.

Tears of the anterior capsule

Uncontrolled and unintentional tears of the anterior capsule can occur while performing the anterior capsulotomy with a blunt cystitome and/or in a relatively hard and rigid anterior capsule. They can also happen during nucleus delivery if the nucleus is much larger than the capsulotomy. Tears of the anterior capsule can extend to the equator of the lens capsule and are not visible behind the iris (**11.4**). Thus it can be difficult during lens insertion to implant the lens haptics into the capsular bag. In those doubtful cases, sulcus fixation should be preferred to avoid an unsafe or half capsular, half sulcus fixation. If large flaps of the anterior capsule are left behind after the lens has been implanted into the capsular bag, the remaining anterior capsule should be removed from the optic zone. The more capsule there is left behind, the higher is the chance of decentration caused by postoperative shrinkage of capsular flaps.

11.4

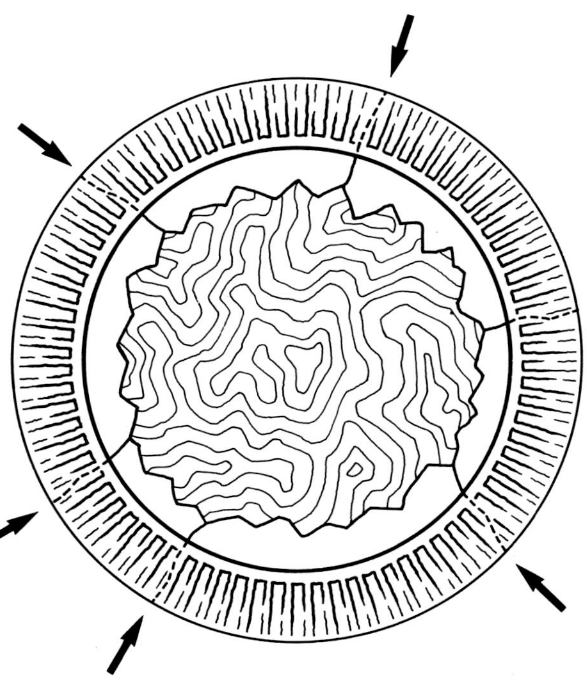

11.4 Tears (arrows) of the anterior capsule produce difficulty in the safe and exact capsular fixation of the lens.

Choroidal hemorrhage

The sudden onset of an expulsive choroidal hemorrhage is well known as one of the most dreaded complications of intraocular surgery. It occurs more frequently with the intracapsular technique and is extremely rare in the extracapsular one.

High risk factors include arteriosclerosis, hypertension, diabetes mellitus, glaucoma, high myopia and choroidal sclerosis. The intra-operative factors that may contribute include sudden decrease of intra-ocular pressure, increased cephalic venous pressure, vitreous loss and sudden rise in systemic blood pressure.

If the posterior capsule is intact, the surgeon must be aware of this complication if the the anterior chamber becomes flattened and the eye hardened. In the case of a rupture in the posterior capsule after nucleus expression, this complication must be suspected if there is increasing vitreous loss. The most important factors in the successful management of expulsive hemorrhage are early recognition, quick closure of the incision and drainage of the suprachoroidal bleeding through a sclerotomy opening. With the use of coaxial illumination the surgeon can recognize the development of an increasing red–brown 'tumor', growing up from the posterior segment and pushing the vitreous forwards. If the hemorrhage is recognized, the eye should be closed immediately with the help of sutures or even with a finger. The injection of a viscoelastic substance into the eye should be performed simultaneously with the trans-scleral drainage of the choroidal bleeding (**11.5**). An intraocular lens is only recommended as a secondary procedure into the anterior chamber some months later.

11.5

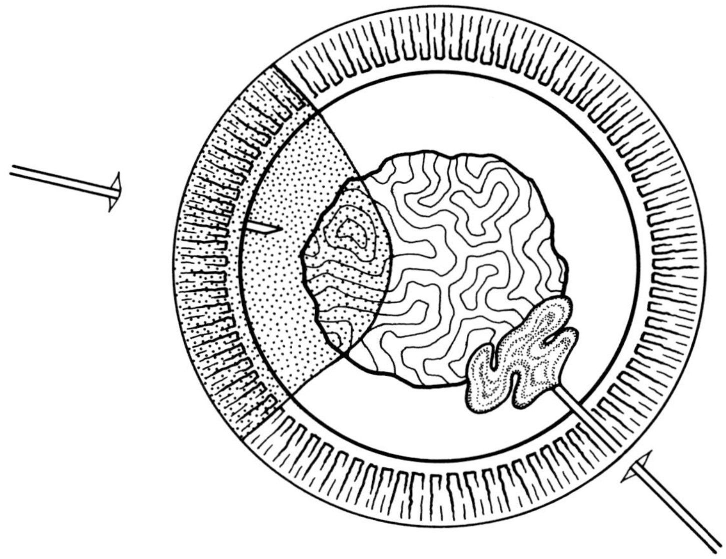

11.5 Expulsive choroidal hemorrhage with intact posterior capsule: trans-scleral drainage of the choroidal bleeding with simultaneous injection of a viscoelastic substance into the eye.

Ruptured zonule

Causes and prevention

The rupture of the lens zonule should be a rare complication, considering the fact that the elasticity of the zonule is nine times higher than that of the lens capsule. An intraoperative rupture can occur in a primary weakness of the lens zonule or its attachments to the ciliary processes, as in the Exfoliation Syndrome. It also can happen from trauma to the zonule during surgery. Depending on the extent of the rupture, an intraocular lens can either be inserted into the capsular bag or placed into the ciliary sulcus or into the anterior chamber angle.

There are several possibilities during surgery for a rupture of the zonule. First, it can happen during the anterior capsulotomy if a blunt cystitome is used or if there is a hard and rigid anterior capsule requiring a considerable force for tearing. An excessive movement during the anterior capsulotomy should alert the surgeon to the possibility of a weakened zonular apparatus. Second, if the anterior capsulotomy is too small in comparison with the size of the nucleus a ruptured zonule can happen during delivery of the nucleus. A careful capsulorhexis with sharp instruments as well as an anterior capsulotomy large enough for the delivery of the nucleus are therefore recommended. Third, a ruptured zonule can happen during intra-ocular lens placement if the loops of the lens are too stiff or if the surgeon is too rough. Too much downward displacement of the lens during insertion of the upper loop may drive the lower loop through the capsule or zonule. The upper loop should not be allowed to snap into the posterior chamber, but should be placed gently. The use of a viscoelastic substance is recommended to expand the capsular bag and thus prevent the lower haptic becoming entangled with the folded posterior capsule.

Management

A zonular dialysis during extracapsular surgery can be recognized with the help of coaxial illumination. The posterior capsule will show corrugation marks at right angles to the ruptured area. For a zonular dialysis of less than one quadrant, a capsular fixation of the intraocular lens is still possible without the risk of a postoperative sunrise syndrome. If the surgeon recognizes a zonular dialysis of one quadrant (**11.6**), a posterior chamber lens should be placed into the ciliary sulcus at right angles to the rupture. An anterior chamber lens may be preferred if the zonular dialysis is between one and two quadrants. If the posterior capsule has zonular dialysis for more than two quadrants (**11.7**), the whole capsule and cortex should be removed, followed by miosis and an anterior chamber lens implantation.

11.6

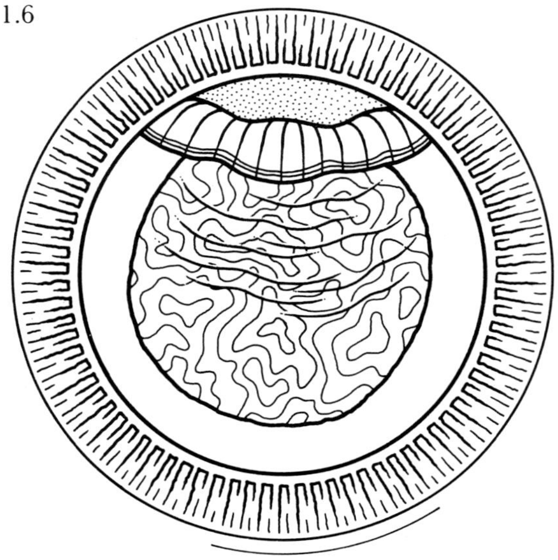

11.6 Zonular dialysis of one quadrant, sulcus fixation preferable.

11.7

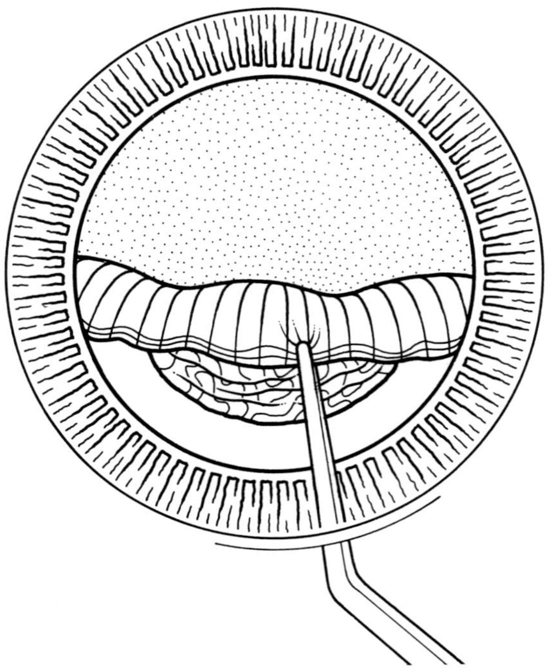

11.7 Zonular dialysis of more than two quadrants merits total removal of the capsule with forceps and anterior chamber implantation.

Ruptured posterior capsule

Causes and prevention

The rupture of the posterior capsule in extracapsular cataract extraction can be a serious complication that forces the abandonment of implantation. It can occur during delivery of the nucleus if the anterior capsulotomy is too small and the nucleus is pressed backwards. This can be avoided by hydrodissection of the nucleus, lifting it out of the capsule with the help of a blunt iris hook, simultaneously with a slight pressure on the scleral wound edge.

During irrigation/aspiration or polishing of the capsule there is a greater risk of rupture. The irrigation pressure should be adapted to surgical conditions. Cleaning and polishing of the posterior capsule should be performed carefully and gently. If there are dense axial plaques on the posterior capsule, which cannot be removed without the risk of a ruptured capsule, the lens should be inserted into the capsular bag, followed by a primary posterior capsulotomy or a postoperative neodymium YAG capsulotomy.

A rupture of the posterior capsule can also happen during the placement of the lower haptics into the capsular bag, if the loop becomes entangled with the posterior capsule and is pushed downwards. This should be prevented by the use of a viscoelastic substance to expand the capsular bag. When the lower haptics and the optics have been placed, the insertion of the upper haptics should be performed slowly, avoiding sudden movement. Direct trauma to the posterior capsule can also be caused by the phaco-instrument or, in very rare cases, after the onset of an expulsive hemorrhage.

Management

In the case of a small ruptured zone of the posterior capsule with an intact vitreous face, the IOL can be placed into the capsular bag after injection of a viscoelastic substance to push the posterior capsule and the vitreous backwards (**11.8**). If a bead of vitreous passes the capsular defect, it can either be pushed backwards by a viscoelastic substance or it can be removed by vitrectomy, still allowing capsular fixation. If the defect is in the pupillary zone, it will be tamponaded by the lens optic, and if in the peripheral zone, by the iris. Larger ruptures of capsule will require sulcus fixation (**11.9**). If after a large rupture there remains sufficient capsule to support a lens, sulcus fixation should be possible, but if not, and the vitreous remains intact, the removal of the whole capsule and cortex may be preferred, followed by an anterior chamber lens implantation. If the rupture is combined with vitreous loss (**11.10**), an extensive vitrectomy is necessary. This should be done in a closed eye by preplacing and tieing sutures, especially if increasing vitreous loss indicates a choroidal hemorrhage.

After the vitrectomy has been performed, it is sometimes difficult to remove the residual cortex lying behind the iris, particularly if the pupil constricts. If much remains, a postoperative phacoanaphylactic reaction is possible. If the removal cannot be performed safely, it is best to remove the whole lens capsule, including the residual cortex, followed by an anterior chamber lens implantation. With the intercapsular technique, however, there is sufficient lens capsule for sulcus fixation of the intraocular lens. If the rupture of the posterior capsule combined with a vitreous loss occurs during lens implantation, it may be possible to continue the insertion and then to perform vitrectomy, often resulting in a successful capsular placement and a round pupil. If this is not achievable, removal of the lens and anterior vitrectomy is indicated, followed by sulcus fixation if sufficient supporting capsule remains or an anterior chamber fixation if there is no support. In cases where the eye has been severely traumatized by surgery it is preferable to abandon the implantation and to consider a secondary implantation some months later.

11.8

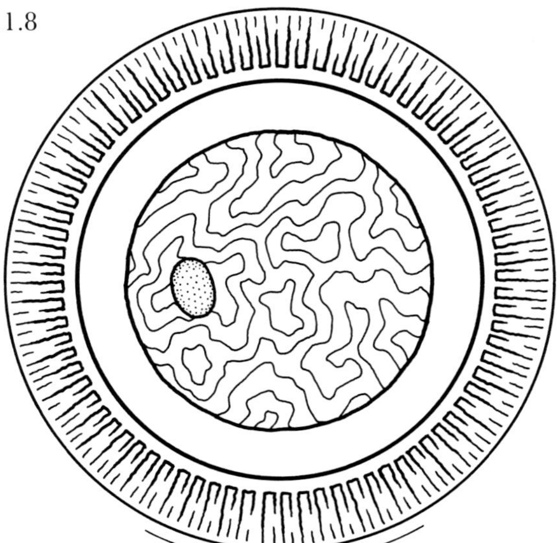

11.8 Small rupture of the posterior capsule with intact vitreous face: capsular fixation is possible.

11.9

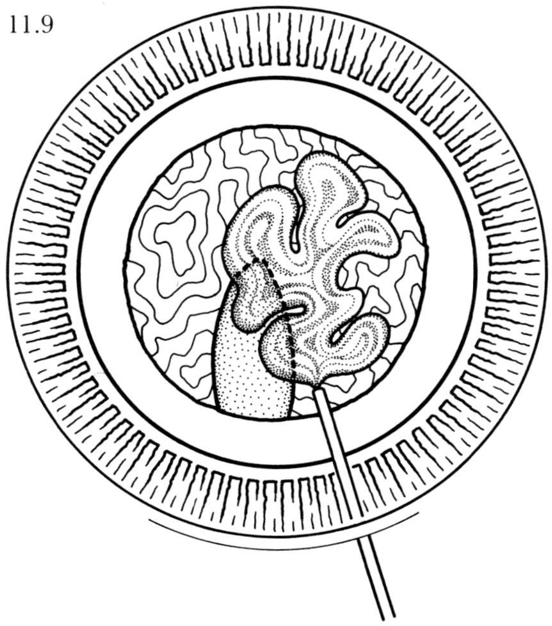

11.9 A moderate capsular rupture without vitreous loss: the opening is sealed with viscoelastic substance injected through a 27-gauge cannula, prior to sulcus fixation of the implant.

11.10

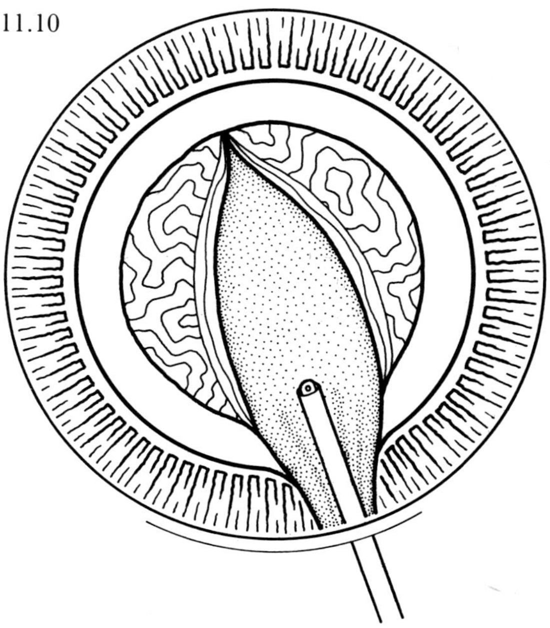

11.10 For a large capsular rupture with vitreous loss, after vitrectomy a sulcus or anterior chamber fixated lens may be implanted or the implantation abandoned.

Further reading

Awan K.J. Intraocular lens implantation following expulsive choroidal haemorrhage. *Am. J. Ophthalmol.*, **106,** 261–263, 1988.

Drews R.C. Management of complications during posterior chamber lens implantation, *Implants in Ophthalmology*, **2,** 175–176, 1988.

Hagan H.C. III. Repair of Descemet's membrane detachment by anterior chamber paracentesis and air injection performed at the slit lamp. *Implants in Ophthalmology*, **2,** 208–210, 1988.

Skuta G.L., Parrish R.K. II, Hodapp, E., Forster R.K., and Rockwood E.J., Zonular dialysis during extracapsular cataract extraction in pseudoexfoliation syndrome. *Arch. Ophthalmol.*, **105,** 632–634, 1987.

Section 2:
LENS IMPLANTATION AND POSTOPERATIVE CARE

12: Anterior chamber lenses

Michael Absolon

Design requirements

For an anterior chamber lens (ACL) to be safe and effective, there should be minimal contact with the drainage angle, stability within the anterior chamber with no micromovement in the angle, no iris chafing and no endothelial touch. To achieve this the lens should incorporate the Choyce principle of four-point fixation with thin footplates. The lens should be one piece and either rigid (**12.1, 12.2**) or have open semiflexible loops using the Kelman principle (**12.3**). There should be a perfect finish to the edges and adequate anterior vaulting.

Other more flexible or closed loop ACLs are not considered suitable because they do not adhere to all the above requirements (see Chapter 37).

12.1

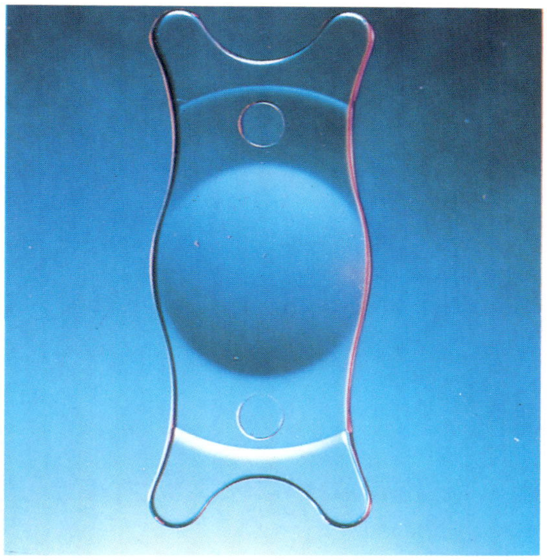

12.1 Choyce Mk IX ACL (Rayner, 496).

12.2

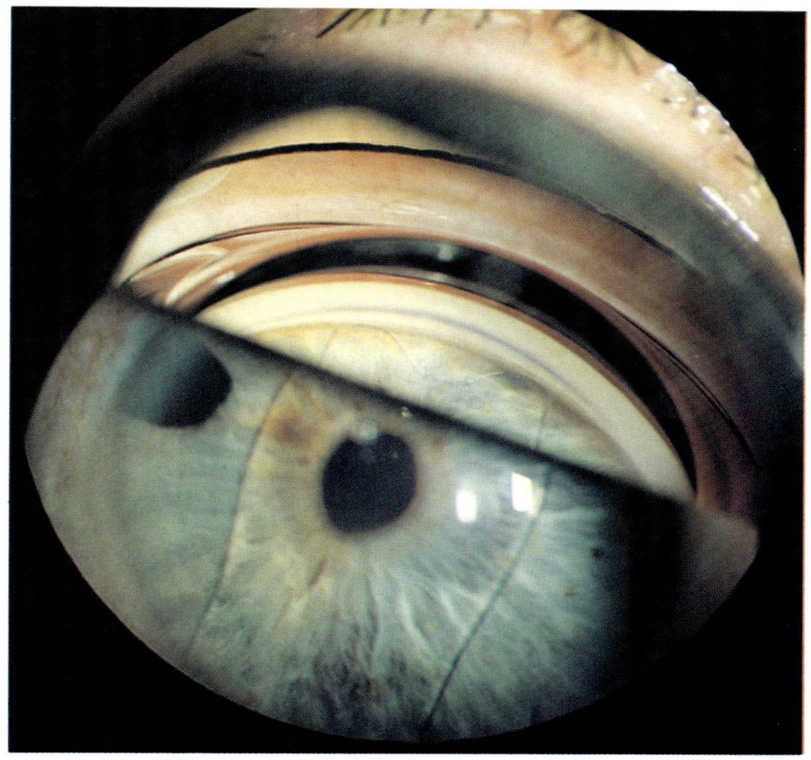

12.2 Gonioscopic view of Mk IX feet 5 years after surgery.

12.3

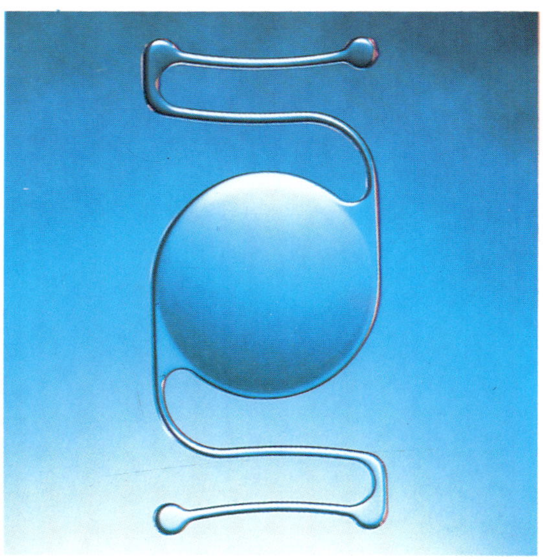

12.3 Open loop semiflexible lens (Rayner, 870).

Technique for primary insertion of Choyce Mk IX ACL

The horizontal 'white-to-white' corneal diameter is measured before the incision is made, using calipers checked against a ruler (**12.4**). The implant should be 1 mm longer than this measurement. If in doubt, it is safer to use an implant that is 0.5 mm shorter than to force in a rigid implant that is too long.

Following intracapsular or extracapsular cataract extraction, miosis is induced by the injection of acetylcholine into the anterior chamber (**12.5**). A gap of at least 6 mm is left in the suture line in the 12 o'clock position (**12.6**). A more lateral position is preferred by some surgeons, particularly for deep-set eyes, in order to achieve a flat approach to the plane of the iris. Two or three peripheral iridectomies are advisable. A small bubble of air is introduced (**12.7**), and then a viscoelastic substance (sodium hyaluronate is preferred) is injected into the anterior chamber, first above and then over the pupil (**12.8**) and finally into the inferior angle (**12.9**). The iris diaphragm should not be made too concave, since this encourages iris tuck.

12.4

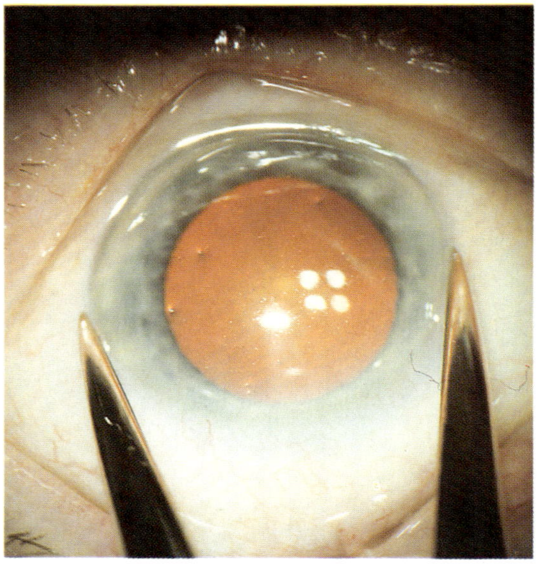

12.4 Measuring 'white-to-white' corneal diameter using inside edges of caliper.

12.5

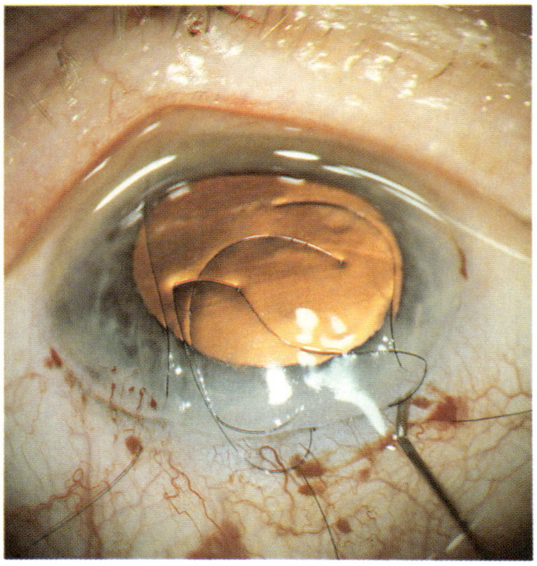

12.5 Injection of acetylcholine.

12.6

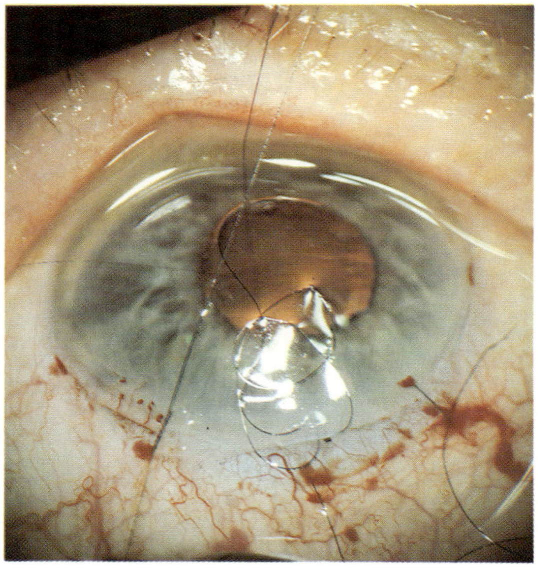

12.6 Gap of 6 mm in suture line.

12.7

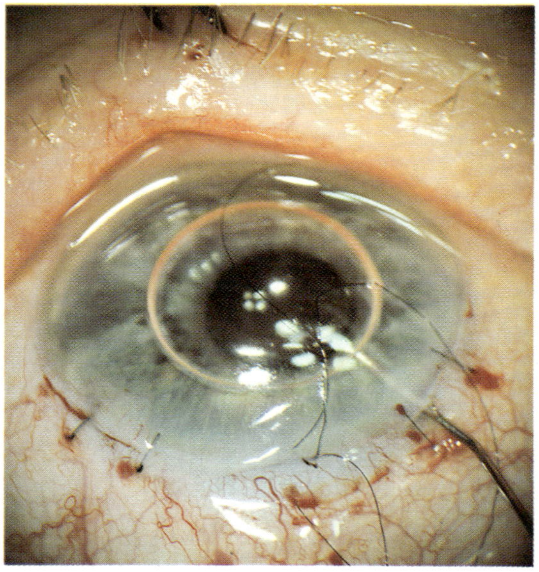

12.7 Injection of air bubble with Rycroft cannula.

12.8

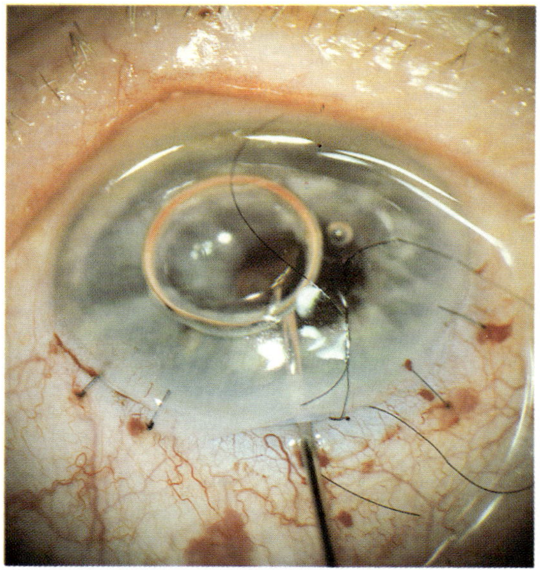

12.8 Injection of viscoelastic over the pupil.

12.9

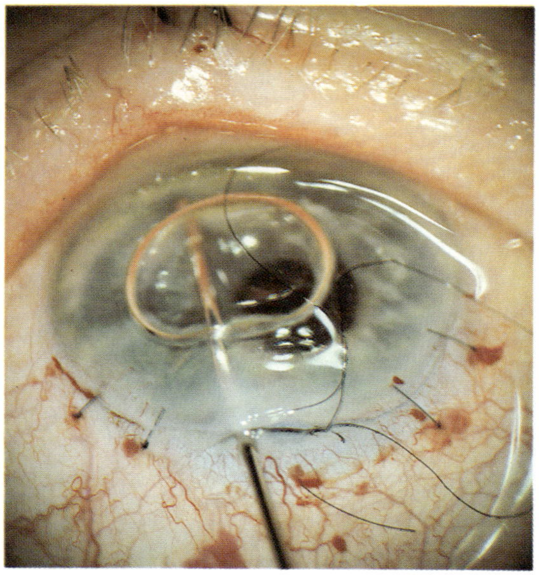

12.9 Injection of viscoelastic into the inferior angle without distending the iris backwards.

The implant is grasped by the two upper feet with suitable forceps, and sodium hyaluronate is applied to the lower feet and optic (**12.10**). The lower feet are then inserted between the lips of the incision with a slight sideways movement, taking care to avoid catching the looped suture (**12.11**). The implant is passed smoothly across the anterior chamber and the lower feet are engaged in the angle. The upper feet are separately inserted beneath the corneoscleral shelf by pulling the scleral incision upwards and applying gentle pressure *posteriorly* (*not* inferiorly) to the footplate (**12.12**).

The middle suture is tied, further sutures are inserted if necessary, the air bubble is removed and the anterior chamber reformed with balanced salt solution. Cyclopentolate 1%, an antibiotic drop, betaxolol 0.5% and an antibiotic and steroid ointment are instilled, and the eye is padded for 24 h.

12.10

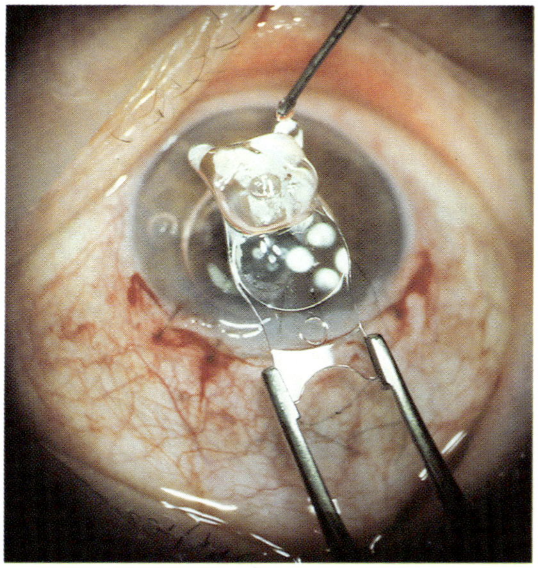

12.10 Sodium hyaluronate applied to the lower feet and optic of Choyce MkIX held by Absolon forceps.

12.11

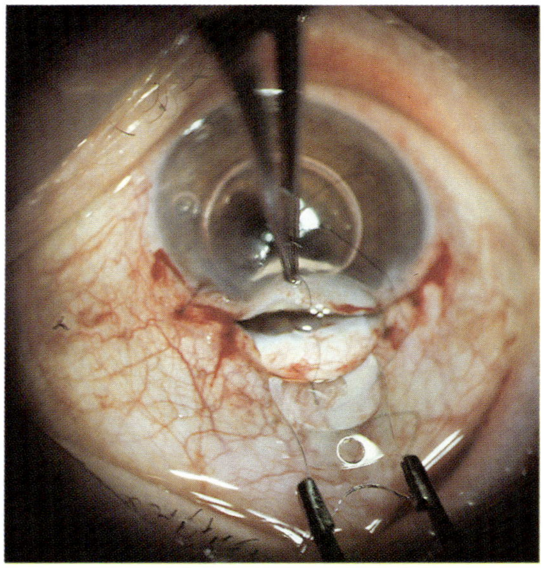

12.11 Insertion of lower feet into incision.

12.12

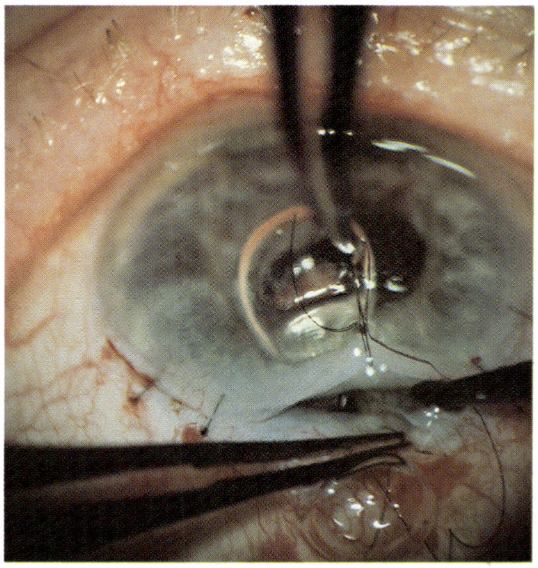

12.12 Insertion of upper foot beneath corneoscleral shelf.

Technique of primary insertion of semiflexible ACL

The horizontal 'white-to-white' corneal diameter is measured before the incision is made, as with the Choyce ACL implantation (**12.4**). For the semiflexible lens, 1.5 mm is added to this measurement, since the lens should be slightly flexed when *in situ* in order to maintain stability. If in doubt, it is safer to use an implant 0.5 mm *longer*.

Following ICCE or ECCE, a gap of at least 6 mm is left in the suture line in the 12 o'clock position. Two peripheral iridectomies are advisable. The injections of acetylcholine (**12.5**), an air bubble (**12.7**) and sodium hyaluronate (**12.8, 12.9**) are carried out, as described for the Choyce Mk IX implantation.

The ACL is held by the inferior haptic with Micra forceps, and Clayman's forceps are placed across the superior haptic (**12.13**) in order to achieve stability during insertion.

Having checked that the implant is being held with the vaulting convex anteriorly, sodium hyaluronate is applied to the lower feet and the optic. The section is minimally opened and the lower feet are inserted between the lips of the incision with a slight sideways

12.13

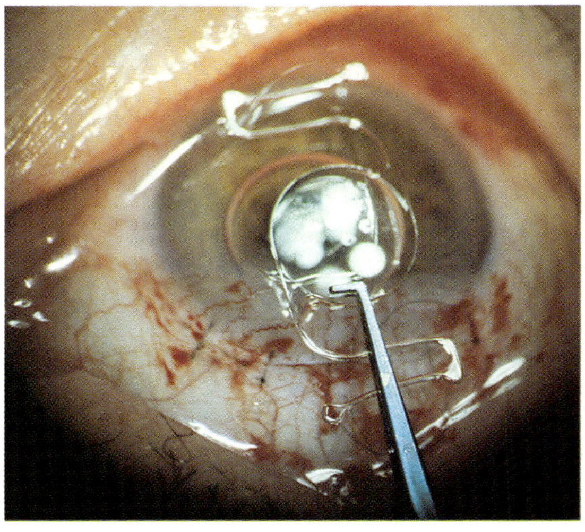

12.13 Method of grasping implant with Clayman's forceps to achieve stability.

movement, taking care to avoid the looped suture. The implant is passed beneath the air bubble (**12.14**) until the Clayman's forceps are just within the lips of the wound, at which point they are removed while steadying the haptic with Micra forceps (**12.15**). The lower feet are now tilted anteriorly by pressing the superior haptic gently posteriorly with Micra forceps, and while maintaining this pressure, the lower feet are placed in the angle by gently nudging the superior haptic (**12.16**). This maneuver avoids tucking the iris with the lower feet. If, despite this, there seems to be a danger of iris tuck, then the implant is withdrawn slightly, sodium hyaluronate is injected beneath each lower foot and the maneuver is repeated.

The upper feet are inserted under the shelf of the incision by grasping the haptic with plain forceps, and flexing the implant while pulling the scleral lip of the incision superiorly with toothed Micra forceps, the incision being opened a little by the assistant (**12.17**). The implant is then allowed to extend gently, and the upper feet pass under the shelf into the angle. The anterior chamber is reformed if necessary, and the pupil inspected to ensure that it is perfectly round. If there is iris tuck below, a Sinskey hook is passed across the anterior chamber to engage the lower haptic. The haptic is flexed to free the iris (**12.18**) and then allowed to extend anteriorly to the iris so that the feet rest against the scleral spur. If the iris is tucked above, a similar maneuver is carried out using a Sinskey hook or plain Micra forceps, the iris moving inferiorly.

The middle suture is tied, and further sutures inserted if necessary. The anterior chamber is reformed with balanced salt solution, pushing the iris diaphragm backwards. Any tendency for the iris to come forwards again around the edge of the optic means that the wound is leaking. It is wise not to aspirate any sodium hyaluronate unless an excessive amount has been used, because this may cause the vitreous face to herniate into the anterior chamber. It is sufficient to remove the air bubble with a Ryecroft cannula (**12.19**).

Cyclopentolate 1%, an antibiotic drop, betaxolol 0.5% and an antibiotic and steroid ointment are instilled, and the eye is padded for 24 h.

12.14

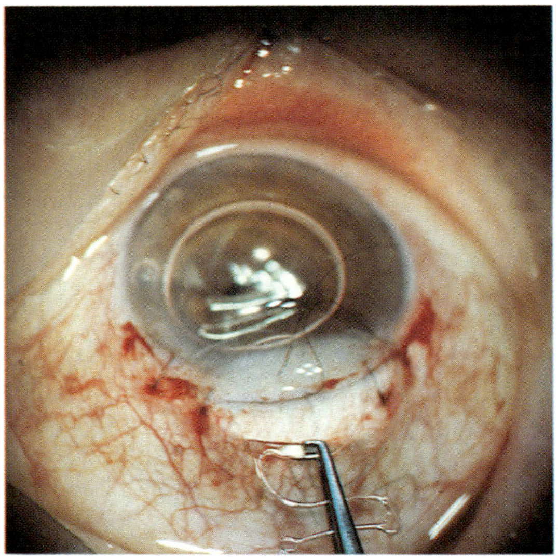

12.14 Implant passed across the anterior chamber.

12.15

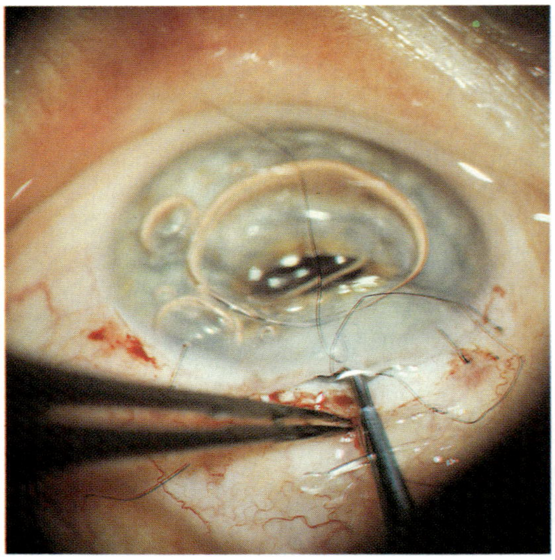

12.15 Clayman's forceps are removed while the lower arm of the upper haptic is held with forceps.

12.16

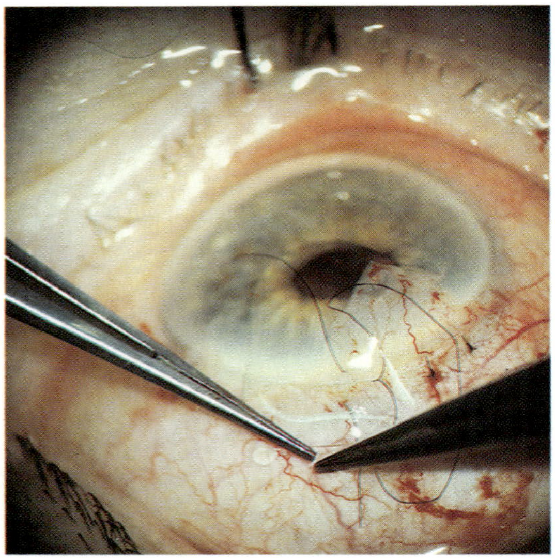

12.16 Placing lower feet in the angle without tucking the iris.

12.17

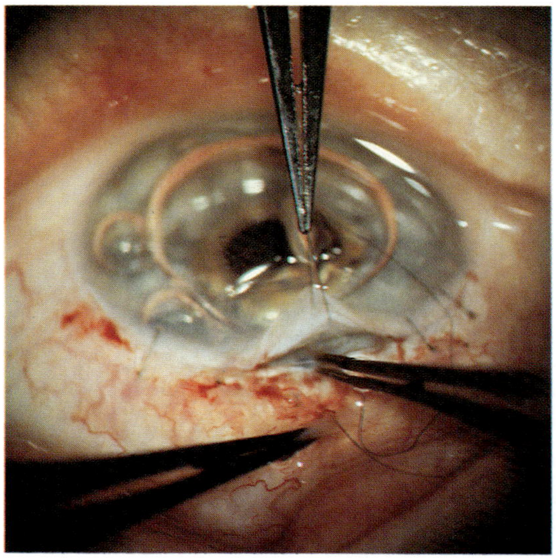

12.17 Insertion of upper feet.

12.18

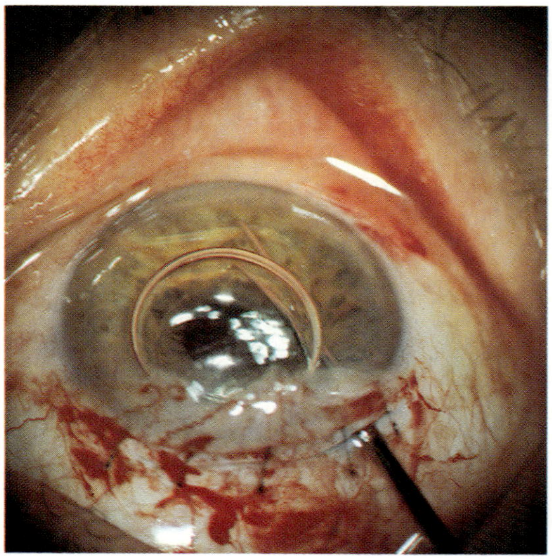

12.18 Correction of iris tuck with a Sinskey hook.

12.19

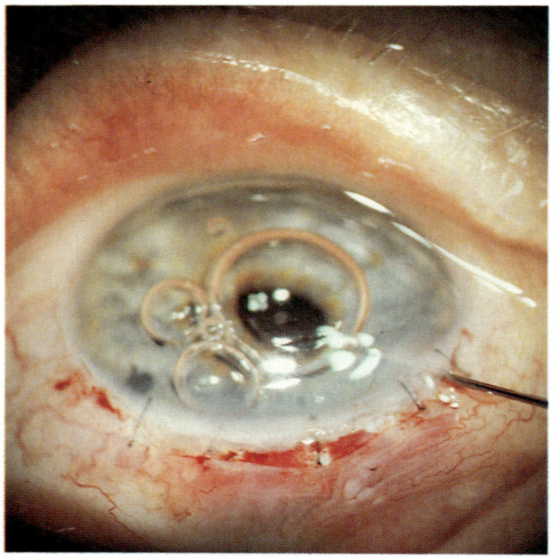

12.19 Aspiration of air bubble.

Postoperative care following ACL implantation

The nonsteroidal anti-inflammatory drug, such as diclofenac, that was used preoperatively is continued postoperatively for 2 weeks, as is the mydriatic with topical betamethasone and neomycin 4 times daily and guttae betaxolol 0.5% twice daily. Thereafter the topical steroid alone is used, in a tapered dosage for 3 months. Subsequent to this, should an episode of anterior uveitis occur, a short course of topical steroids is given, together with systemic diclofenac if CME appears. For a comprehensive account of the complications that may be associated with these lenses, see Chapter 37.

Further reading

Apple D.J. *et al.*, Anterior Chamber Lens Part I: Complications and pathology and a review of designs. Part II: A Laboratory Study. *J. Cataract Refractive Surgery*, **3,** 157–189, 1987.

Engelstein J.M. *Cataract Surgery, Current Options and Problems*, Grune & Stratton Inc, 1984.

13: Iris-fixated lenses: evolution and application

Jan Worst

The evolution of the various lens types proposed in the course of 40 years shows an interesting line, from which a number of biophysical deductions can be made, helpful in the evaluation of present day lenses. Various proposed systems have become obsolete because of early or late complications, while other systems have remained in constant use, never disappearing completely from the pseudophakic 'scene'. Great differences of opinion on the various modalities of fixation exist.

The original Ridley lens was of rigid design and implanted behind the iris, after extracapsular surgery.

The second generation of lenses was initiated by Ridley and modified by Strampelli and Choyce; the lenses were rigid and supported by the anterior chamber angle. It was thought that the rigidity of the Choyce lens, an apparently negative factor, could be overcome by the introduction of flexible loops. However, instead of being an improvement, loop flexibility proved a negative factor and long-term results with the early lenses were universally bad.

However, an interesting clinical phenomenon can be noted from the early flexible loop lenses placed in the anterior chamber, as many resulted in a partial penetration of the supramid loops into the chamber angle. The supramid loops tended to disintegrate through erosion and were finally transformed into long straight spikes, which lodged in the ciliary body. Such lenses became enveloped by a cocoon of connective tissue, which resulted in great stability with an improvement in long-term tolerance.

At the present time an untold but huge number of corneal dystrophies exist that have resulted from instability of lenses in the anterior chamber. Only lenses associated with no movement in the chamber angle have a chance of long-term survival, unless the angle support is transformed into uveal support where the haptics rest against the ciliary processes with interposition of the iris base. Unfortunately, this interposition in turn may endanger the sectorial vascular supply of the iris, leading to ischemic iridopathy, sectorial iris atrophy, ectropion pupillae, neovascularization, uveitis glaucoma hyphema (UGH) and late corneal dystrophy.

The third generation of lenses, independently introduced by Epstein and Binkhorst, used the pupillary part of the iris diaphragm for anatomical fixation. This system worked, but led to luxation if the pupil dilated unexpectedly. Several antiluxation methods were practiced, but each was associated with further unacceptable morbidity, and pupillary fixated lenses of all descriptions may now be considered obsolete. Complications were minimized by the introduction by Binkhorst of iridocapsular fixation.

A second development was the use of a Medallion lens (**13.1**) fixed to the iris by a perlon suture. Due to biodegradation of the perlon suture, unexpected late luxations occurred and, to overcome this, stainless steel, which is biochemically inert, was introduced. To facilitate the introduction of the steel suture, a triangular part of the lens haptic was removed.

13.1

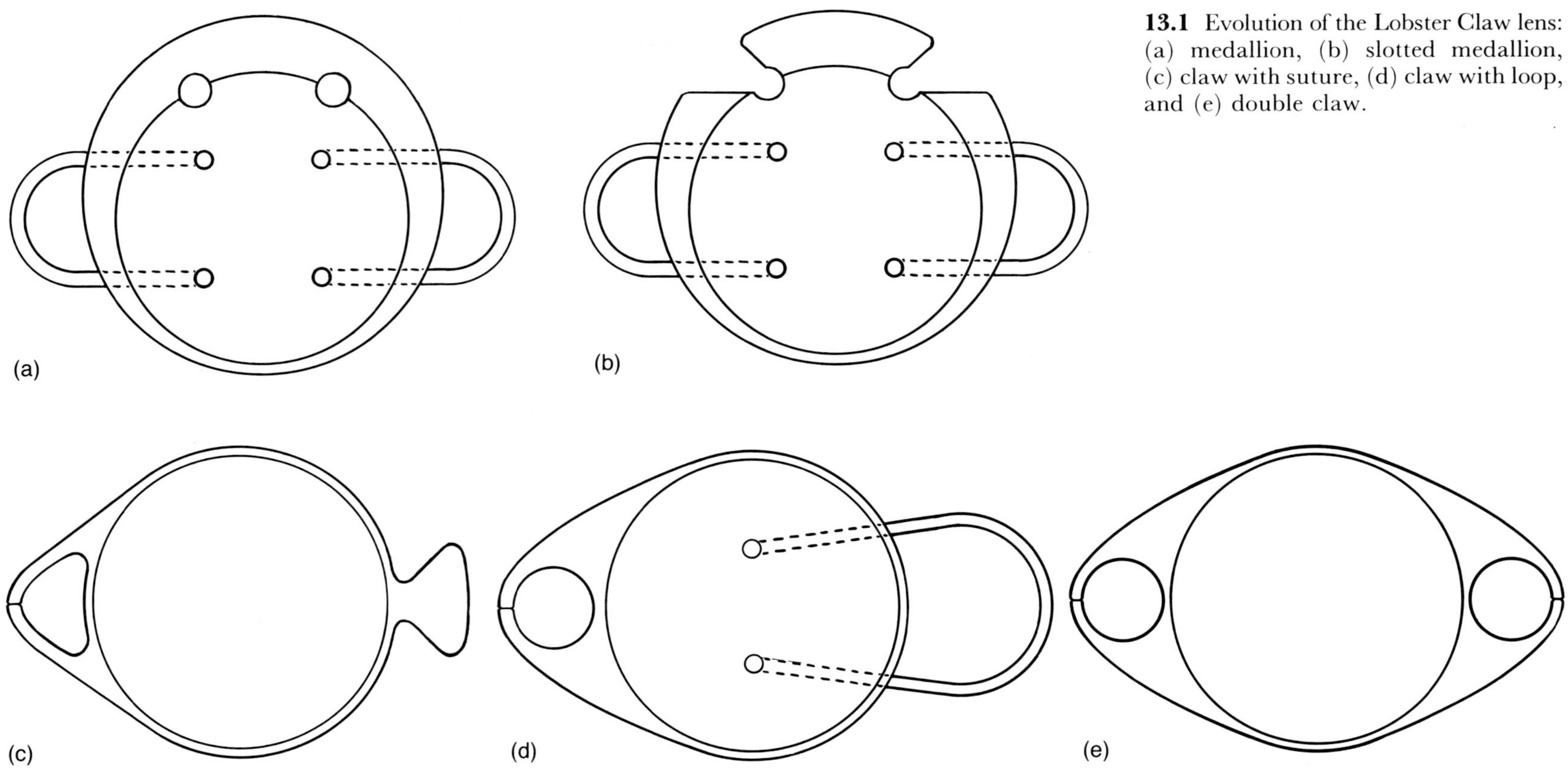

13.1 Evolution of the Lobster Claw lens: (a) medallion, (b) slotted medallion, (c) claw with suture, (d) claw with loop, and (e) double claw.

It was observed sometimes that *iris tissue was accidentally captured in these hand-made slots*. This 'iris pinching' serendipitously *provided an interesting new possibility for stable fixation*. In the lens models that followed, this fixation was used for further stabilization and it was soon realized, with advantage, that both haptic loops and sutures could be abandoned.

All surgical and clinical experiments and experience with peripheral iris stroma fixation finally converged to the design of the Lobster Claw lens (**13.2**), with a fixating mechanism based on the enclavation of a fold of iris tissue, which would remain viable with a normal vascular and nerve supply. The lens was partly developed in Taxila Hospital, Pakistan, for use in developing countries, because it could be manufactured with intermediate technological means. The lens design is simple (one piece, one material, no loops) and can be applied to all types of surgery.

As to manufacturing, some important points should be kept in mind: *the claw mechanism must function optimally*, since iris fixation is totally dependent on it. The claws should have *enough flexibility* to bend without breaking. Since the haptics are fixated to the immobile part of the iris, *full mobility of the pupil* is permitted (**13.3, 13.4**). The lens body makes contact with some areas of iris tissue and, in order to prevent UGH syndrome, a smooth edge finish is of paramount importance.

Over a period of 11 years many Lobster Claws have been implanted and interest is steadily rising. The total number of Lobster Claw lenses in Europe is estimated to be about 8000 and in Asia about 40,000.

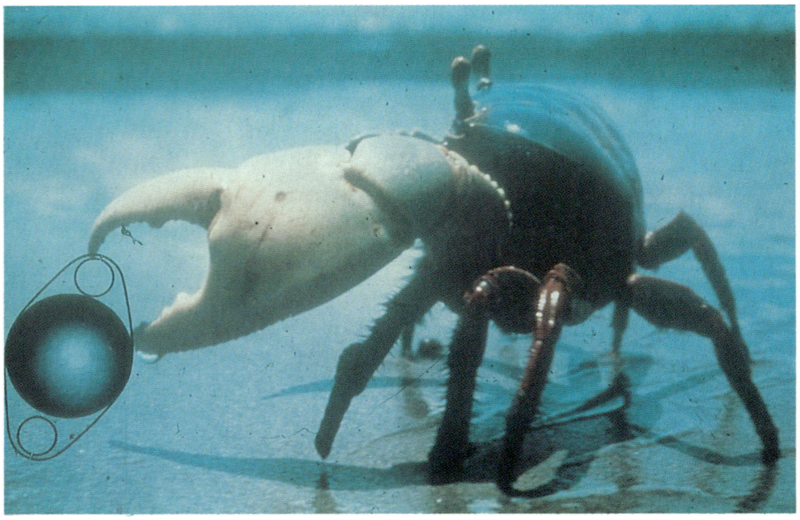

13.2 The lobster and its claw.

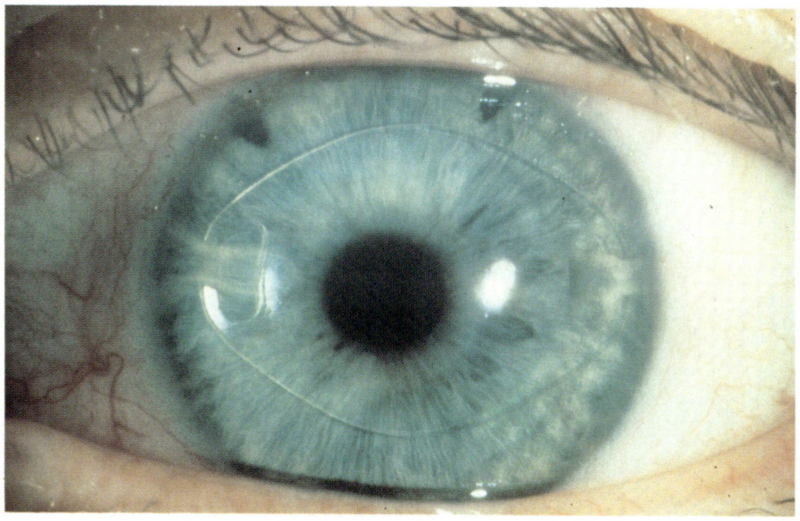

13.3 A horizontally implanted Lobster Claw lens with miosed pupil.

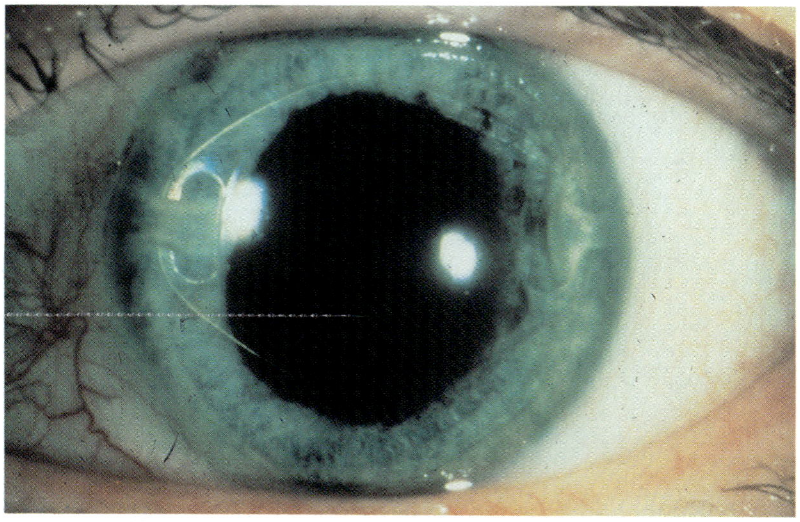

13.4 Same eye as in **13.3** under full mydriasis.

Implantation technique

Special instruments are required for the technique of Lobster Claw implantation:

- The straight or the curved Lobster Claw implantation forceps*.
- Iris enclavation forceps*.
- Iris 'crochet' needles†.

After intra- or extra-capsular cataract extraction, the section is closed with a preplaced 12 o'clock suture. With ECCE the capsulectomy can be made maximally large, as no 'capsular bag' is required. Cortical remnants are washed out. A viscoelastic substance (sodium hyaluronate or methylcellulose) is inserted into the anterior chamber to protect the corneal endothelium.

Another possibility is to keep the anterior chamber filled with balanced salt solution through a cannula, but then an iridectomy must be made before entering the anterior chamber with the Lobster Claw, otherwise pressure in the anterior chamber may increase, causing iris prolapse.

* Manufactured by Moria, France; distributed by Ophtec, Holland.
† Manufactured by Ophtec, Holland.

A third possibility is the 'open sky' method of Pramila Lall (Pakistan). The cornea is lifted and the lens is introduced under direct visual control.

The Lobster Claw is held with the special implantation forceps well over the optical part to guarantee optimal stability of grasp (**13.5**). After entering the anterior chamber, the Lobster Claw is placed horizontally (or in any other orientation if so required).

To determine the correct position of the lens it is helpful to depress it temporarily on the iris surface, 'marking' the enclavation site. After careful centering of the lens, the iris fold below the claw is grasped with enclavation forceps (**13.6**). While firmly grasping the lens optic with the implantation forceps, depress the lens onto the iris enclavation forceps (**13.7**). During this procedure the iris enclavation forceps are not moved. (If this step is not performed correctly, there is a danger of pulling the iris from its base, causing an iridodialysis.) After formation of an iris bridge, the implantation forceps are retracted before the iris bridge is released (**13.8**). The procedure is repeated on the opposite side.

13.5

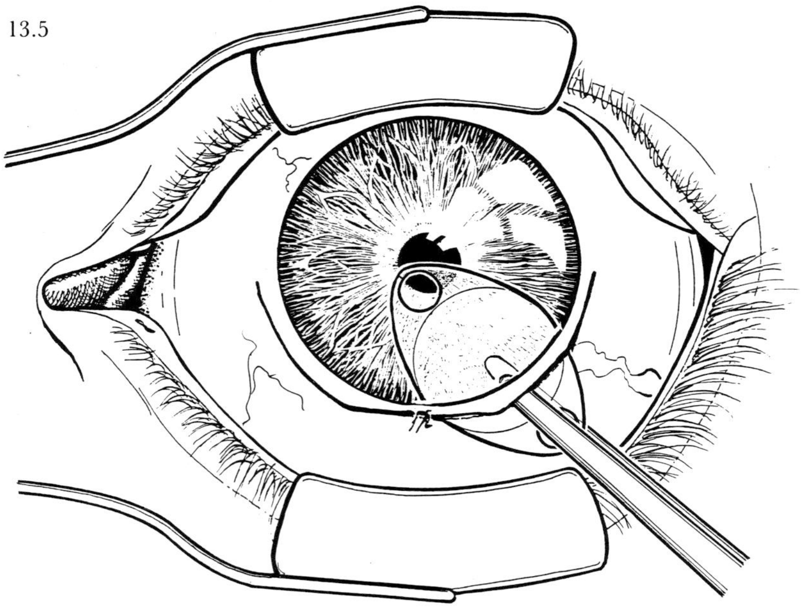

13.5 Insertion of the Lobster Claw lens. Note the special implantation forceps.

13.6

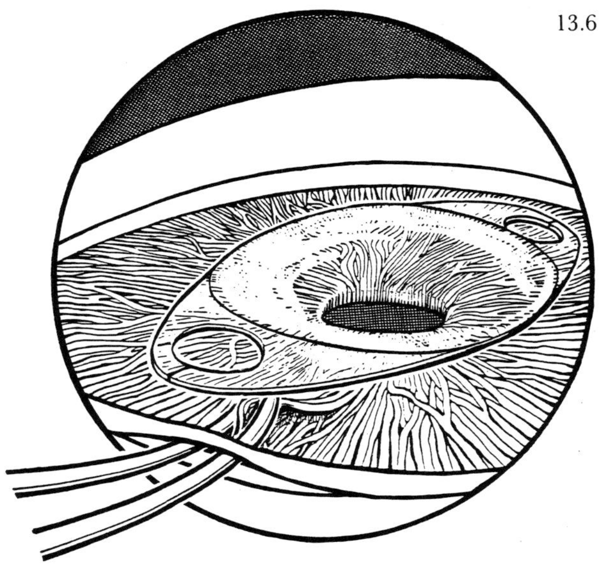

13.6 A fold of iris is grasped in the iris enclavation forceps.

13.7

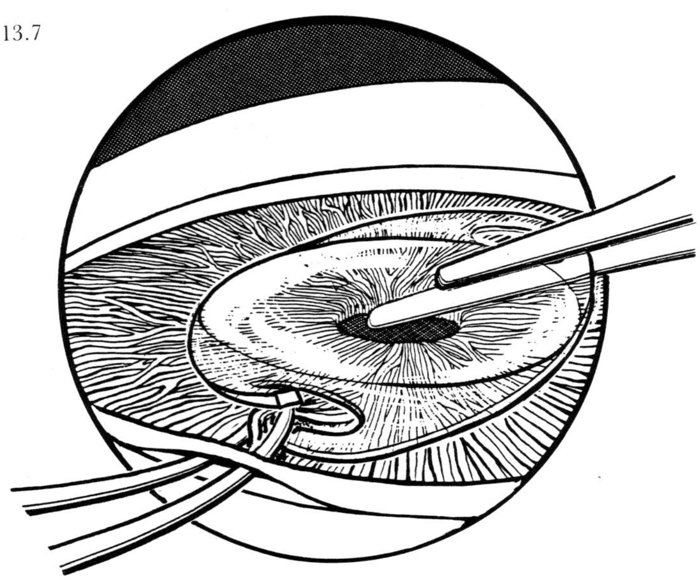

13.7 The lens is *depressed* onto the claw with the implantation forceps, *without moving the iris enclavation forceps.*

13.8

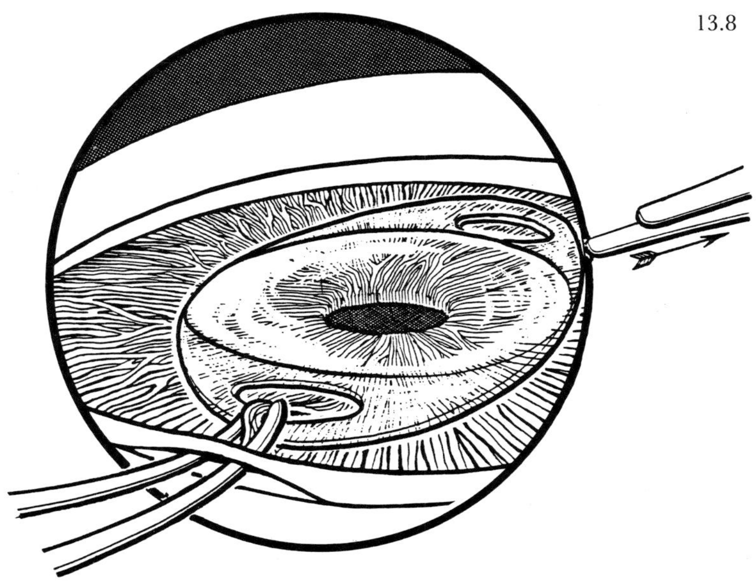

13.8 The implantation forceps are retracted (arrow) before the iris bridge is released.

After this a peripheral iridectomy is made, the wound is partially closed, the viscoelastic substance is replaced by balanced salt solution or air and wound closure is completed.

An alternative procedure for fixation is the iris 'crochet' needle method (Rubingh procedure). A pair of doubly bent 30-gauge needles is used (**13.9**), i.e. separate needles for enclavation of the right and left claw. The needle can be connected to an irrigating system, which partially replaces the use of a viscoelastic substance. The needle can be bent by the surgeon. After formation of an iridoplastic bridge (**13.10**), the hook-like needle should be retracted carefully, avoiding any hooking onto the iris surface (**13.11**).

13.9

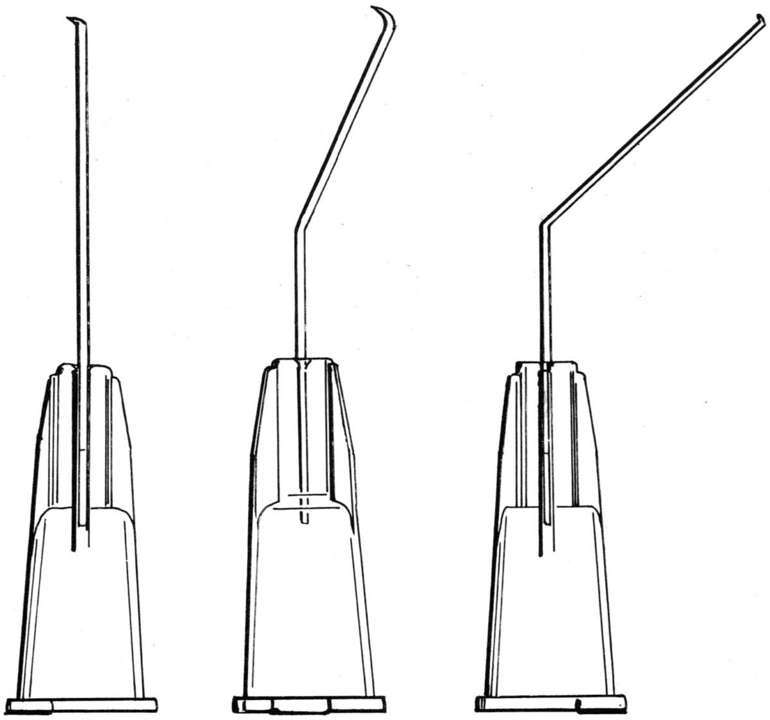

13.9 'Iris crochet' needles.

13.10

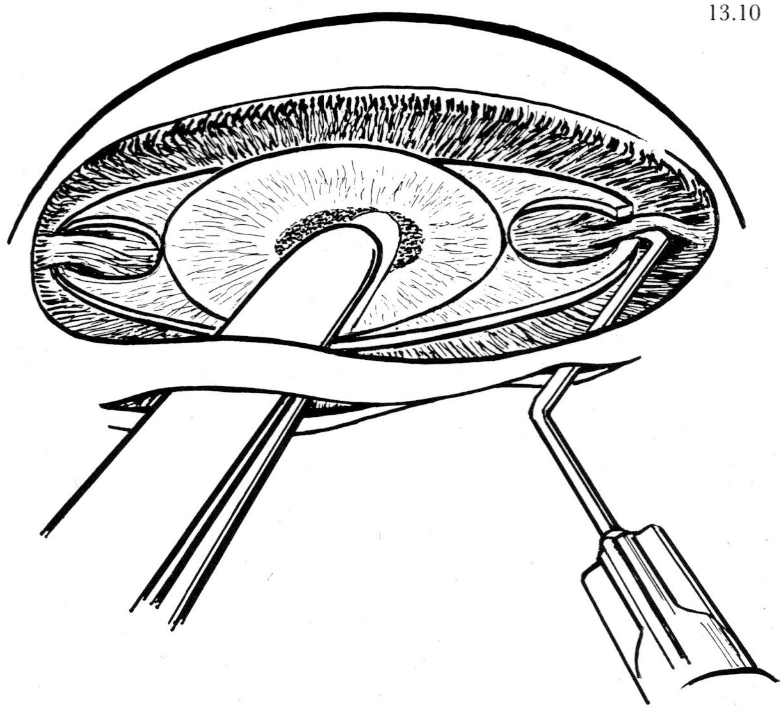

13.10 Enclavation with right 'iris crochet' needle.

13.11

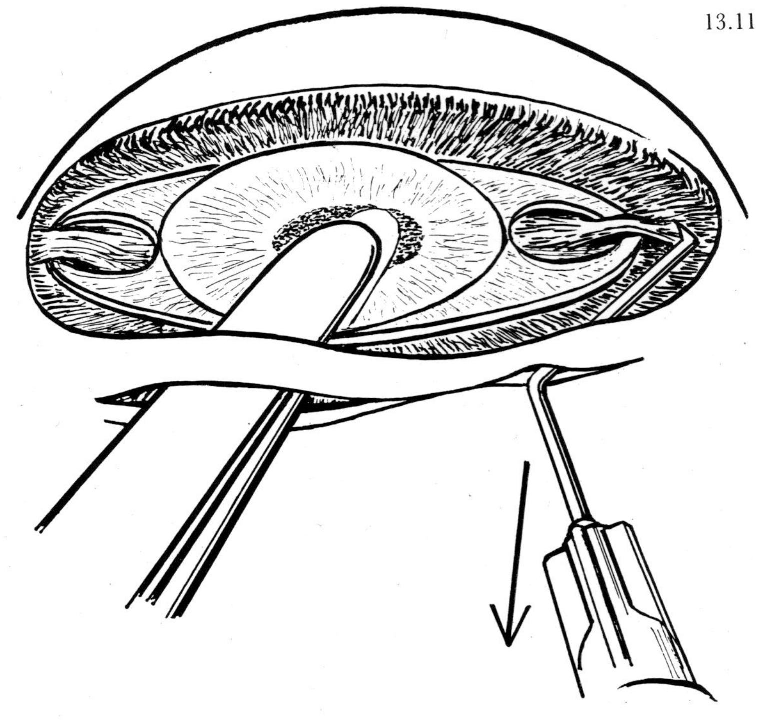

13.11 An iridoplastic bridge is formed. The hook-like needle should be carefully retracted without damaging the iris surface (arrow).

Special indications for the lobster claw lens

Traumatic cataracts with loss of iris stroma

The only requirement for Lobster Claw fixation is the anatomical presence of two diametrically opposite parts of the peripheral iris for fixation (**13.12**). If no diametrically opposite peripheral iris is present, the position of the claws may be modified. Where there is eccentricity of the pupil, a third claw for additional fixation may be added (**13.13**).

After trauma, individualized versions of the Lobster Claw may be made according to the anatomical situation of the remaining iris. As the Lobster Claw avoids chamber angle fixation, capsular bag fixation and sulcus fixation, there is wide application.

Asymmetric fixation: A special type of eccentric placement of the Lobster Claw 'arms' is the Worst–Singh version (**13.14**), in which the eccentricity of the arms facilitates enclavation. A further advantage is the increased flexibility of the lower arm, due to its greater length. Optimal flexibility has been obtained by maximum reduction of the thickness of the arms. A Worst–Singh lens may be implanted after standard cataract surgery, as well as in cases with large iris defects (**13.15**). However, it may be less stable within the eye than the Worst lens (**13.3**).

13.12

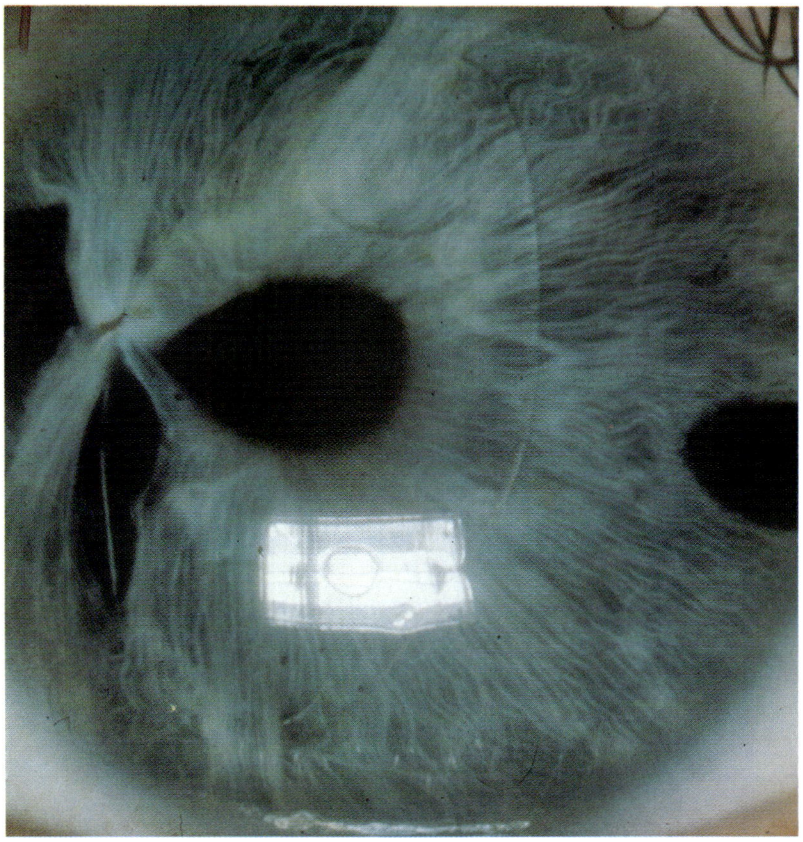

13.12 Lobster Claw placed vertically in an eye with traumatic iris coloboma. Note the iris suture for coloboma repair.

13.13

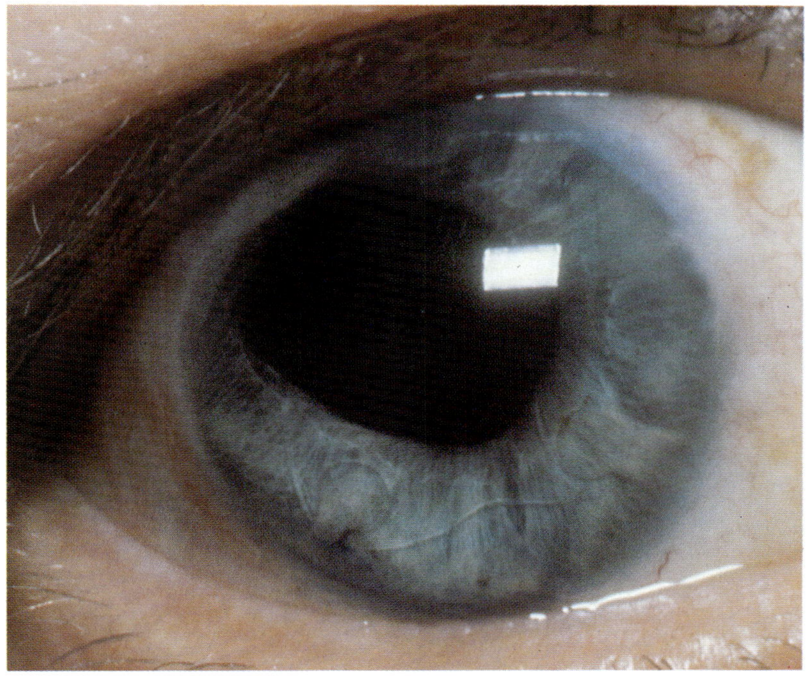

13.13 Worst Tripod Claw lens.

13.14

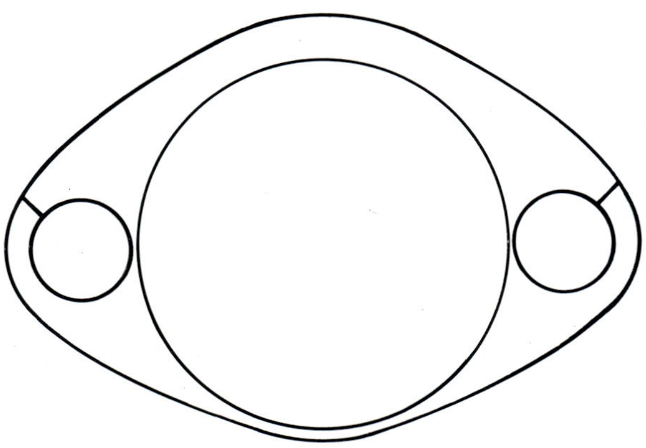

13.14 Worst–Singh Claw lens.

13.15

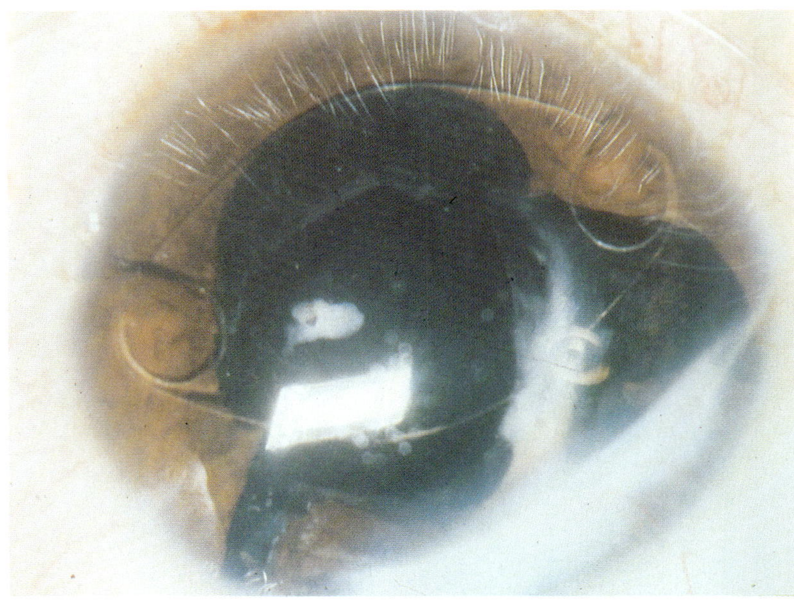

13.15 Worst–Singh Claw lens in a large traumatic iris defect.

Aniridia

A special Lobster Claw lens has been designed for replacing the lost iris in cases of total loss of the lens and iris diaphragm, or in cases of aniridia with cataract (**13.16**). The circular artificial iris carries a 4 mm optic in its center. The fixation is made with a Strampelli suture of 50μ stainless steel (**13.17–13.20**).

13.16

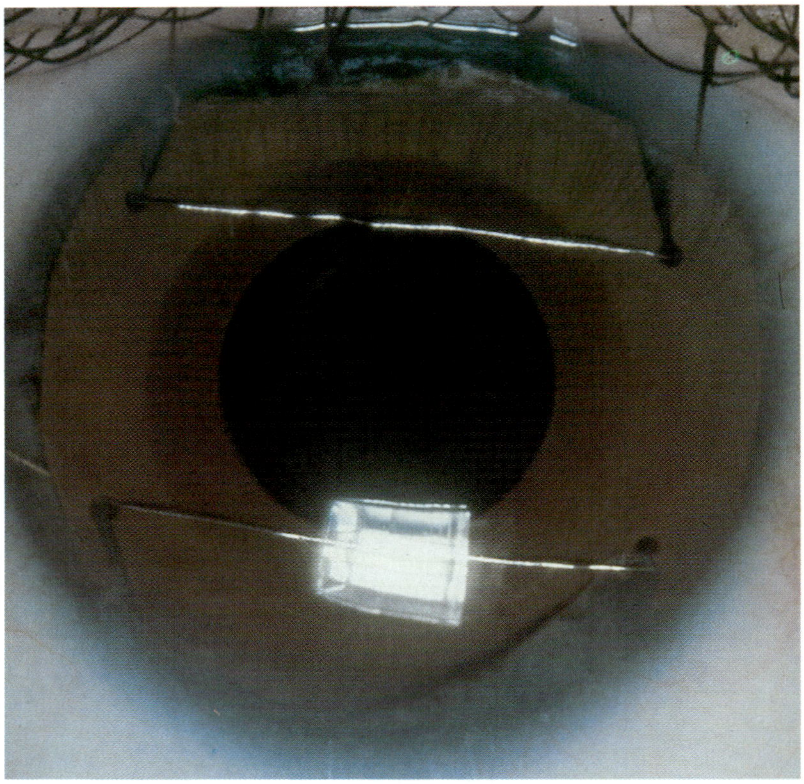

13.16 Artificial iris implantation.

13.17

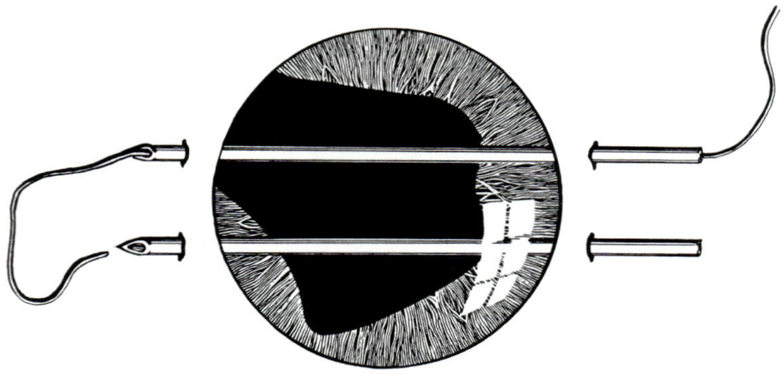

13.17 Two broken-off 24-gauge needles crossing the anterior chamber to guide a 50μ stainless steel suture.

13.18

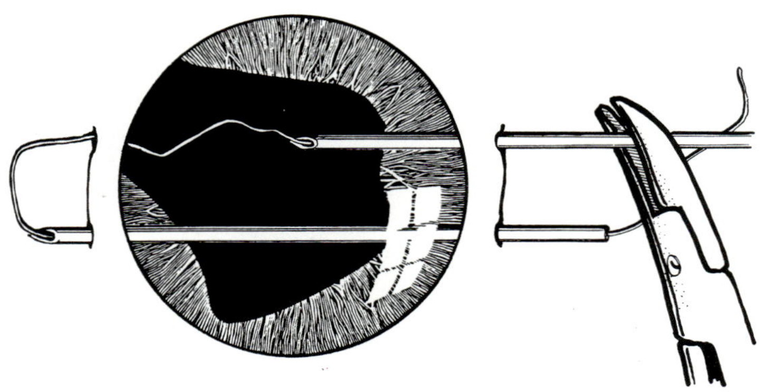

13.18 After passage of the steel suture the needles are retracted one by one.

13.19

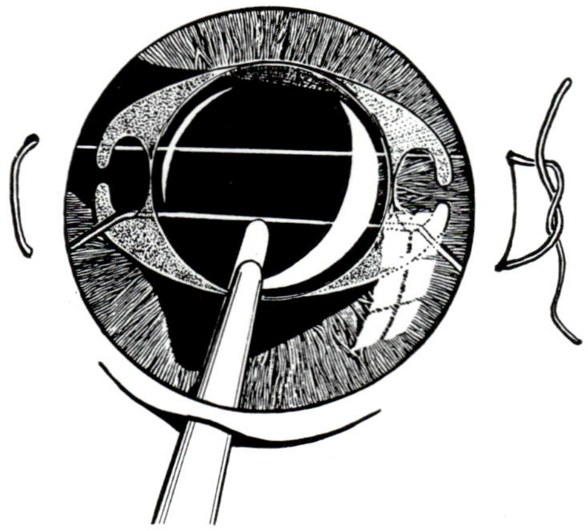

13.19 A specially designed lens with an oblique slot is inserted onto the slack steel sutures (the diagram shows the use of a standard lens).

13.20

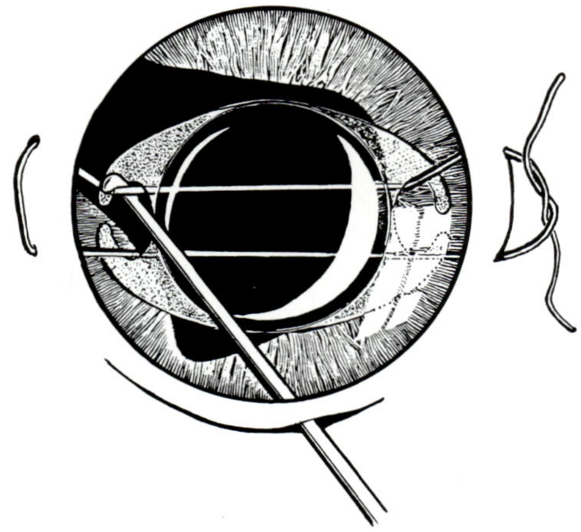

13.20 The slack sutures are brought through the slot between the tips of the claws.

Children

Traumatic cataract and congenital cataract form a specially favourable group for *secondary* lens implantation of the Lobster Claw lens (**13.21**) which is simple, safe and effective. Smaller sized lenses have been designed for microphthalmic eyes. It must be noted, however, that children are prone to cystoid macular edema when the posterior capsule is open. If the capsule is intact and epithelial ingrowth occurs, it is recommended that the capsule be cleaned rather than opened by discission (**13.22**).

In cases of capsule fibrosis, the posterior capsule is separated from the anterior hyaloid in order to preserve the compartmentalized state of the posterior segment. YAG laser treatment in children may lead to cystoid macular edema and even retinal detachment. Surgical posterior capsulotomy, sparing the anterior vitreous membrane, is therefore preferred.

13.21

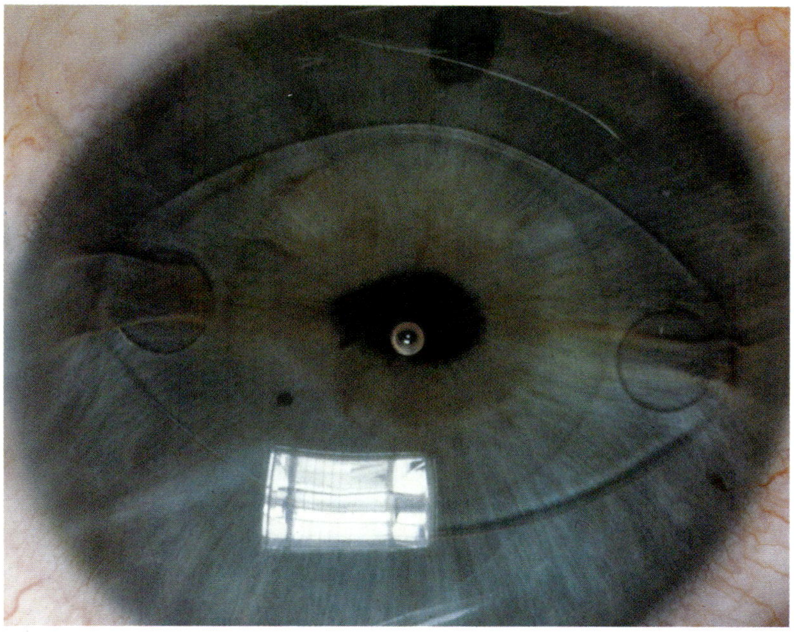

13.21 Lobster Claw lens in a child of 4 years.

13.22

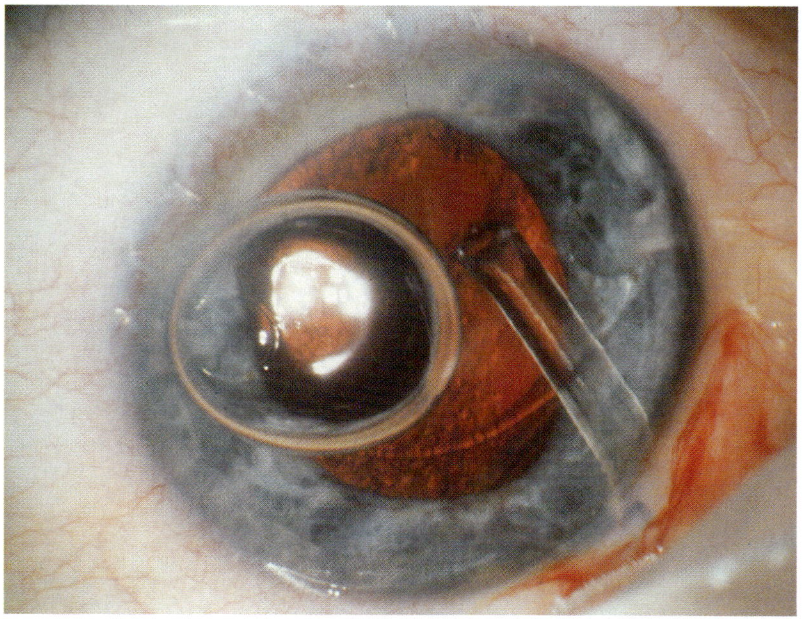

13.22 Cleaning by aspiration of the secondary cataract under sodium hyaluronate using a glass cannula. The Lobster Claw lens leaves enough space for this procedure.

Glaucoma

Owing to the universal applicability of peripheral iris support, indications have been extended to glaucoma eyes with cataract after ICCE or ECCE, including those where sector iridectomies are necessary (**13.23**). In cases of coexisting glaucoma and cataract, a fistulizing procedure can be combined with Lobster Claw implantation, and if the anterior chamber shallows postoperatively, the iris bridges will protect the cornea from contact with the lens.

13.23

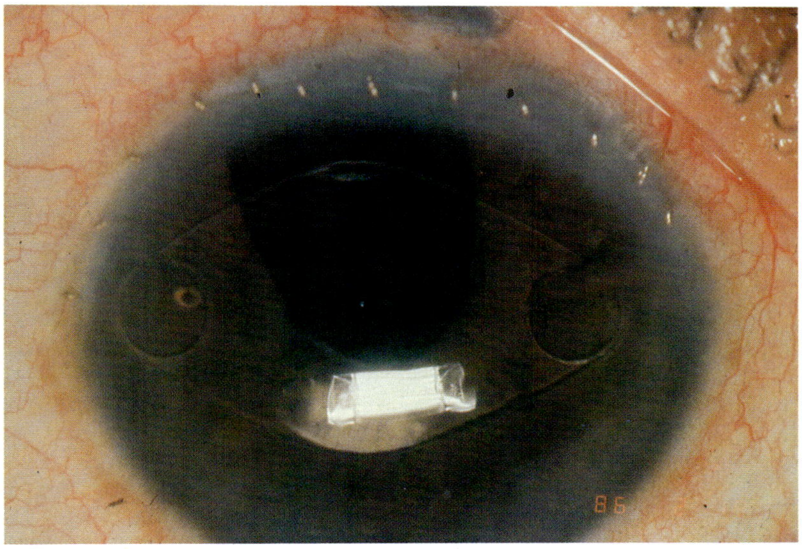

13.23 Worst–Singh lens after glaucoma surgery (wide coloboma).

High myopia

The highly atraumatic and stable fixation on the iris periphery has made it possible to apply negative power Lobster Claw lenses of a vaulted type for phakic myopic eyes (**13.24–13.26**). Fechner and Worst have between them performed 100 cases, but the follow-up period is relatively short (3 years) and this treatment of high myopia is not yet advised as a routine procedure.

13.24

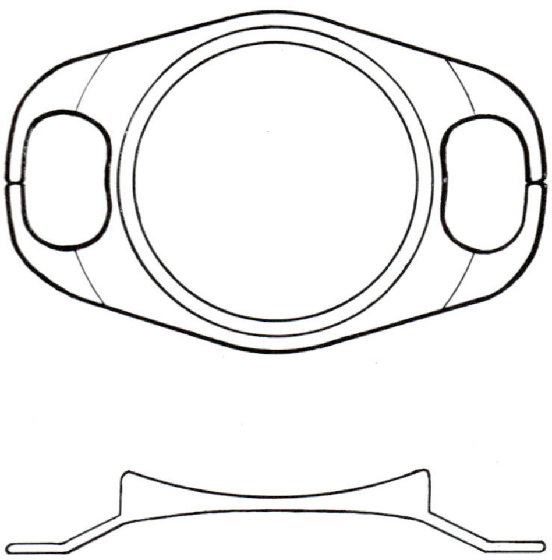

13.24 A vaulted lens for high myopia.

13.25

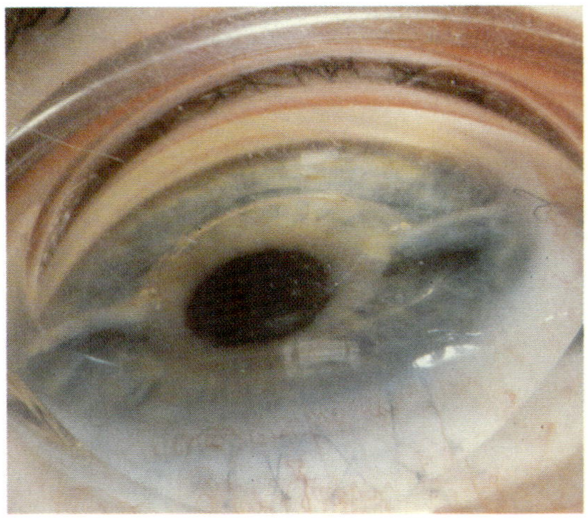

13.25 Vaulted negative power lens showing iris bridges.

13.26

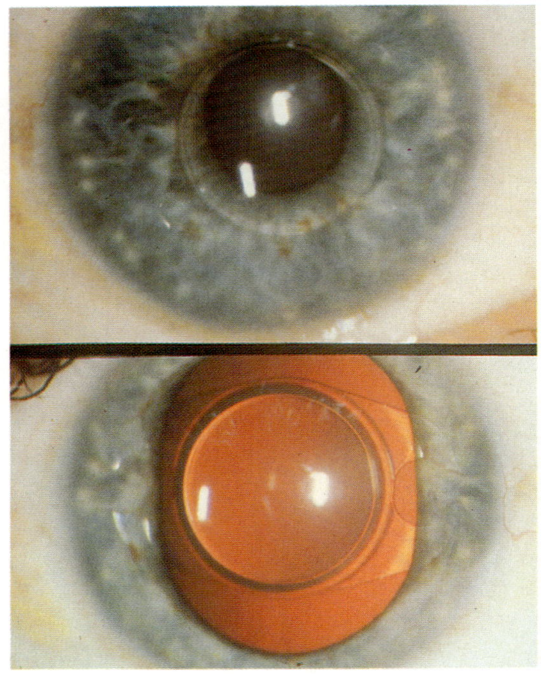

13.26 Vaulted negative power lens showing miosis (top) and mydriasis (bottom).

Albinism

In cases of extreme photophobia, as in the albino patient with cataract, the lens haptic may be tinted (**13.27**).

13.27

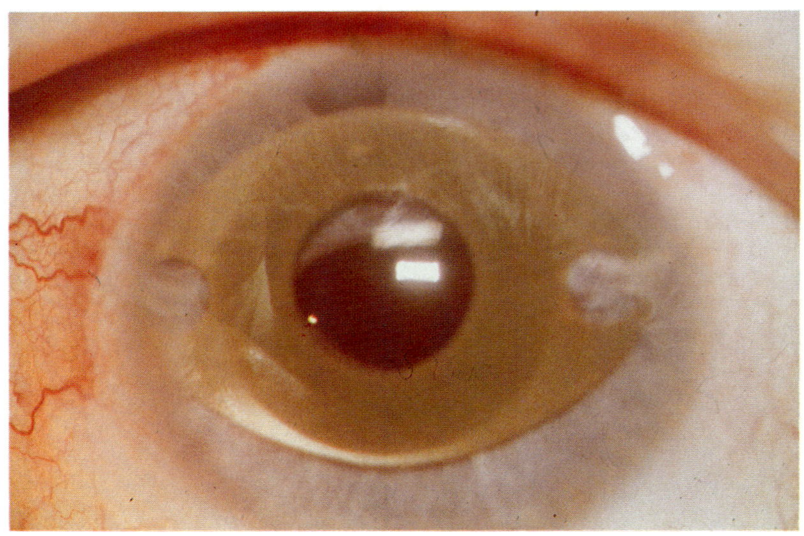

13.27 Colored haptic for treatment of photophobia in an albinotic eye.

Summary of advantages and disadvantages of the Lobster Claw lens

Advantages

- One piece, one plane, loopless construction suitable for modification in special situations.
- Lightweight and physiological as the fixation does not interfere with the mobility of the pupil or the blood supply of the iris (**13.28**).
- There is reduction of iridodonesis in intracapsular cases.
- Fixation is stable with no late decentrations or dislocations.
- The lens may be removed easily and replaced.
- Suitable for coloboma closure by means of the claw mechanism (**13.12**).
- Fixation not dependent on an intact iris, the lens being suitable when much of the iris tissue is missing (**13.15**).
- For maximum surgical visibility and accessibility, a wound of only 6 mm is sufficient.
- Universal application.

Disadvantages

- Lens implantation technique requires surgical skill and learning time.
- A bimanual procedure is necessary.
- High demands are made on manufacturing quality to guarantee claw function, resilience and absence of iris chafing.

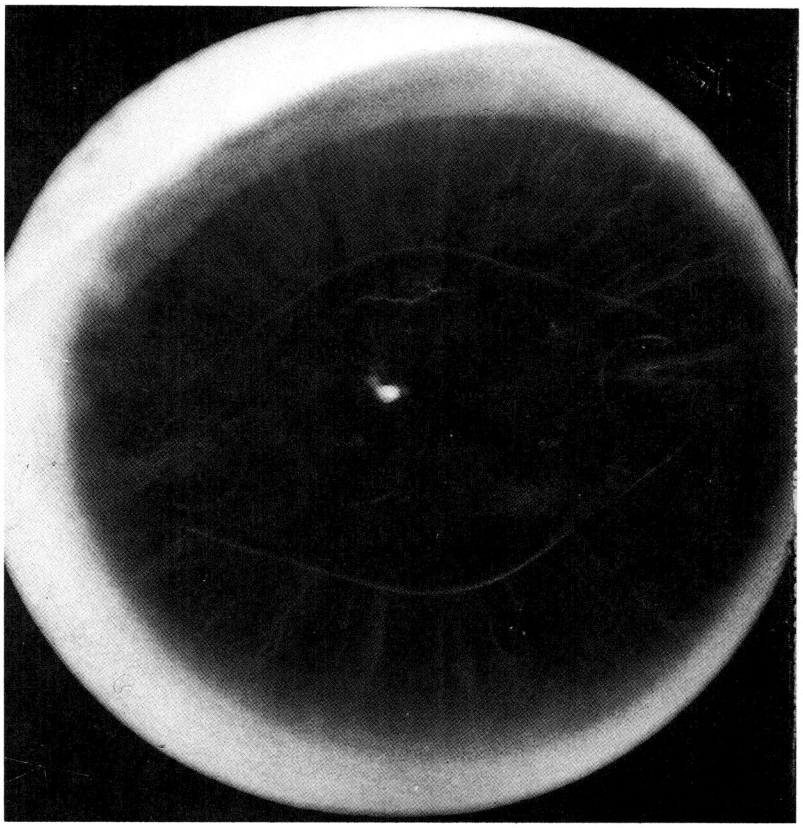

13.28

13.28 Angiography of iris showing no leak of fluorescein.

Further reading

Fechner P.U., van der Heyde G.L., and Worst J.G.F. Intraokulare Linse zur Myopiekorrektion des phaken Auges. *Klin Mbl Augenheilk,* **193,** 29–34, 1988.

Worst J.G.F. Biotoxizitat des Kammerwassers. Eine vereinheitlichende pathologische Theorie, begrundet auf hypothetische biotoxische Kammerwasserfaktoren. *Klin Mbl Augenheilk,* **167,** 376–384, 1975.

Worst J.G.F. The single loop single claw lens. In: *Cataract Surgery and Visual Rehabilitation.* III International Congress Florence, 9–12 May 1984. Kugler Publications, 1985.

14: Ciliary sulcus fixation

William Simcoe

The ciliary sulcus is that area of the posterior chamber bounded anteriorly by the peripheral iris, laterally by uveal tissue in apposition with the inner scleral wall and posteriorly by the most anterior ciliary process. Intraocular lens (IOL) haptics placed in this region ('sulcus fixation') therefore employ uveal fixation. Sutured and unsutured posterior chamber lenses with open-ended loops were first implanted by the author in the capsular bag and also outside the bag in 1975 (**14.1**). However, experience has shown that the uveal fixation of sulcus placement leads to many complications: loops may erode (**14.2**) or become adherent to any of the surrounding structures or zonular fibres (**14.3**) or to the pars plana surface (**14.4**). Sometimes loops erode through the iris and into the anterior chamber (**14.5**). These complications contrast with placement inside the capsular bag ('bag fixation'), which is the natural location of the crystalline lens and where the implant is isolated from contact with any vascular tissue. If a decentered IOL must be removed or at least freed from its eccentric position, the risk of tissue injury is less with capsular fixation than with loops

14.1

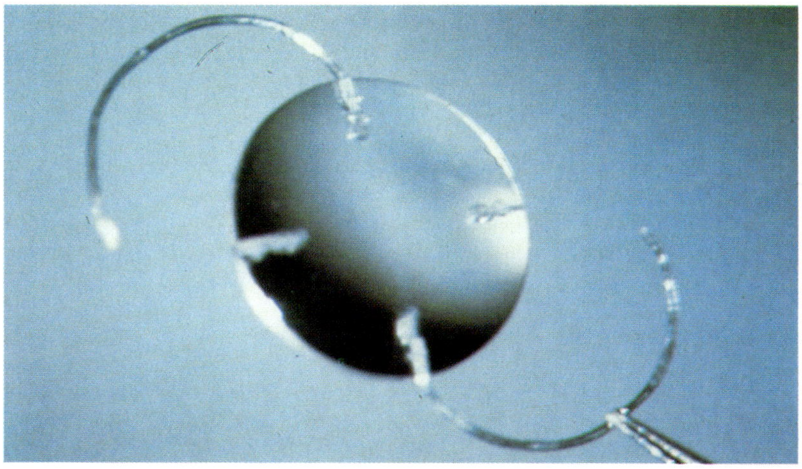

14.1 Prototype open loop compressible posterior chamber lens made from 4-loop Binkhorst iris clip lens.

14.2

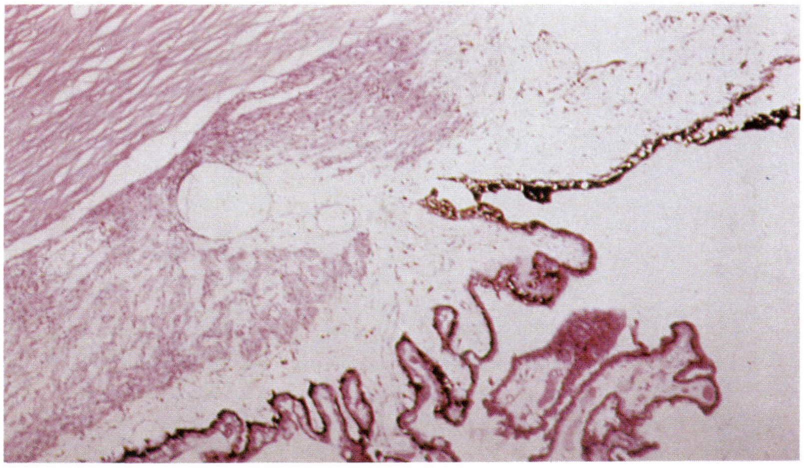

14.2 IOL loop erosion into sulcus uveal tissue (courtesy Prof. David Apple, USA).

14.3

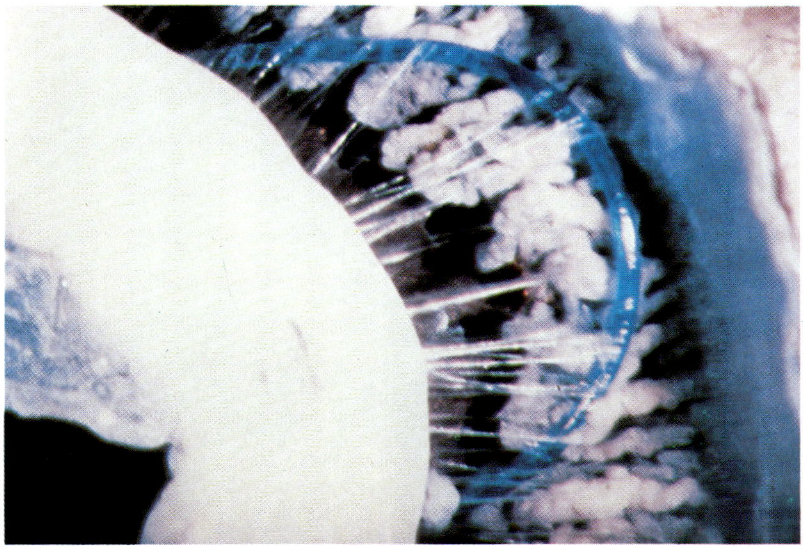

14.3 Adherence to zonular fibers (courtesy Prof. David Apple, USA).

14.4

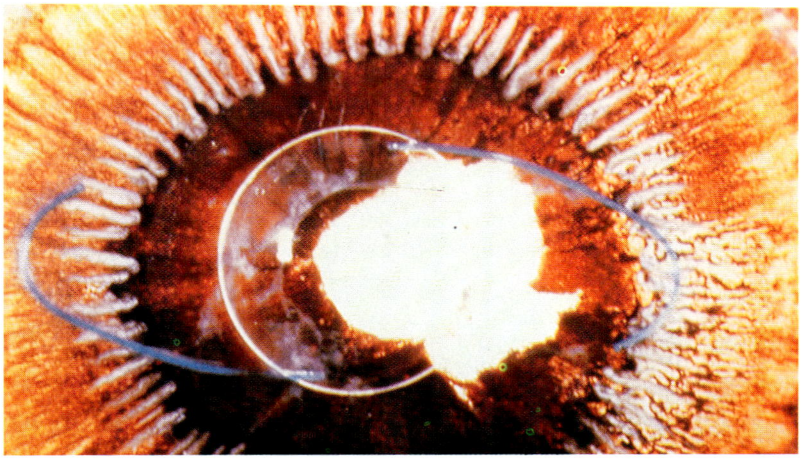

14.4 Decentration with pars plana fixation (courtesy Prof. David Apple, USA).

14.5

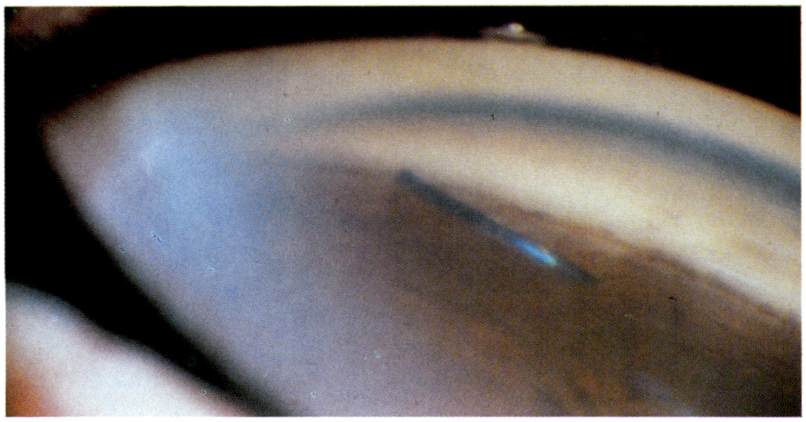

14.5 J-loop erosion through the iris into the anterior chamber (courtesy Dr. John Alpar, USA).

adherent to or buried in uveal tissue. Loops with notches or eyelets at various places or recurved tips to facilitate insertion are not now recommended, as they may compound the difficulty if a malpositioned IOL has to be removed (**14.6**). Only a clean, unencumbered, C-type loop can be safely and atraumatically dialled out of capsular or uveal fixation (the use of two hooks can be helpful).

Other complications of sulcus fixation include pupil capture, iris chafing and late uveitis, glaucoma and hemorrhage. With the present level of skill and experience, surgeons are increasingly confident of placement in the bag, but sometimes it may be difficult to determine that both loops are in, especially with small pupils or high vitreous pressure.

In these circumstances, viscoelastic substances will help to prevent asymmetric placement. One loop may be in the bag and one loop out, resulting in decentration (**14.7**). Both loops may be in the bag and then one may escape postoperatively, also causing decentration. This can be due to the anterior capsule leaf being torn during nucleus removal. Another cause may be that postoperatively the anterior capsule leaf fuses to the posterior capsule progressively from the capsule fornix towards the center and to one side before the other, with a 'zip' effect pushing the IOL laterally until the loop opposite the 'zip' is forced out of the bag. To remedy these situations, an asymmetrical 'differential haptic' posterior chamber lens concept is possible (**14.8, 14.9**). One previous proposal was for one prolene loop to go into the bag with a larger PMMA loop for the sulcus, but this had limited appeal. Designs in the late 1970s included smaller equal-size loops for bag placement as well as larger equal-size loops for sulcus fixation (**14.9**), but it became expedient for companies to market only the larger size as a suitable style for both places. The present lengthy loop spans (overall lens diameters) may contribute to postoperative escape of one loop.

The concern that capsule-fixated lenses might later spontaneously or traumatically subluxate into the vitreous, as is occasionally seen with hypermature cataracts, is largely unfounded. The IOL is much lighter in weight than a cataract and, although this situation is possible, it is not an argument for sulcus fixation. It is now widely accepted that bag fixation is safer than sulcus fixation. However, primary sulcus fixation is preferable to primary implantation into the anterior chamber.

14.6

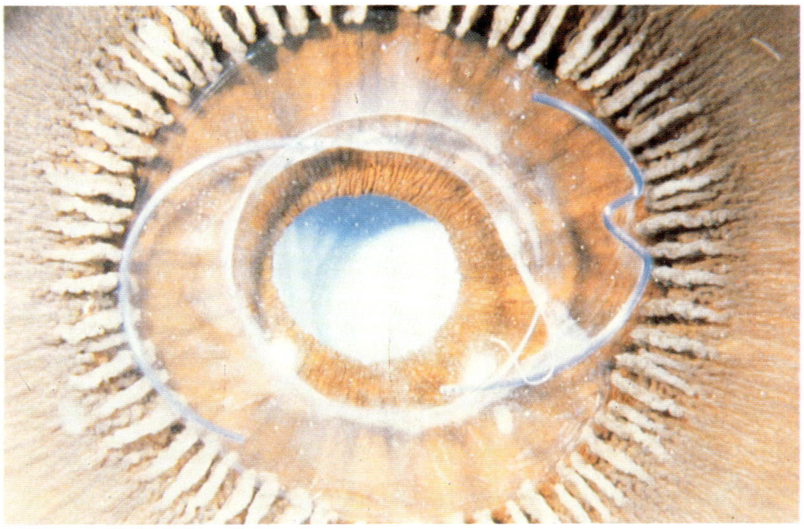

14.6 Embedded loops with notches or circles (not shown) can injure tissue during removal (courtesy Prof. David Apple, USA).

14.7

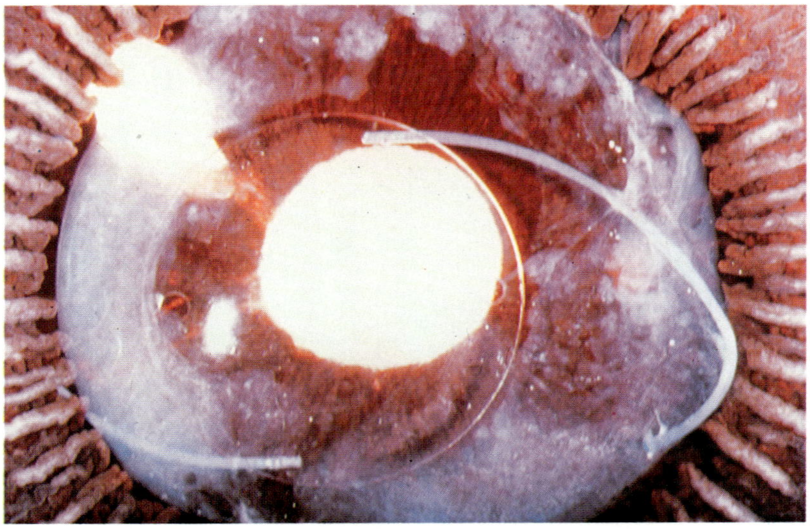

14.7 Decentration with one loop in the bag, one loop in the sulcus (courtesy Prof. David Apple, USA).

14.8

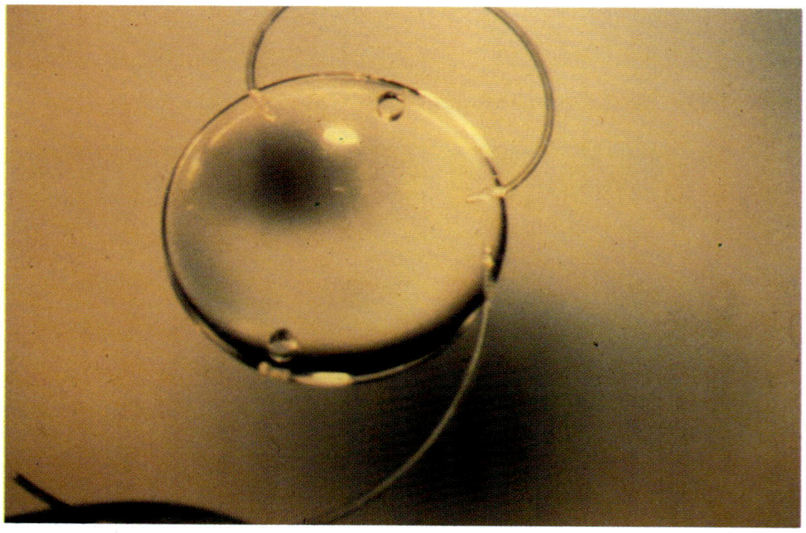

14.8 Asymmetrical Simcoe lens for a closed loop in the bag, and an open loop in the sulcus.

14.9

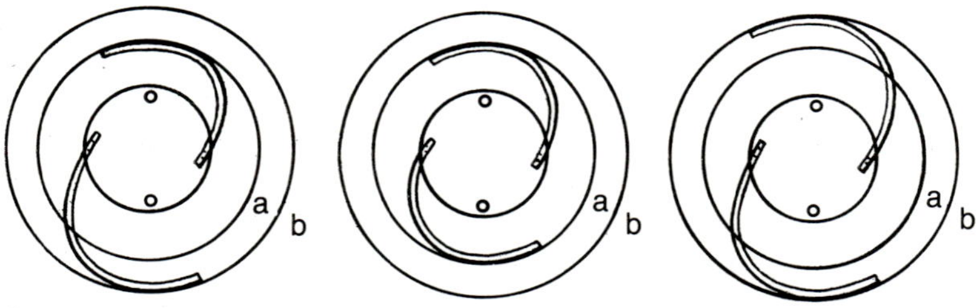

14.9 Open loop asymmetrical lens (left), lens for bag placement (center), lens for sulcus placement (right). (a) Capsular fornix ring; (b) ciliary sulcus ring.

Technique

Technique should include the injection of viscoelastic substance behind the iris to open the iridociliary space and to occlude the fornix of the lens capsule. The lens haptic should be of a flexible soft 'C' style. Many surgeons prefer the use of all-PMMA haptics.

Indications for sulcus fixation

- ECCE with rupture of the posterior capsule yet retention of sufficient anterior capsule to support a posterior chamber lens.
- ECCE with rupture of zonule for less than one third of the circumference: loops should be placed at 90° to the site of rupture.
- Secondary implantation in trauma cases or when implantation has been postponed because of high vitreous pressure or other reasons: in such cases the capsular fornix will be obliterated by fusion of the anterior capsule leaf to the posterior capsule, precluding bag fixation.
- Surgical difficulty with capsular flaps: a well-centered lens placed totally in the sulcus is preferable to an asymmetrically placed lens, which will later decenter.
- Secondary implantation after ICCE when most of the iris tissue is missing or the angle of the anterior chamber has been damaged, and so anterior chamber implantation is contraindicated. Needles 13–16 mm long are used to carry sutures across the anterior chamber, through the pupil and uveal tissue for trans-uveal or trans-scleral fixation (**14.10–14.12**). This method may also be used for any secondary posterior chamber implantation in the absence of a posterior capsule or in the event of a wide rupture of zonule or capsule dehiscence during ECCE (see also p. 257).

4.10

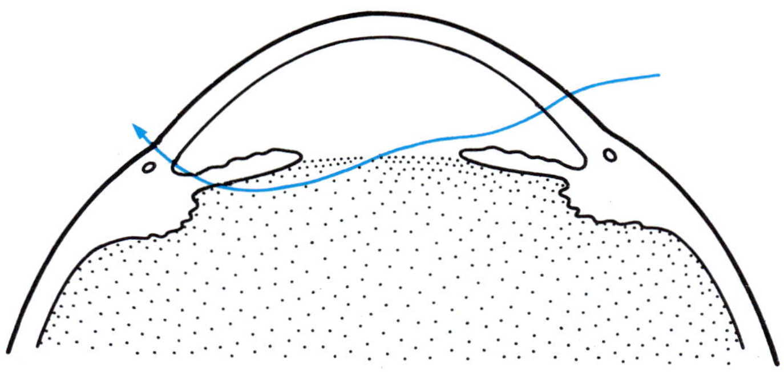

14.10 A double-armed polypropylene suture attached to a posterior chamber lens haptic is passed with 16 mm needles through the posterior chamber and distal iris to exit through a stab incision at 6 o'clock.

14.11

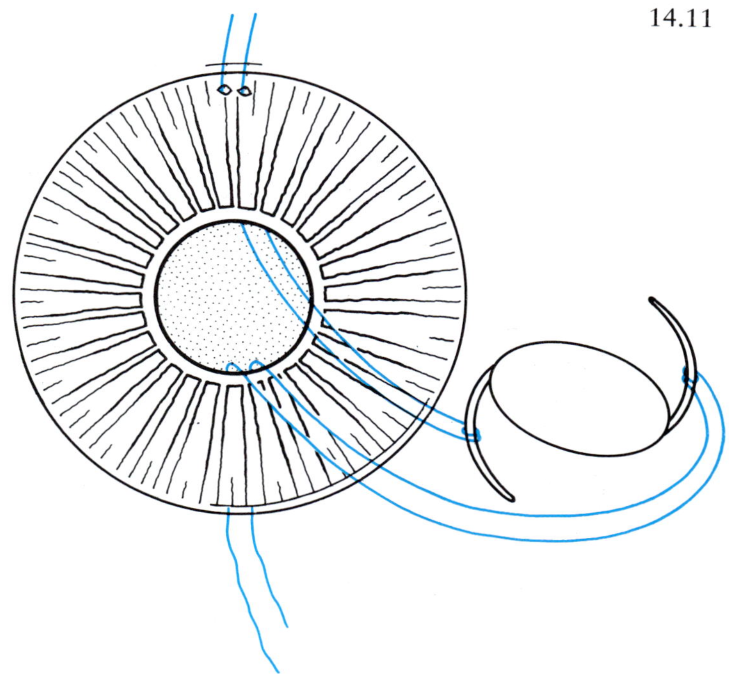

14.11 The polypropylene previously looped around and/or fixed to the upper lens haptic is also passed under the iris to exit through a limbal wound at 12 o'clock.

14.12

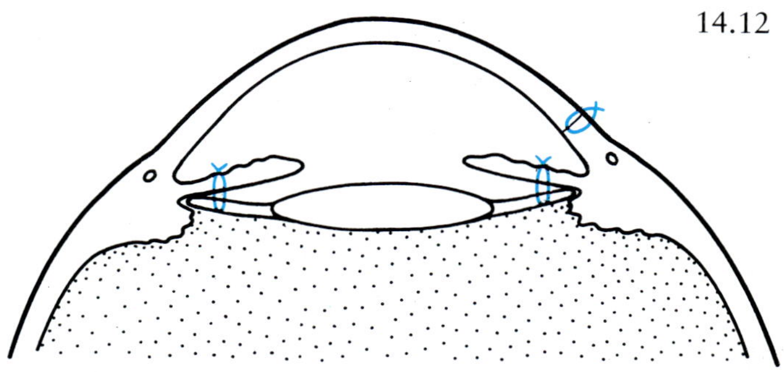

14.12 Sutures are tied and placed in the anterior chamber to fix the haptics to the peripheral iris.

Postoperative care

Topical steroid, combined with an antibiotic, may be recommended for three to four weeks. Indomethacin, if used, should be continued for three months. In cases of iritis, care should be taken not to allow excessive mydriasis, as this will invite the complication of pupil capture. A note should be made of any surgical transillumination defects. If vitreous has herniated in front of the lens optic, no particular treatment is required. Small beads of vitreous, provided they are not adherent to the section, will often be found to retract behind the iris in the course of time. Postoperative visits are recommended, at least on an annual basis, in order to monitor the intraocular pressure and assess the possibility of complications from iris chafing.

15: Capsule fixation

Kensaku Miyake

Advantages of capsule over sulcus fixation

Using an aqueous fluorophotometric technique to compare the postoperative sequelae of several IOL fixations, it has been demonstrated that capsular fixation of the posterior chamber lens is the method least traumatic to the blood–aqueous barrier (**15.1**). The safety of capsular fixation has been demonstrated by observing the intraoperative behavior of the haptics using the Miyake posterior video simulation technique with human cadaver eyes (**15.2–15.8**).

15.1

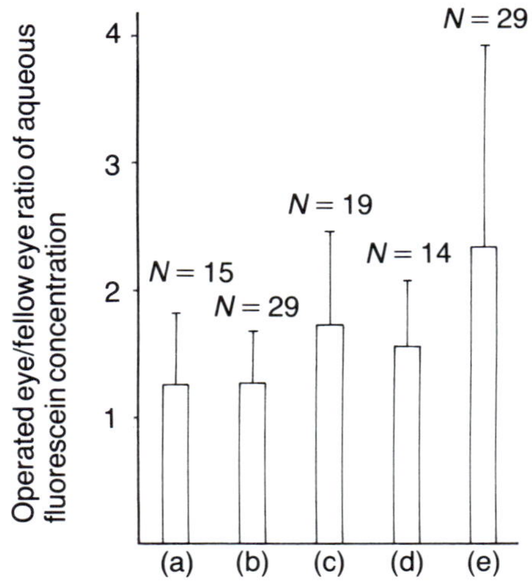

15.1 Ratio of aqueous fluorescein concentration in the treated *vs* the fellow eye in five groups: (a) Aphakia without implants (1.26 ± 0.55); (b) PCL with capsular fixation (1.27 ± 0.41); (c) PCL with ciliary sulcus fixation (1.73 ± 0.73); (d) ACL with open flexible loops (1.56 ± 0.52); (e) ACL with closed semiflexible loops (2.35 ± 1.56). (Miyake, with permission from *Am. J. Ophthalmol.)*

15.2

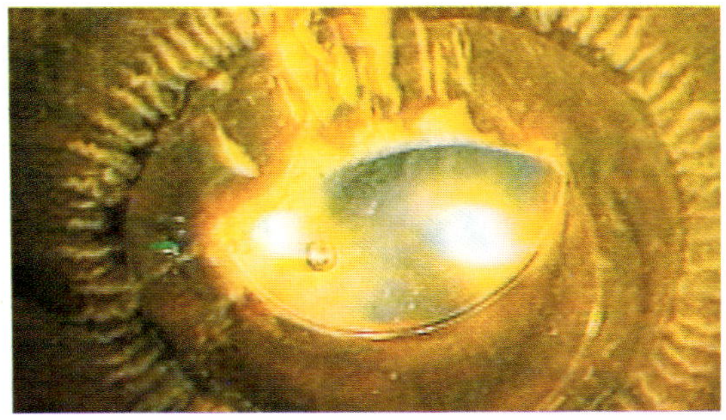

15.2 The capsular bag is well-ballooned with a viscoelastic material and the inferior half of the IOL entering into the bag. (Courtesy of Prof. David Apple, USA.)

15.3

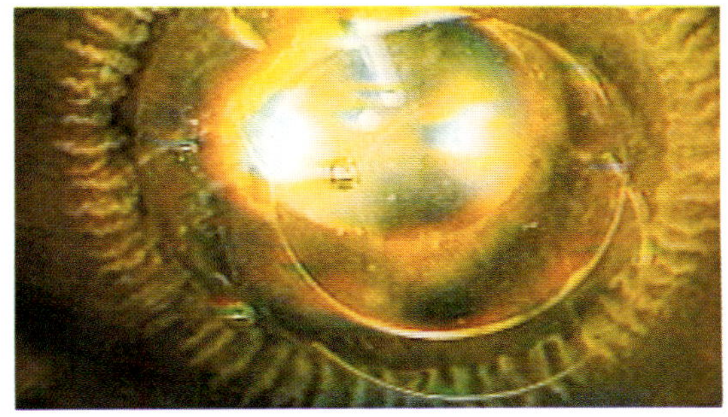

15.3 The capsular bag tolerates the lens implantation maneuver well. The capsule prevents trauma, which could occur to the surrounding tissues from the lens haptics. (Courtesy of Prof. David Apple, USA.)

15.4

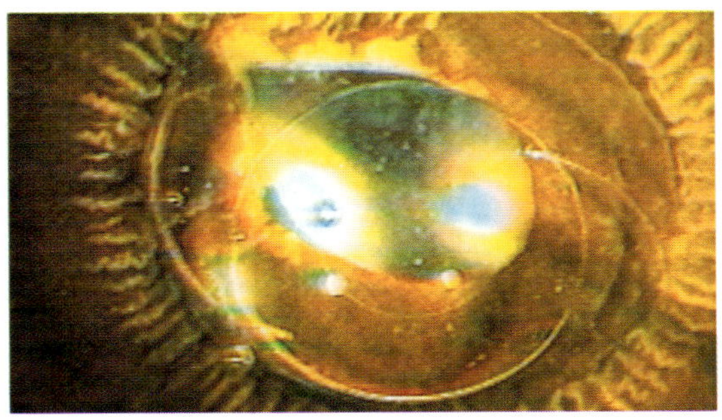

15.4 The capsular bag is acting as a barrier between the haptics and the surrounding uveal tissues. (Courtesy of Prof. David Apple, USA.)

15.5

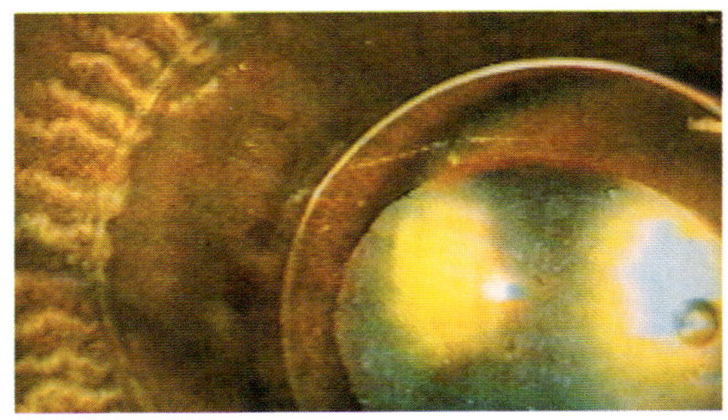

15.5 The configuration of short C loops is suitable for capsular bag fixation. Note the linear contact of these to the capsular bag. (Courtesy of Prof. David Apple, USA.)

15.6

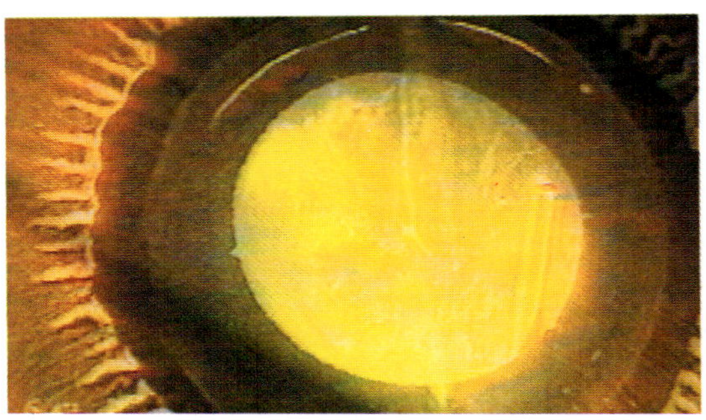

15.7

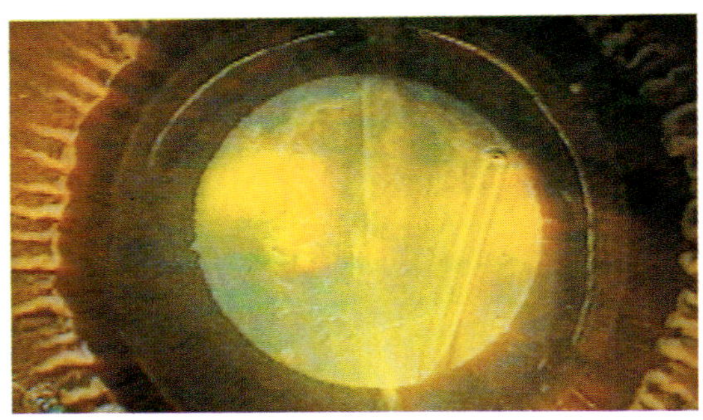

15.8

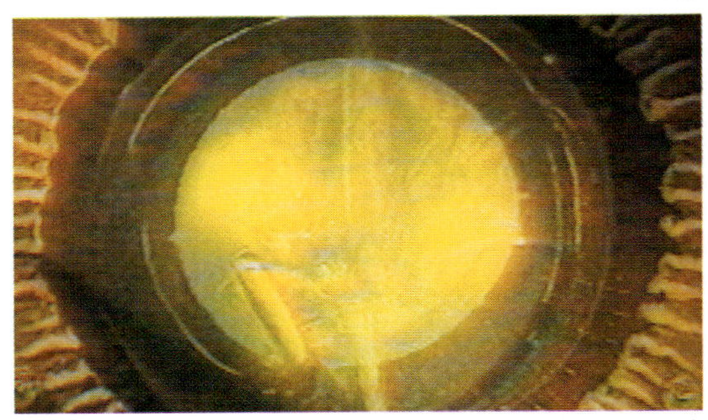

15.6–15.8 The Miyake posterior video simulation technique shows hydrodissection of the nucleus and formation of the 'golden ring' peripheral to the iris margin as the nucleus and cortex separate. (Courtesy of Prof. David Apple, USA.)

Apple and his colleagues, by studying a large number of histopathological specimens from pseudophakic eyes, have confirmed that capsular fixation of posterior chamber lenses is more secure and that the haptics are less likely to undergo biodegradation than with sulcus fixation. Finally, there are several reports of iris chafing with unwanted sequelae of intermittent uveitis and late pigment dispersion glaucoma associated with sulcus fixation.

These biological, morphological, histopathological and clinical findings are the reasons for the current trend towards capsular fixation of posterior chamber lenses.

Preparation of the capsule and removal of the nucleus

Although the advantages of capsular placement of the lens haptics have been demonstrated, methods for preparation of the capsule and for precise fixation need further consideration. The integrity of the capsule–zonula unit is essential in order to prevent decentration or malpositioning of the lens. This integrity depends on the shape and the nature of the anterior capsulectomy, the condition of the zonula, and the amount of lens remnants. The capsule opening should be round, with a diameter of 5–6 mm, because the diameter of the zonule-free area in elderly patients may be only 6 mm. The anterior capsular rim should not have accidental radial tears. Ruptures of the zonule should be avoided during surgery. The amount of residual lens material or cells should be minimal.

Table 15.1 shows the recommended methods of anterior capsulectomy and nucleus delivery. The new method of continuous tear capsulotomy with a smooth edge or capsulorhexis is called continuous circular capsulectomy (CCC), and was independently suggested by Gimbel and Neuhann. In cases with a soft nucleus, CCC and posterior chamber phacoemulsification are recommended. In cases with a hard nucleus, CCC may also be used with a single (or double) purposely made radial tear at the rim. In cases with large and hard nuclei, mature or hypermature cataracts, scarred anterior capsule, or poor mydriasis, the envelope technique may be recommended with capsule punch or forceps capsulorhexis after the implantation.

Table 15.1 Flow chart of methods recommended by Miyake in 1990

Nucleus condition	*Anterior capsulectomy*	*Nucleus delivery*
Soft →	CCC	→ Phacoemulsification
Small hard →	CCC with relaxing incision	→ Expression or vectis
Large hard, mature, hypermature, scarred ant. capsule, poor mydriasis →	Linear capsulotomy (envelope method) with capsule punch *after* lens implantation	→ Expression or vectis

Continuous circular capsulectomy (CCC) and posterior chamber phacoemulsification

The CCC technique of Gimbel and Neuhann is suitable for posterior chamber phacoemulsification. The capsulectomy is initiated at the 5 o'clock position, where a precise, linear, 2 mm opening is made with two or three contiguous punctures using a 25-gauge needle (**15.9**). The tear is then extended circumferentially inside the margin of the pupil (**15.10**) in a clockwise direction around to the original puncture (**15.11**). The needle is withdrawn and the disc of anterior capsule is removed with forceps or later by phacoemulsification. Hydrodissection

15.9

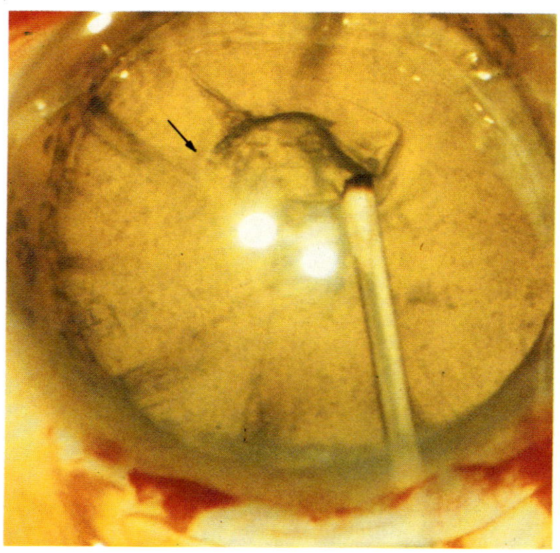

15.9 Initiation of CCC at 5 o'clock (arrow).

15.10

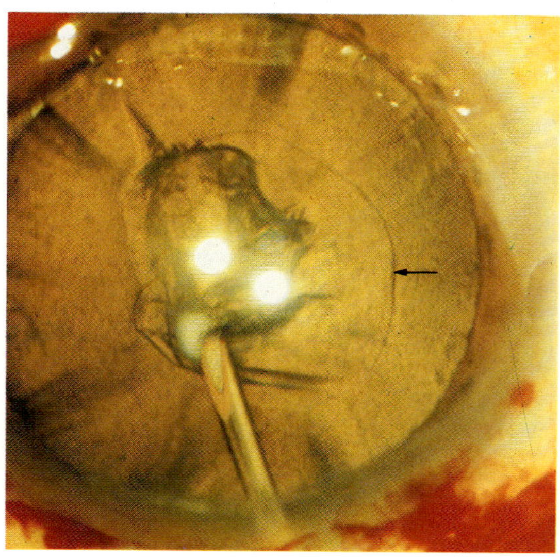

15.10 CCC is extended parallel to the pupil margin at 9 o'clock (arrow).

15.11

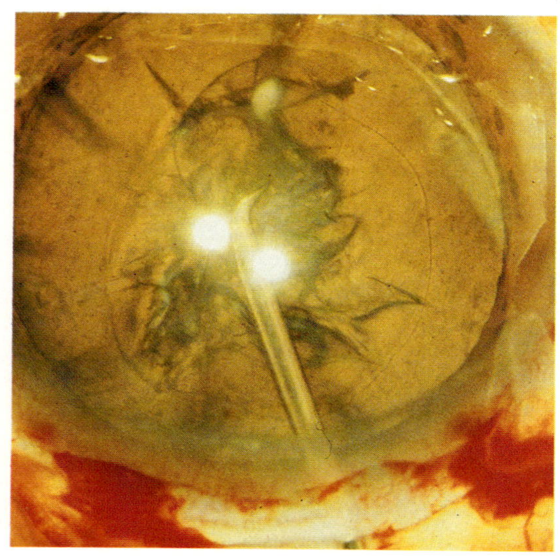

15.11 Completion of CCC.

of the nucleus is then performed; in many cases, completion of this is recognized by the appearance of the 'golden ring' (**15.6–15.8**).

One-handed phacoemulsification begins with central sculpturing (**15.12**). By rotating the nucleus in the posterior chamber (made easy by prior hydrodissection), the inner core of the nucleus is removed (**15.13**). The thin outer shell of the nucleus remaining in the posterior chamber is emulsified by low-power ultrasound (**15.14**). The power must be reduced, otherwise hard fragments will be bounced away from the tip of the probe. Finally, in most cases, a thin, plate-like or flexible U-shaped structure is left in the capsular bag. This is removed with minimal power and with the pointed bevel tip downwards (**15.15**).

During these maneuvers, precise control of the ultrasonic power is essential. Machines are available with linear power control to allow selection according to the type of nucleus. The use of minimal amounts of ultrasonic power is important because too much power will reduce the ease of aspiration. An irrigation/aspiration (I/A) tip is used to aspirate the cortex. Then the capsule vacuum mode, with a low flow and vacuum, is used to clean the capsule (**15.16**).

15.12

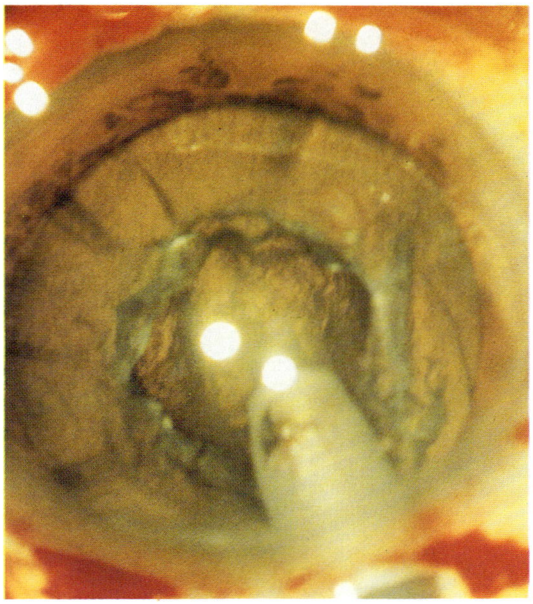

15.12 Central sculpturing in posterior chamber phacoemulsification.

15.13

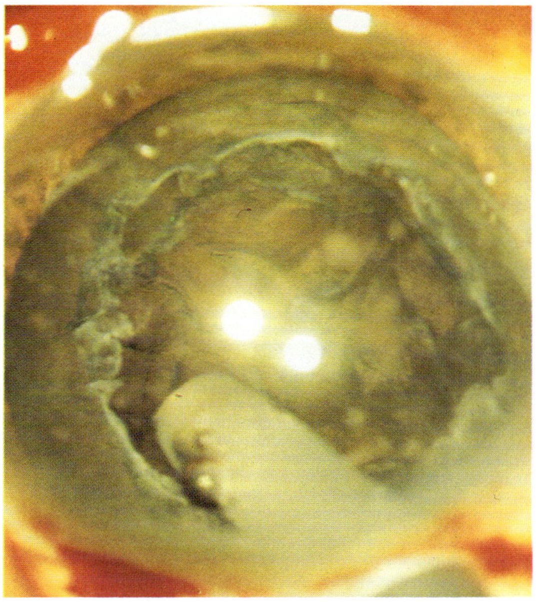

15.13 Most of the nucleus has been removed.

15.14

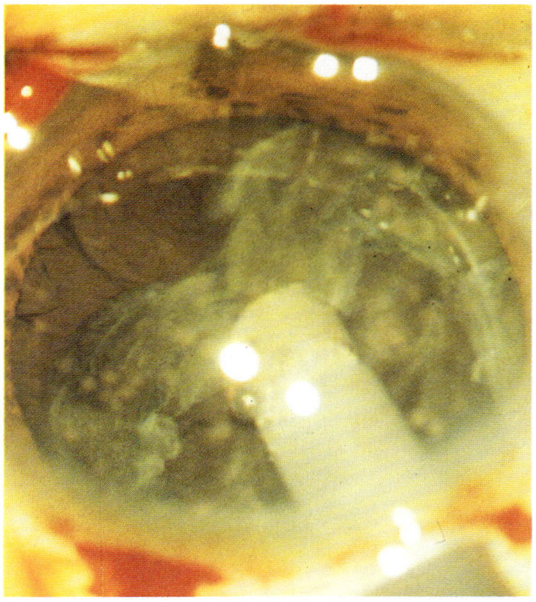

15.14 Outer shell of the nucleus is emulsified.

15.15

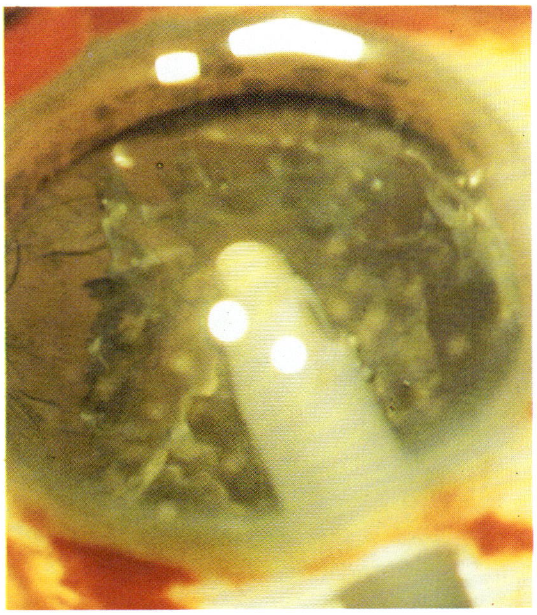

15.15 The thin plate-like structure left in the capsular bag is being emulsified by the bevel-down technique.

15.16

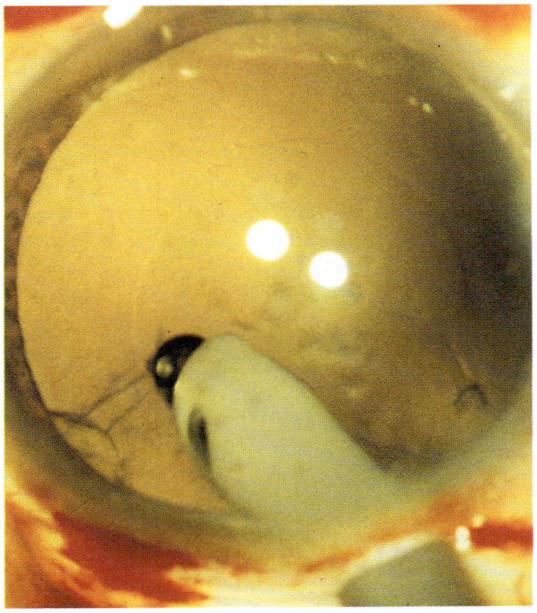

15.16 A low flow and vacuum is being used to clean the capsule.

The capsular bag is ballooned by injection of a viscoelastic material (**15.17**), and a posterior chamber lens is introduced into the anterior chamber. First, the inferior haptic is placed inside the capsule (**15.18**); then the superior haptic is placed inside, with the use of a compression technique. The superior haptic is grasped with Miyake forceps, compressing it inferiorly with the right hand, while the optic is pressed downwards towards the capsule with a Sinskey hook (**15.19**). By this maneuver, the round opening is stretched into an oval without trauma to the zonule, and it is not difficult to place an optic with a 6.5 or 7 mm diameter through a capsule opening of 5–6 mm.

15.17

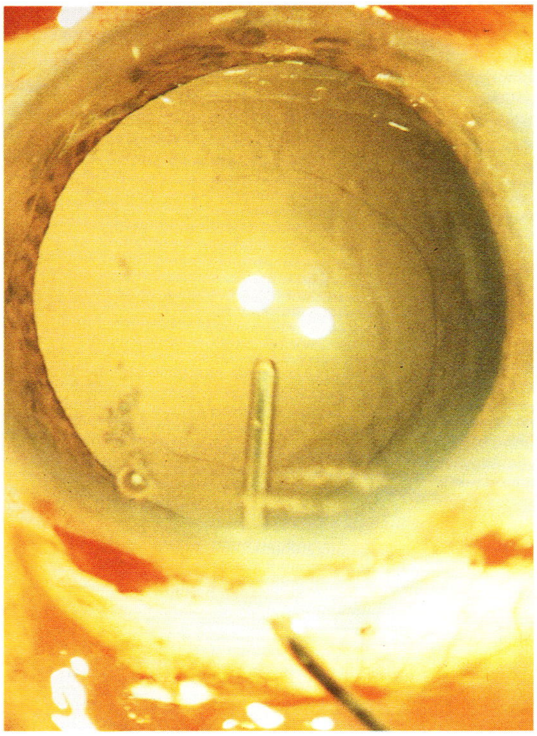

15.17 The capsular bag is being ballooned with a viscoelastic material. Note the 6 mm diameter opening in the anterior capsule.

15.18

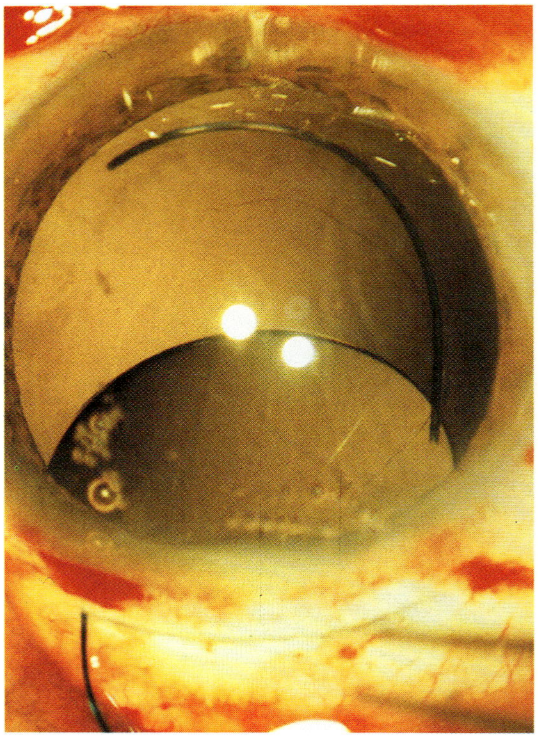

15.18 The inferior haptic is being placed inside the capsule.

15.19

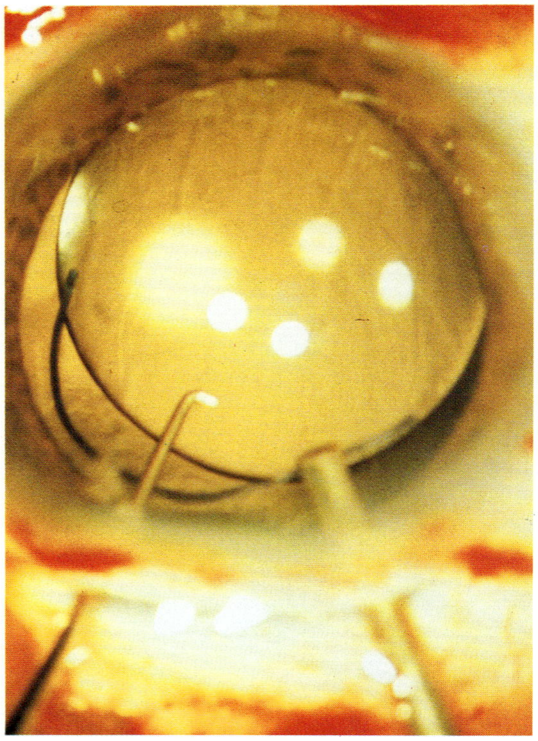

15.19 By using Miyake forceps and the Sinskey hook, an IOL with a 7 mm optic is placed entirely inside the capsular bag.

CCC, relaxing tear and ECCE

In cases of ECCE with nucleus extraction, a single or double relaxing radial tear is made in the capsule rim following the CCC (**15.20**). The nucleus is then removed by conventional methods, such as expression, and the residual lens cortex is aspirated. The IOL is inserted as before.

15.20

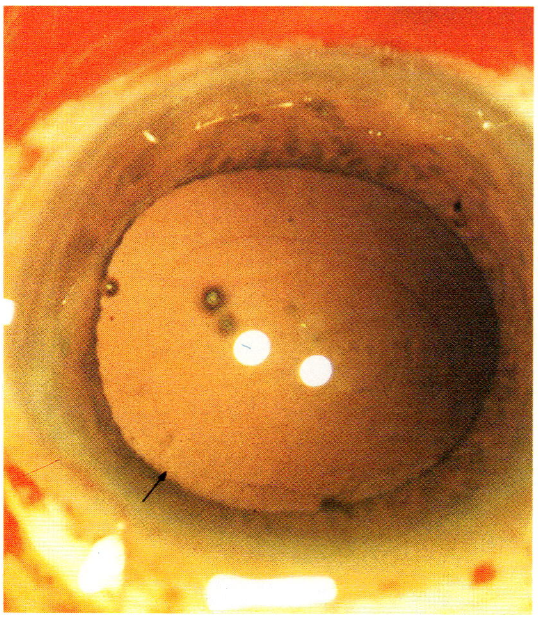

15.20 Preparation of the capsular bag in cases for ECCE. Note the relaxing radial tear at 1 o'clock (arrow).

Envelope technique and capsule punch

A special punch for excision of the anterior lens capsule (**15.21**) has been designed for use in combination with the envelope technique (**15.22**).

15.21

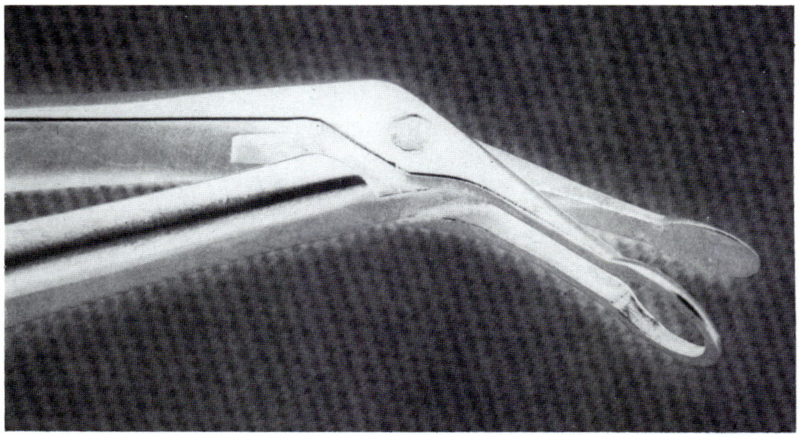

15.21 A special punch for excision of the anterior lens capsule (Miyake).

15.22(a)

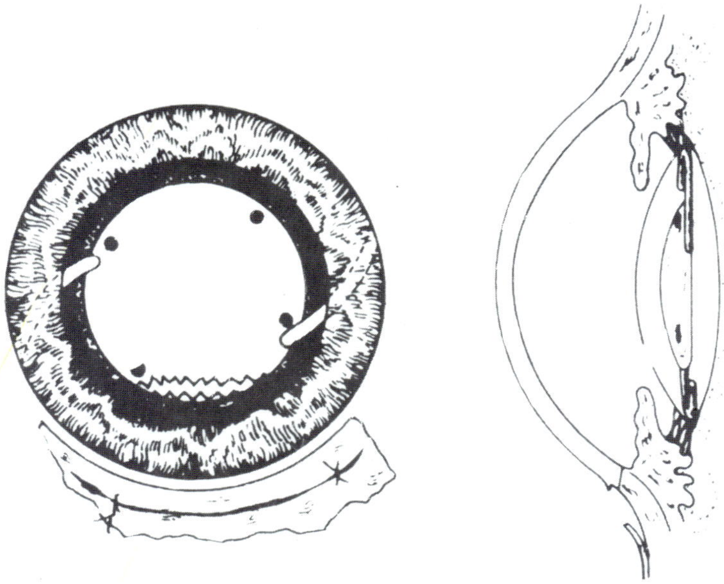

15.22(b)

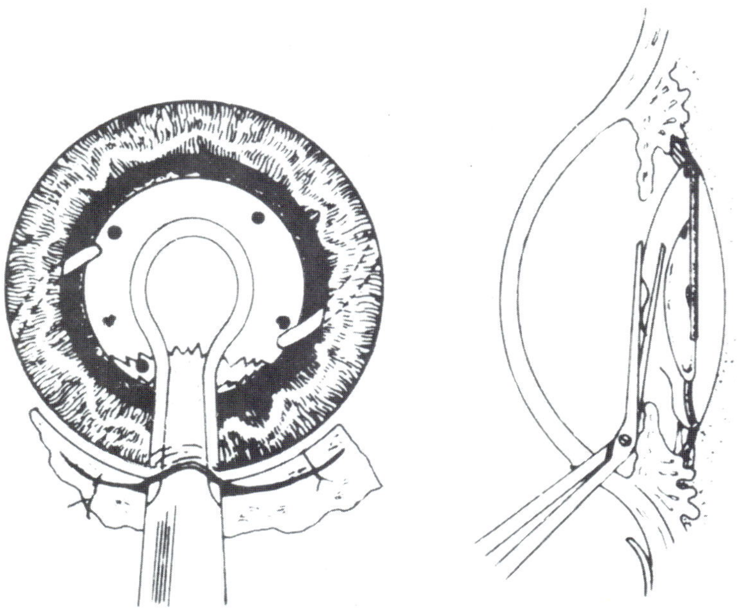

15.22(c)

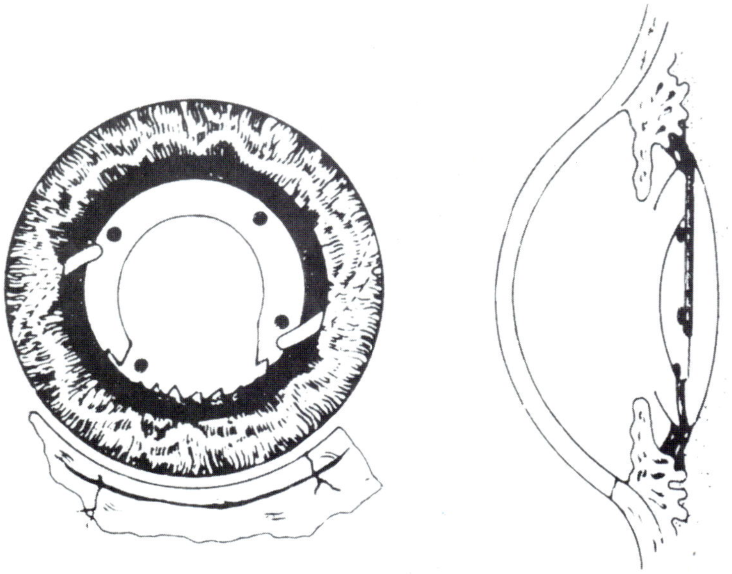

15.22 (a) A posterior chamber lens has been placed inside the lens capsule through a horizontal anterior incision. (b) The lower blade of the punch is introduced into the space between the anterior lens capsule and intraocular lens and an anterior capsulectomy is then carried out. (c) A tongue-shaped opening is left in the anterior capsule (Miyake, with permission from the *Arch. Ophthalmol.*).

The nucleus is removed through a horizontal incision in the anterior portion of the capsule (**15.23**), and the residual cortex is aspirated (**15.24**). Following injection of a viscoelastic material to balloon the capsule and the anterior chamber (**15.25**), a posterior chamber lens is placed inside the lens capsule through the horizontal incision by use of the technique previously described (**15.26**). The punch is introduced into the anterior chamber with the blades close together; the blades are then opened slightly, and the lower blade is inserted between the anterior capsule and the intraocular lens (**15.27**). (This space has been maintained by the viscoelastic material.) After the position of the punch at the center of the pupil has been confirmed, a tongue-shaped piece of the anterior capsule is grasped and extracted (**15.28**), leaving behind a well demarcated capsular opening of constant diameter. Before removing the punch, ensure that the piece of tissue being removed is free from the remaining lens capsule by slightly opening the two blades. If the piece of capsule has been cut free, it can be extracted on the lower blade of the punch. If it does not come with the blade, it is still attached and must be punched again.

15.23

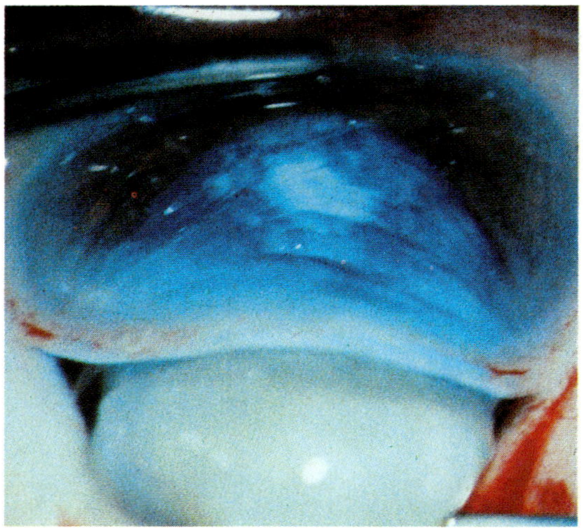

15.23 Nucleus delivery.

15.24

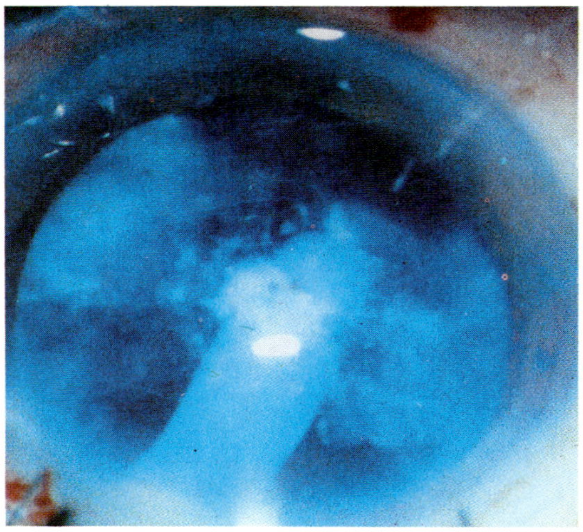

15.24 Aspiration of the residual cortex with an I/A cannula.

15.25

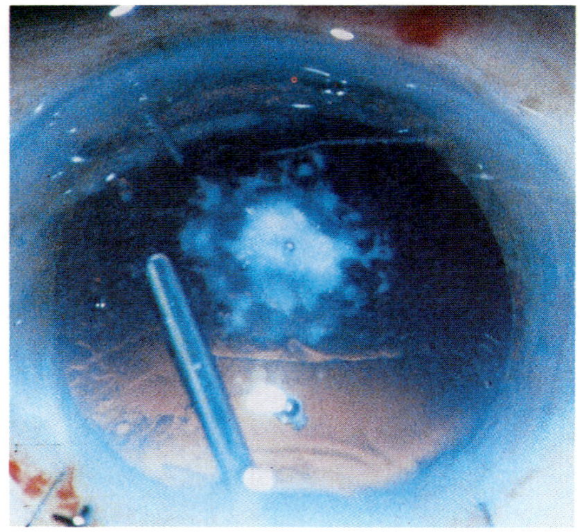

15.25 Ballooning of the capsular bag with a viscoelastic material. Note the plaque on the anterior capsule.

15.26

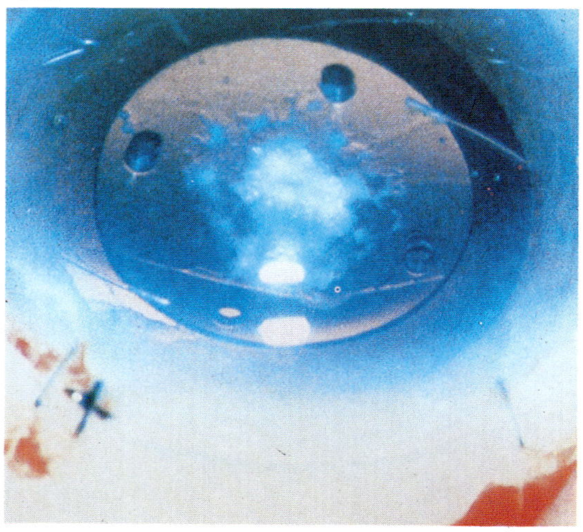

15.26 Placement of an IOL through a horizontal anterior incision. The upper edge of the anterior capsule is easily seen.

15.27

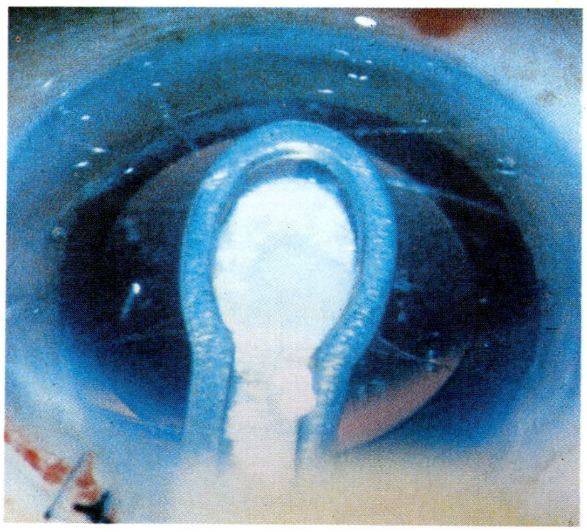

15.27 The punch is being inserted between the anterior lens capsule and intraocular lens.

15.28

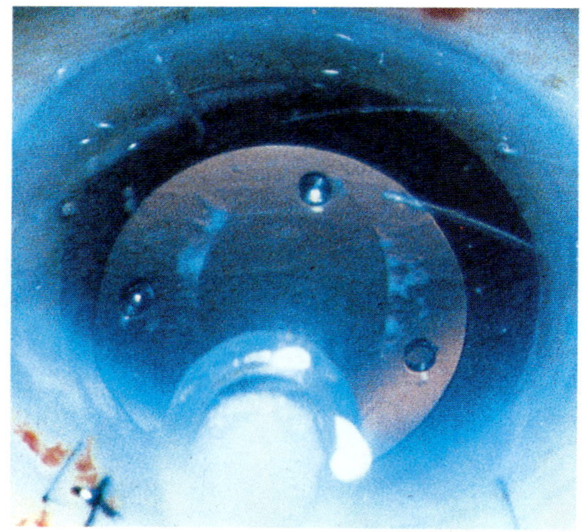

15.28 A tongue-shaped piece of anterior capsule is grasped and extracted.

Alternative procedures

The can-opener technique of anterior capsulotomy is *not* recommended, because the multiple tags of residual anterior capsule make aspiration of the cortex more difficult, because the wider opening interferes with the more anterior insertions of zonule, and because the residual anterior capsule has no rim and is less stable. Placement into the bag for capsule fixation becomes less certain, particularly if the pupil constricts. Asymmetric placement of haptics (one in the capsular bag and one in the sulcus) and lens malpositioning may result because the unstable flaps of anterior capsule may be rucked into a fold during haptic insertion, they may unfurl or move posteriorly postoperatively, or they may be torn during the aspiration technique so that they are of insufficient size to support the haptic. Further, while the dialling method of implantation may be preferred sometimes (**15.20**), dialling after the can-opener method can lead to asymmetric placement if one haptic is allowed to move through an unseen radial tear. Dialling may also further compromise the integrity of the zonule.

The intercapsular or envelope method (**15.23–15.26**) of Galand has the advantages that linear capsulotomy is easier than circular capsulorhexis and that there is greater protection of corneal endothelium and iris during surgery. However, it is less easy to avoid unwanted splits or tears in the capsule. With the wider opening, implantation of the inferior haptic is easy and similar to that shown in **15.18**; the upper haptic may then be pronated under the upper flap (or rim if after CCC) with a one-handed technique (**15.29**). This is preferred to the dialling method (**15.30**), which may damage the zonule, but care must be taken during pronation to avoid folding of the upper capsular flap and other problems associated with the can-opener method. The dialling method is most useful when loops are very flexible and of a soft 'C' configuration. Capsule placement is easy to confirm for solid haptics, but for looped haptics it is sometimes necessary to lift the iris (**15.31**) to

15.29

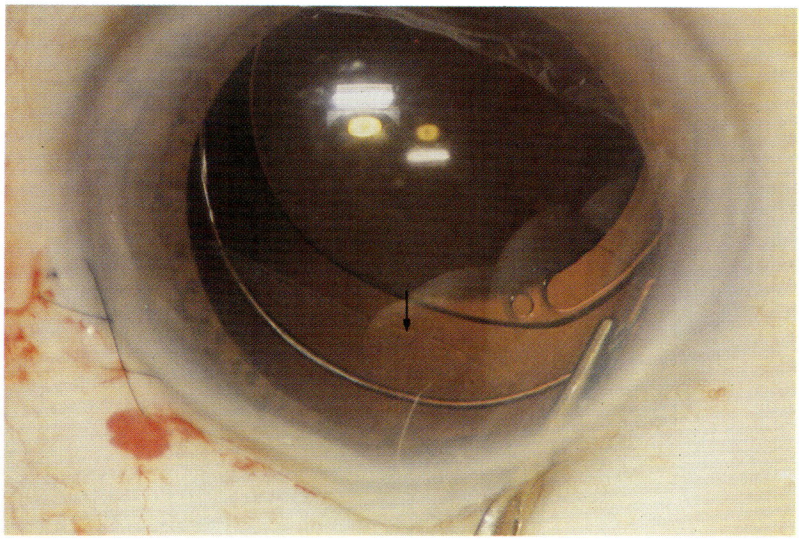

15.29 *Pronation:* the upper loop, grasped at its tip with Kelman–McPherson forceps in the right hand, is flexed downwards towards the rim of the optic. The hand is then gently pronated so that the bend in the loop flexes backwards to lie behind the superior flap of capsule (the inferior edge of which (arrow) can be seen running from the 11 o'clock to the 3 o'clock meridian).

15.30

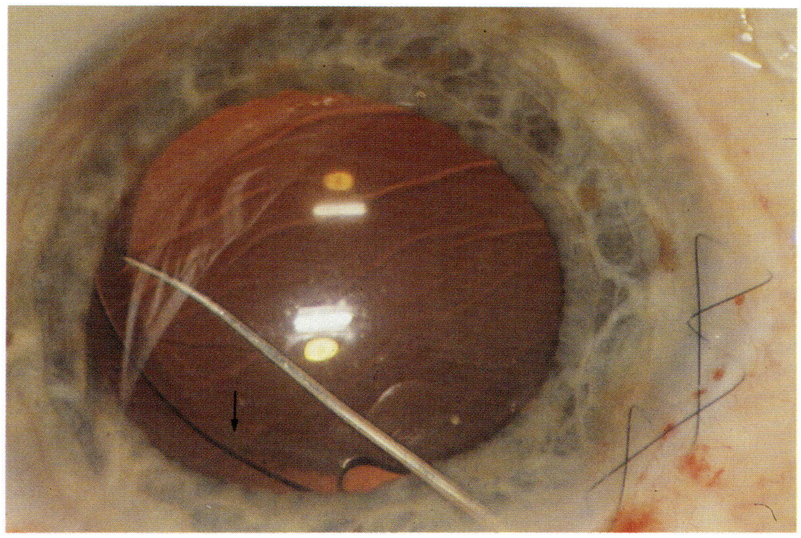

15.30 *Dialling:* as the upper loop is dialled clockwise into the capsular bag, care is taken to ensure that the proximal part of the inferior loop rotates underneath the superior flap of the capsule (the inferior edge of which (arrow) can be seen running horizontally from the 10.30 o'clock to the 2 o'clock meridian).

15.31

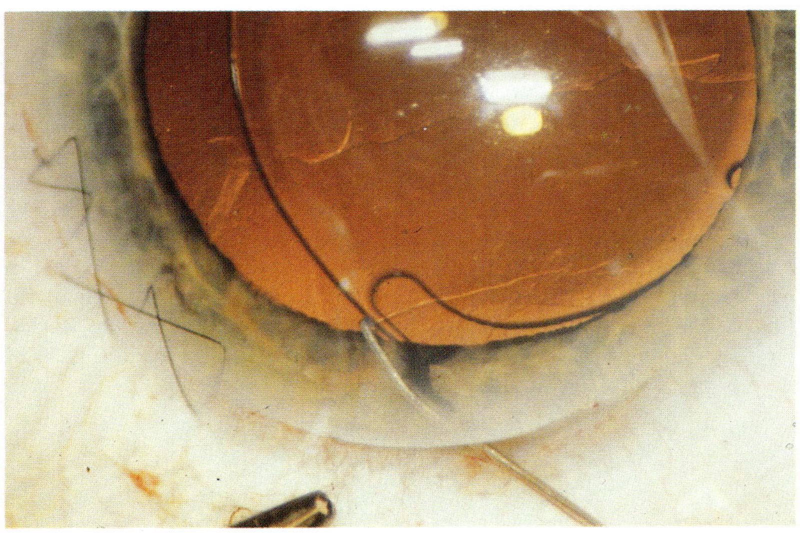

15.31 Confirmation of bag placement is made by lifting the edge of the upper anterior capsule with a Sinskey hook in front of the proximal arm of the loop.

ensure that the upper loop lies behind the flap of the capsule. Closed loop lenses are best inserted using a two-handed technique (**15.32, 15.33**). If a punch is not available, the final U-shaped capsulorhexis is made by cutting the inferior flap with fine long-bladed scissors (**15.34**), then grasping the flap at the apex of the cut with Kelman–McPherson forceps and gently tearing in a circumferential direction (**15.35**).

15.32

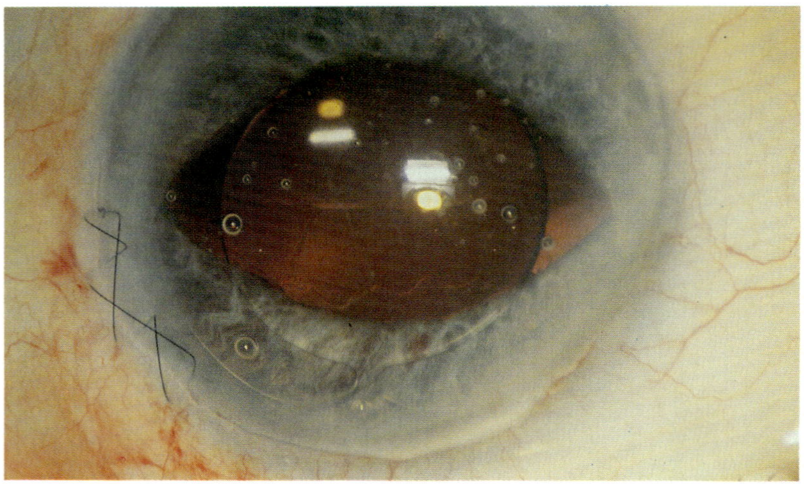

15.32 Intercapsular surgery showing insertion through a 7 mm wound of a 9.0 mm compressible disc lens in an eye with poor mydriasis. Dialling holes are present in the rigid part of this lens, lying here at 6 o'clock and 12 o'clock.

15.33

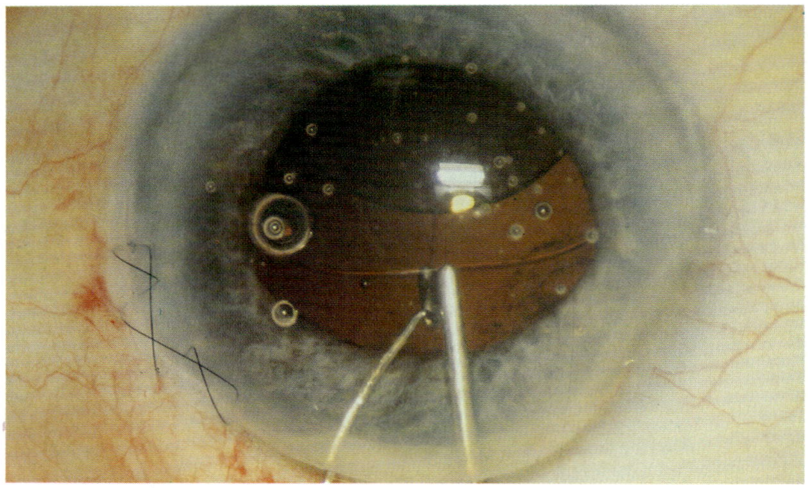

15.33 After rotation of the lens through 90°, the flexible upper rim is compressed downwards with a Hirschman hook (or Lester manipulator) in one hand while the edge of upper capsule is lifted with a Sinskey hook in the other.

15.34

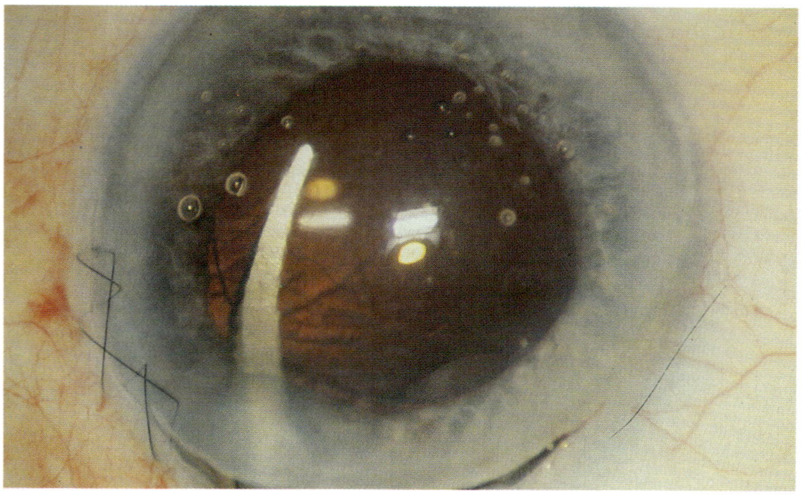

15.34 The lens springs back into position. Fine long-bladed scissors are used to cut into the inferior part of the anterior capsule.

15.35

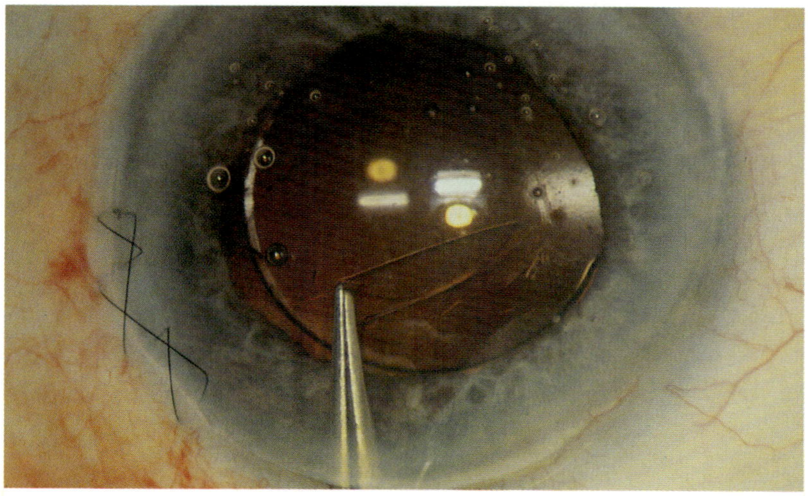

15.35 Final U-capsulorhexis as a disc of anterior capsule is removed with Kelman–McPherson forceps.

Choice of lens for capsule fixation

From observing the video simulation technique using human cadaver eyes (**15.5**), short C-loop lenses (loop span of around 12 mm) are considered the most suitable for capsular fixation. Owing to the possibility of glare, any positioning holes should be placed outside the central 6 mm zone. The recommended optic diameter is 6.5 or 7 mm.

Occasionally haptics may be dislodged by proliferation of lens epithelial cells, and although experience so far is limited, the use of biconvex flexible disc lenses (**15.32–15.33**), which exert an even pressure throughout the circumference of the lens capsule, appears promising.

Further reading

Apple D.J., *et al.* A comparison of ciliary sulcus and capsular bag fixation of posterior chamber lenses. *Am. Intra-Ocular Implant Soc. J.*, **11,** 44–63, 1985.

Postoperative care

After capsular fixation the postoperative course is straightforward. A healthy gap should be seen between the iris and lens on the slit lamp, and uveitis is minimal. Topical indomethacin is recommended three times daily for two months. Routine antibiotics are sometimes appropriate. Topical steroids (intensively at first) and mydriatics should be added only in the presence of active uvetis or synechia formation. Contraction and tightening of the capsule generally leads to a slight forward movement of the implant during the first two weeks. Thereafter, refraction should stabilize and following the prescription of any necessary glasses, further visits are usually unnecessary.

Miyake K. *et al.* Effect of intraocular lens fixation on the blood-aqueous barrier. *Am. J. Ophthalmol.*, **98,** 451–455, 1984.

Miyake K. *et al.* Intraoperative posterior chamber lens haptic fixation in the human cadaver eyes. *Ophthalmic Surg.*, **16,** 230–236, 1985.

16: Secondary implantation and anterior chamber reconstruction

Bruce Noble and Michael Hayward

There is a wide range of aphakic eyes in which the ophthalmologist may wish to consider secondary lens implantation. At one end of the spectrum lies the uncomplicated eye with either an intact capsule or a vitreous face lying behind the pupillary margin (**16.1**), and, at the other end, a traumatized eye, aphakic with a tough cyclitic membrane, lens remnants and probably vitreous incarcerated in the scar tissue of the anterior chamber (**16.2**). The techniques demanded will vary according to the state of the eye but the basic principles are the same.

Careful preoperative examination and planning are required. It is especially important to anticipate the need for specialized cutting and vitrectomy instruments because vitreous must be removed from the anterior chamber. Traction on the vitreous base by vitreous ensnared by anterior chamber structures is an invitation to retinal detachment (**16.3**).

The relative risks and benefits must be discussed with the patient. The improvement in vision to be expected in an eye requiring an anterior segment revision and lens implantation is relatively greater than in the 'uncomplicated eye' where the corrected vision may already be of the order of 20/20. The risks of a reduction in corrected visual acuity are higher in the uncomplicated case, even though the surgical techniques are more straightforward.

16.1

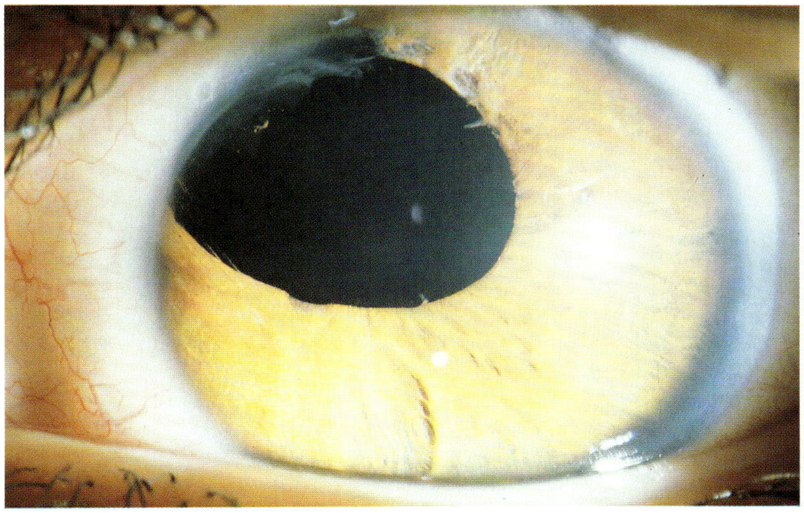

16.1 Aphakic eye with vitreous face well back.

16.2

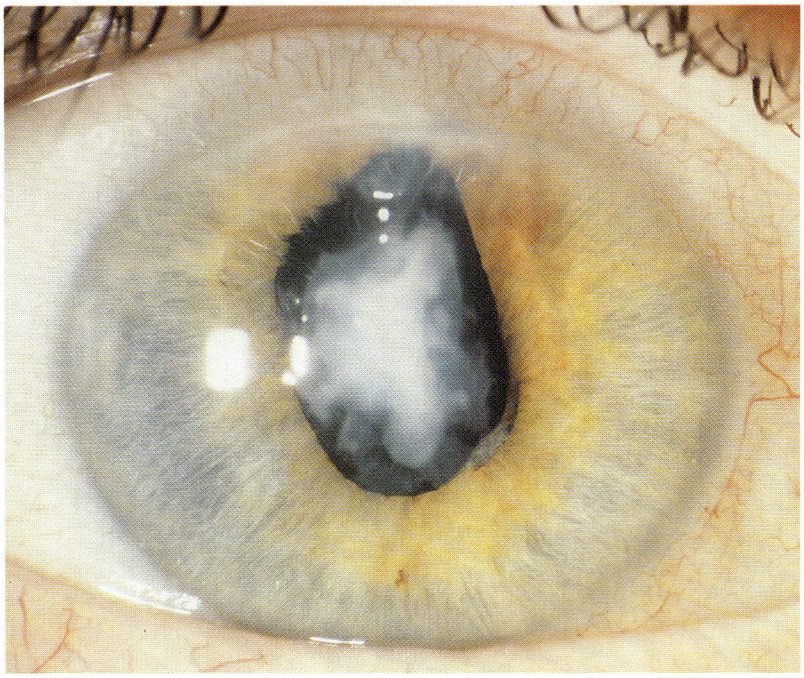

16.2 Aphakic eye with complicated pupil membrane. Note vitreous drawing iris up to an old wound.

16.3

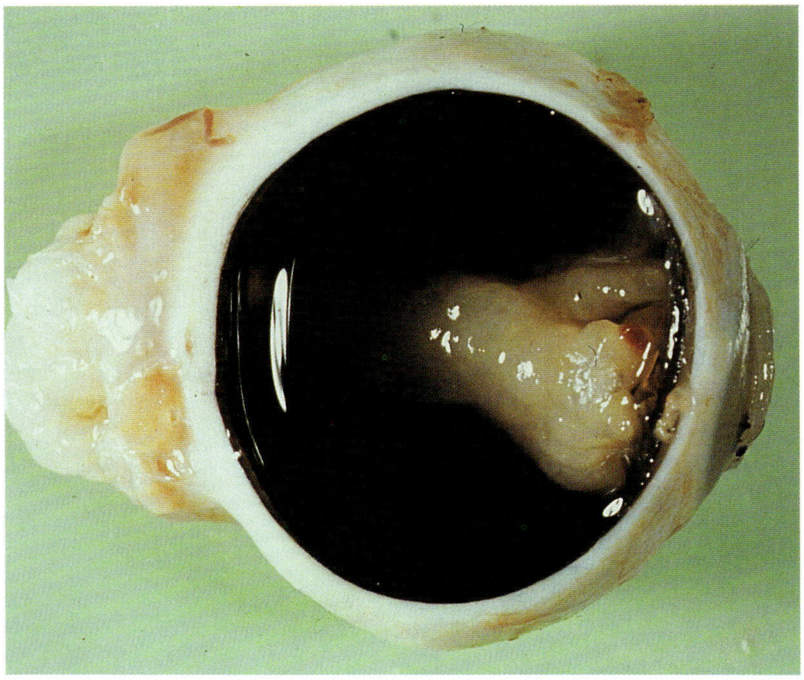

16.3 Funnel (D3) retinal detachment.

Indications for secondary intraocular lens insertion

Optical problems: The distortion and magnification produced by aphakic spectacles and the problems of contact lens intolerance and complications are well recognised.

Prevention of amblyopia: There is a high incidence of amblyopia in children with aphakic eyes that have been corrected with contact lenses following trauma.

Problems of fusion: Many adults who have had a traumatic cataract extracted experience problems with fusion when using a contact lens. Some discard their contact lenses and secondary divergence then develops (**16.4**).

External disease: Severe vernal conjunctivitis, eczema and lid margin disease may prevent the successful wearing of contact lenses (**16.5**).

Legal standards: In some countries it may be necessary for a person to have an intraocular lens *in situ* to meet driving licence requirements. For example, in the United Kingdom, it is not possible to hold a Heavy Goods Vehicle (HGV) licence following cataract surgery unless an intraocular lens has been inserted.

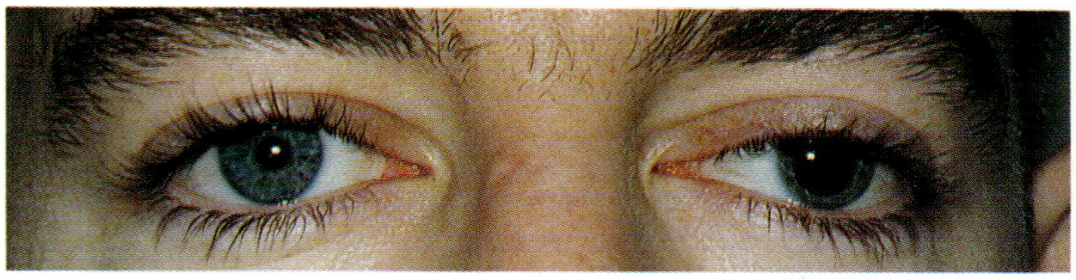 16.4

16.4 Divergent aphakic eye following extraction of the traumatic cataract.

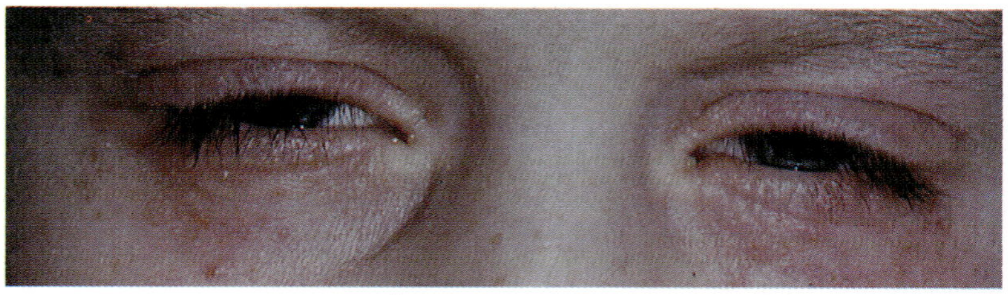 16.5

16.5 Severe atopy.

Preoperative evaluation

Visual acuity: The aphakic refraction must be assessed.

Relative afferent pupillary defect: Should contraindicate surgery.

Slit-lamp examination of the anterior segment: Care must be taken to note the state of the cornea and look for the presence of anterior chamber inflammation or damage to the drainage angle. The presence of an intact posterior capsule will protect the anterior chamber from vitreous prolapse. If vitreous is seen in the anterior chamber, it must be noted whether this is adherent to any previous surgical or traumatic scars (**16.2**). Examine the iris and pupillary margin and look for the presence of any cyclitic membranes that will require particular techniques and that may bleed during surgery (**16.6, 16.7**).

16.6 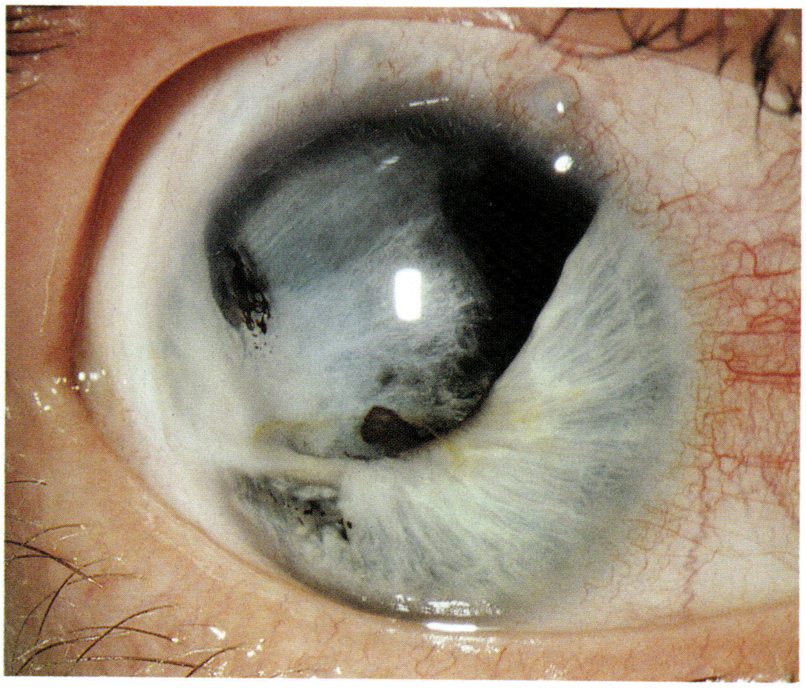

16.6 Previous surgery for penetrating injury and traumatic cataract. Surgical problems included: broad iridectomy (dictated horizontal orientation of AC IOL), a vascularized cyclitic membrane extending from the original laceration, temporal PAS which required angle revision to allow horizontal placement of IOL, and vitreous in the anterior chamber.

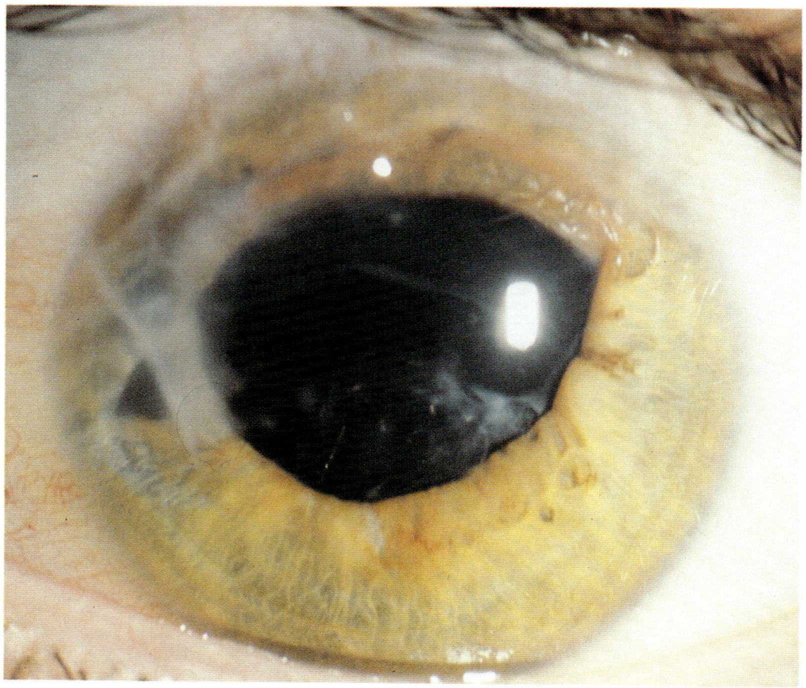 16.7

16.7 The vitreous face is well back but there is an adhesion between a capsular remnant and an old corneal scar that will need to be divided.

Fundal examination: If media opacity precludes this by visual means, then a B-scan ultrasound should be performed to exclude the possibility of retinal detachment (**16.8**). In some cases of previous trauma, an X-ray or CT scan may be valuable to exclude the possibility of an intraocular foreign body (**16.9**).

16.8

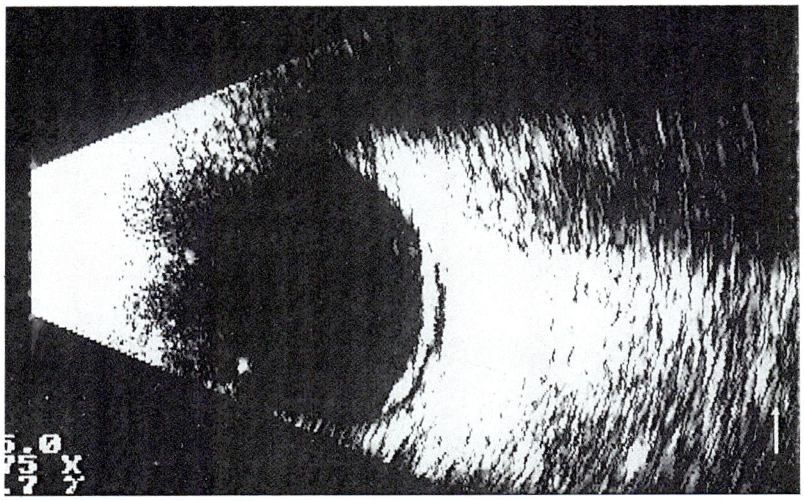

16.8 Retinal detachment shown on ultrasound B-scan.

16.9

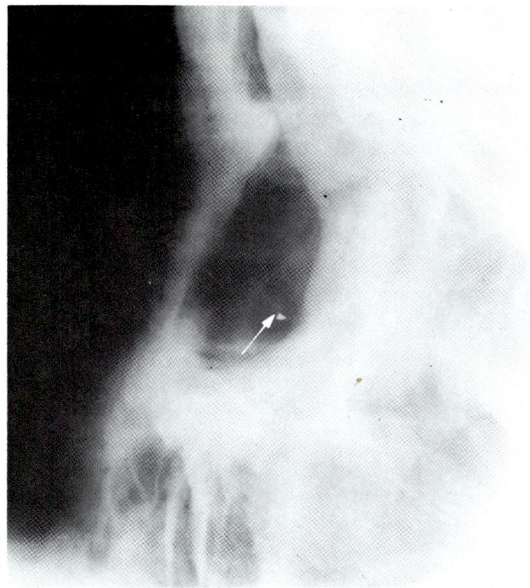

16.9 Small radio-opaque intraocular foreign body (arrow).

Fundal examination: If media opacity precludes this by visual means, then a B-scan ultrasound should be performed to exclude the possibility of retinal detachment (**16.8**). In some cases of previous trauma, an X-ray or CT scan may be valuable to exclude the possibility of an intraocular foreign body (**16.9**).

Orthoptic assessment: The potential for binocular single vision and the likelihood of postoperative diplopia should be determined

Assessment of intraocular lens power: This can be determined by conventional biometric techniques (with A-scan ultrasound and keratometry). Alternatively, it can be roughly estimated by using the spherical equivalent of the patient's aphakic correction and adding +7D for an anterior chamber lens and +9D for a posterior chamber lens. The surgeon should aim for a postoperative refraction of about 1D of myopia (not emmetropia) as, in general, patients prefer to focus on a mid distant rather than a far distant object.

The patient's refraction will also reveal if there is a high cylindrical component, which may be partially corrected by choosing the position of the incision for the secondary IOL. For example, if the patient has a plus cylinder on the 90° axis, then a temporal incision (based at 180°) should be chosen (**16.10**).

Consent: The patient must be fully informed of the risks of cystoid macular edema, retinal detachment and persistent postoperative uveitis.

16.10

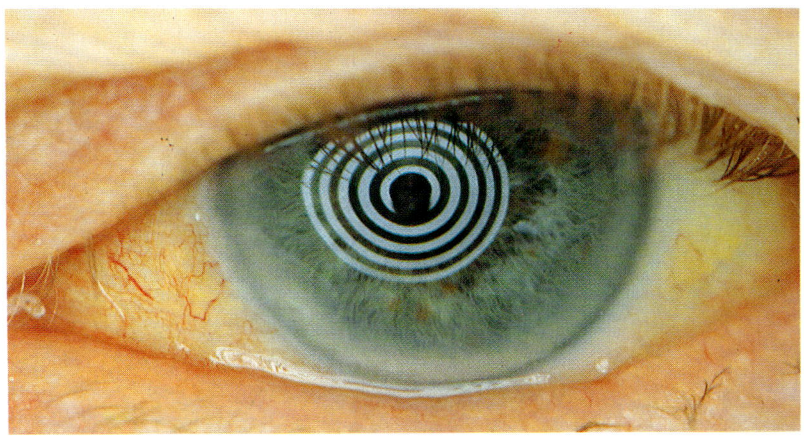

16.10 Keratoscope showing astigmatism with 'plus' axis at 90°. A temporal incision should be used if possible.

Equipment

Basic microsurgical tray, calipers and steel rule, diamond knife (**16.11**).

16.11

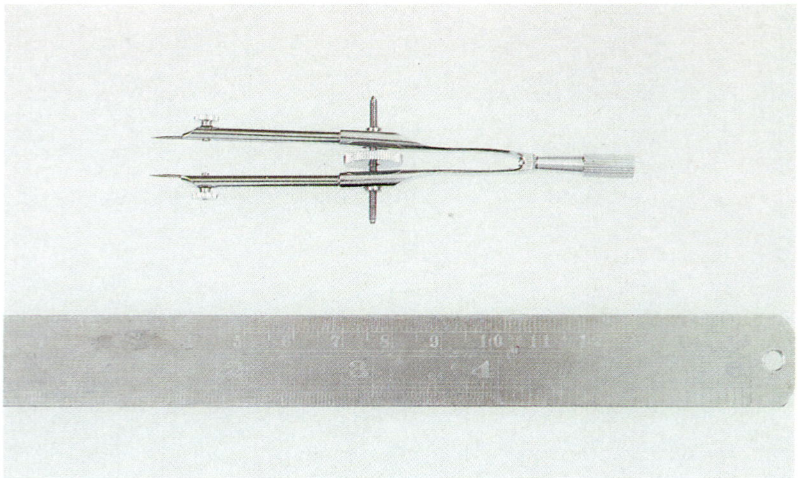

16.11 Calipers and steel rule.

Closed microsurgical vitreous cutter (**16.12**): This is to be preferred to disposable cutters such as the Kaufman vitrector as the instruments are fine enough to be used in the closed eye rather than having to use an open-sky technique. Sponges and scissors can be used for the final iris and wound toilet, but they are inadequate for anterior vitrectomy.

Special scissors: The Greishaber forceps and microscissors (**16.13**) have been designed for use through a common 20-gauge port and they are extremely useful tools for cutting membranes inside the anterior chamber. Capsulotomy scissors (**16.13**) are also useful once the eye has been opened.

Spatulas and hooks: A range of fine cyclodialysis spatulas are required (for synechia dissection and angle reconstruction), as are IOL manipulating hooks (**16.14**).

16.13

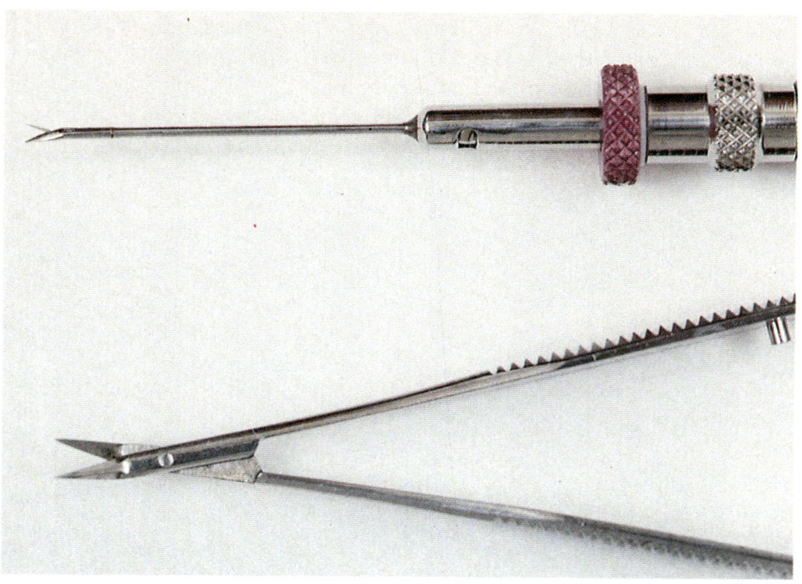

16.13 Above: Grieshaber microsurgical scissors. Below: Ong capsulotomy scissors.

16.12

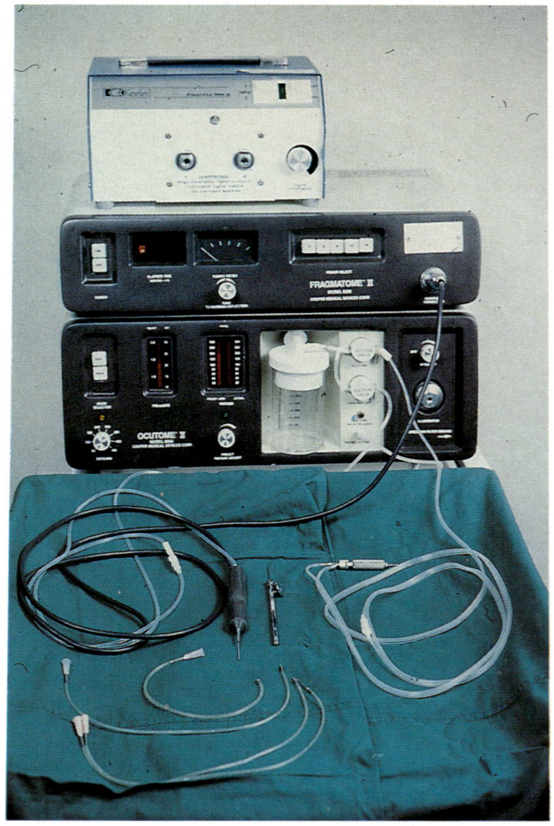

16.12 The Ocutome® closed microsurgical vitreous cutter and aspiration system. (Here shown with infusion, fragmatome and flute needle for pars plana vitrectomy.)

Viscoelastic and other space maintaining agents: A viscoelastic agent such as sodium hyaluronate is essential for splinting the anterior chamber, defining structures and dissection. However, vitreous is not easily seen when viscoelastic agents fill the anterior chamber and air injected through a fine cannula will allow clear definition of the presence of vitreous. This is particularly useful during lens insertion when vitreous may easily become entangled with the implant.

16.14

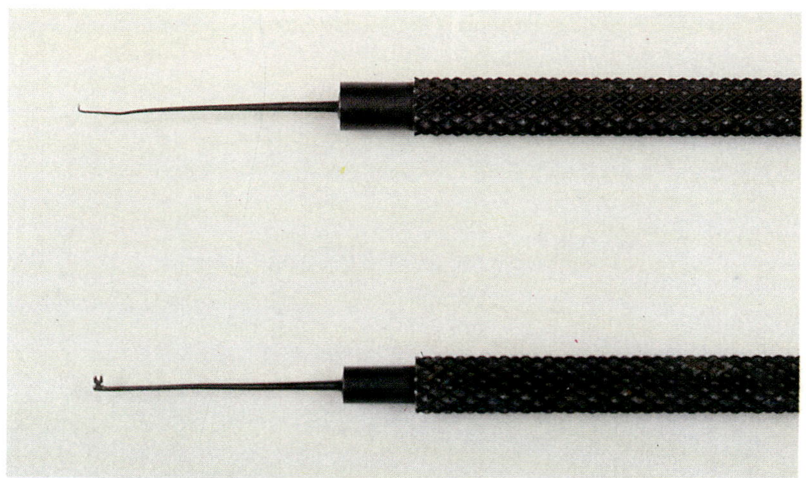

16.14 Above: Sinskey hook. Below: Kuglan hook.

Technique

Uncomplicated anterior chamber secondary lens implantation (vitreous posterior to pupillary margin)

The eye should be prepared according to the surgeon's own preference. The use of adhesive plastic draping totally isolates the lid margins and lashes from the procedure. The surgeon may prefer a lateral orientation. A superior rectus fixation suture may or may not be required to allow good surgical exposure. The corneal diameter should be measured 'white-to-white' horizontally (**16.15**) and 1 mm added to this measurement to give the size of the required anterior chamber IOL.

The incision of a 6.5 mm chord length (**16.16**) should, unusually for a corneal section, be anteriorly sloping both for ease of entry of the implant and so that there is a small shelf to prevent extrusion of the implant feet through the section. Air is introduced and retained inside the anterior chamber by the use of a dam of sodium hyaluronate (**16.17**). The lens is then inserted using forceps of the surgeon's choice (**16.18**). A Sheet's glide may be used to guide the lens across the anterior chamber. It is important that the distal (leading) feet are aimed anteriorly towards the cornea on the opposite side of the eye because of the problem of apparent depth. Iris tuck will then be avoided. To insert the proximal feet the haptic is grasped centrally between the feet and pushed towards the opposite side of the eye and finally slightly backwards. It is important to check that the feet are clear of the wound.

The pupil should then be inspected and, if there is any iris tuck, the lens repositioned. This is often difficult to achieve on the side of the eye opposite the incision, but may be carried out using a Kuglan hook under sodium hyaluronate and air (**16.19**). If a small vitreous prolapse occurs at the time of lens implantation the Ocutome® should be used to perform a limited pupil-clearing anterior vitrectomy. The pupil margin is carefully checked for vitreous strands before closing the section. If not already present, a peripheral iridectomy should be performed at this stage. The wound is then sutured (remembering that, because it is anteriorly sloping, it has no intrinsic watertight properties), and the anterior chamber reconstituted with balanced salt solution. The pupil should be dilated postoperatively.

16.15

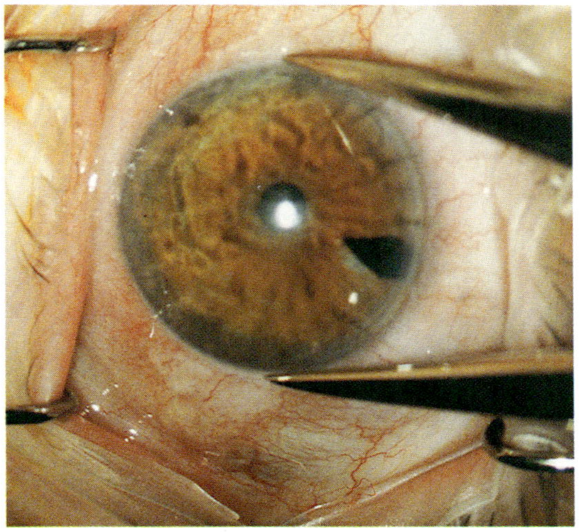

16.15 Measuring horizontal corneal diameter 'white-to-white'.

16.16

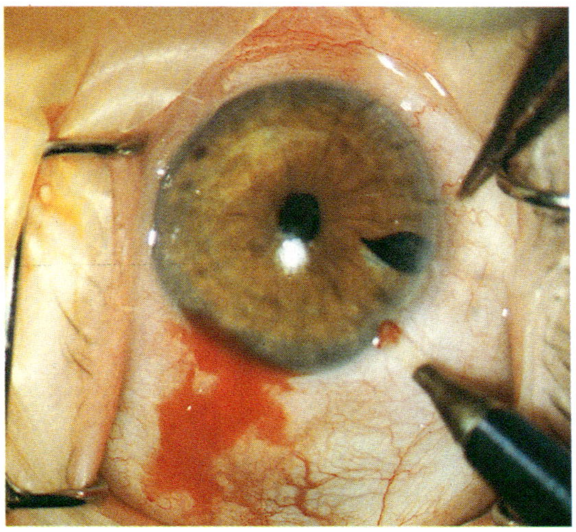

16.16 Temporal anteriorly sloping corneal section with diamond knife.

16.17

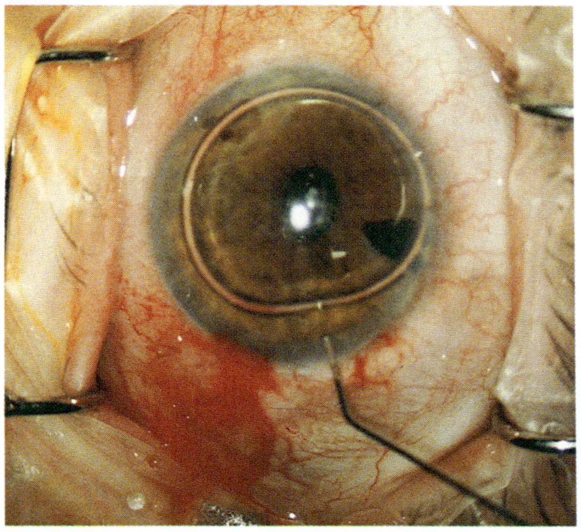

16.17 Air retained with a 'dam' of sodium hyaluronate.

16.18

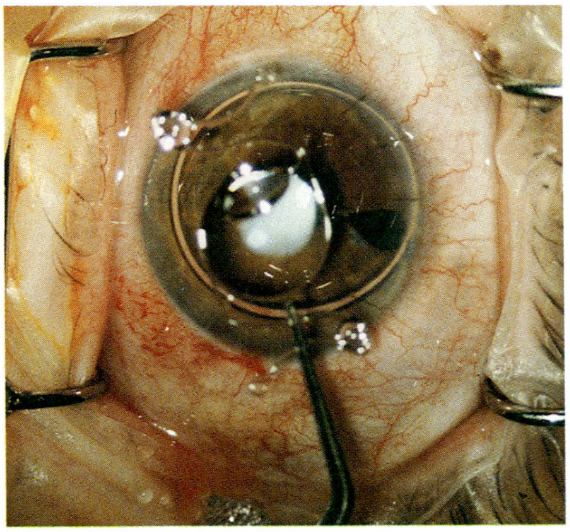

16.19

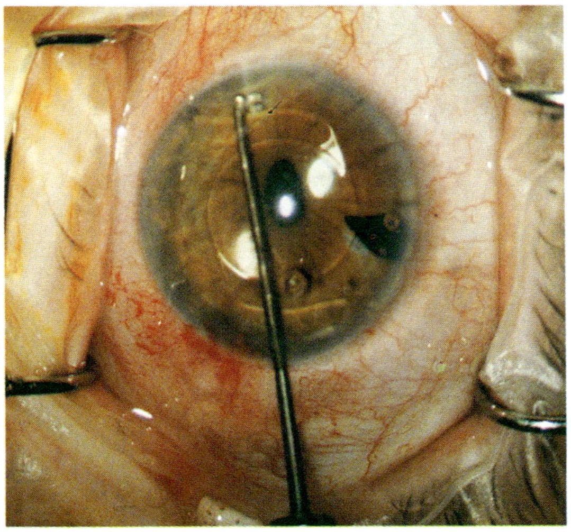

16.18 Kelman multiflex style semiflexible anterior chamber IOL being held above the eye with a pair of McPherson forceps.

16.19 Adjusting distal foot position with a Kuglan hook. The anterior chamber must be filled with sodium hyaluronate.

Secondary posterior chamber lens implantation

The post-iris space should be swept with the cyclodialysis spatula to free any iris capsule adhesions, or be distended and swept whilst injecting sodium hyaluronate. Attempts to open up the capsular bag to allow 'in the bag' fixation are not recommended as vitreous prolapse invariably results. Therefore the lens has to be placed in the ciliary sulcus. If there are soft lens remnants on the posterior capsule, these should be removed with an irrigation/aspiration cannula before lens insertion (for scleral fixation techniques, see p. 257).

Anterior segment reconstruction

If possible, a bimanual closed microsurgical technique should be used. Cut a partial thickness groove at the site chosen for lens insertion. Two ports are prepared in a comfortable and appropriate position for the surgeons hands (not too close together or too superior) and the surgical task.

Inflate the anterior chamber with sodium hyaluronate and explore carefully the scar tissue, using the sodium hyaluronate to place it under tension (**16.20**). If necessary the vitrectomy lancet or 20-gauge hypodermic needle may be used to initiate the segmentation of the scar tissue, which can then be further cut with microscissors (**16.21, 16.22**) or the Ocutome®.

The infusion cannula (which is simply made with a Butterfly infusion needle held in Spencer Wells forceps) is introduced and then, through the other port, the Ocutome®. Cutting of solid tissues requires moderately high suction pressures and a slow cutting speed (1 Hz). Conserve all or most of the iris tissue if possible and control hemorrhage by increasing the height of the infusion bottle or by bipolar cautery attached to the Ocutome® and infusion needle.

Vitreous cutting requires higher cutting speeds and lower suction pressures, so the surgeon must aim to completely clear the vitreous from the anterior chamber, away from the pupil margin (**16.23**), dividing all the anterior–posterior traction elements. The surgeon should never aspirate vitreous without cutting and should always beware of vitreous strands drawn out of the eye by instrumentation (**16.24**).

16.20

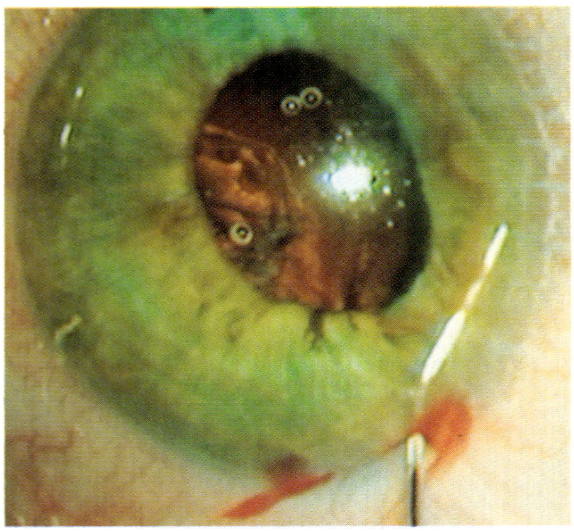

16.20 Using sodium hyaluronate to put adhesions under tension.

16.21

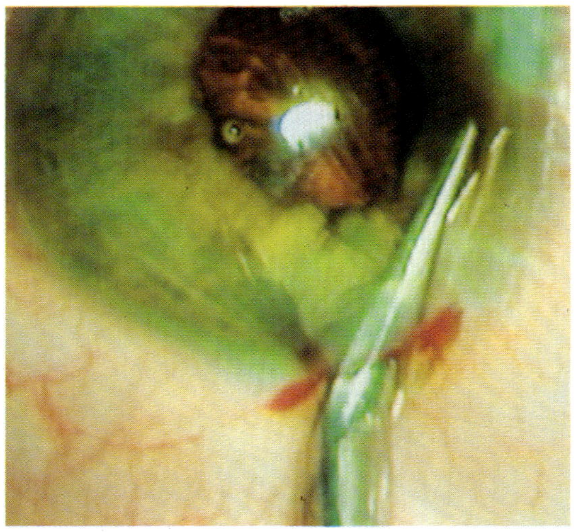

16.21 Using capsulotomy scissors (Ong) to cut an iris adhesion.

16.22

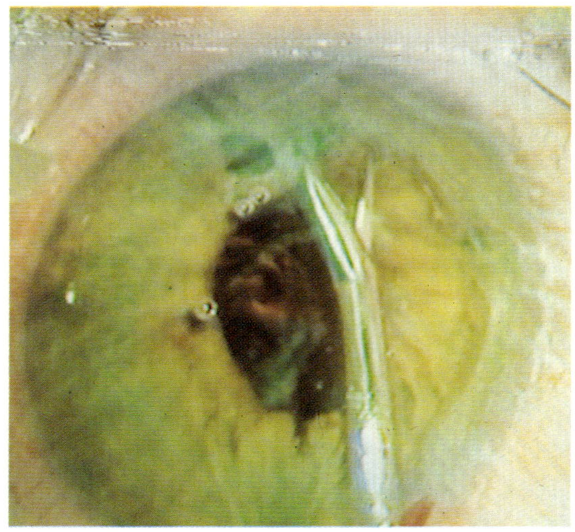

16.22 Using the microscissors (Grieshaber) to cut adhesions; note how much less corneal folding takes place than in (**16.21**).

16.23

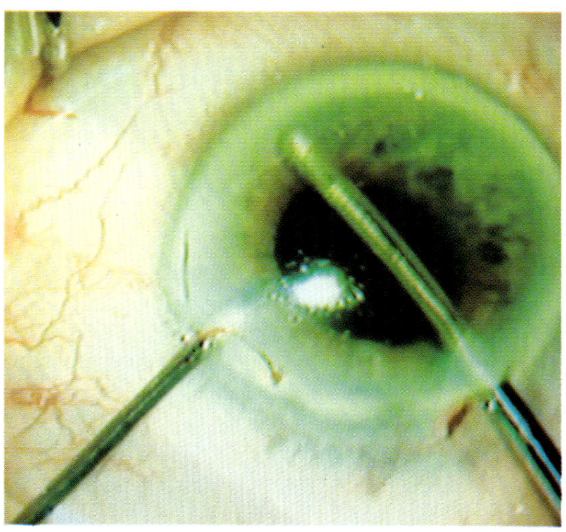

16.24

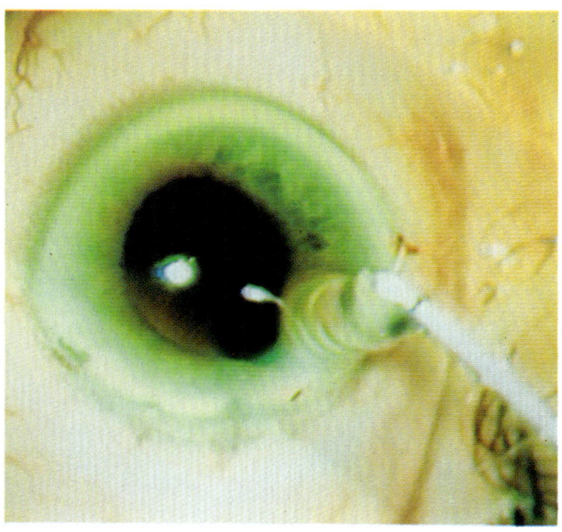

16.23 The anterior pupillary margin is cleared of vitreous using the two ports of entry into the eye.

16.24 Vitreous presenting as infusion cannula withdrawn.

The positions of infusion and cutting instruments may be reversed if this allows better access to the scar tissue and remaining incarcerated vitreous. Air is then introduced and the anterior segment carefully checked for the presence of vitreous (**16.25**). When the 'reconstruction' is complete, lens implantation can proceed as previously described.

At the end of the operation, cyclopentolate drops and a subconjunctival injection of antibiotic and steroid are given.

KEY POINTS FOR ANTERIOR SEGMENT RECONSTRUCTION
• At all times be aware of the extent and spread of vitreous: Leave no trace of vitreous in the anterior chamber. • Inadequate management of vitreous raises the incidence of CME and retinal detachment. • Pre-cut a partial groove for the lens implant section before fully entering the eye. • Use a closed microsurgical technique for anterior segment toilet and reconstruction. Use a bimanual technique and be prepared to interchange the instrumentation through the ports. • Maintain and define fluid compartments with viscoelastic agent and air. • Check intraocular lens position and ensure no tuck either of vitreous or iris.

16.25

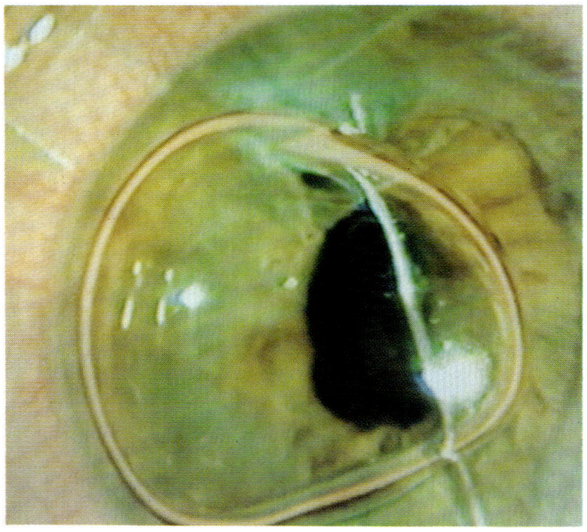

16.25 Use of air to inspect the anterior chamber and pupillary margins for the presence of vitreous.

Follow-up and complications

Topical steroids, such as betnesol and dexamethasone are used in combination with topical antibiotics. The pupil should be dilated postoperatively to prevent pupil block and iris bombé (**16.26, 16.27**).

During the first two postoperative months the steroids can be reduced in strength and frequency. Patients may require topical steroid for 4–6 months and many require one drop of predsol indefinitely.

16.26

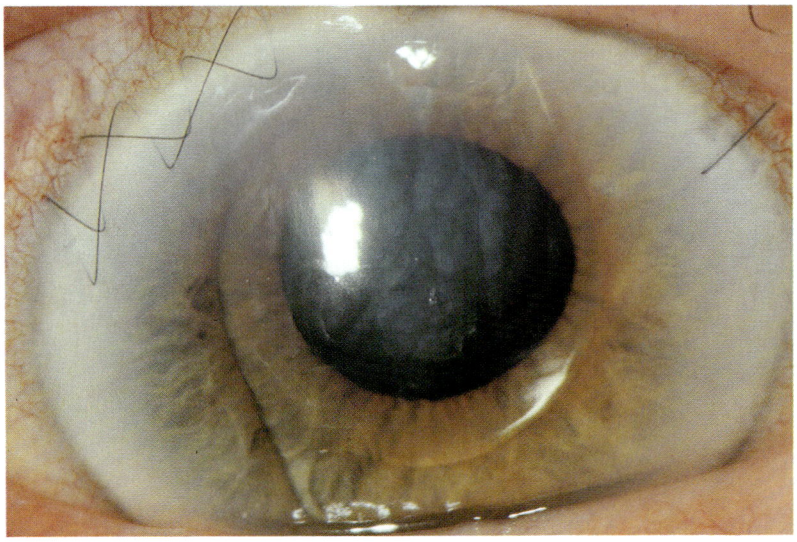

16.26 Pupil block and iris bombé.

16.27

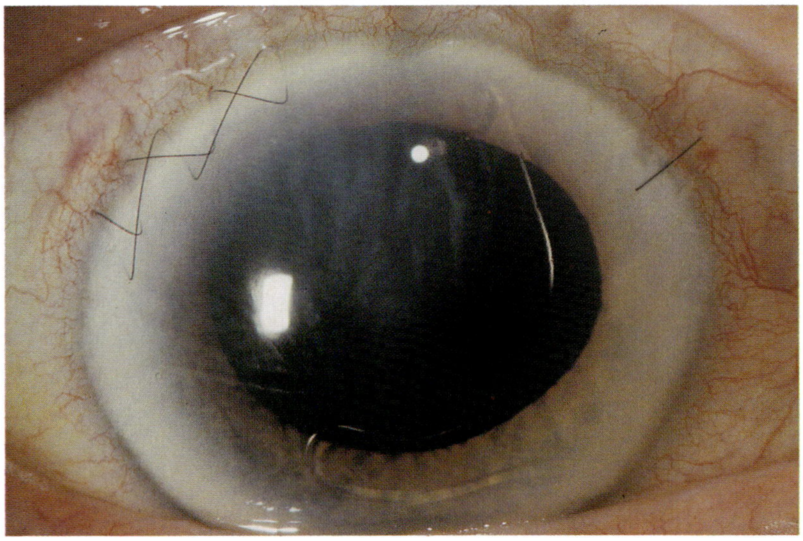

16.27 Same eye as in (**16.26**). The pupil block and iris bombé have been relieved by pupil dilation.

Continuing intraocular inflammation may lead to lens precipitates and these should be treated either by increasing the frequency or potency of topical steroid drops (**16.28**).

Retinal detachment is significantly increased by anterior–posterior vitreous traction and most commonly occurs when vitreous is incarcerated with anterior segment structures. Very fine vitreous threads may be easily divided by the neodymium YAG laser, although larger vitreous strands are not so easy to treat by this method.

Cystoid macular edema (CME) (**16.29**) may occur in any eye postoperatively, but vitreous incarceration, poor lens fit and chronic uveitis are important predisposing conditions. CME is a major cause of reduced vision in these patients. If a patient's visual acuity with a pinhole deteriorates, then they should be refracted. A demand for increased 'plus' suggests CME; funduscopy should confirm this. The use of acetazolamide is recommended by some to treat this condition. If this fails, systemic steroids may be worth trying. However, by anticipating the problem (e.g. treating a grumbling uveitis or dividing a vitreous strand) it may be prevented.

Glaucoma may develop because of pre-existing iris root and angle damage or pigment fall-out in the angle: But it can also be iatrogenic, very often steroid induced. If it persists despite curtailing steroid drops and is not adequately controlled on topical antiglaucoma therapy, then trabeculectomy may be considered. An anterior chamber IOL is not a contraindication to trabeculectomy, but sodium hyaluronate should be left in the eye at the end of the operation to help prevent lens–cornea touch if a shallow anterior chamber develops. A paracentesis should be carried out immediately prior to the trabeculectomy so that there is easy access into the anterior chamber should it become shallow postoperatively.

Immediate postoperative glaucoma may be due to pupil block if an anterior vitrectomy has not been performed (**16.30**) and the peripheral iridectomy is either imperforate or also blocked by vitreous. A neodymium YAG laser iridotomy is the treatment of choice once the intraocular pressure has been controlled medically and corneal clarity restored (**16.31**). If the iris is seen to be billowing around the IOL and the pressure is low, suspect a wound leak.

Ocular motility and fusional difficulties: Orthoptic treatment and assessment may be necessary. If binocular vision is a possibility prisms may be useful, but any previous squints will probably require surgical correction, preferably with the use of an adjustable suture.

Corneal decompensation: Any implant that is unstable and mobile may aggravate or cause corneal damage. The lens should be removed or

16.28

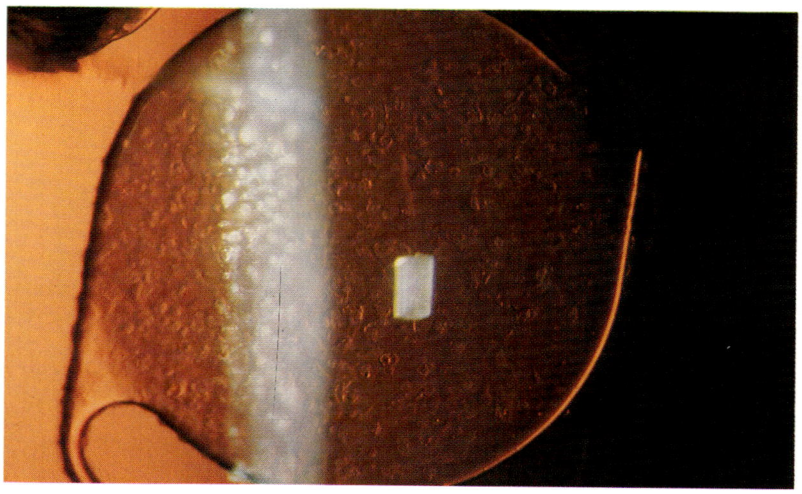

16.28 Lens precipitates requiring increasing frequency or potency of topical steroid.

16.29

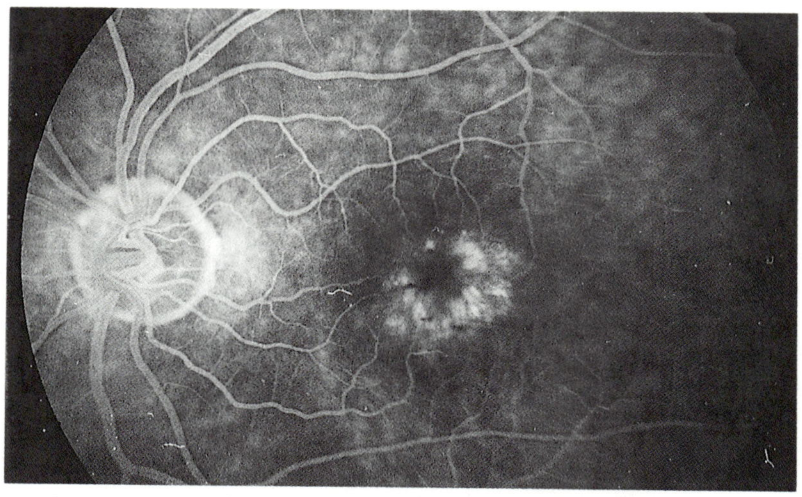

16.29 Fluorescein angiogram showing cystoid macular edema.

16.30

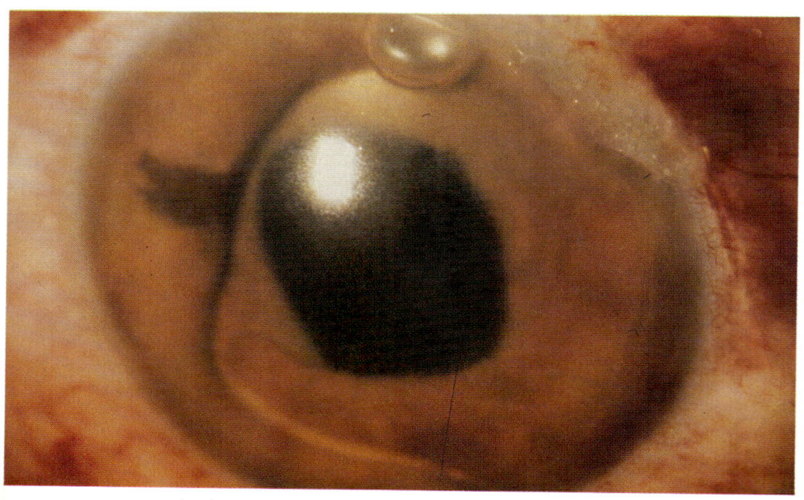

16.30 Postoperative glaucoma with corneal edema due to pupil block.

16.31

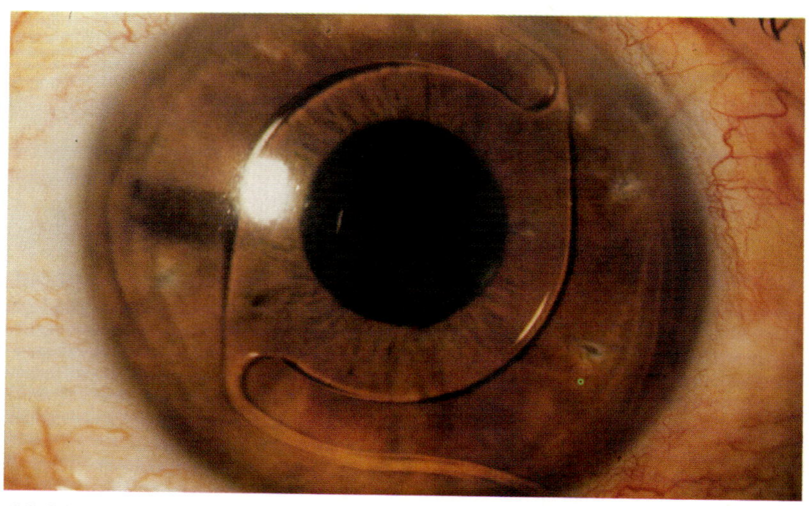

16.31 Same eye as in (**16.30**). Pupil block relieved by neodymium YAG iridotomies.

exchanged at the time of penetrating keratoplasty. Pseudophakic bullous keratopathy is often associated with CME and once the cornea has decompensated, penetrating keratoplasty, lens exchange and anterior vitrectomy (if necessary) should be undertaken without delay.

Prolonged postoperative pain is usually only a problem following implantation of an anterior chamber lens with rigid haptics. There is no specific treatment apart from instructing the patient not to rub the eye. Severe and persistent pain may require removal of the implant.

Results

The techniques described give good visual results (**Table 16.1**) with a lower serious complication rate, even in the disorganized eye, provided the vitreous is adequately managed. Not only may the quality of vision be improved compared with the use of other methods of correcting aphakia, but also the removal of membranes, capsule, etc., at the time of surgery, may substantially improve visual acuity (**16.32, 16.33**). The most frequent complication is long-term low-grade uveitis. However, secondary lens implantation should not be undertaken lightly, but by surgeons who are prepared to study and develop the microsurgical techniques outlined above.

16.32

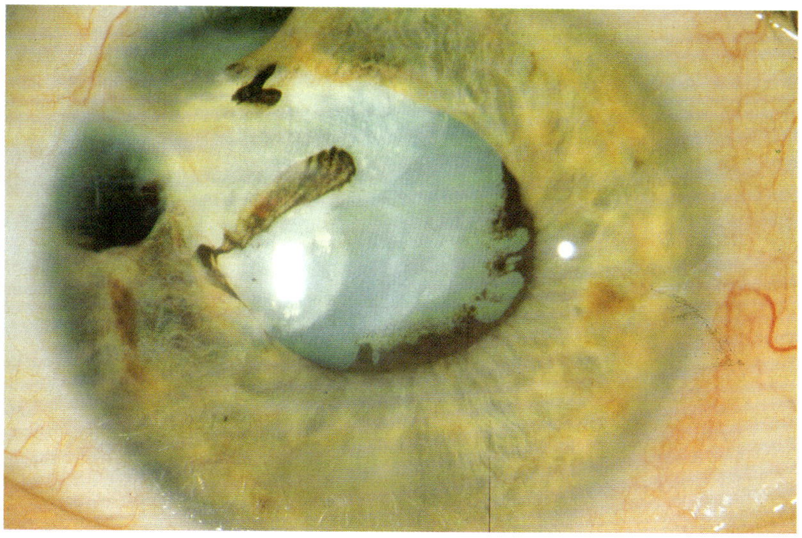

16.32 Traumatic cataract; initial penetrating injury has been repaired.

16.33

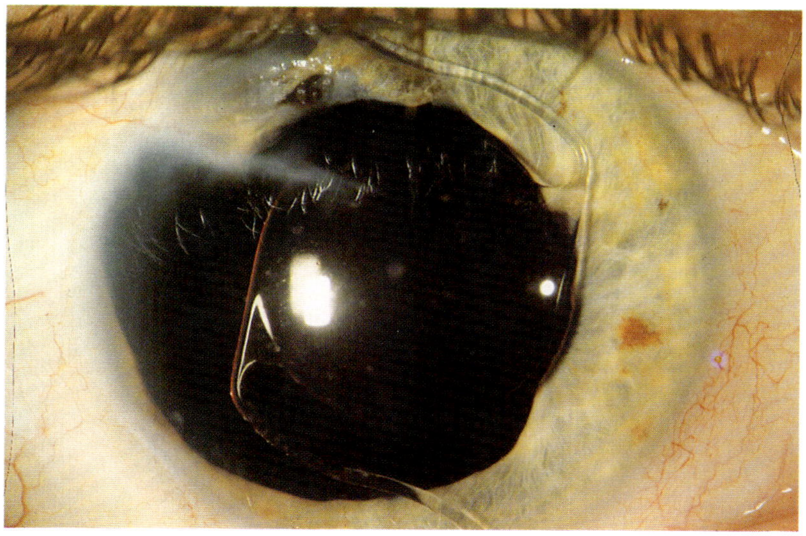

16.33 Same eye as in **16.32** after anterior segment reconstruction and secondary anterior chamber IOL implantation 15 years later.

Table 16.1 The change in visual acuity following surgery

Visual acuity (lines of Snellen)	*Noble*	*Kraff (1983)*	*Wong (1987)*	*Lindstrom (1984)*	*Shammas (1983)*	*Leather barrow (1988)*
Worse by 2 lines	7.8%	5%	4%	8.5%		
Worse	18.3%				3%	
No change	26.4%				42%	
Same ± 1 line	63.3%		72%	65.4%		
Better or within 1 line	92.2%	87%				83%
Better	55.3%				55%	
Better by 2 lines or more	28.9%		24%	26.1%		

Further reading

Kraff M.C., Lieberman H.L., and Saunders D.R. Secondary intraocular lens implantation: Rigid/semi-rigid versus flexible lenses. *J. Cataract Refract. Surg.*, **13,** 21–26, 1987.

Leatherbarrow B., Trevett A., and Tullo A.B. Secondary lens implantation: Incidence, Indications and Complications. *Eye*, **2,** 370–375, 1988.

Lindstrom R.L. and Harris W.S. Secondary anterior chamber lens implantation. *CLAO J.*, **10,** 133–136, 1984.

Shammas H.J.F. and Milkie C.F. Secondary implantation of anterior chamber lenses. *Am. Intra-ocular Implant Soc. J.*, **9,** 313–316, 1983.

Wong S.K., Koch D.D., and Emery J.M. Secondary intraocular lens implantation. *J. Cataract Refract. Surg.*, **13,** 17–20, 1987.

17: Looped posterior chamber lenses

Peter Agapitos and Richard Lindstrom

When choosing an implant style, a surgeon must utilize a lens that conforms well to his or her own operating technique. This is largely a personal choice. Different lens styles may be more appropriate for certain situations. For example, in the case of a zonular disinsertion or capsular rupture that may require sulcus fixation, some surgeons prefer the less flexible looped style of a single piece all polymethylmethacrylate (PMMA) implant and 13.5 mm loop span. When using the intercapsular technique, one may prefer lenses with closed or totally encircling loops, or short C-loop types with a loop span of less than 13 mm (**17.1, 17.2**).

The J-looped posterior chamber lens (PCL) was introduced by Shearing in 1977. This was a major advance in design because the loops could be compressed on insertion, yet re-expand within the posterior chamber to take up stable fixation. Initially, the lenses were uniplanar, but problems with pupil capture led Mazocco to suggest forward angulation. Other modifications were introduced by Simcoe, Sinskey, Kratz and others. Closed-loop posterior chamber implants were introduced by Anis (**17.3**), Harris, Galand, Knolle and Sheets for placement in the capsular sac. Lindstrom introduced the reversed or posterior convex optic with loops made of extruded PMMA. Up to this point, loops were made of polypropylene.

17.1

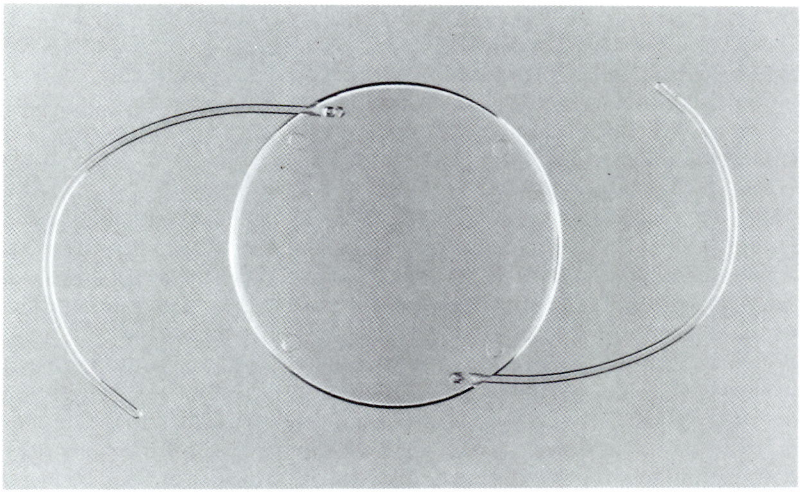

17.1 Three-piece biconvex PMMA lens with angulated short C-loops, 6.5 mm optic and 12.5 mm loop span for capsular fixation (courtesy of Dr Spencer Thornton, USA).

17.2

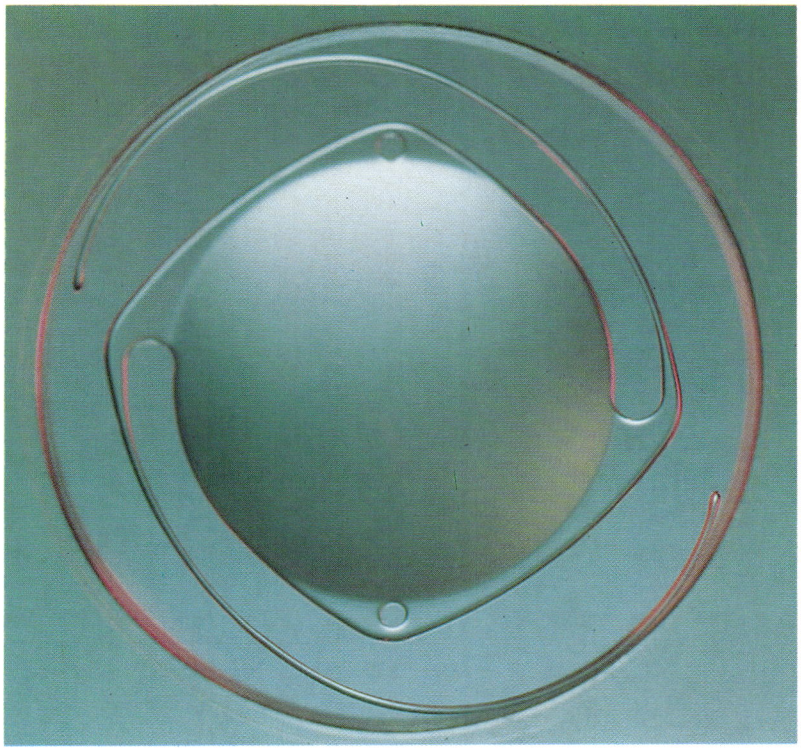

17.2 Lens with 6.5 mm optic and 12.5 mm loop span shown within a 10 mm ring indicating the smooth haptic spread within a space of this diameter (courtesy of Rayner Intraocular Lenses Ltd).

17.3

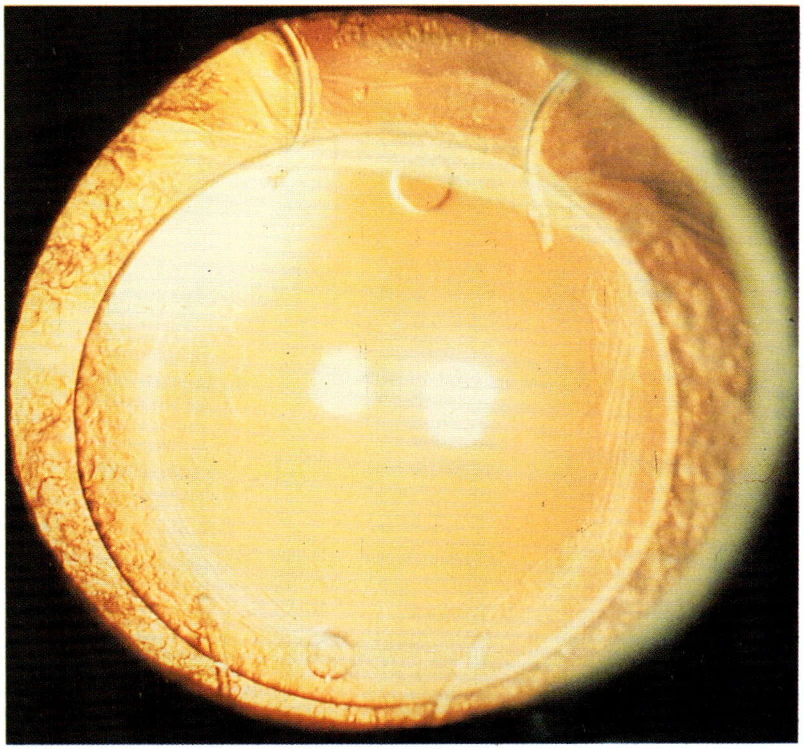

17.3 Convex posterior lens with closed-loop encircling haptics within the capsular bag. Note that the ingrowth of epithelium stops at the edge of the optic (right-hand border) and at the fibrous ring (inside left-hand border); see also p. 282. (Courtesy of Dr Aziz Anis, USA).

The broad group of implants comprising the J- and C-loop styles and their modifications are the most commonly used implants today. Arnott introduced a single piece, all-PMMA, posterior chamber implant with totally encircling loops, which facilitates implantation into the capsular sac and gives a broad fixation with more even pressure within the capsular fornix. Binkhorst has advocated the use of a 'Moustache lens' with the two haptics adjoining the same side of the optic for use with the intercapsular technique. Looped designs of soft intraocular lens implants, including silicone and hydrogel, have been introduced for small incision surgery and Kelman designed a 'phakofit' PMMA lens with collapsible wings. Charleux and Apple have proposed disc lenses with totally encircling haptics.

Intraocular lens design features

Loop design

The major issue in loop design is the type of material used. The use of polypropylene was advocated because of its flexibility and ability to conform to the space in which it was placed. Surgeons implanting in the ciliary sulcus felt that polypropylene would not exert undue pressure on the delicate tissues of the ciliary sulcus; however, polypropylene has been shown in autopsy eyes to erode into adjacent tissues despite the flexibility and apparent loss of memory of shape. In contrast, PMMA loops are more rigid and tend not to lose their memory, so theoretically are more likely to give rise to undue pressure and erosion when placed in the ciliary sulcus. Erosion of PMMA loops into the ciliary sulcus has not, however, been shown to be more common compared to polypropylene. Autopsy studies and clinical experience have shown that for capsular fixation, polypropylene loops are readily deformed (**17.4**) and more subject to the stresses of capsule contraction than PMMA, suggesting that the more rigid PMMA loops may be the more desirable and are less likely to be associated with decentration.

Newer manufacturing methods, using extruded PMMA and compression moulding technology, have improved the flexibility of PMMA loops. A wide range of flexibility now exists among the loops of one piece PMMA lenses and the more flexible one piece lenses have tended to supplant the three piece PMMA lenses. Laboratory studies have suggested that these single piece lenses have the least propensity for decentration. For comparison of the more flexible PMMA lenses now available, see **32.10** (p. 207).

Angulation of the loops is another design feature. Forward angulation by approximately 10° is desirable to increase the distance of the optic from the iris, so decreasing the incidence of pupillary capture and iris chafing. Forward angulation of the loops will also exert more pressure on the posterior capsule and, when associated with posterior vaulting of the optic, will increase IOL surface contact with the posterior capsule so decreasing the incidence of late opacification.

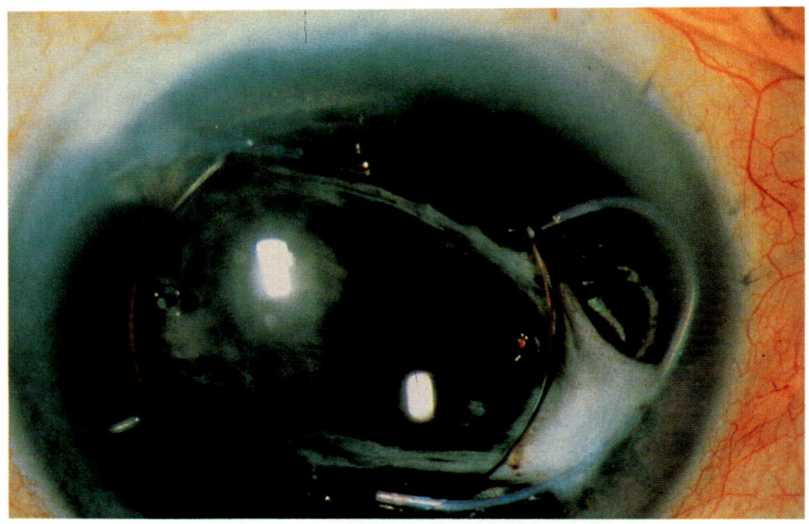
17.4

17.4 Clinical photograph of a PCL with modified J loops showing contraction forces from the capsular fibrosis, causing bending of the haptics towards the optic (courtesy of Dr James McCulley, USA).

Optic design

The configuration of the lens optic may be convex plano, plano convex (reverse optic), biconvex or meniscus. In terms of optical quality, the least amount of image degradation with decentration or tilt will occur with biconvex designs. Biconvex or plano convex implants offer a greater distance between the iris and the optic of the implant and require the highest *A* constants in the SRK formula for power calculation. By virtue of their contact with a posterior capsule, convex posterior or biconvex optic implants have been shown to retard capsular opacification (**17.3**). However, use of the YAG laser is more difficult with these lenses because there is a higher chance of pitting of the lens surface, although these pits are generally not visually significant.

The size of the optic may vary from 4.5 mm to 7 mm in diameter. A large optic may be ideal for patients with large pupils and offers more leeway in cases of minor decentration. However, this type of optic may be more difficult to insert, requiring a larger anterior capsulotomy and a two-handed maneuver for placement into the capsular sac. Optics smaller than 6 mm may lead to lens edge glare when the pupil dilates and should not be recommended for younger patients.

Holes, notches and ridges

Various types of control tips, such as that of Osher and Fenzel and that of Hunter, have been introduced to facilitate loop insertion. Loop indentations or notches have also been incorporated to aid insertion of the superior loop. Dialling holes on the optic may vary in number from one to four. When the optic is of small diameter, these may give rise to glare, particularly if the lens is decentered (**17.5**). The drilling of holes can often lead to polishing or manufacturing defects (**17.6**), allowing sites for iris incarceration or development of synechias. To obviate these problems it is recommended that all holes be placed exterior to the optic zone or at the optic haptic junction, or be omitted altogether. Various techniques for creating a central space between the posterior capsule and the IOL and, hopefully, at the same time creating a barrier to migration of lens epithelial cells, have been advocated. Meniscus optics and circumferential ridges were designed for this purpose, but have not been shown conclusively to retard capsular opacification. In fact the space will allow a more rapid proliferation of epithelium so that, while laser treatment may be facilitated, these modifications do incur a higher need for treatment and therefore are of doubtful benefit.

17.5

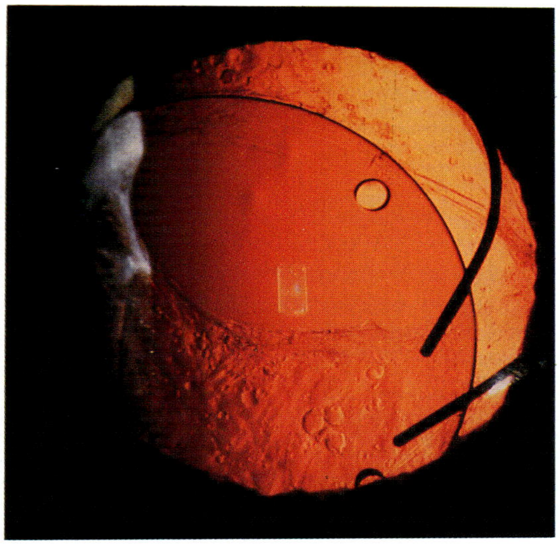

17.5 A decentered PCL with a positioning hole visible. In this patient, under normal conditions, the pupil was between 4 and 5 mm diameter. This positioning hole could cause glare.

17.6

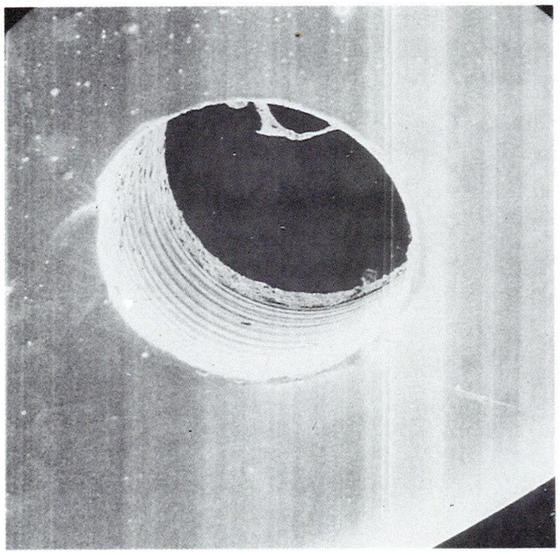

17.6 This modern PCL has surface roughness present, as seen by examining the positioning hole using scanning electron microscopy. This is a common manufacturing defect and, with present technology, should be avoidable (courtesy of Dr Douglas Cameron, USA).

IOL design and capsular opacification

It is believed that biconvex intraocular lens optics, by virtue of their broad and tight contact with the posterior capsule, can retard capsular opacification, thus decreasing the necessity for YAG capsulotomy. However, fibrotic changes can occur even with broad areas of contact and there is some evidence that biconvex or convex posterior lenses are associated with a higher incidence of fibrosis.

Pharmacological agents, such as the antimetabolite methotrexate or daunomycin, which is less toxic, are currently being evaluated in research laboratories as a means to prevent epithelial cell proliferation. Another experimental approach is to use a lens coating with cell-specific monoclonal antibodies conjugated to an epithelial cell toxin, which would cause cell lysis in the presence of complement, so destroying viable epithelial cells. Crosslinking the antibodies with a cytotoxic agent such as methotrexate would allow cell lysis without complement activation. It is also possible that a pharmacological agent could be bound to IOL surfaces.

IOL material

The advantages of PMMA as a material for both optic and haptic are that PMMA induces a minimal inflammatory response, is not adversely affected by ultraviolet (u.v.) light and is not biodegradable within the eye. Because of this, it maintains a smooth surface even when in contact with vascular and metabolically active tissue. Its disadvantage is that it is hard and hydrophobic. Chronic low grade inflammation can occur following posterior chamber intraocular lens implantation, the pathogenesis of which is unknown. One potential pathway is the activation of complement by the plastics themselves. Studies of the capability of PMMA to activate inflammation as measured by complement cascade activation and chemotaxis of PMNs have demonstrated that PMMA is less inflammatory than polypropylene. It also promotes less giant-cell reaction. Another factor is the effect of u.v. light, and it has been shown that polypropylene is sensitive to u.v. light exposure, which may cause a progressive reduction in tensile strength; a reason that this material has now been discarded for the haptics of lenses to be placed in the anterior chamber. Polypropylene is also subject to oxidative biodegradation, which may be enhanced by u.v. radiation and in turn can result in a rough surface with fissures and cracks (**17.7**), which may contribute to ocular inflammation.

Our experience with silicone implants in the laboratory has shown that they are also more reactive than PMMA. Hydrogel implants, which are hydrophilic, have been less reactive in the laboratory and current clinical studies are encouraging.

17.7

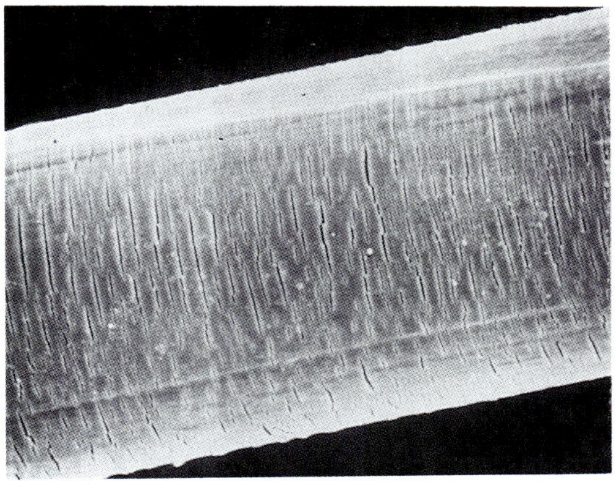

17.7 Polypropylene loop of a PCL which was removed for incorrect power, demonstrating haptic fissures and cracks, indicative of biodegradation (courtesy of Dr Douglas Cameron, USA).

Ultraviolet absorbing chromophores

The cornea absorbs u.v. radiation up to a wavelength of 300 nm, and the crystalline lens absorbs u.v. radiation between 300 and 400 nm. When cataract surgery is performed, the retina loses its natural protection from u.v. radiation, since PMMA transmits most of the u.v. energy between 300 and 400 nm. Concern about light-induced maculopathy from the operating room microscope has led to the availability of u.v. filters in ophthalmic microscopes.

U.v. filtration would seem to be desirable for the pseudophakic patient. Several animal studies have shown the damaging effects of u.v. radiation on the posterior segment, but there is little clinical evidence for this in humans. The incidence of angiographic cystoid macular edema has been shown to be lower in u.v.-filtered pseudophakic patients; however, there are no clinical trials that demonstrate a significant difference between u.v.-filtered and non-u.v.-filtered patients in terms of visual acuity.

There are two approaches to the process of incorporating u.v.-absorbing chromophores into PMMA. One is to prepare a mixture of the u.v.-absorbing additive with PMMA resin (additive system) and the second approach uses chemical bonding in which the chromophore is bound to the PMMA polymer. The chemical bonding system is technically more difficult. The additive method is prone to loss of the chromophore during different stages in the manufacturing process, and the possible slow migration or loss of the additive over time, once it is in the eye, is a potential concern.

The chromophores are either hydroxyphenylbenzotriazoles or hydroxybenzophenones. By a process called phototautomerism, u.v. light energy is absorbed and converted into heat, which in an IOL would cause a temperature change in the range of a fraction of a degree. The long-term stability of these materials appears to be good. There does not appear to be significant loss of the chromophore over time or with YAG laser damage.

At present, over 80% of ophthalmologists in the United States use IOLs with u.v.-absorbing chromophores, but surgeons should be aware that the absorption characteristics vary with different IOL manufacturers, and that the long-term effects are still unknown.

Manufacturing techniques

Two types of PMMA are currently used in IOL manufacture. Perspex CQ has a high molecular weight in the range of 1,200,000–1,600,000 and this is the PMMA which Ridley used for his early IOLs. In this state, the PMMA can be prepared by lathe-cutting, compression-casting or cast-molding techniques. Injection molded PMMA is of a lower molecular weight (80,000–140,000) and is used to produce IOL optics as well as extruded PMMA loops.

In order for the IOL surface to be smooth, a manufacturing method is used called tumble polishing. The sterilization process usually consists of ethylene oxide gas sterilization, since PMMA cannot be autoclaved.

Manufacturing defects have been found to occur in modern IOLs inspected from the shelf. Most of the defects, which included surface roughness (polishing defects) and sharp burrs present at the loop optic junction in IOLs with staked haptics, are evident on inspection with the operating microscope. It is important for each surgeon to inspect the quality of implants prior to insertion and to discard those with defects. In our laboratory explanted IOLs have been shown to have manufacturing defects in 40% of cases (**17.8**).

17.8

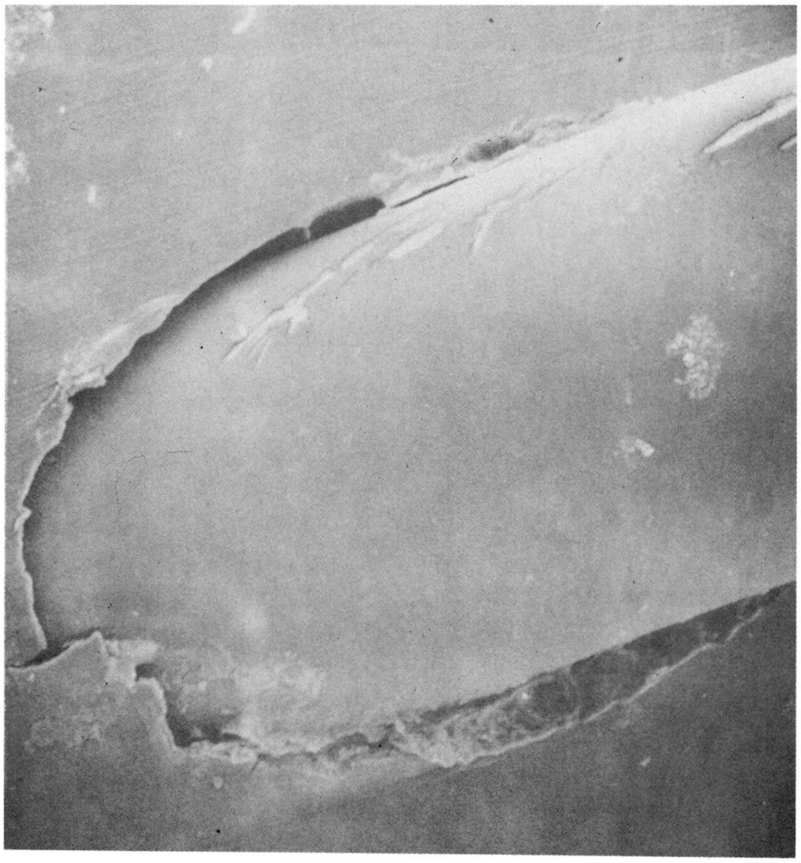

17.8 An explanted PCL showing, on scanning electron microscopy, manufacturing faults at a loop optic junction (courtesy of Dr Douglas Cameron, USA).

Surface modification of implants

In an effort to decrease surgical trauma to tissues in contact with IOLs during insertion and to prevent ongoing damage to tissues in contact with IOLs after insertion, various methods of surface modification of PMMA have been proposed. These include plasma fluorination of the IOL surface, surface passivation and the binding of various substances to the IOL surface (chondroitin sulfate, hydrogels, heparin, viscoelastics). Some of these methods are designed to make the IOL hydrophilic (e.g. addition of hydrogel or heparin), and some have been designed to make the IOL hydrophobic and oleophobic (surface passivation).

Although PMMA has not been found to degrade within the eye, inflammatory cell precipitates are often seen on the anterior surface after implantation (**17.9**) and, although postoperative inflammation may be related to factors other than IOL material or surface characteristics, surface modification may be useful in cases where inflammation may be expected, as in uveitis or glaucoma patients (**17.10**).

Surface passivation is a proprietary process designed to modify the IOL so that it is oleophobic and hydrophobic, thus repelling lipids, including cell membranes and ocular tissues. This process has been designed to decrease surface irregularity of tumble polished PMMA by reorienting the IOL surface molecules through the sequential exposure of chemical reagents. This modification, which is not supposed to change the PMMA and not add any molecules or substances to the PMMA, decreases surface energy and increases the contact angle with water.

Hydrogels, such as polyvinylpyrolidone (PVP), have been covalently bonded to PMMA in order to make the IOL surface more hydrophilic. The surface coating is 5 μ in thickness and designed to be permanent, but there is concern that PVP may be released from the IOL surface with the passage of time and lead to toxic effects.

Plasma grafting of polyacrylic acid and chondroitin sulfate onto PMMA in a permanent fashion has also been proposed.

In heparin surface modification of PMMA, the PMMA is subjected to oxidative treatment which adds negative charges to the surface. Polyethylenimene is then electrostatically adsorbed to the negatively charged PMMA, and heparin is bound by a secondary amine linkage. This type of chemical bond is permanent. These lenses are hydrophilic; however, in the dry state, they are hydrophobic and need to be soaked for several minutes prior to insertion.

It is also possible for the IOL to be used as a vehicle for drug release: antibiotics and anti-inflammatories may be mixed with a biocompatible viscoelastic agent and reversibly bound to an implant. This may be useful in patients not able to use postoperative medications. The potential for use of inhibitory drugs to prevent capsular opacification has also been proposed.

17.9

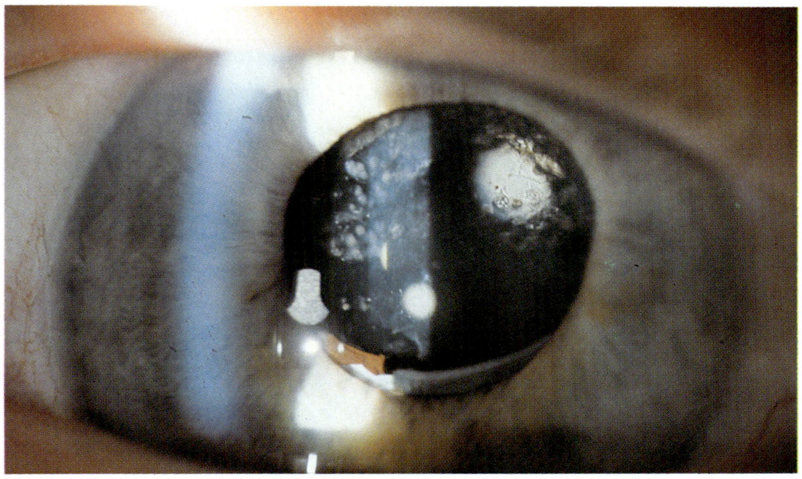

17.9 Slit lamp photograph of a standard one piece PMMA lens implanted in the capsular sac. The pupil has been dilated to show precipitates on the anterior surface of the optic and a posterior synechia at 7 o'clock. This eye showed no overt iridocyclitis, either preoperatively or postoperatively.

17.10

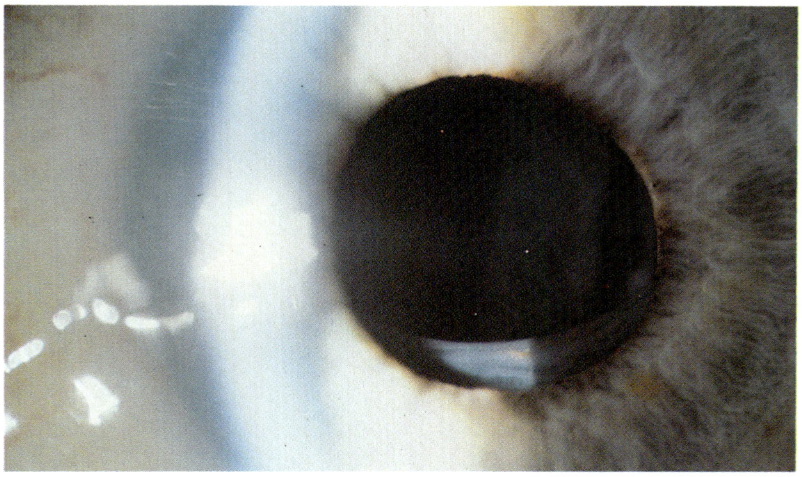

17.10 Slit lamp photograph of the fellow eye of the same patient as in **17.9**. There had been six episodes of iridocyclitis during the five years before surgery. The photograph was taken six months after implantation of a heparin-modified lens (covalently bonded). Note the space between the iris and lens capsule, and the absence of precipitation on the lens surface.

Choice of posterior chamber lens implant

Our preferences are for all-PMMA implants, of either three piece or single piece constuction, with flexible modified C-loops (**17.11**). The flexibility of a single piece implant depends not only on the haptic material but also on the haptic junction area. A large biconvex optic without positioning holes is also preferred. The type of implant that a surgeon will use is largely one of personal choice. The larger the optic, the more difficult it is to insert into the capsular bag. We prefer an optic size of 6.5 mm and, in order to manipulate the optic and haptic in the capsular bag, it is usually necessary to use a second instrument to tip the optic posteriorly (**17.12**). Not every surgical case is alike and the occurrence of a complication may necessitate a change of style. The principles listed in this chapter should give the implant surgeon a thinking framework within which a rational decision can be made as to the most suitable style to use.

17.11

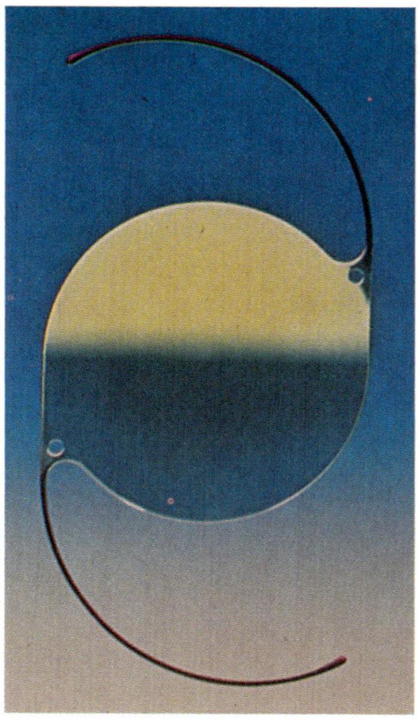

17.11 Preferred style of 6.5 mm biconvex optic, all-PMMA implant with modified C loops, single piece construction, and a loop span of 13.5 mm (photograph courtesy of Iolab).

17.12

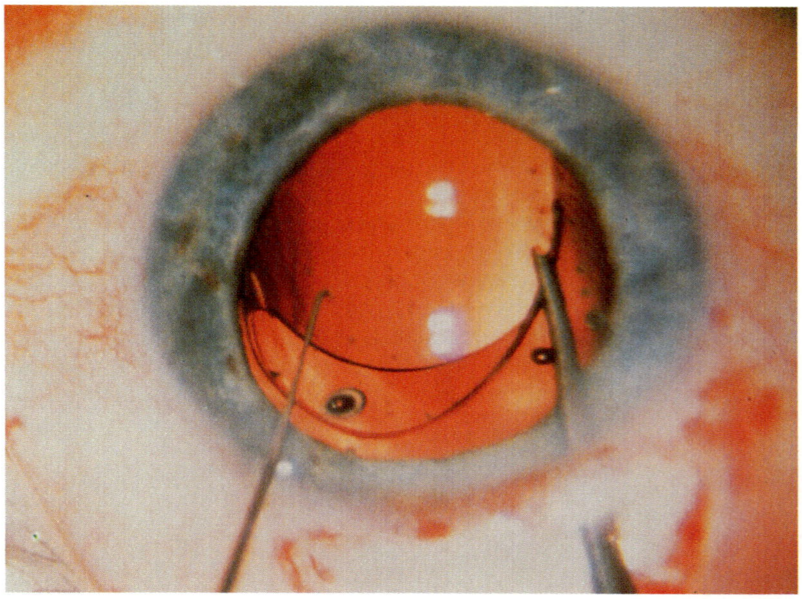

17.12 When using an optic of 6.5 mm or larger, a two-handed maneuver is usually necessary to insert the optic and haptic into the bag.

18: The disc lenses

Albert Galand

The concept of disc lenses for capsular bag fixation evolved from the author's consideration of 14 different lens models during a four year period using the intercapsular envelope technique. The principal complication from this study was clinical decentration. The lowest rates of decentration were obtained with the Anis implant, which has an almost circular shape with closed loops, and the Pearce tripod lens, which is totally rigid, suggesting that a circular configuration with a rigid structure would lead to an improvement of centering in the long term.

The inherent disadvantages of loops are:

- Two points of attachment to the optic that create an axis around which the optic may pivot. This may lead to iris capture or, more commonly, to capture of the anterior capsule.
- A 'spring-like' force acting against a capsule that has a thickness of only 10 μ, and that may lead to compression of adjacent structures. Without this force, the implant may rotate in the bag leading to the possible exit of one loop into the sulcus and to decentration.
- Highly flexible loops may not compress adjacent structures, but also do not permit the implant to resist postoperative forces in the capsular bag without some displacement (**18.1, 18.2**).

Standard lens implants are seven or eight times lighter in water than the human crystalline lens. It appears that this is unnecessary and that the PMMA disc lenses, which are 3 to 4 times lighter in water, provide a sufficient margin of safety. The zonular system has less to support after the operation than before. Although the original Epstein implant was placed in the posterior chamber, the disc lens is designed only for capsular fixation. The diameter of the disc (**18.3**) was chosen by taking into account the exact measurements of the sac on 49 cadaver eyes, which showed a mean diameter of 10.32 mm and a range of measurements from 9.25 to 11.25 mm.

18.1

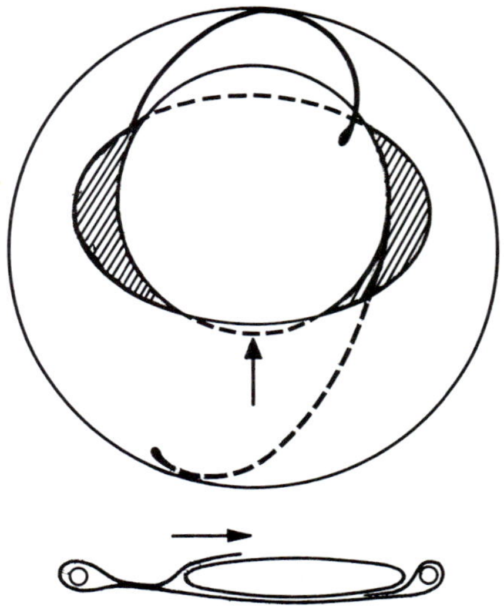

18.2

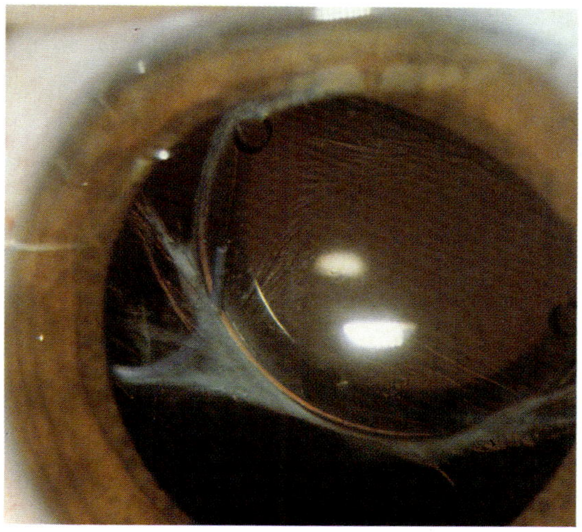

Several advances since the beginning of the 1980s have made it possible to take advantage of the simplicity of the disc implant:

- The envelope technique (**18.4**) permits a precise pupillary zone capsulectomy, leaving adequate anterior capsule over the implant. Loops are not needed to fix or maintain the implant in position.
- The use of viscoelastic agents to expand the capsule prior to implantation.
- The YAG laser for posterior capsule opacification, because, as disc implants completely fill the pupillary zone even in mydriasis, they make surgical capsulotomy a difficult procedure.

18.3

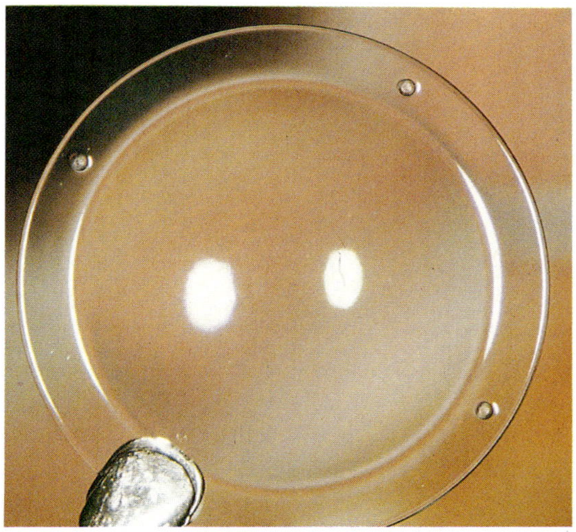

18.4

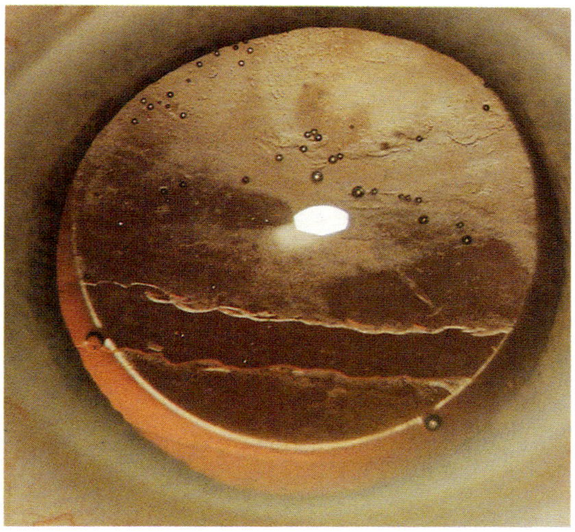

18.1 A cause of decentration (arrows) with soft loops is the squeezing or 'peapodding' effect resulting from fusion of leaves of the capsule.

18.2 Decentration of flexible closed loop implant caused by 'peapodding' effect.

18.3 The 9 mm rigid disc lens.

18.4 A 9 mm rigid disc inside the envelope, before making a U-capsulectomy. Note the wide mydriasis to improve visibility.

Results

The experiences resulting from insertion of 1,737 disc implants (**18.4, 18.5**) are summarized below. An advantage is:

- Consistent centration whether the disc is of 8 or 9 mm diameter (**18.6**).

However, there are several inherent disadvantages:

- A wide incision of 9 mm is necessary for insertion.
- Fixation is directly dependant on the conservation of a significant portion of anterior capsule. If the capsulotomy is too large, retraction of the anterior leaflets may lead to pupillary block (**18.7, 18.8**), which occurred in 0.3% of cases.
- A back-up lens is required in cases of posterior capsule rupture.
- The complete separation of anterior from posterior capsule (**18.9**) inhibits Soemmering ring formation and opacification of the posterior capsule is more common (**18.10**) than with regular implants using smaller optics (**18.11**).

18.5

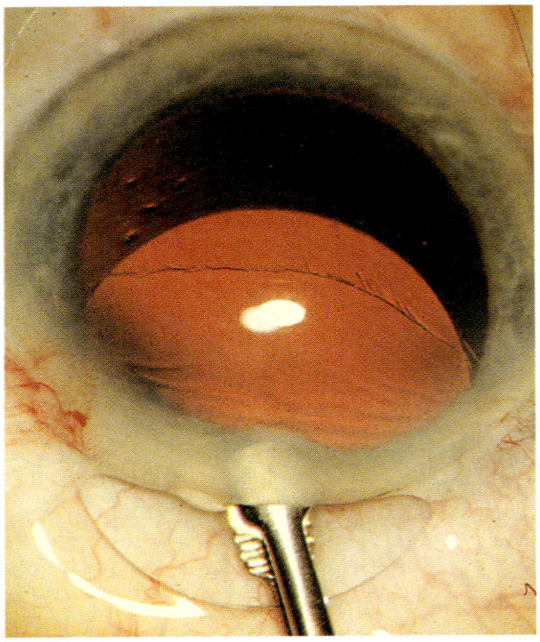

18.5 Insertion of the 8 mm rigid disc into the bag of the lens capsule.

18.6

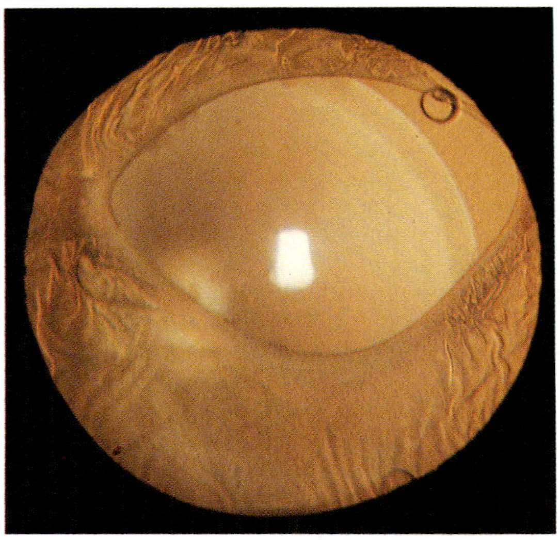

18.6 Rigid disc lens, well-centered despite asymmetrical capsular flaps.

18.7

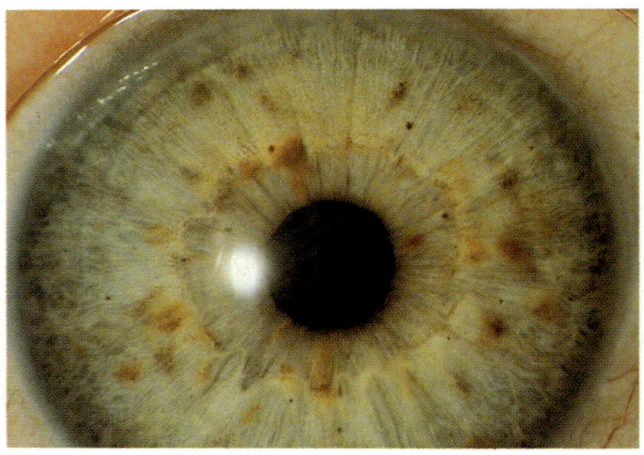

18.7 Pupillary block due to retraction of the capsular flaps behind an 8 mm rigid disc lens.

18.8

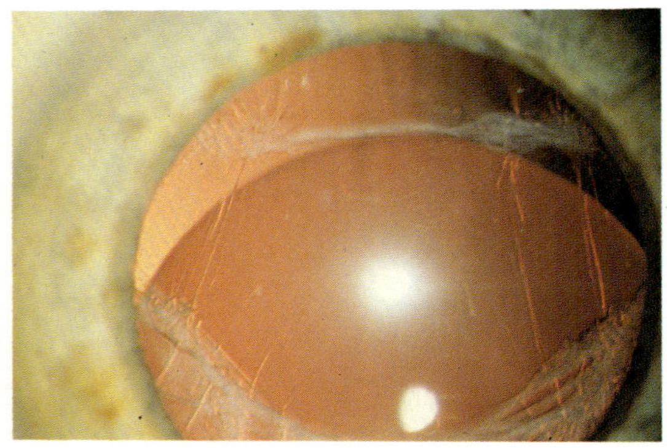

18.8 Same eye as in **18.7**. Slit lamp examination on mydriasis showed anterior capsular flaps behind the implant.

18.9

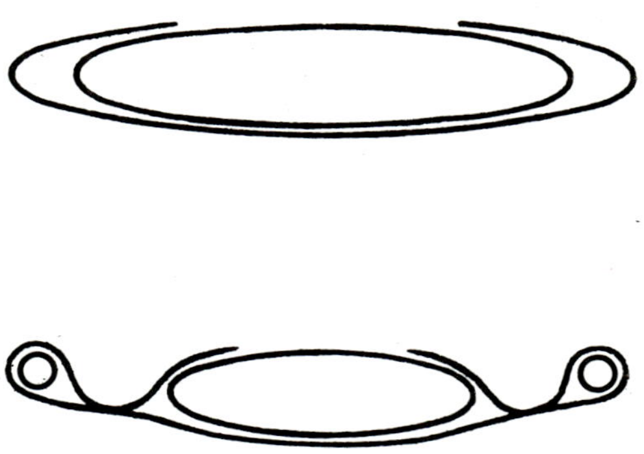

18.9 Large optics separate the capsules. Small optics permit fusion of the anterior capsule margin with the posterior capsule, which often results in a Soemmering ring. Adhesion of the anterior capsule margin with the optic edge will give space for a Soemmering ring only when the optic is small.

18.10

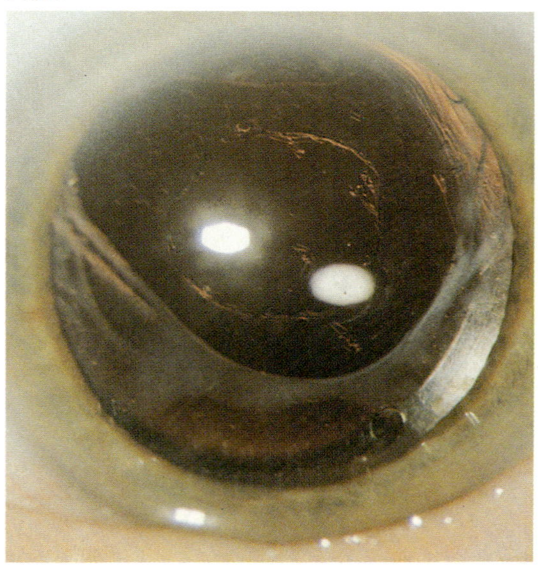

18.10 Rigid disc lens. The posterior capsule was opened by a neodymium YAG laser.

18.11

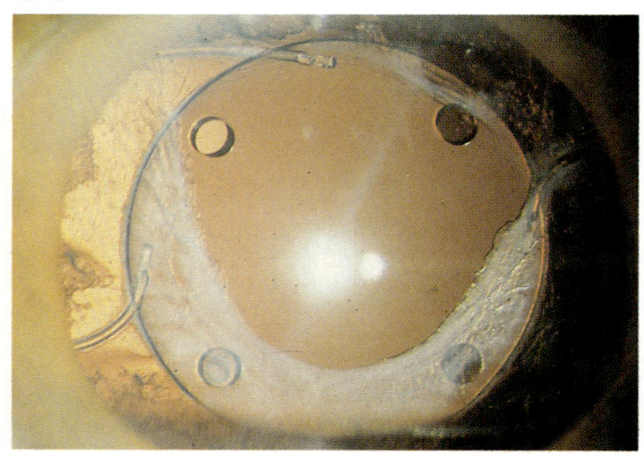

18.11 Closed loop implant three years after surgery. Note the proliferation of epithelium imprisoned in a Soemmering ring. The central posterior capsule remains clear.

The compressible disc

The above observations led to development of the Compressible Disc (CD) lens. The basic CD design (**18.12**) consists of a 6 mm biconvex optic attached by 2 'bridges', one each at 6 and 12 o'clock, to a flexible continuous ring (**18.13**). CD construction comprises single-piece PMMA with a total diameter of 9 mm, although wider diameters are possible.

For insertion, the CD is held with forceps at either point where the optic is 'bridged' to the haptic. The implant is slid through the limbal incision, towards the linear capsulotomy and then into the capsular bag (**18.14**). Once inside, the CD is pushed in the direction of 6 o'clock until it just reaches the inferior equator.

The next step is passage of the implant behind the superior capsular flap. A Rycroft cannula, attached to a perfusion line, is held in the dominant hand and a Sinskey hook is held in the other. The tip of the hook is placed in a positioning hole and the implant is lowered towards 6 o'clock. Simultaneously, the Rycroft cannula, using its irrigation, is slid under the superior capsular flap. Moving the cannula tip upwards and towards the front slips the superior capsular flap over the edge of the implant (**18.15**).

18.12

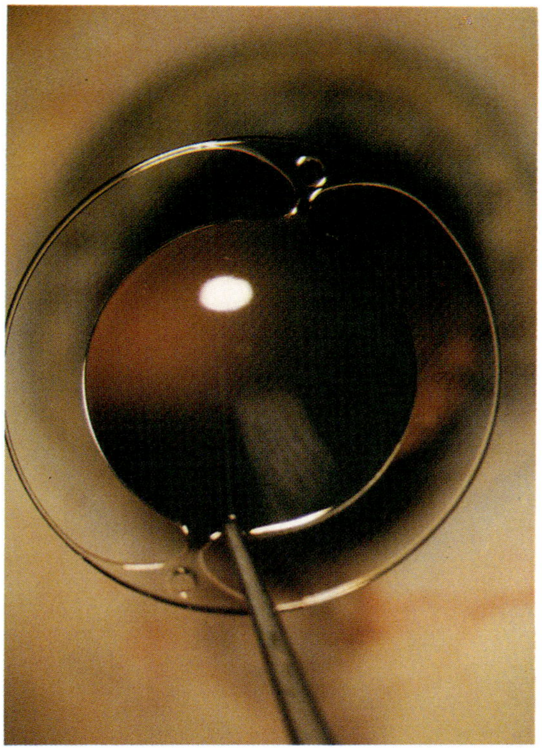

18.12 The compressible disc.

18.13

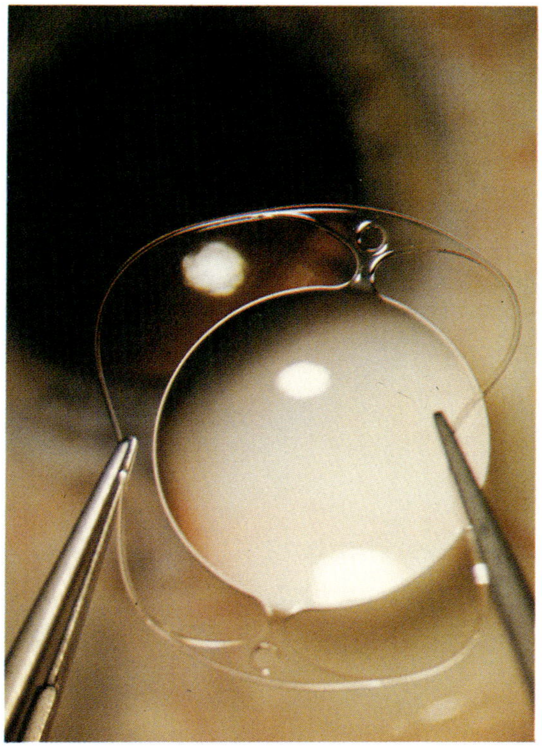

18.13 Shows flexibility of the CD lens, which can be inserted through a 6 mm incision. However, the rigidity is sufficient to resist 'peapodding' forces.

18.14

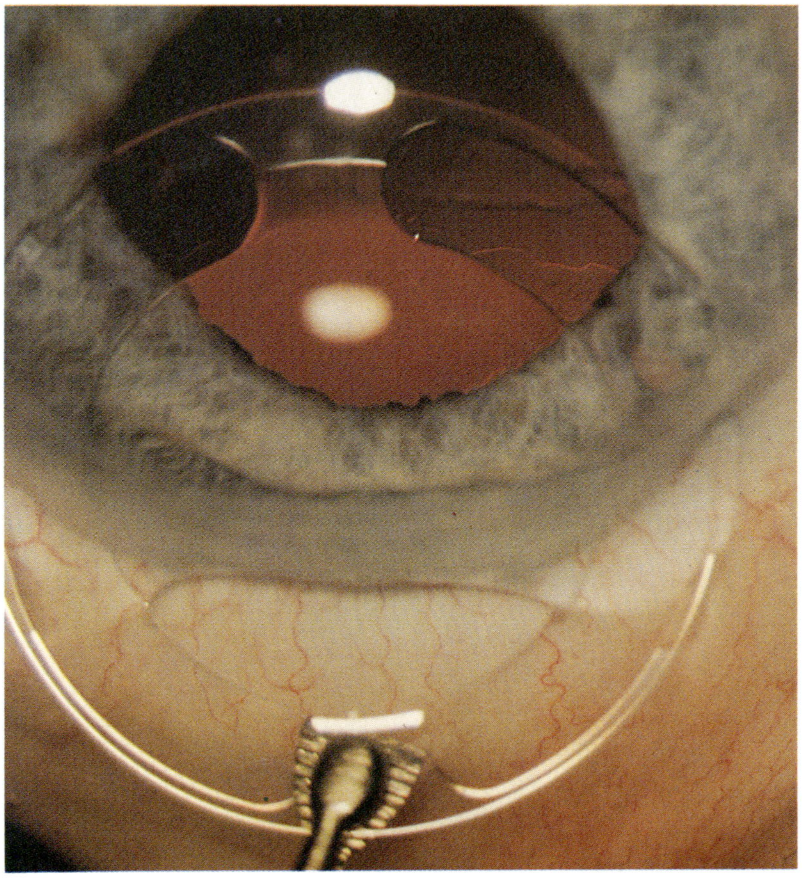

18.14 Insertion of a CD lens, held with Shepard forceps, into the envelope of the lens capsule in an eye with poor mydriasis.

18.15

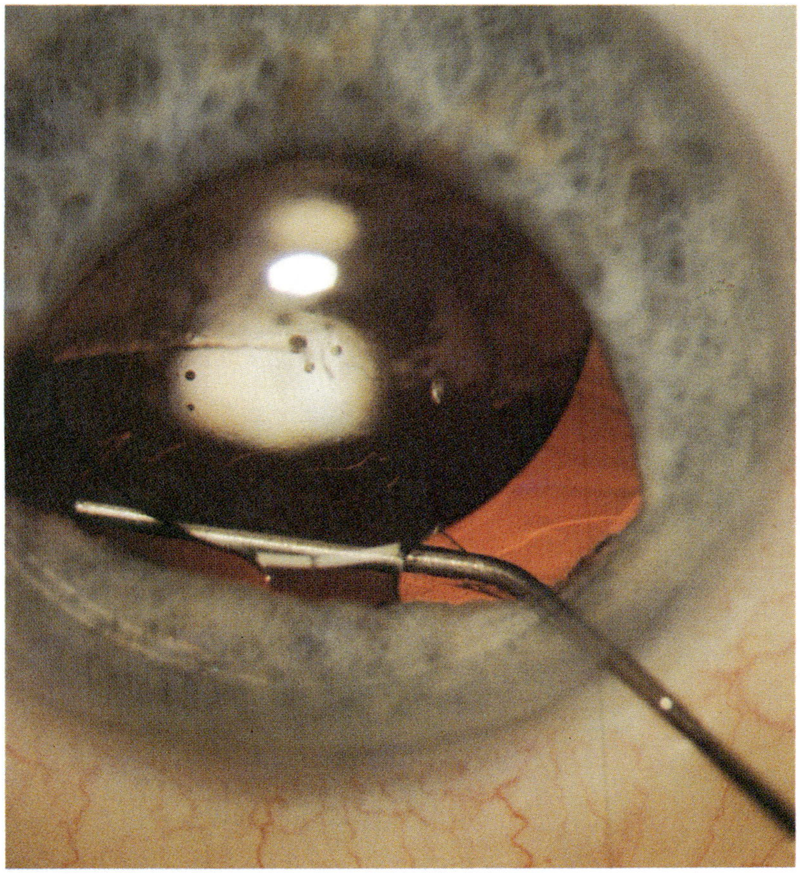

18.15 Same eye as in **18.14** showing placement of the superior capsular flap over the upper pole with a Rycroft cannula.

The Sinskey hook may be replaced with a 'Y' hook set against the edge of the optic. If there is excellent mydriasis, it may be possible for the superior flap to be correctly placed single-handed with a 27- or 30-gauge cannula. An alternative is to rotate the lens with a dialling hook 90°, then compress the outer flexible ring of the lens downwards with a notched probe in one hand using a capsule retractor in the other (p. 100).

More than 600 CD lenses have now been inserted without the occurrence of implant-related complications. The lens appears to provide a good compromise between the advantages of rigid discs and the advantages of implants with loops (**18.16**).

18.16

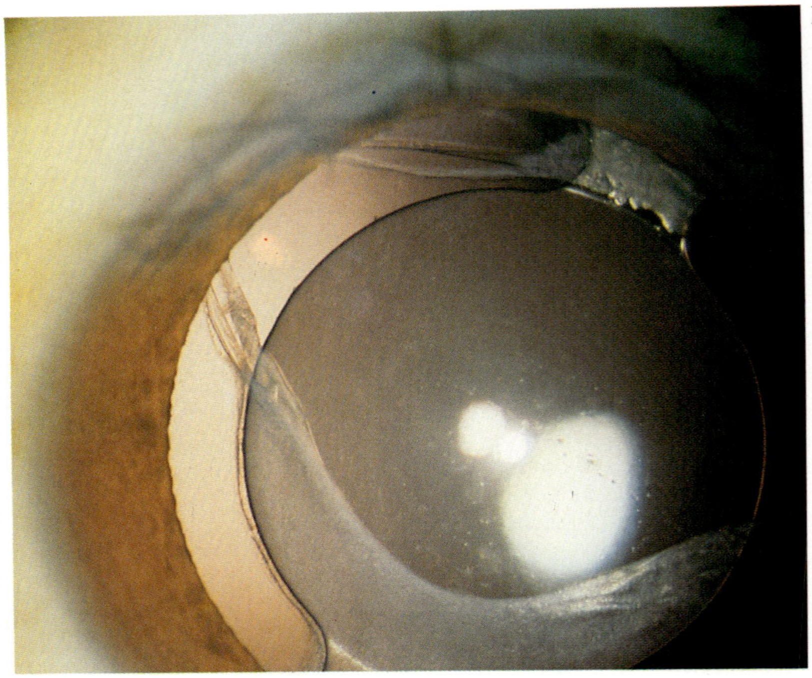

18.16 CD lens 3 months postoperatively. The inferior capsular flap may clasp the optic, but there is sufficient space outside the optic for a Soemmering ring to form.

Further reading

Galand A., Bonhomme L., and Collee M. Direct measurement of the capsular bag, *Am. Intra-ocular Implant Soc. J.* **10,** 475–476, 1984.

Tetz M., O'Morchoe D., Gwin T., Wilbrandt T., Solomon K., Hansen S., and Apple D. Posterior capsular opacification and intraocular lens decentration. Part II: Experimental findings on a prototype circular intraocular lens design. *J. Cataract Refract. Surg.* **14,** (6), 614–623, 1988.

19: Soft intraocular lenses: evolution and potential

Michael Blumenthal and Varda Chen

Polymethylmethacrylate (PMMA) was and still is the major plastic material used for intraocular lenses (IOLs). The main concerns for biocompatibility are: lens material, optical properties, loop material, lens design, and manufacturing. PMMA has been proven to have excellent optical properties but, in spite of its acceptance, there is ongoing research for IOL coating materials, and different lens materials in order to improve biocompatibility and, in particular, to find a material that would reduce or abolish the harmful effect on endothelium caused by the touch of PMMA.

In the mid 1970s the concept of intraocular lenses composed of soft materials was explored by Epstein (hydrogel posterior chamber implants), followed by Mehta and Parker with hydrogel iris supported implants. In the late 1970s Blumenthal started basic research with hydrogel material and its effect on the eye tissue and, later, with clinical studies on humans, to be followed by Barrett (hydrogel implant) and Mazzocco (silicone implants). Hydrogel and silicone implants are both considered as soft lenses, but except for their softness they do not share any other biological or chemical characteristics. Hydrogel, which is hydrophilic, was the first soft material to be investigated, and was found to be more biocompatible with the endothelium. However, it did not gain popularity since sodium hyaluronate had already been introduced to overcome the possible endothelial damage from PMMA touch. The enthusiasm for hydrogels subsided, but rose again with the interest in small incision surgery.

A small incision has a variety of benefits, but the size of the lenses negated the advantages, since the wound has to be enlarged to allow IOL insertion. Lenses made of soft materials, such as silicone (which is hydrophobic) and hydrogel (which has variable size and physical properties according to the state of hydration), are compressible and foldable, and therefore may be suitable for small incision surgery.

Utilizing the physical property of hydrogels, which are water swollen polymers, enables the production of a lens design that is much smaller when dry than a conventional PMMA lens. The dehydrated hydrogel lens can be inserted through a small incision and, on subsequent hydration within the eye, will become larger and more flexible, taking up its ideal position within the capsular bag.

From our relatively short clinical experience with soft lenses, both silicone lenses and hydrogel lenses have good biocompatible qualities. Besides being suited to small incision surgery, they are less irritant to iris pigment epithelium and less pigment dispersion occurs in cases of direct touch with this tissue. In cases of eye trauma or eye rubbing, the soft lenses are more pliable than PMMA lenses, owing to their softness and flexibility.

It seems that in some cases a soft implant may be more favorable than the traditional rigid PMMA lens. For example, in a patient with a low grade uveitis where a minimum foreign body reaction will lead to a greater tolerance to the implant, in young patients who may be expected to have an implant for many years, and in the presence of a posterior capsule rupture where the implant can still be implanted utilising the Sheet's glide effect of the plated lens. Soft IOLs may decrease the potential for pigmentary glaucoma and also provide an added margin of safety for patients with blood dyscrasias and other disorders because of their nonadhesive properties. Theoretically, all soft lens materials have the potential for intraocular torque by fibrosis of the lens capsule, iris distortion or synechia formation. Clinical experience will show whether this produces changes in lens power, astigmatism, or optical aberrations.

Silicone lenses

Silicone elastomers (elastic polymers) are composed of highly cross-linked polysiloxane chains to which organic functional groups have been appended. The most common silicone elastomers used in medicine are cross-linked polydimethylsiloxane (PDMS) polymers, which are obtained from a chemical process that begins with a heat-catalyzed reaction involving silica and graphite. Silicone devices are biologically inert. They are coplanar in profile with web-like haptics (**19.1**) or prolene haptics (**19.2**).

19.1

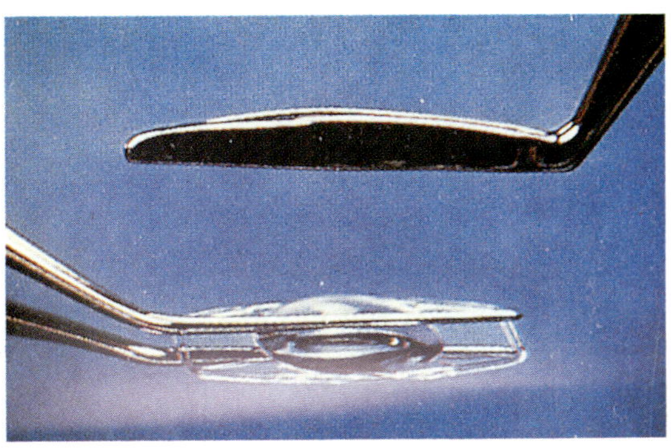

19.1 Silicone IOL with web-like haptics and Faulkner folder (courtesy of Implants in Ophthalmology).

19.2

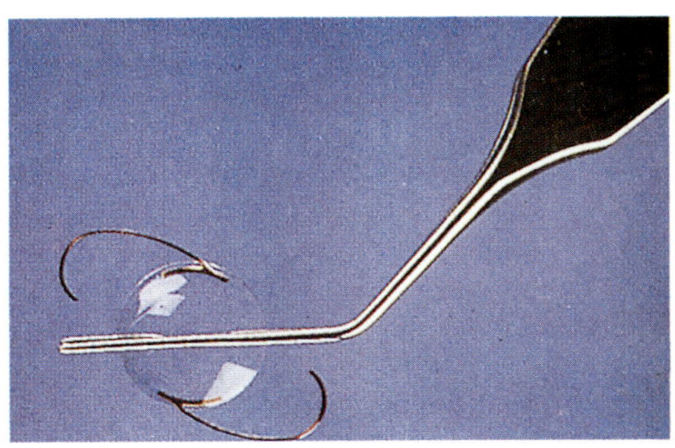

19.2 Silicone IOL with prolene haptics in the Sinskey–Kratz style (courtesy of Implants in Ophthalmology).

The silicone implant's great advantage is that it is compressible and can be inserted through a small incision by folding (**19.3–19.6**) However, silicone has a lower refractive index than PMMA, hence the lens is thicker, and this may be an impediment to a very high power. Silicone lenses are homogeneous, heat resistant, autoclavable, moldable and compressible. The silicone lens is highly transparent to visible light (except for the 200–400 nm wavelength range when an u.v. blocking agent is incorporated). The specific gravity of the material is low and therefore the lens is nearly weightless in aqueous. It also has excellent tensile and tear strength, and is extraordinarily flexible. It is stable in heat, organic solvent and in accelerating models of hydrolytic and u.v. degradation.

Although the silicone lens is transparent to neodymium YAG laser radiation, the lens can be pitted when hit by the laser beam. However, the extent of the damage is smaller than that observed in similarly treated Perspex CQ lenses, and there is neither radial cracking nor the release of any toxic products as a consequence of this damage.

The major disadvantage of the silicone implant is that it is a hydrophobic material that can damage contiguous ocular tissue. Endothelial cell loss with silicone lenses appears to be comparable to that observed with conventional IOLs. However, Kassar and Varnell noted that surface-modified silicone lenses produce less damage than do unmodified lenses.

19.3

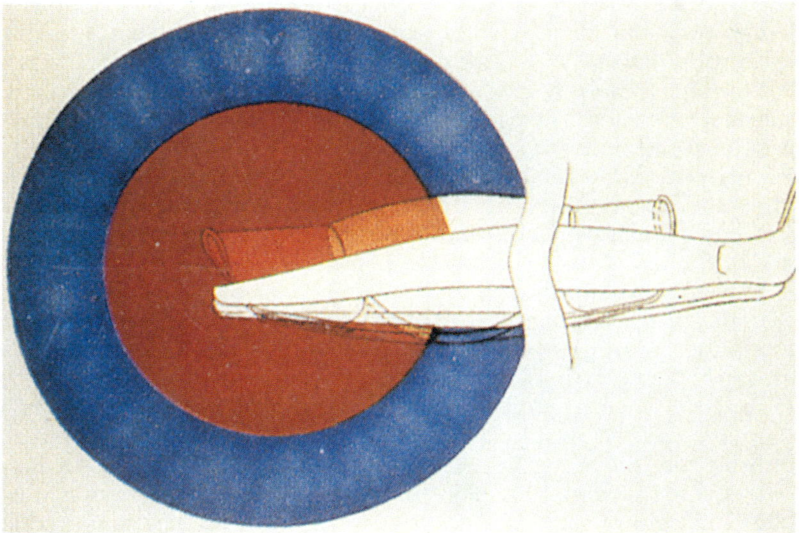

19.3 Folded silicone implant with web-like haptics being inserted through a small incision (courtesy Implants in Ophthalmology).

19.4

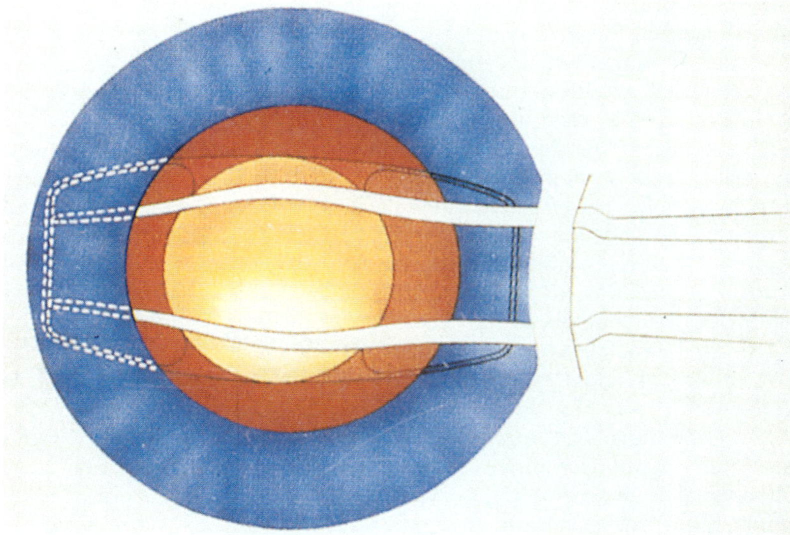

19.4 Release of implant after insertion through a small incision (courtesy of Implants in Ophthalmology).

19.5

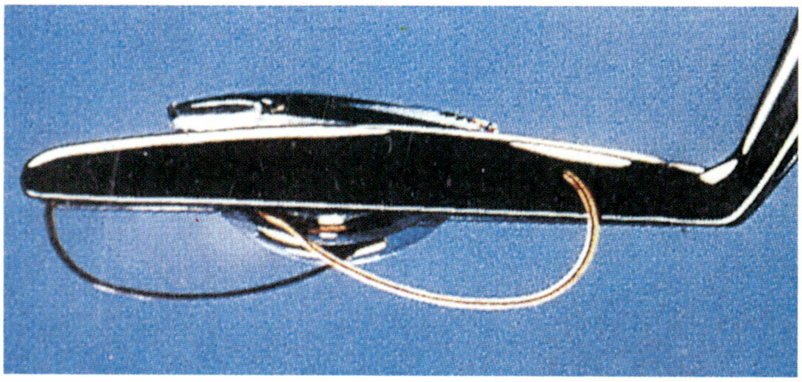

19.5 Silicone implant with prolene haptics held with Faulkner folder (courtesy of Implants in Ophthalmology).

19.6

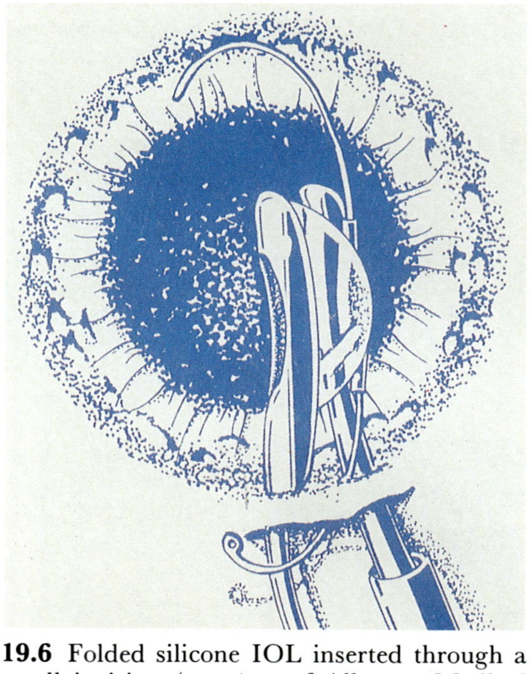

19.6 Folded silicone IOL inserted through a small incision (courtesy of Allergan Medical Optics).

Hydrogel lenses

Hydrogels include a broad class of polymer materials that swell extensively in water but are not water soluble. Such a hydrogel is polyhydroxyethylmethacrylate (PHEMA), which contains 38% water. High water-content hydrogels are cross-linked polymers based on a hydrophilic monomer (such as acrylonitrile, methacrylonitrite, vinyl pyrrolidone, vinyl caprodactan and similar derivates). They may be composed of one or more hydrophilic monomers or may contain hydrophilic and hydrophobic monomers in order to obtain a variety of water contents (from 50% to 90%) in equilibrium. High water-content hydrogel intraocular lenses have some important advantages over other lenses. They are soft and resemble living tissue in their physical properties, since most human organs have a high water content. Because of their soft, smooth and hydrophilic nature, they minimize mechanical friction with ocular tissues, reduce endothelial cell loss on contact, prevent unnecessary irritation and contribute to superior biocompatibility.

The hydrophilic nature of the lens surface causes low interfacial tension (wettability) of the hydrogel in aqueous solution and reduces the tendency of proteins to denature on the surface of the polymer, thus preventing or reducing biological rejection mechanisms. It also prevents fibrosis or adhesion formation at the interface between the lens and contiguous ocular tissue; therefore it is possible to recenter or remove a lens easily from the capsular bag. Hydrogels expand after hydration, thus allowing thorough extraction of contaminants, such as residual monomers, initiators and solvents. This renders hydrogels more biocompatible than rigid material (which may contain contaminants that can leach out *in vivo* and cause undesirable side effects). The dimension of the high water-content hydrogel lens changes in direct proportion to the degree of water saturation (**19.7**). This special characteristic enables implantation of a semihydrated lens through a small limbal incision and small capsulotomy. Introducing the small lens into the capsular bag is easily performed without traumatizing the zonule.

While proceeding with wound closure, the lens diameter increases to a size where luxation to the anterior chamber is improbable (**19.8**). The low reflection factor of the lens surface and the internal reflection of hydrogels minimize glare and discomfort to the patient. Hydrogels are permeable and heat sterilizable. The PHEMA intraocular lenses can accumulate fluorescein from the anterior chamber, but it disappears within 48 h. Whether they will accumulate topical or systemic medications has yet to be established.

Barrett reported a relatively low incidence of capsular fibrosis after PHEMA lens implantation and suggested a barrier effect from the close apposition of the posterior convex surface of the lens to the posterior capsule. The posterior surface of the optic and flanges of the lens have a single continuous arc of curvature, which maximizes the contact with the capsule. Several studies have clearly demonstrated the excellent compatibility of hydrogel lenses with YAG lasers. When there is a direct impact on the lens, mild to moderate localized pitting can be seen (**19.9**) without the typical radial fracturing seen on a PMMA implant (**19.10**). This is due to the resilience of the material and its ability to act as a 'shock absorber' rather than cracking under stress.

19.7

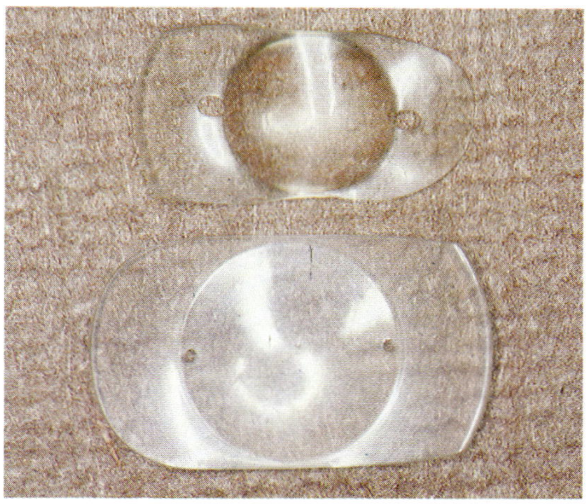

19.8

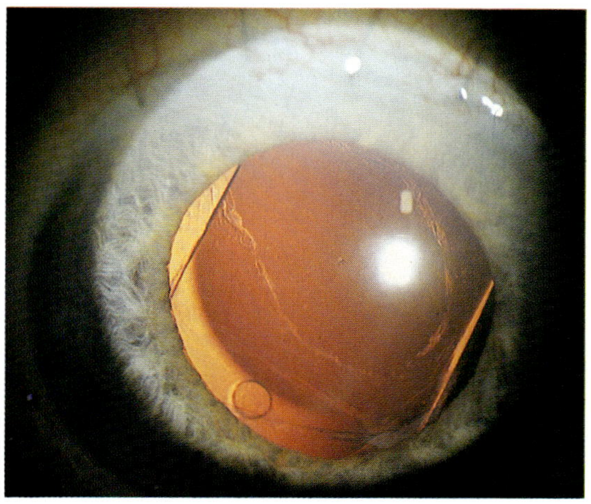

19.7 High water-content hydrogel lens in a dry (top) and wet (bottom) state.

19.8 Hydrogel lens in the bag. The diameter increases on hydration, preventing luxation to the anterior chamber.

19.9

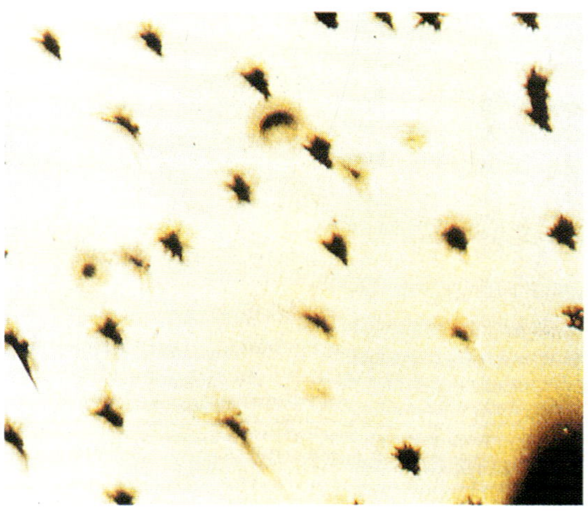

19.10

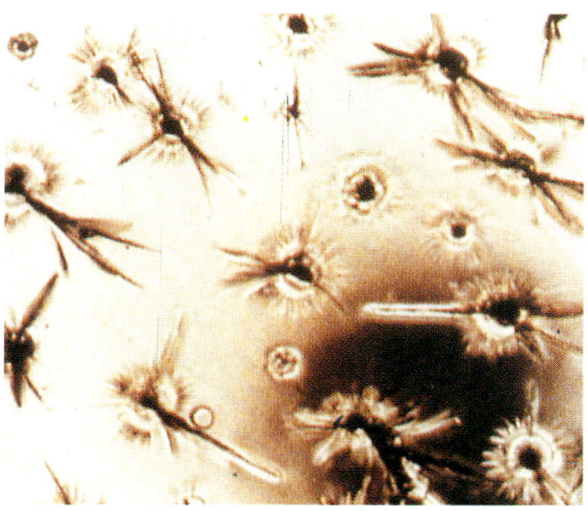

19.9 Mild YAG laser marking on the surface of a hydrogel implant (courtesy of Alcon Ltd).

19.10 Severe YAG laser marking on the surface of a PMMA implant with typical radial fractures (same magnification and power as in **19.9**; courtesy of Alcon Ltd).

Although high water-content polymers are usually mechanically weak, the hydrogel can be very strong owing to certain changes of the polymer itself produced during the process of polymerization. The tensile strength can reach 15.10 kg cm^{-2} and elongation to break 138%. *In vitro* measurements of the adhesive forces between the corneal endothelium and IOLs (**19.11**) indicate that the adhesive forces between the endothelium and hydrogel lenses are small, amounting to less than 20% of the adhesive forces generated between the endothelium and PMMA lenses.

Scanning electron microscopy of cats' corneas following intended touch between the endothelium and various IOLs during the implantation (*in vivo* study), revealed numerous microvilli (**19.12**), but no damage to the cell membranes after hydrogel lens touch, compared with extensive damage after PMMA lens touch. Following implantation of hydrogel material into the anterior chamber of aphakic cat and rabbit eyes, there was no damage to the corneal endothelium or the pigment epithelium of the iris and ciliary body. In many cases a monolayer of fibroblasts encapsulated the lens (**19.13**).

19.11

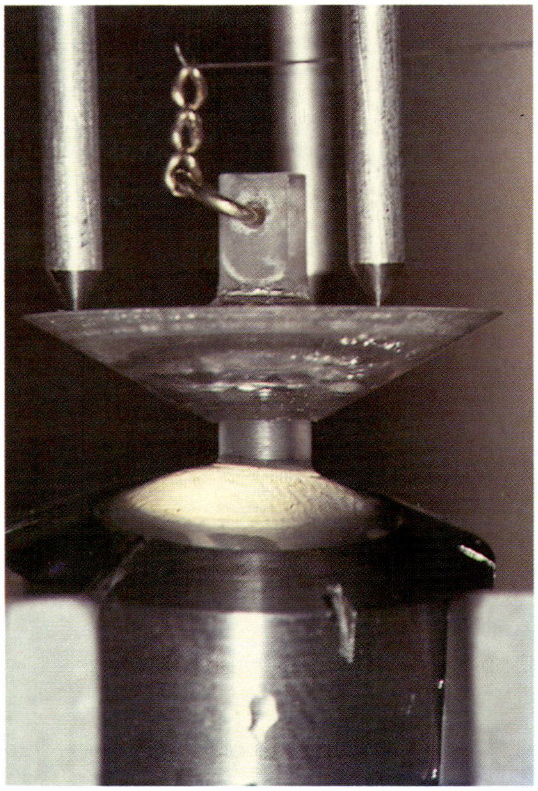

19.11 Inverted cornea from an adult rabbit placed on a plate (endothelium upward) showing the experimental apparatus for measuring disengagement forces after contact between the endothelium and the tested lens.

19.12

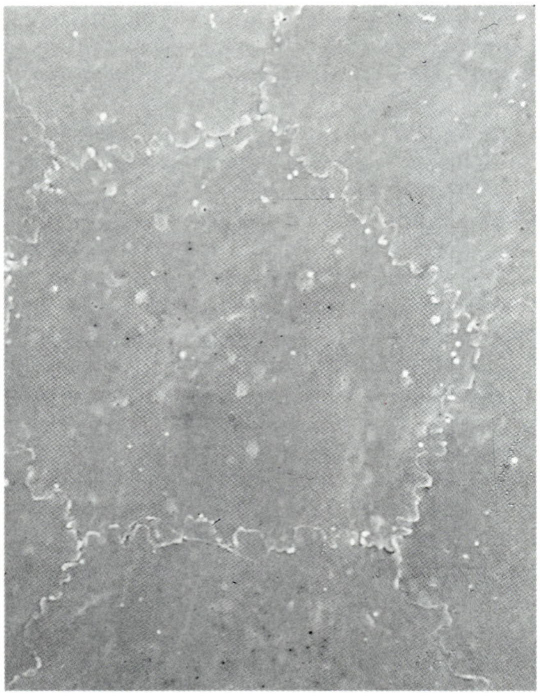

19.12 Scanning electron microscopy of a cat's cornea showing numerous microvilli in the endothelium following hydrogel lens touch, without damage to the cell membranes.

19.13

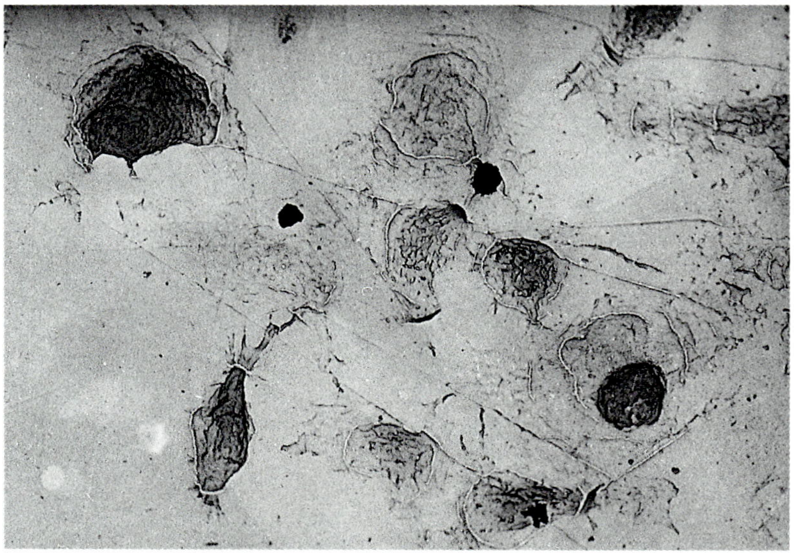

19.13 High magnification showing fibroblasts on the hydrogel surface.

Experimentally, removing the hydrogel lens from the eyes of a cat or rabbit at an interval of up to 2.5 years did not reveal any mechanical or physical changes in the lens, nor the transparency, dioptric power and resolution. Scanning electron microscopy after IOL explantation demonstrated a smooth lens surface. No biodegradation process could be documented and no deposits were seen on the hydrogel lenses.

Lens design and size are important factors to be considered when introduction in the dry, reduced state is intended. In order to prevent the possibility of soft lens torque and decentration due to fibrosis of the capsule and asymmetric compression, a new style, full-size hydrogel lens has been designed, of 6 mm diameter and 2 mm thickness in the dry state, and 9 mm diameter and 4.5 mm thickness in the hydrated state (**19.14**). After hydration this style occupies most of the capsular bag and imitates the natural crystalline lens (**19.15**). It prevents postoperative capsular fibrosis and contraction and provides stable fixation in the capsular bag.

19.14

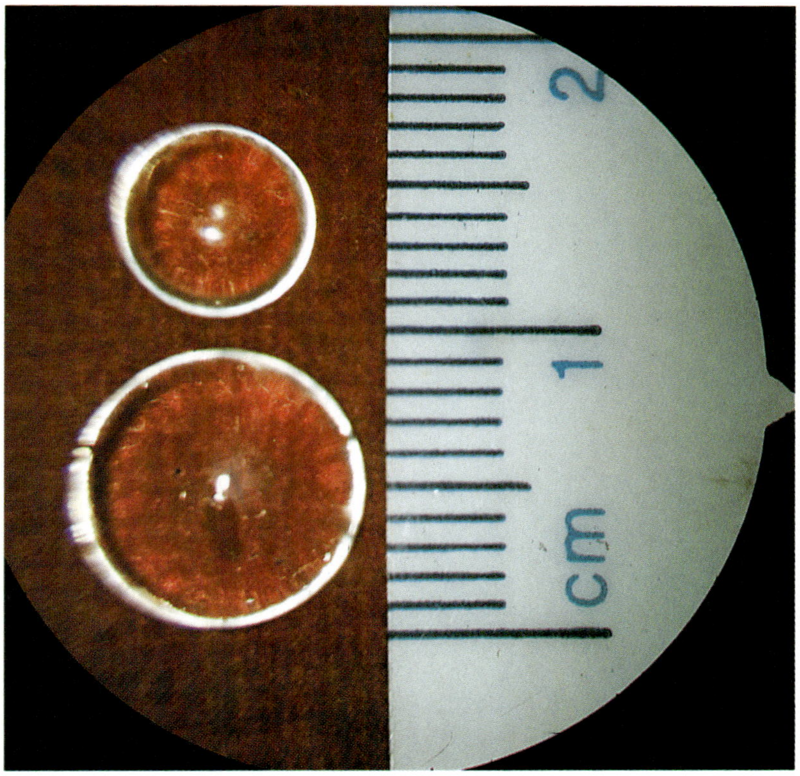

19.14 The full-size round hydrogel lens in its dry (top) and wet (bottom) state.

19.15

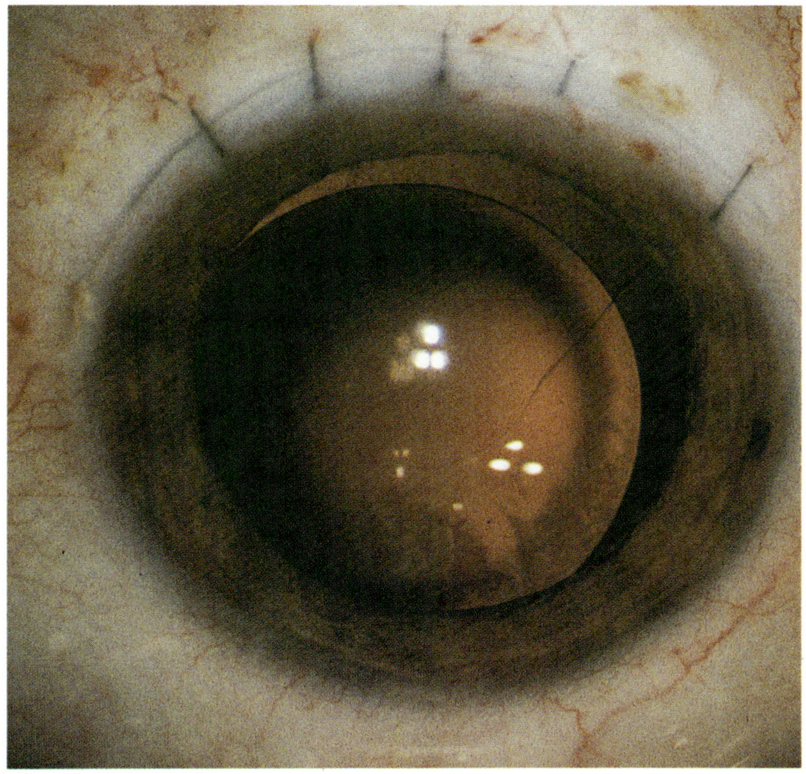

19.15 In the bag implantation of the full-size hydrogel lens, imitating the natural crystalline lens.

The future

As evolution of cataract surgery develops towards the removal of all lens material through a small hole in the lens capsule it will be appropriate for replacement with a soft injectable plastic material. This could mold within the capsular bag to a predetermined optical power and possibly preserve the power of accommodation.

Further reading

Allarakhia L., Knoll R.L. and Lindstrom R.L. Soft intraocular lenses. *J. Cataract Refract. Surg.*, **13,** 607–620, 1987.

Barrett G.D., Constable I.J. and Stewart A.D. Clinical results of hydrogel lens implantation. *J. Cataract Refract. Surg.* **12,** 623–631, 1986.

Blumenthal M. The use of high water content hydrogels as intraocular lenses. In: *Soft Implant Lenses in Cataract Surgery*, Mazzocco, T.R., Rajacich, G.M. and Epstein, E. (Eds), Slack Inc., pp 107–117, 1986.

Blumenthal M. and Yalon M. Interaction of soft and hard intraocular lenses with cat cornea endothelium. *Cornea,* **1,** 129–132, 1982.

Kassar B.S. and Varnell E.D. Effect of PMMA and silicone lens materials on normal rabbit corneal endothelium: An *in vitro* study. *Am. Intraocular Implant Soc. J.,* **6,** 344–346, 1980.

Silva M. Soft lenses – an overview. *Implants in Ophthalmol.,* **2,** 132–134, 1988.

20: Hydrogel lenses: technique

Graham Barrett

Although soft intraocular lenses and particularly hydrogel lenses have only recently become available to ophthalmic surgeons, the first hydrogel intraocular lens was inserted by Edward Epstein in 1977. Currently this is an active area of research and surgeons are evaluating several designs composed of hydrogel materials. These designs include disc hydrogels which may be inserted in the hydrated state or dehydrated state, and three piece dehydrated hydrogel implants with conventional loops. The implantation techniques of these different lens designs will vary dramatically. Here we confine ourselves to a description of the surgical techniques useful with the IOGEL® intraocular lens, which at present is the only widely available hydrogel implant.

The IOGEL® lens is a single piece posterior chamber lens developed by the author and first implanted in August 1983. The lens was developed from a more biocompatible material than polymethylmethacrylate (PMMA) and is composed of polyhydroxyethylmethacrylate (PHEMA) with a water content of 38%. It is a soft hydrophilic material with several properties dissimilar to conventional implants composed of PMMA.

Besides the inherent properties of the material, the lens design is different (**20.1**). The lens has an asymmetrical biconvex optic supported by flanges rather than loops of PMMA or polypropylene. The single posterior convex arc of curvature of the optic and flanges allows the lens to vault posteriorly and accommodate the contracture of the capsular bag (**20.2**). Owing to its different design the technique of insertion of the lens differs from that of conventional implants.

Many different surgical techniques are possible with the IOGEL® lens, including the standard extracapsular, intercapsular and phacoemulsification techniques. Whatever the technique of implantation, it is important to understand that a single piece soft implant, such as the IOGEL® lens, has different fixation characteristics and is less tolerant of malposition than flexible loop implants. IOGEL® implants placed in the capsular bag show excellent centration, but if placed in the sulcus the centration may not be perfect and there is a higher incidence of pigment dispersion. Asymmetric placement may result in significant decentration and produce flexion or a C-shaped flange deformation (**20.3**). The latter situation should therefore be avoided if possible. C deformities may also arise after placement in the capsular bag if the lens is too long. Ideal measurements for bag placement are a length of 11.25 mm with a 3 mm width to the haptic tips. The ideal length for sulcus placement is 12.5 mm. The Iogel® lens should only be implanted if the posterior capsule is intact. Owing to the lack of fibrosis and the adhesion of the flanges to the capsule, large YAG laser capsulotomies should be avoided for up to three months after surgery, as in these circumstances it is possible for the lens to be dislocated posteriorly by contracture of the capsular bag.

20.1

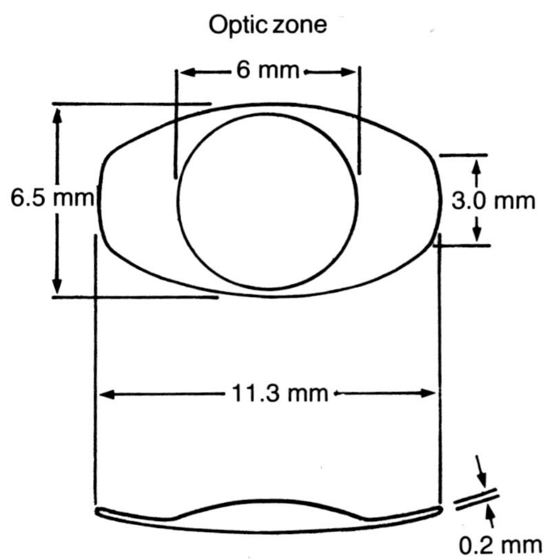

20.2

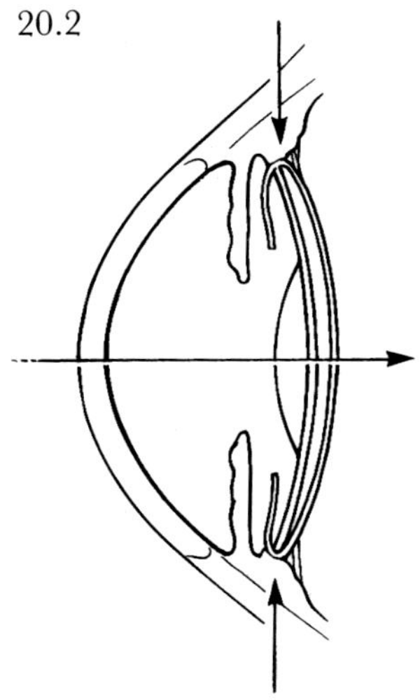

20.3

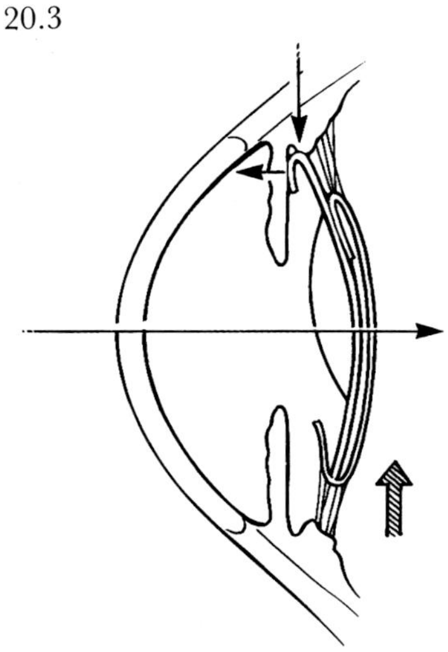

20.1 IOGEL® lens dimensions for model no. 1103.

20.2 Side view of IOGEL® lens fixated in the capsular bag. Note the close apposition of the posterior convex surface of the lens to the posterior capsule. The vertical arrows indicate symmetric forces from capsular contraction.

20.3 The IOGEL® lens placed asymmetrically with the lower flange in the bag and the upper one in the sulcus, resulting in decentration and a C-shaped deformity of the upper flange. The vertical arrows indicate asymmetric forces from capsular contraction.

Surgical technique

It is possible to damage a soft implant by the use of inappropriate instrumentation. Surgeons should avoid instruments with teeth or sharp edges when implanting hydrogel lenses. A series of instruments that allow safe and easy handling of the IOGEL® lens have been designed and could be used for other soft implants, as described below.

Soft lens forceps

Soft lens forceps (**20.4**) differ from conventional smooth-jawed lens forceps in that the inner aspects of the jaws have a rounded rather than flat surface. When pressure is applied the soft material simply moulds to the jaws and cannot be cut when excessive pressure is applied, as with conventional forceps. Similarly, the handles are not cross-actioned, which tends to increase the mechanical advantage and the pressure applied to the lens. The jaws are delicate and have a curve that conforms to the optic–flange junction. The forceps can be used to remove the lens from the fluid-filled vial and to insert the lens without changing forceps. The same principles also allow the forceps to grasp soft tissues, such as capsule or iris, without injury.

20.4

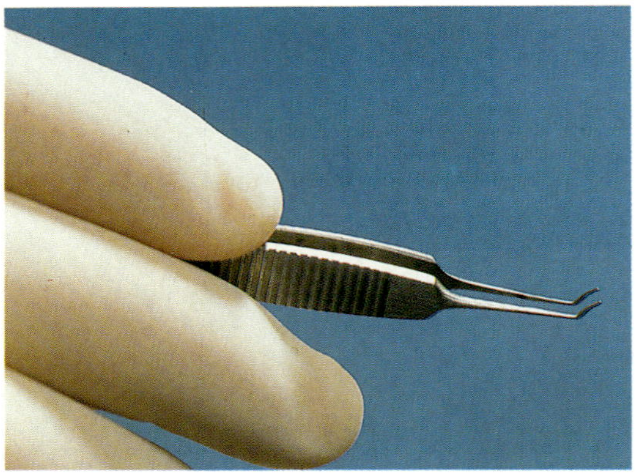

20.4 The lens forceps designed for soft hydrogel implants.

Soft lens manipulator

Conventional intraocular lens manipulators or hooks, though not considered sharp, may pierce a soft hydrogel implant. The surface of the IOGEL® lens has a rubbery texture and therefore does not require manipulating holes. The soft lens manipulator (**20.5**) has a smooth convex tip in the shape of an inverted mushroom, with which the surgeon can safely apply pressure on the surface of the lens, with no risk of penetrating the material. The lens can then be manipulated in any desired direction.

The manipulator consists of the inverted mushroom on the end of a fine spatula and is also very useful as an atraumatic iris retractor or as a second instrument to manipulate the nucleus during phacoemulsification. In cases with relatively small pupils, two micromanipulators are well suited for simultaneous retraction of the iris and insertion of the lens.

20.5

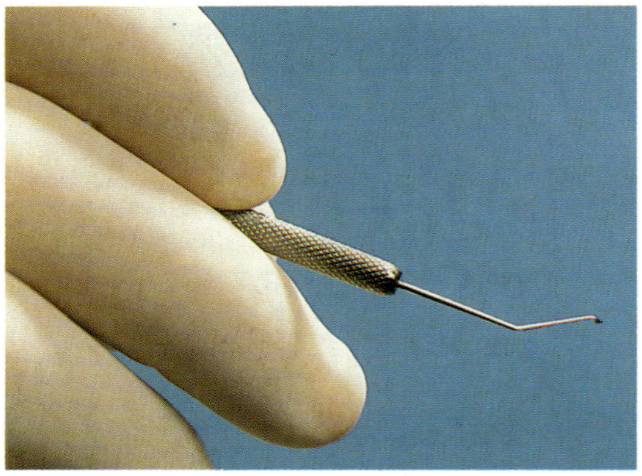

20.5 The 'mushroom' manipulator designed for soft hydrogel implants.

Folding forceps for small incision

The folding forceps (**20.6**) are designed to fold the IOGEL® lens prior to a small incision insertion following phacoemulsification. The forceps have two outer supports and a central rod. There is no floor or gutter so that the lens is not compressed when folded. The design also allows the lateral supports to expand slightly when the lens is folded, minimizing the stress on the folded lens and avoiding damage.

20.6

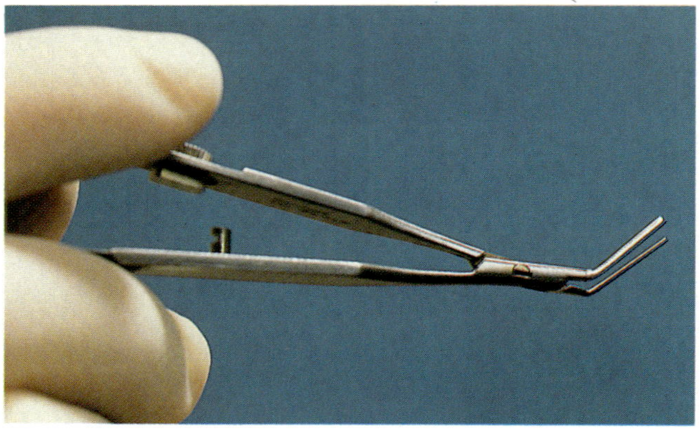

20.6 The folding forceps to be used in conjunction with the holding forceps for implanting the hydrogel implant through a small (3.5 mm) incision following phacoemulsification.

Implantation of the IOGEL® lens following extracapsular cataract extraction

To ensure capsular bag fixation, it is necessary to visualize the anterior edges of the anterior capsule during insertion of the lens and a relatively small capsulotomy is recommended.

Two sutures approximately 6 mm apart are utilized. Interestingly, due to its flexibility it is possible to insert a hydrogel lens through a smaller incision than that necessary for a PMMA lens of comparable diameter with less risk of damaging Descemet's membrane.

The IOGEL® lens is provided in a crimped 'V'-shaped vial filled with balanced salt solution. The 'V' configuration ensures that the lens always has a semivertical orientation to facilitate ease of removal from the vial. The lens should be removed from the vial with the soft lens forceps and held at the junction of the flange and the optic zone for maximum stability (**20.7**). The inner surfaces of the jaws are smooth and rounded and are designed to grasp soft implants without the risk of damage, which can occur with conventional forceps. The lens should be rinsed with fresh balanced salt solution, but does not require soaking. The surgeon should check that the lens is being held in the correct orientation with the curvature and angulation of the flanges facing upwards.

The lower flange and optic are then inserted into the anterior chamber, but the tip of the upper flange is left protruding (**20.8**). One of the advantages of the lens design is that it acts as a 'Sheets glide' upon insertion and the lower flange is inserted with ease behind the iris into the capsular bag. Since the IOGEL® lens is hydrophilic, viscoelastic agents are generally not necessary either to expand the capsular bag or to protect the corneal endothelium. If a viscoelastic material is being used the surgeon should aim to insert the lens behind rather than through the bulk of viscoelastic material. A second instrument, such as a fine spatula, may occasionally be necessary to guide the lower flange into the desired position inferiorly if the flange is flexed anteriorly by the viscoelastic agent (**20.9**). Large quantities of viscoelastic material may hinder rather than facilitate implantation. If the chamber is only moderately shallow, air may be found to be more helpful than a viscoelastic substance. If the chamber is flat a Sheet's glide can be inserted into the bag inferiorly, sodium hyaluronate injected in front of the glide and the implant inserted behind the glide.

Insertion of the upper flange can be accomplished by grasping the upper flange with the soft lens forceps at the top edge and rotating the tip of the flange posteriorly beneath the iris into the capsular bag. Alternatively, a blunt manipulator may be placed at the junction of the upper flange and optic, and pressed gently inferiorly and posteriorly until the upper flange slips into the capsular bag above (**20.10**). The lens manipulator has an inverted mushroom-shaped button and the vector of insertion is between 6 o'clock inferiorly and the optic nerve posteriorly. With this technique the lens is guided inferiorly below the edge of the iris and then allowed to recoil so that the upper flange slides behind the iris into the capsular bag above.

If the pupil is not well dilated, a second mushroom manipulator is used to engage the iris at 12 o'clock. The superior anterior capsular flap as well as the iris may be retracted as an additional maneuver to facilitate capsular bag placement, especially with a small circular capsulotomy produced by capsulorhexis.

Once the iris has been satisfactorily engaged and retracted to 12 o'clock, the rest of the lens is inserted into the anterior chamber and the upper flange placed into the capsular bag with the other mushroom manipulator as described above (**20.11**).

20.7

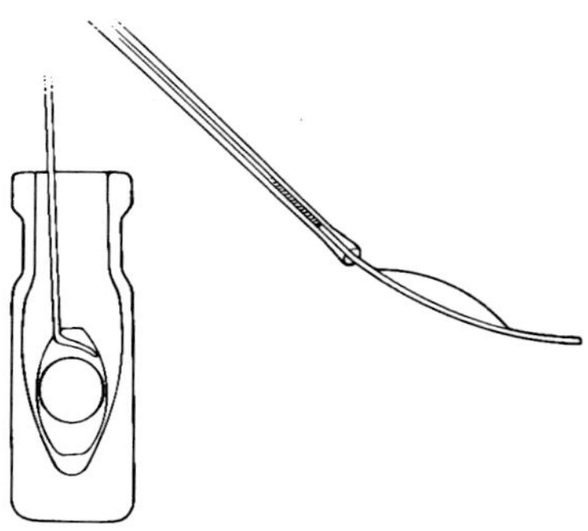

20.8

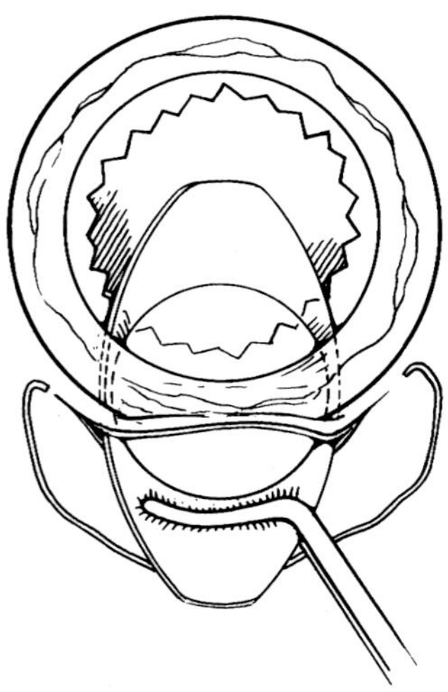

20.9

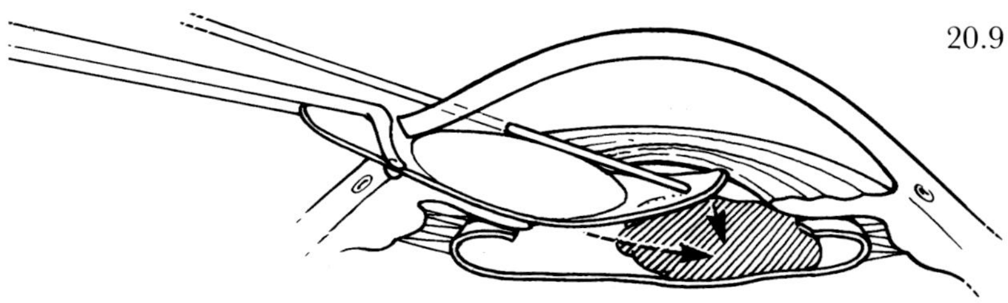

20.10

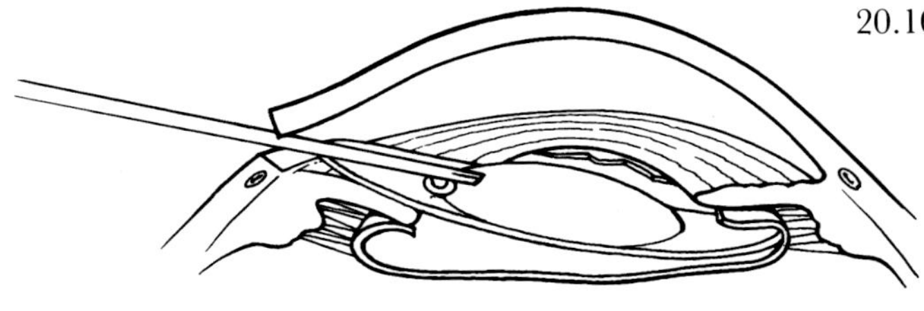

20.11

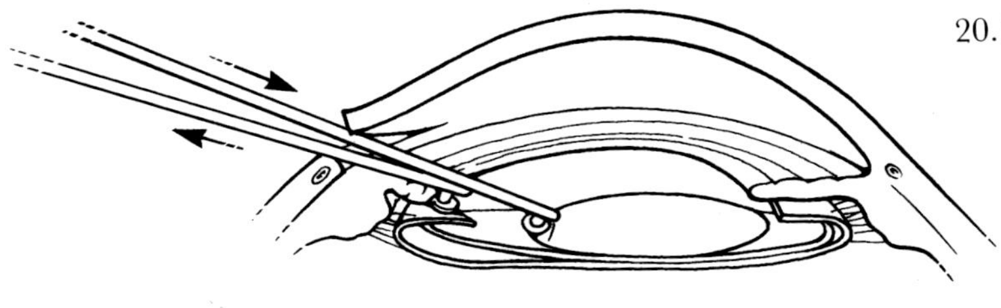

20.7 The IOGEL® lens as supplied in a vial and held in the forceps in the correct orientation for implantation.

20.8 The IOGEL® lens being inserted into the anterior chamber after a standard ECCE.

20.9 Flexing of the inferior flange by a bolus of viscoelastic material, necessitating positioning of the lower flange with a second instrument.

20.10 The preferred method of inserting the upper flange by pressure directed posteriorly and inferiorly using the mushroom manipulator placed at the junction of flange and optic.

20.11 Simultaneous retraction of the iris with a second mushroom manipulator for cases with poor mydriasis.

Further balanced salt solution can then be injected as this tends to center the lens, relieve any possible iris tuck and ensure that the lens is correctly situated in the posterior chamber.

The viscoelastic material, if present, is then removed and the position of the lens checked using the lens manipulator. There is sufficient purchase on the surface of the lens with a cannula to manipulate the lens and ensure that it is correctly centered without the use of positioning holes. No attempt is made to rotate the lens and in the vast majority of cases the lens centers itself with no alteration of its position being necessary. A vertical orientation is preferred to a horizontal position. Pupil capture is highly unlikely and it is not necessary to constrict the pupil with miotic agents at the end of surgery.

Implantation of the IOGEL® lens using the intercapsular technique

The anterior capsule will be left intact until after the intraocular lens has been implanted. A horizontal capsulotomy is performed in a curvilinear fashion from 10 to 2 o'clock, with the convexity of the capsulotomy positioned inferiorly and extended to approximately one third of the pupil diameter below the pupil margin.

The IOGEL® lens is inserted between the leaves of the anterior and posterior capsule (**20.12**), so that the entire lens except for the upper flange is now in the capsular bag. The upper flange is then inserted by rotating the lens with the mushroom manipulator through approximately 45° in a clockwise direction (**20.13**). In so doing, the angle formed by the lateral extent of the capsular incision acts as a fulcrum, which flexes the upper flange into the capsular bag (**20.14**). A vertical position is preferred. A single vertical incision (**20.15**) is then performed in the anterior capsule and a Simcoe cannula used to engage and tear the anterior capsular flap. The cannula maintains the anterior chamber whilst tearing. Viscoelastic substances are usually unnecessary.

20.12

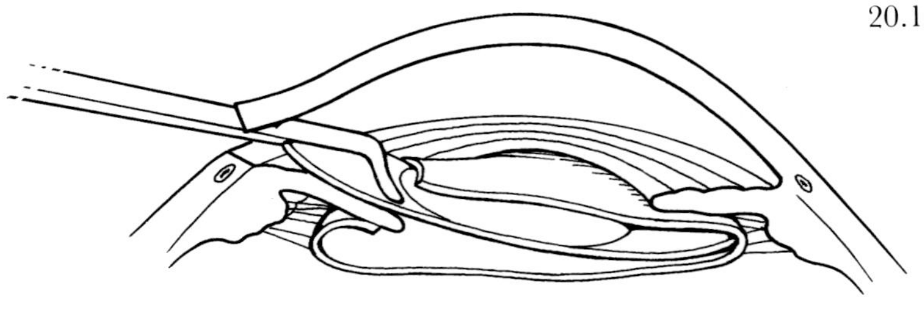

20.12 Insertion of an IOGEL® lens between the anterior and posterior capsule following an intercapsular cataract extraction.

20.13

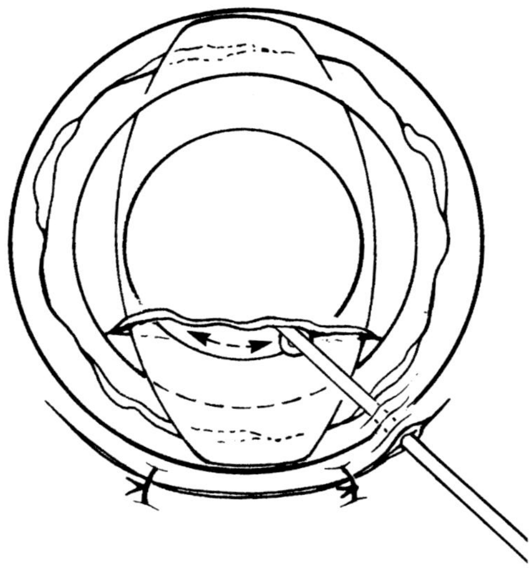

20.13 Insertion of the upper flange by rotating the lens with a manipulator through approximately 45° with a simultaneous slight posterior pressure. Once the upper flange is inserted then the lens should be returned to a vertical orientation and the surgeon should check that the superior flap of the anterior capsule is in front of the flange.

20.14

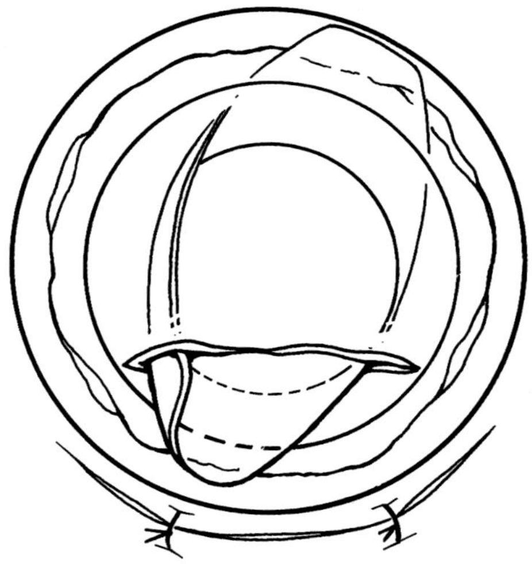

20.14 The mechanism of flange flipping into the capsular bag by the angle of incision in the anterior capsule. Note that if the anterior capsular flap is torn, then the lens should be rotated in the other direction towards the intact capsular edge.

20.15

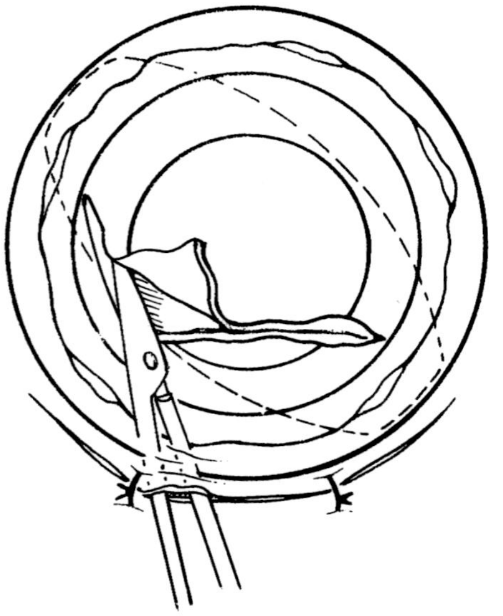

20.15 Anterior capsule incision with fine scissors.

Implantation of the IOGEL® lens following phacoemulsification

One of the unique characteristics of this type of implant is its capability of being folded for small incision surgery (**20.16**). Folding the IOGEL® implant following phacoemulsification enables one to perform cataract surgery through a 3.5 mm incision.

A 3.5 mm two-plane incision is made 1 mm posterior to the surgical limbus with a multifaceted diamond knife. A 6 mm capsulotomy is then done in a rectangular fashion with a bent 25-gauge needle, leaving more capsule above and below than laterally. It is important that plenty of capsule is visible when inserting the lens. The lens is also ideally suited to continuous circular capsulorhexis, which should be performed in a horizontally oval rather than a circular fashion.

The section is then opened with the same diamond blade and the nucleus phacoemulsified using a mushroom manipulator as a second instrument, so that the phacoemulsification is performed in the posterior chamber.

The wound is then left at 3.5 mm and the anterior chamber filled with a viscoelastic material, simultaneously expanding the capsular bag.

The IOGEL® lens is then folded posteriorly with the folding forceps (**20.6**). The lens is placed horizontally between the central folding rod below and the two lateral supports above, with the anterior surface facing upwards. The long axis of the lens should coincide with the long axis of the instrument so that the folding rod lies along the longitudinal midline of the lens. The handle should then be closed, folding the lens symmetrically (**20.17**). The lens is next grasped with a separate holding forceps and the folding forceps removed (**20.18**). The lens is inserted on its side into the anterior chamber (**20.19**) and rotated anteriorly (**20.20**). The inferior folded flange is directed into the capsular bag inferiorly and the forceps gently opened. The lens then

20.16

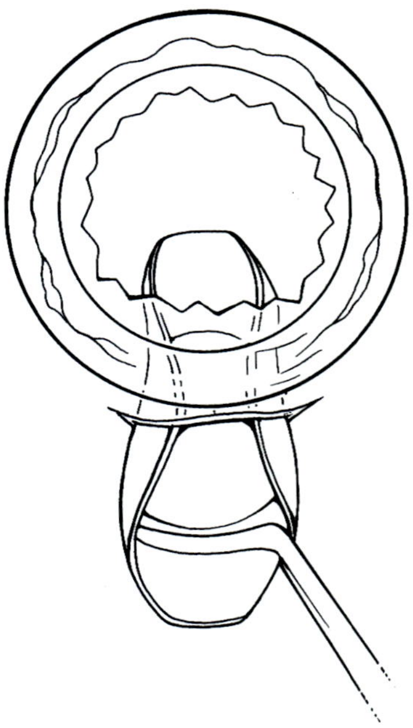

20.16 Illustrating insertion of the lens through a 3.5 mm incision. The edges of the lens are folded by the scleral incision to produce a 'winging' effect.

20.17

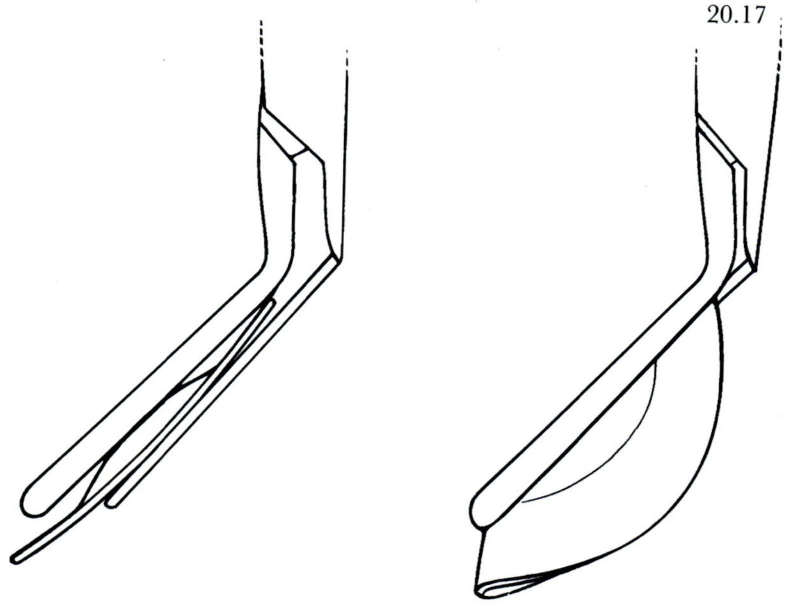

20.17 Folding of the lens posteriorly by the folding forceps.

20.18

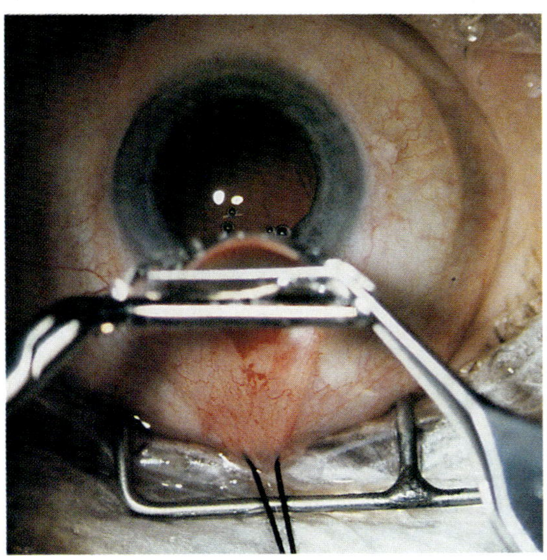

20.18 Transfer of the lens from the folding forceps to the holding forceps.

20.19

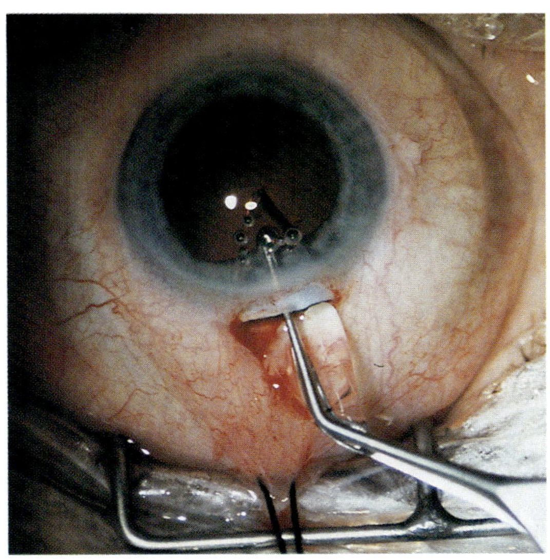

20.19 Insertion of the lens on its side with the holding forceps held approximately 20° to the line of incision.

20.20

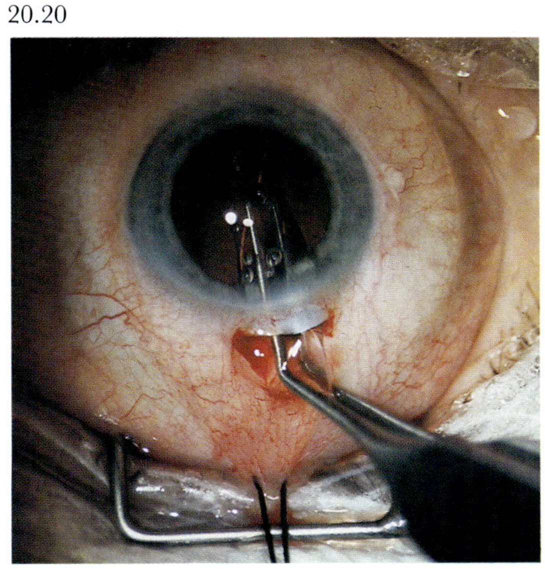

20.20 Anterior rotation of the forceps perpendicular to the line of incision.

unfolds, opening posteriorly (**20.21**). The forceps are removed and the upper flange inserted by placing the mushroom manipulator at the junction of the upper flange and optic, and pressing gently inferiorly and posteriorly as before (**20.22**). The remaining viscoelastic material is then removed.

The wound is closed with a single cruciate 10/0 nylon suture. A qualitative keratoscope may be used to adjust suture tension and minimize astigmatism.

20.21

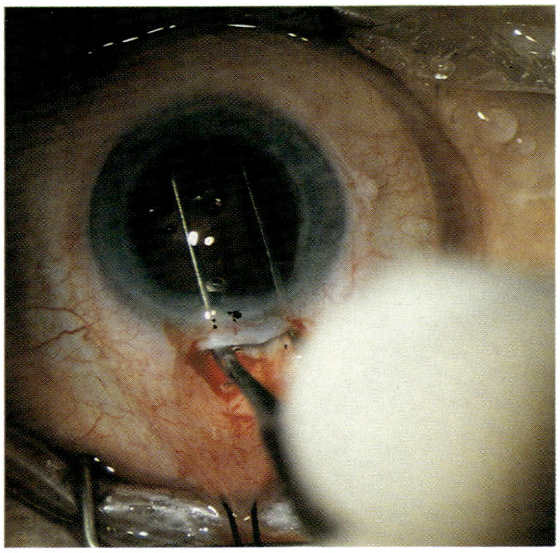

20.21 Opening of the forceps and unfolding of the lens with the lower flange in the capsular bag.

20.22

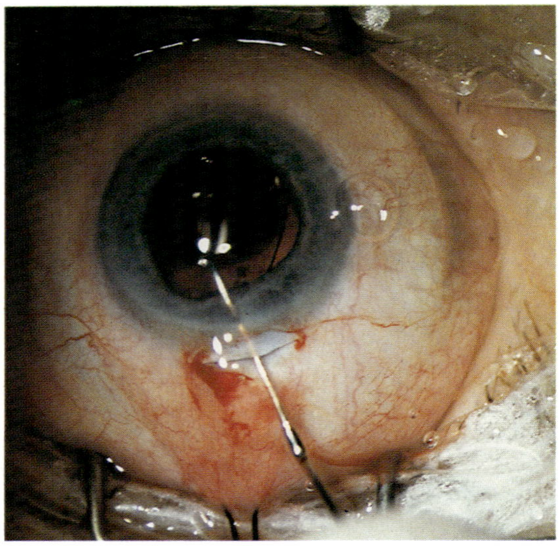

20.22 Insertion of the upper flange into the superior capsular bag with the mushroom manipulator.

Editor's Note: Hydrogel lenses, although they show an improved biocompatibility and are useful for small incision surgery, show no adherence to the posterior capsule. Dislocation into the vitreous following posterior capsulotomy has been reported. Surgical capsulotomies are, therefore, not recommended after such implantations, and laser capsulotomies should be limited to 2 mm in diameter.

Further reading

Barrett G.D., Constable I.I. and Stewart A.D. Clinical results of intraocular hydrogel lens implantation. *J. Cataract Refract. Surg.* **12,** 623–631, 1986.

Mazzoco T.R., Rajacich G.M. and Epstein E. (eds). *Soft Implant Lenses in Cataract Surgery.* New Jersey, Slack Inc., 1986.

Percival S.P.B. Prospective study comparing Hydrogel with PMMA lens implants. *Ophthal. Surg.,* **20,** 255–261, 1989.

21: Multifocal intraocular lenses

Richard Duffey, Ralph Zabel and Richard Lindstrom

Accommodation in the healthy eye

The normal eye is constructed so that the various refracting surfaces and ocular media focus parallel rays of light from a distant object upon the retina. The eye can also adjust its dioptric power through the accommodative process to bring near objects into focus. In an analysis of the Purkinje images during accommodation, Helmholtz has shown that the posterior lens surface remains fixed in position and undergoes a slight increase in curvature, but the major dioptric shift during accommodation results from the forward movement and marked increase in the convexity of the anterior pole of the lens.

The cortex of the young lens is a soft, easily moulded material contained in an elastic capsule. The traction of the zonular fibers opposes the natural tendency of the lens to assume a spherical shape. During accommodation, however, contraction of the ciliary muscles pulls the zonular attachment sites inward towards the lens equator, reducing the tension on the zonules and lens capsule and thereby allowing the lens to passively increase its convexity. The resultant steepening of the anterior and posterior poles of the lens effects the accommodative process.

The amplitude of accommodation is greatest in childhood and slowly decreases until it is lost in middle age. The loss of accommodation, although fairly uniform in the population, fluctuates with the demands of the visual task, the level of illumination, drug effects, pupillary size, and a person's general health. When the inability to carry out prolonged near-vision tasks due to fatigue, headache, and other symptoms of asthenopia occurs, the condition is called presbyopia. Duane's standard curve of accommodative amplitude versus age reveals that by the age of 60 all accommodation has generally been lost. Thus, although presbyopia is defined as the vision of old age it is a poor term relative to today's lifespans. Several explanations have been suggested for the development of presbyopia: that the lens nucleus grows and scleroses with age and that the plasticity of the cortex is lost; that the ciliary muscle weakens and is no longer able to adequately relax the zonules; and that the elasticity of the lens capsule decreases. Experimental results both support and contradict these various theories.

Without exaggeration, the difficulties in adapting to bifocal glasses are often considerable. As the reading addition is increased in strength or the patient requires trifocal or multifocal reading segments there is often frustration and discouragement.

Intraocular lens implantation surgery has overcome the loss of vision associated with the formation of cataracts. Since standard IOLs are monofocal the loss of accommodation becomes absolute with surgery and the need to correct the resultant presbyopia is apparent. In what may be considered an evolutionary step, bifocal and multifocal IOLs of several different designs have been introduced. They differ from conventional monofocal IOLs in that they offer the potential for providing both distance and near vision without additional spectacle correction.

Multifocal intraocular lens designs

Multifocal IOL designs to date incorporate either refractive and/or diffractive optical principles to achieve simultaneous distance and near visual acuity. Although most are of bifocal design the lenses are termed multifocal because of their ability to function at more than two foci, often with a satisfactory acuity for distant, near and intermediate vision. Refractive optics can be broken down further into spheric and aspheric designs. The anterior and/or posterior IOL surface can be utilized for single or combination designs.

There are, at present, four different designs about which information has been released. Others surely exist but so far remain unavailable. Some designs have already been incorporated into lenses that have been implanted clinically while others are still in the early manufacture stage. The different designs are discussed below with no critical evaluation intended.

Two or three zone bifocal refraction

This involves the combination of two or more different anterior spheric refractive surfaces for distance and near correction (the Iolab Nuvue™ bifocal IOL and Pharmacia Ophthalmics bifocal). The Iolab IOL (**21.1**) has a 2 mm diameter central optic for near vision. The remainder of the lens, which is lower in power by 4D, is a ring-shaped zone for distance correction. When the pupil size is 2.8 mm the light distribution between near and distance focus on the retina is even, when 4 mm the distribution is 1/4 for near and 3/4 for distance, assuming that the lens is perfectly centered. The Pharmacia design (**21.2**) has a central circular distance zone (2.1 mm diameter) surrounded by a ring-shaped near zone of 0.7 mm width, which is then surrounded by another peripheral ring-shaped zone for distance correction. Both of these designs effect their dioptric changes for distance and near by refractive spheric curvature changes on the anterior surface of the IOL.

21.1

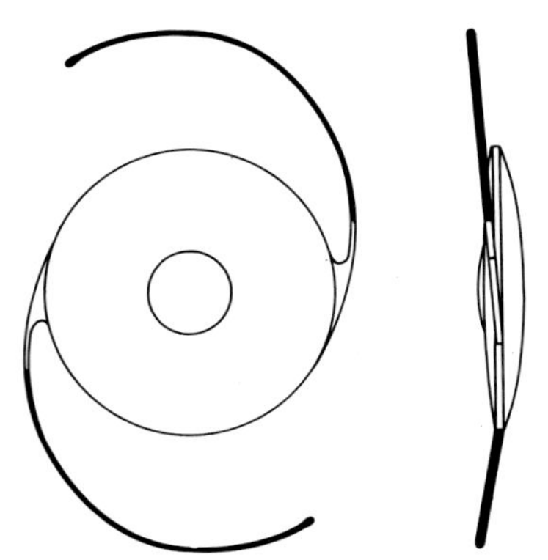

21.1 Two zone bifocal design (courtesy of Iolab). The lens is biconvex with a 2 mm central button for near vision.

21.2

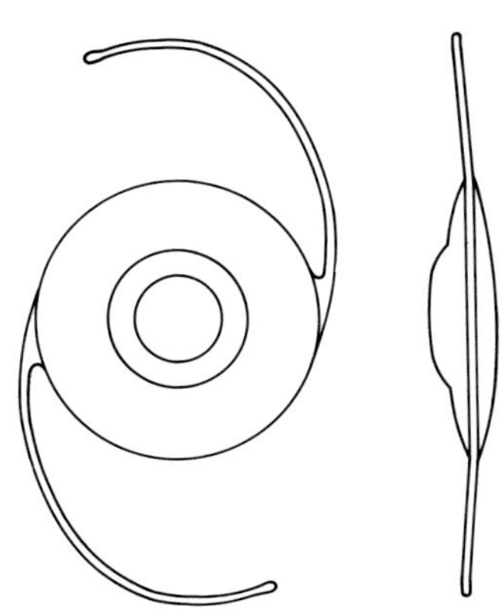

21.2 Three zone bifocal design (courtesy of Pharmacia).

Combination of spheric and aspheric surfaces for multifocal refraction

This involves the combination of an anterior spheric and an anterior aspheric refractive surface as designed by Lee Nordan for true multifocal refraction (Wright Medical, Inc. and Ioptex aspheric multifocal lenses). As it is not necessary to involve the entire visual axis for a multifocal design the Nordan IOL made by Wright Medical (**21.3**) incorporates a spheric and aspheric combination on a one half segment of the anterior surface of a biconvex lens. The radius of curvature of this aspheric segment constantly changes, thus incorporating a smooth increase in power towards the midperiphery of the lens of up to 3D (**21.4**). A second design is used by Ioptex which combines spheric and aspheric curves concentrically (**21.5**) for a progressive power increase of 4D. The smooth transition minimizes aberration and ensures a truly multifocal function (**21.6**). The dioptric power changes that occur as the more peripheral optical zones are reached are shown in **21.7**. The mid zones represent the anterior aspheric refractive surfaces for near correction.

21.3

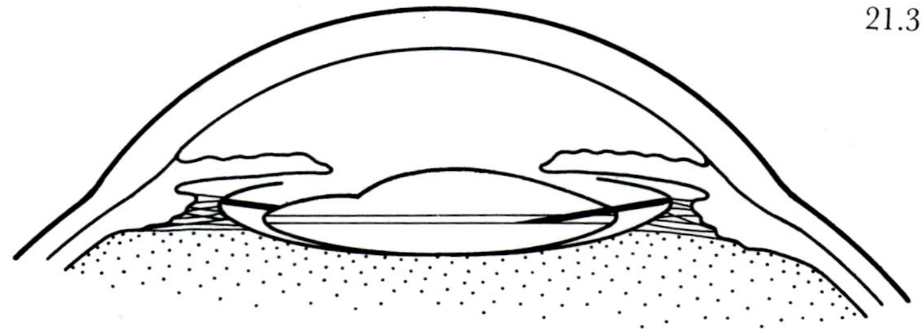

21.3 Silicone small incision varifocal Nordan lens from Wright Medical *in situ*, with a 6 mm optic. The aspheric curve on the one half segment of the anterior surface creates a 3.0 D addition at a distance 1.5 mm from the center of the optic (courtesy of Dr Lee Nordan, USA).

21.4

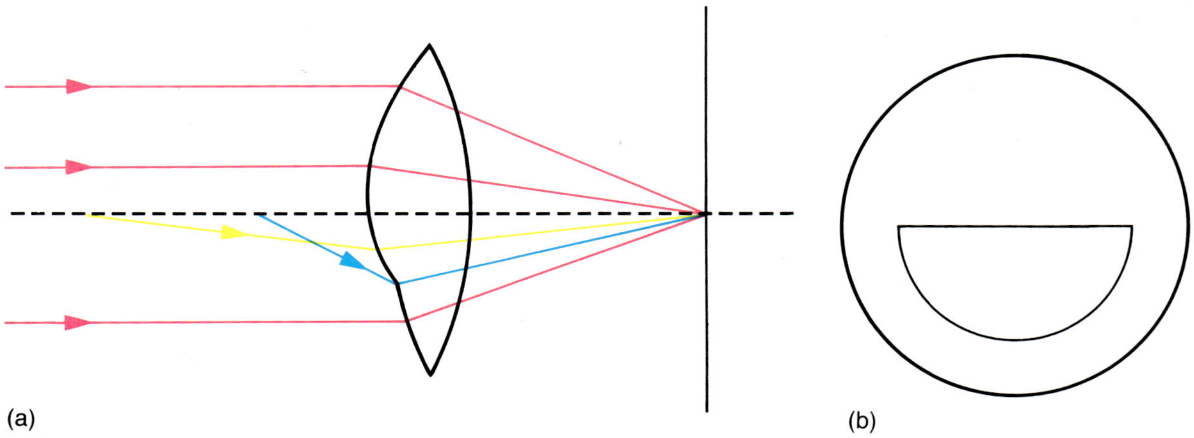

21.4 (a) Ray diagram of light (red, distant; yellow, intermediate; blue, near) entering the aspheric lens of (**21.3**). At least half the visual axis is for distance vision. (b) The semicircle for intermediate and near is aspheric in both horizontal and vertical directions. The peripheral 1 mm is for distance.

21.5

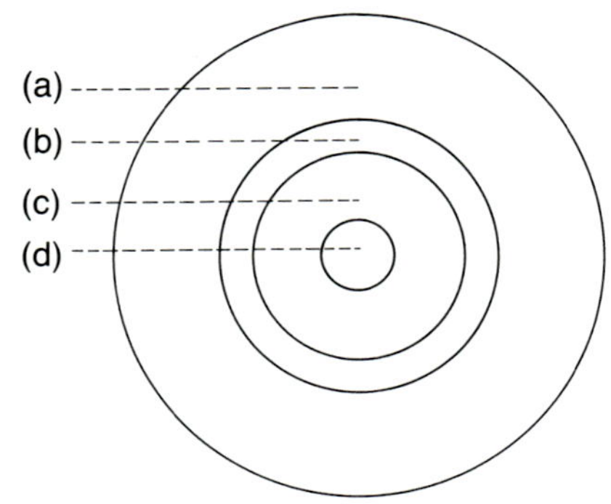

21.5 The Ioptex lens optic combining aspheric and spheric zones on the anterior surface: (a) spherical distance zone; (b) aspheric flattening zone; (c) aspheric steepening zone; (d) spherical distance zone.

21.6

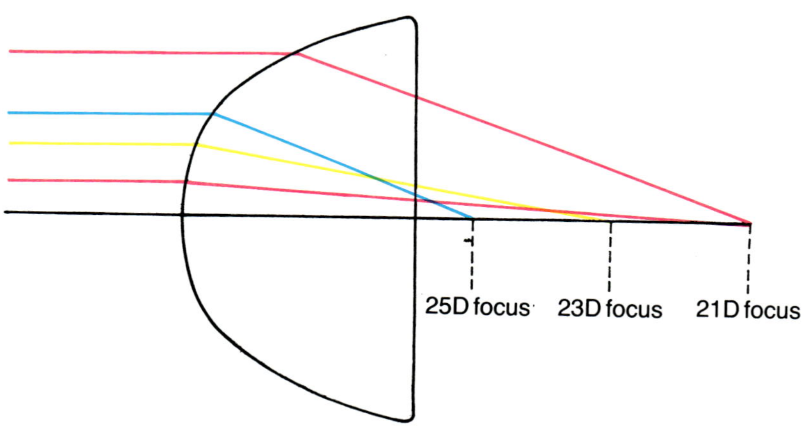

21.6 Ray diagram of light entering the concentric aspheric system of (**21.5**): The lens thickness is exaggerated and the focal lengths are shortened for clarity (courtesy of Dr Lee Nordan, USA).

21.7

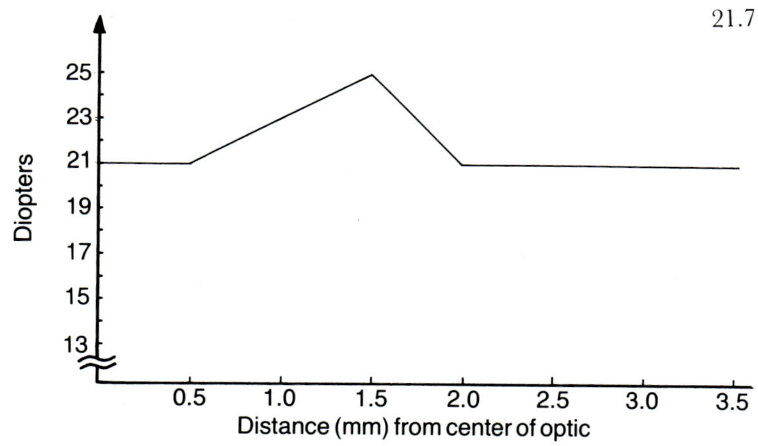

21.7 Dioptric power changes that occur with increasing distance from the center of the optic seen in (**21.5**) and (**21.6**).

Multiple zone refraction multifocals

These are a combination of a posterior spheric refractive surface and multiple anterior spheric refractive surfaces for distance, intermediate and near correction (Allergan Medical Optics: Array design). The front surface of the Array design has five zones (**21.8**), each of which progressively adds from 0 to 3.5D to the overall lens power. All distances from infinity to the near point would be expected to be focused by each zone of this IOL. Theoretically, the multifocal function should not be compromised by decentration or pupillary abnormalities.

21.8

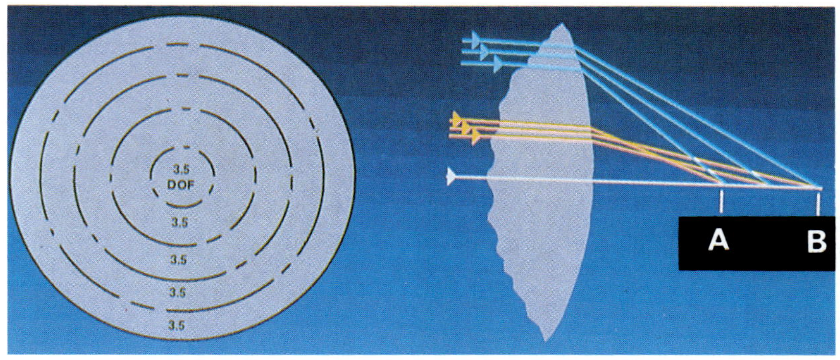

21.8 Array refractive design showing the five zones of progressive power addition, and a ray diagram of light entering two such zones: A, Near 23.5D; B, Far 20.0D (courtesy of Dr Tim Willis, USA).

Multiple zone diffraction bifocals

These are the combination of an anterior spheric refractive surface and multiple posterior diffractive plate surfaces for distance and near correction (3M: microslope design). The 3M IOL combines both conventional refractive (on the anterior IOL surface) and diffractive (on the posterior IOL surface) optical principles. The combination can be reversed with the diffractive plates worked onto the anterior surface if a smooth refractive surface is required posteriorly. By choosing suitable dimensions for 20 to 30 concentric zones, each bounded by stepped discontinuities on the posterior surface (**21.9**), light is diffracted towards two foci (**21.10**). Diffraction can be interpreted as a spreading of wave fronts (**21.11**). After encountering discontinuities, if the waves are in phase they summate, and if they are out of phase, there is destructive

21.9

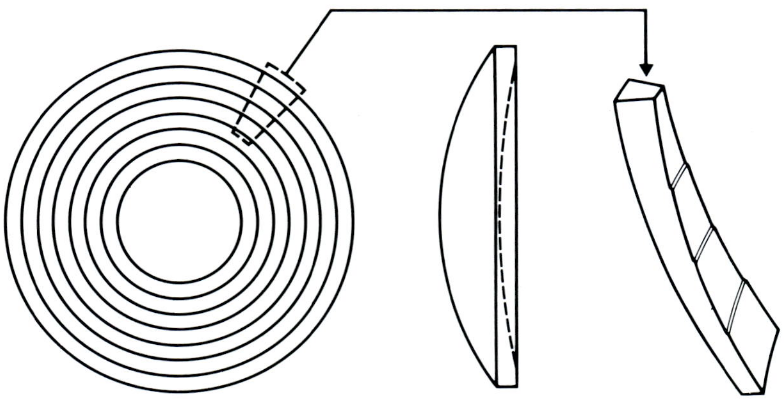

21.9 Diagram of diffractive optic showing microslope rings, edge on representation of the optic and exaggerated detail of the stepped discontinuities.

21.10

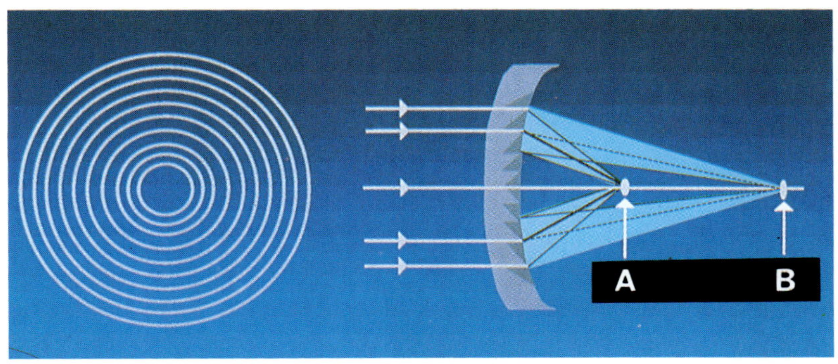

21.10 Diagram of light entering zones of the optic shown in **21.9**: A, Near image; B, Distance image.

21.11

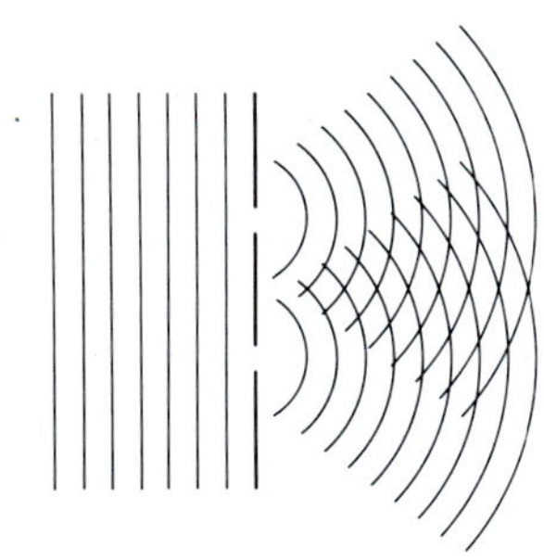

21.11 Diffraction grating.

interference. The design allows approximately 41% of light to be in phase and focussed for distance, 41% to be in phase and focussed for near and 18% to be permanently out of focus (**21.12**). Both foci receive light from every zone so the bifocal function is independent of pupil size and lens centration (**21.13**).

Simplified ray tracings for the Pharmacia, Iolab, Wright Medical (**21.14**) and Ioptex, Allergan Medical Optics, and 3M (**21.15**) multifocal IOLs are illustrated diagramatically. Theoretically, each of these lenses will focus both distance and near objects on the fovea simultaneously, but often by sacrificing contrast and therefore resolution. At either object location, two or more images are formed on the retina; one is in focus and the other is out of focus. The degree to which the contrast at the focussed image is reduced by the out of focus images will characterize, in part, the performance of each lens design.

21.12

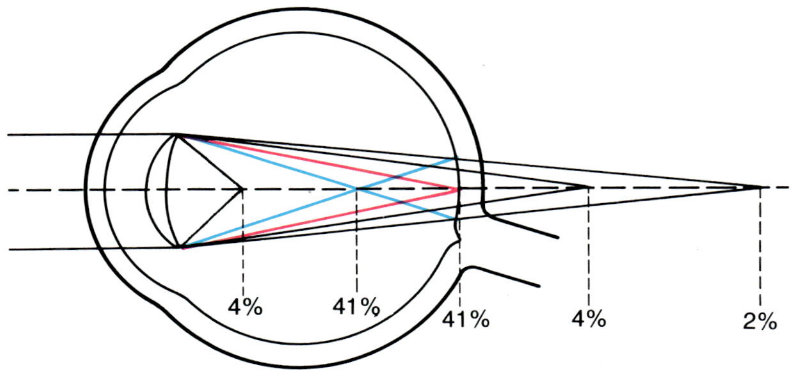

21.12 3M depiction of the proportions of light split into different foci: most of the energy is divided amongst two lens powers. The rest (although not all foci are indicated) is highly defocussed at the retina.

21.13

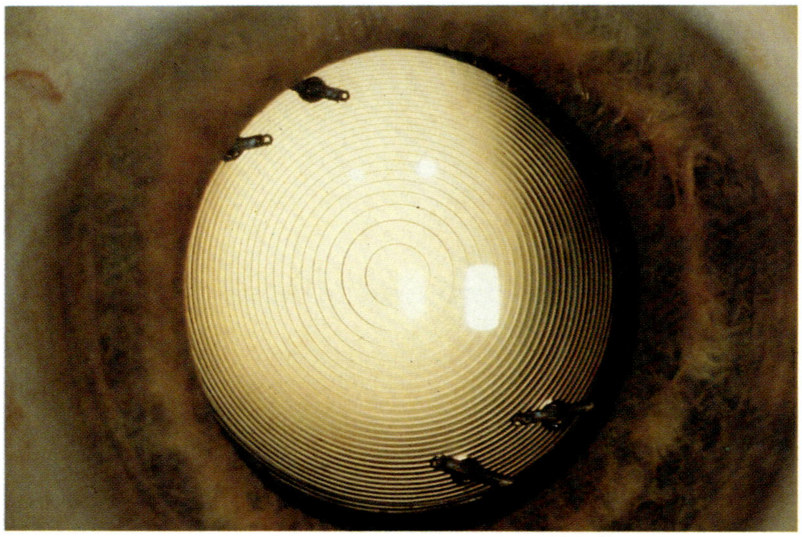

21.13 Diffractive IOL *in vivo* showing microslope rings on its posterior surface.

21.14

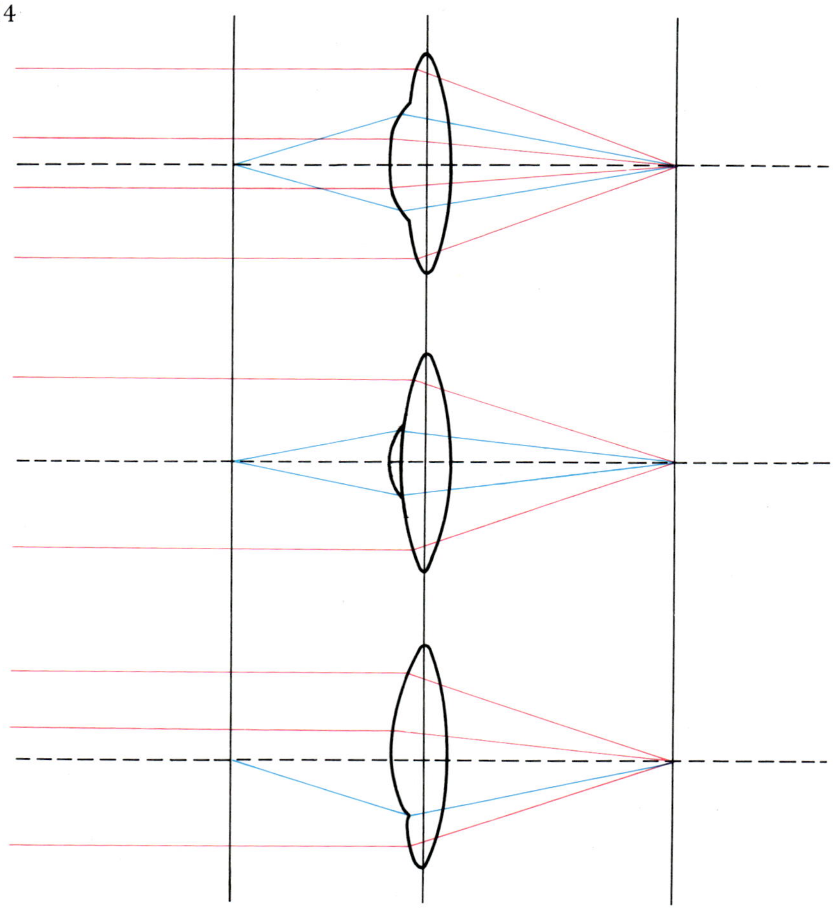

21.14 Simplified diagrams of Pharmacia (top), Iolab (center) and Wright Medical (bottom) multifocal lenses.

21.15

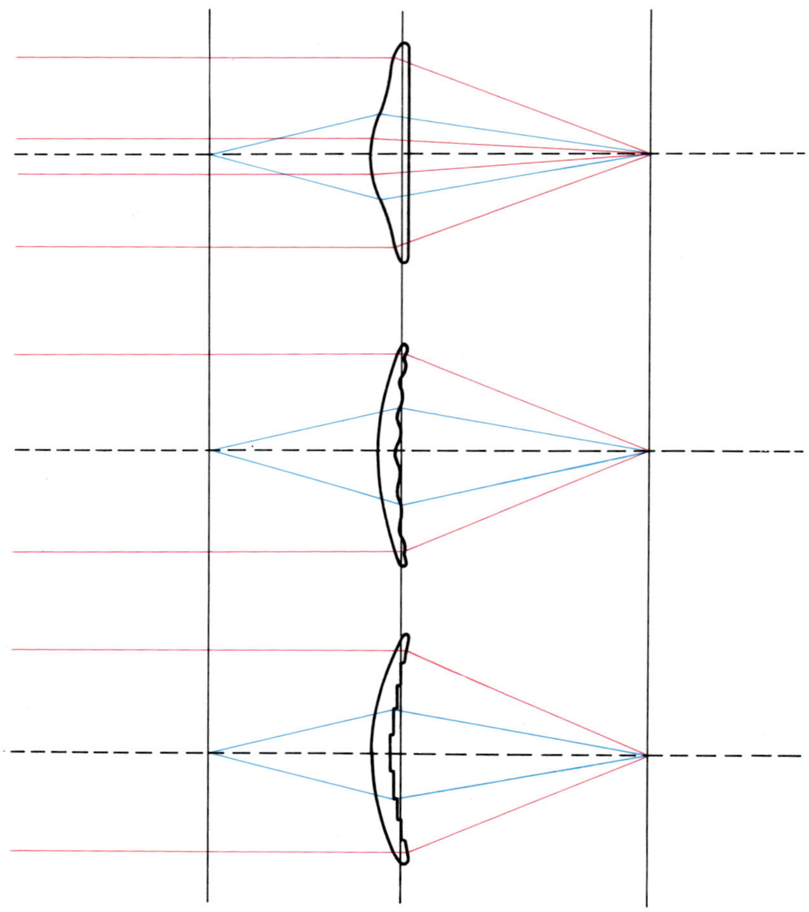

21.15 Simplified diagrams of Ioptex (top), AMO (center) and 3M (bottom) multifocal lenses.

Clinical results from implanted multifocal IOLs

Multifocal IOLs are in their infancy at this time, with only two manufacturers having accumulated and released clinical data from human studies. Core study results at 4–6 months follow up with the 3M diffractive IOL and the Iolab two-zone refractive IOL are available in 167 patients and 119 patients respectively (**Table 21.1**).

Best-case uncorrected distance visual acuity (excluding patients with preoperative pathology or macular degeneration) was 20/40 or better in 50.6% of Iolab-implanted patients, improving with correction to 92.8%. Implantation with the 3M lens produced 57.9% of best cases seeing 20/40 or better uncorrected, and 98.4% with correction.

Uncorrected near acuity was J3 (N6) or better in 79.4% of the 97 best-case Iolab-implanted patients. Equivalent data are not available from 3M, but Percival found that 71% of 55 cases implanted with the 3M lens could see both J3 *and* 20/40 without any aid. With the distance correction in place, the figures for reading J3 improved to 79.3% for the 3M core study best cases and to 80.4% for Iolab cases. 79 of the 97 Iolab best-case patients and 98 of the 121 3M best-case patients did not require any reading addition over their distance correction (**Table 21.1**). There remained a small percentage in both groups who could not read J3.

Brightness acuity testing was performed and no significant decrease in visual acuity was noted in either group of implanted patients. One theoretical drawback of the Iolab lens is dependence on visual axis centration. Decentration greater than 2 mm in eyes with pupillary apertures of less than 2 mm, could result in loss of near acuity requiring a corrective lens in the form of spectacles. The 3M lens theoretically allows any part of the optic to be located behind the pupil and still preserve adequate distance and near visual acuity.

Further 3M data on 41 paired multifocal/monofocal implanted patients showed no significant difference between the two eyes in contrast sensitivity or in subjective complaints of flare, glare, halo, distance and near distortion, monocular diplopia, and night vision problems. Kinetic testing of the visual field did not reveal defects related to the multizone design.

The 3M multifocal has a focus difference of 3.5D (equivalent to a 2.3D spectacle addition) and, although different additions may be available in the future, Percival has found that 3.5D produces commendable results, with 52% requiring no reading addition for a near point of J2 at 25 cm and 80% requiring an addition of less than 0.8D. The mean reading addition for this near point was 0.3D. However, he also found that some patients noted their reading vision to be shadowy, being unable to read J2 at a comfortable distance whatever addition was provided and that, for some, this loss of quality may be a price that has to be paid for the obvious advantage of lessening the dependence on glasses.

Table 21.1 Core study results released by Iolab and 3M in percentage and actual patient numbers

Distance	*20/40 or better*		*20/41 – 20/80*		*20/81 or worse*	
	Iolab	3M	Iolab	3M	Iolab	3M
Overall corrected distance visual acuity	86.6 103/119	95.2 159/167	7.5 9/119	4.2 7/167	5.9 7/119	0.6 1/167
Best-case*uncorrected distance visual acuity	50.6 49/97	57.9 70/121	24.7 24/97	32.2 39/121	24.7 24/97	9.9 12/121
Best-case*corrected distance visual acuity	92.8 90/97	98.4 119/121	5.2 5/97	1.6 2/121	2.0 2/97	0 0/121
Reading	*J3 or better*		*J4 – J7*		*J8 or worse*	
	Iolab	3M	Iolab	3M	Iolab	3M
Overall corrected near visual acuity	93 105/113	88 147/167	3.5 4/113	9.6 16/167	3.5 4/113	2.4 4/167
Best-case*near visual acuity without near or distance correction	79.4 77/97	NA	4.1 4/97	NA	16.5 16/97	NA
Best-case* near visual acuity with distance correction for those who do not require reading additions	78/79	96/98	0/79	2/98	1/79	0/98
Best-case* near visual acuity for those who require reading additions	15/18	19/23	3/18	3/23	0/18	1/23

* Best case excludes patients with preoperative pathology or macular degeneration at any time.

Looking ahead

In the near future the multifocal IOL will provide the advantage of simultaneous distance and near visual acuity correction for many, if not the majority, of pseudophakic patients. Early clinical results with multifocal IOL implantation have established the effectiveness and patients' acceptance of the multifocal concept. Newer designs and further improvement and refinement of these 'first generation' multifocal IOLs will doubtless occur, built on the foundations already established.

It was held in the past that aphakia represents the first complication of cataract surgery. We have been able to overcome this 'complication' with pseudophakic correction, but until recently have had to consider presbyopia as the first complication of pseudophakia. Since 1949 ophthalmology has made great strides in the evolution of intraocular lens implantation to correct aphakia and the multifocal IOL represents yet another step in that evolutionary process.

Accompanying multifocal IOL technology will be an increased realization of the significance of residual surgical or idiopathic astigmatism and ametropic distance visual acuity, caused by less than precise IOL power formulas and calculations. Multifocal IOLs require greater accuracy in power calculation and greater surgical ability to resolve existing ametropia or astigmatism if the need for postoperative glasses is to be avoided. Preliminary results suggest that it is already possible to achieve satisfactory unaided vision for both distance and near in over 70% of patients. It is to be hoped that future modifications will lead to even greater achievements.

Further reading

Percival S.P.B. Prospective study of the new diffractive bifocal intraocular lens. *Eye*, **3**, 571–575, 1989.

22: Viscoelastics

Richard Keates and Richard Erdey

Viscoelastics are a group of agents used to manipulate and protect ocular tissues. The solutions are nontoxic, sterile, pyrogen free and extremely viscous (up to 500,000 times greater than water). In their present form, they are used to maintain anterior chamber depth and visibility and to help minimize interaction between tissues. By coating the surface of the delicate corneal endothelial cell lining during cataract surgery, these viscoelastic substances can also serve to minimize cellular damage during the insertion of an intraocular lens (IOL). Coating of the IOL prior to insertion may also help minimize this type of damage. These solutions must demonstrate not only suitable viscoelastic properties, but superior coatability as well.

When clinically comparing the behavior of these solutions, it is important to consider such parameters as chemical composition, molecular weight, osmolality, wettability (how thoroughly the agent spreads over the surface), coatability (the thickness of the surface coat), viscosity (the measure of resistance towards flow of a solution), and elasticity (the measure of the capacity of a solution to resist deformation) (**22.1, 22.2**).

Generally, as the concentration increases, there is considerable increase in the viscosity of the solution. The viscosity is the property that inversely influences the ability of the solution to percolate through the drainage channels of the trabecular meshwork. Viscoelastic agents are miscible; that is, they will gradually dissolve in aqueous and eventually drain out of the eye through the chamber angle. Viscosity is also dependent on the chemical structure and molecular weight of the substance. Solutions with higher viscosities are better at maintaining chamber depth during surgery.

The current viscoelastics available include: sodium hyaluronate (NaHA), chondroitin sulfate (CS), hydroxypropylmethylcellulose (HPMC) and other carbohydrate polymers in a variety of commercial preparations, including collagen IV (**Table 22.1**). Solutions of NaHA are extracted from rooster combs. NaHA is a high molecular weight polysaccharide that exhibits excellent viscoelastic and lubricating properties. These properties have made NaHA the first widely

22.1

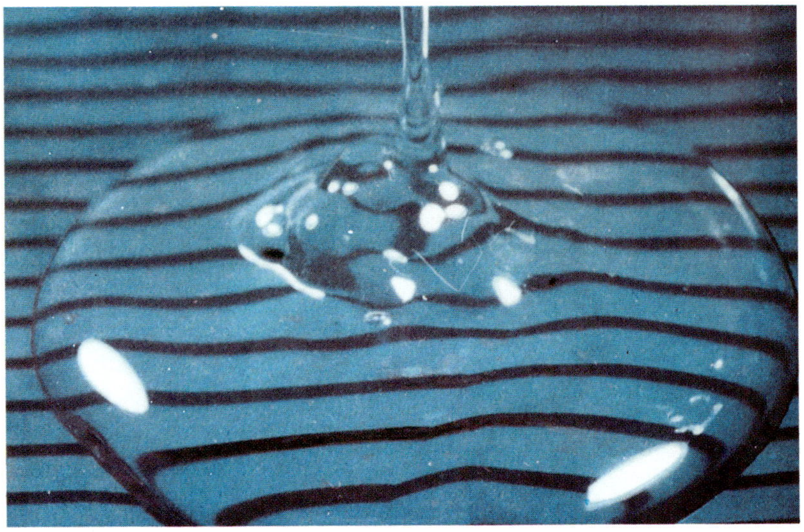

22.1 The viscous and elastic properties of sodium hyaluronate.

22.2

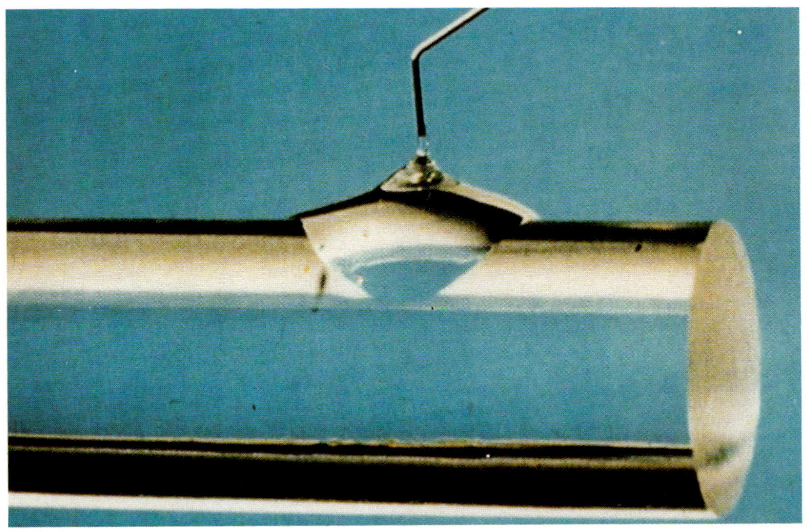

22.2 Coating of a glass rod by sodium hyaluronate injected through a 25-gauge cannula.

Table 22.1 Viscoelastic agents currently available (figures released by manufacturers)*

Viscoelastic	*Manufacturer*	*Solution*	*Osmolality (mOsm l^{-1})*	*Mol. Wt. (Daltons)*	*Viscosity (centistokes)*	*Coatability (mm)*	*Wettability (dynes)*
Amvisc®	Medchem/Iolab	1.2% NaHA	318	2.04×10^6	41,000	0.51	70
Amvisc plus®	Medchem/Iolab	1.6% NaHA	340	1.43×10^6	55,000	0.54	NA
Healon®	Pharmacia	1.0% NaHA	302	2.43×10^6	47,271	0.36	70
Occucoat®	Stortz	2% HPMC	319	8.00×10^5	2,500–5,500	NA	50
Viscoat™	Alcon	4% CS, 3% NaHA	366	5.5×10^5 CS 5×10^6 NaHA	20,000–60,000	NA	60
Cellugel™	Vision Biology/ Rayner	2% Polycarbonate	305	1.0×10^5	14,000	NA	NA
Ial®	Fidia	1.2% NaHA	301	$5–7 \times 10^5$	35,000	NA	NA
Collagel®	Domilens	Collagen IV	300	14.3×10^6	15,000	NA	NA

* NA = not available.

accepted surgical aid in a variety of anterior and posterior segment procedures. CS is similar in regard to chemical and physical composition to NaHA. Each molecule occurs as a large unbranched chain of repeating disaccharide subunits. It is commercially prepared with sodium hyaluronate, hence the preparation combines the characteristics of possibly better endothelial protection (CS) with the benefit of high viscosity and space maintenance (NaHA). HPMC is a cellulose polymer synthesized from natural materials and composed of D-glucose molecules linked together by ß-glycosidic bonds. Although not very viscous, studies have demonstrated improved wettability over other agents. An alternative agent, considered more viscous than HPMC, is a synthetic carbohydrate polymer marketed as Cellugel™ (**Table 22.1**).

NaHA, CS and HPMC molecules are noninflammatory, nonantigenic, nontoxic, and protective of the corneal endothelium (**22.3–22.5**). They are well tolerated in human eyes and, provided preparation has ensured they are free from impurities, they do not cause postsurgical intraocular inflammation.

Viscoelastics are commercially supplied in a sterile disposable syringe and are available in different volumes: 0.25 ml, 0.5 ml and 0.8 ml (Amvisc®/Amvisc plus®), 0.5 ml (Viscoat™), 0.4 ml, 0.75 ml and 2.0 ml (Healon®), 1.0 ml (Occucoat®), 1.5 ml (Cellugel™), 1.0 ml and 2.0 ml (Ial®), and 0.5 ml Collagel®. The volume selected depends on the quantity to be used. For example, 0.25–0.50 ml would need to be used if only instillation of viscoelastic into the anterior chamber is planned. A larger volume may be necessary if additional viscoelastic is needed to coat surgical instruments, for additional corneal protection, or after rupture of the posterior capsule.

The ophthalmic applications of viscoelastics include cataract surgery and IOL implantation, secondary IOL implantation, penetrating keratoplasty, glaucoma filtration surgery, and intraocular injection in conjunction with scleral buckling procedures for retina reattachment. The first three are discussed below.

22.3

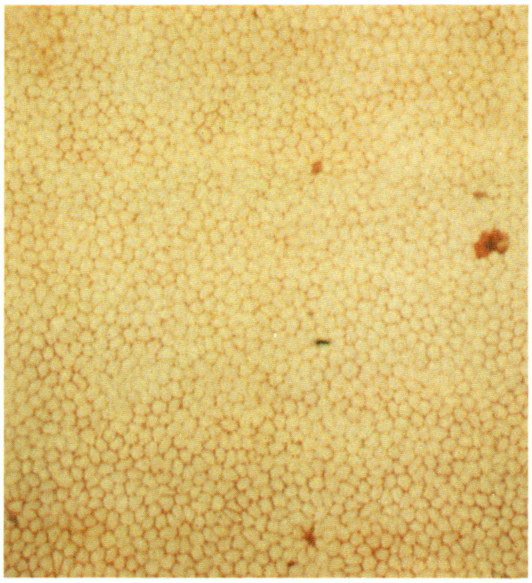

22.3 Normal rabbit corneal endothelium, x80.

22.4

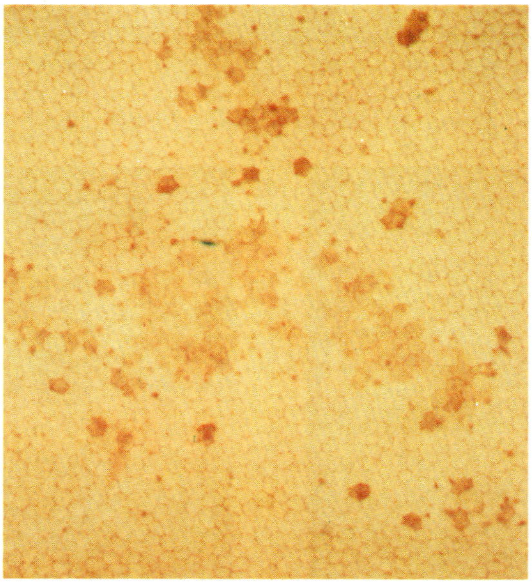

22.4 1.3 g static weight applied to a cornea previously coated with sodium hyaluronate showing minimal endothelial damage, x80.

22.5

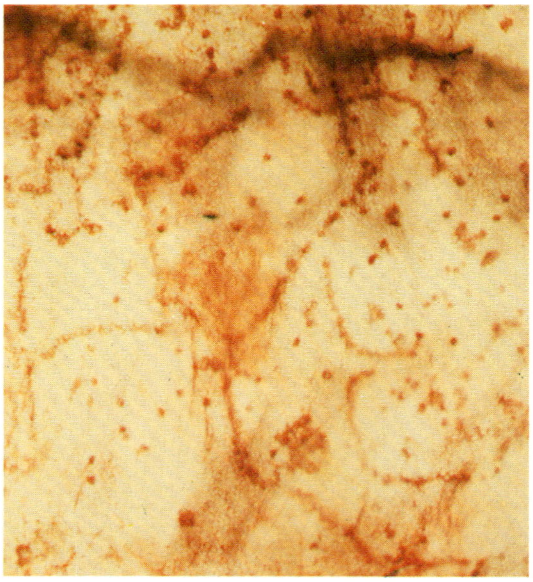

22.5 1.3 g static weight applied to an unprotected cornea showing severe endothelial damage, x80.

Cataract extraction with intraocular lens implantation

A viscoelastic is used to protect the endothelium prior to capsulotomy. The endothelial cells are coated and protected from surgical trauma. Further, viscoelastic aids in the dilation of the pupil. Additionally, the anterior chamber depth is maintained during the capsulotomy by the viscoelastic, replacing the need for anterior chamber stabilization with air or salt solution (**22.6**). It is important not to overinflate the anterior chamber with viscoelastic since increased intraocular pressure could result (**22.7**). This should particularly be avoided in patients with glaucoma.

22.6

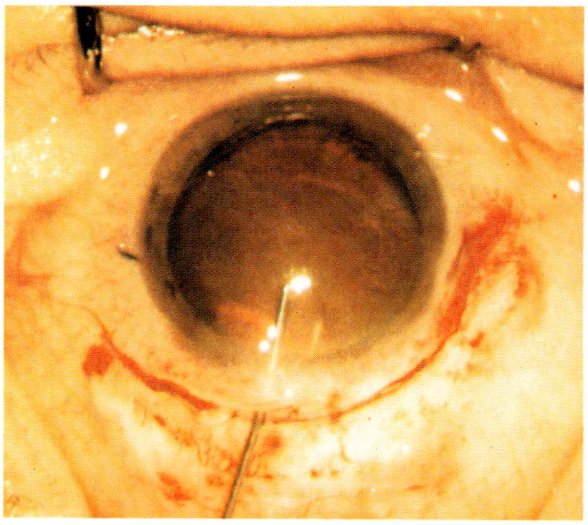

22.6 Instillation of viscoelastic through a fine bore cannula into the anterior chamber before anterior capsulotomy.

22.7

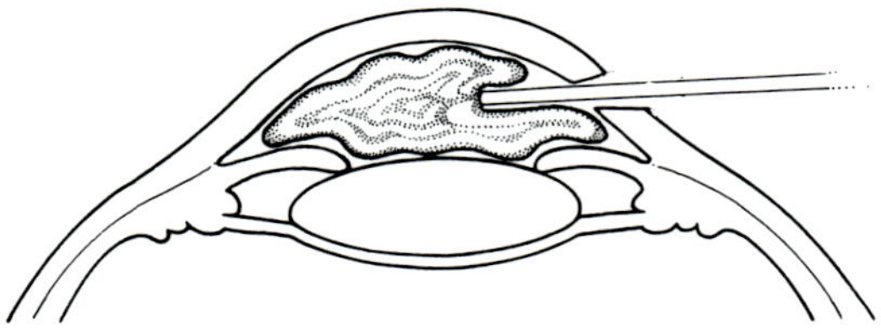

22.7 Aqueous may be replaced, but the anterior chamber should not be overfilled with viscoelastic.

Infiltration under the anterior capsular flap during continuous circular capsulorhexis facilitates the grasping of the anterior capsular leaf with forceps when initiating the capsulorhexis (**22.8**).

After the nucleus has been subluxed into the iris plane, viscoelastic can be used to manipulate it into the proper position for phacoemulsification. This may also afford some protection of the posterior capsule (**22.9**). For nucleus extraction techniques, viscoelastics may be infiltrated behind the nucleus in cases where difficulty occurs in prolapsing it.

Viscoelastics can be used to manipulate the iris away from a keratome incision to allow the introduction of the phacoemulsification instrument into the anterior chamber. Additionally, this may help prevent iris prolapse. Viscoelastics may also be used to prevent iris prolapse during suturing of a hard eye. After cortical material has been removed, viscoelastics are used to inflate the capsular bag, separating the posterior capsule from the anterior leaves. The IOL can now be placed in the capsular bag, while visualizing the anterior capsular leaves (**22.10, 22.11**).

In the event of a small posterior capsule rupture with minimum vitreous prolapse, viscoelastic may be layered over the tear to prevent further vitreous prolapse, without extending the tear (**22.12**). Coating of the anterior surface of the IOL will protect the corneal endothelium during insertion (**22.13**).

After the IOL has been positioned and the limbal incision partially closed, the viscoelastic should be removed using irrigation/aspiration (**22.14**). This has two purposes: first, it will reduce the postoperative intraocular pressure rise secondary to trabecular meshwork occlusion; second, it allows any intraocular miotics to work without viscous impedance.

22.8

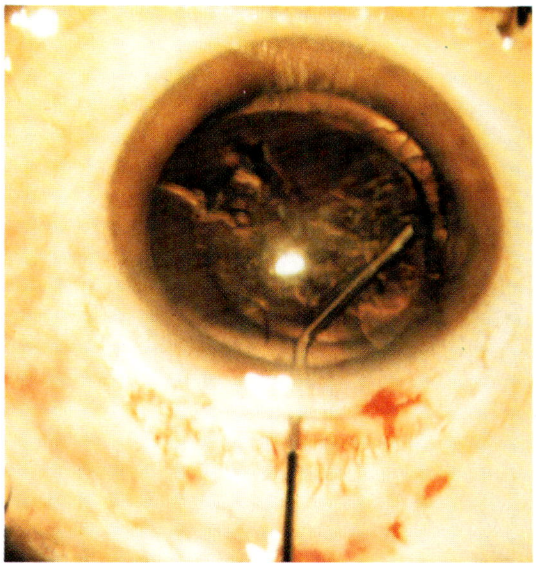

22.8 Infiltration under flap of anterior capsule during continuous circular capsulorhexis.

22.9

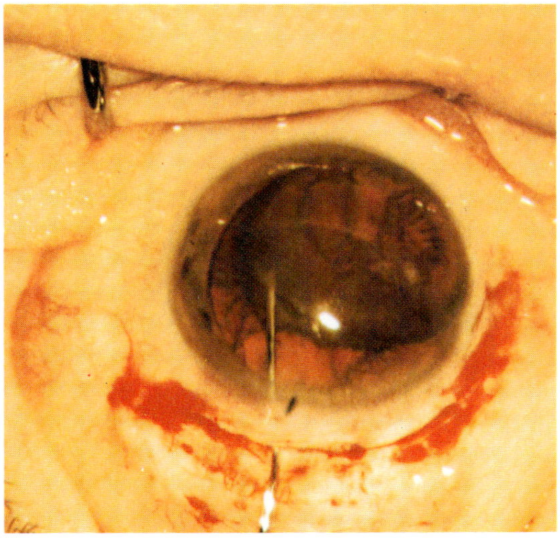

22.9 Subluxation of the nucleus forwards.

22.10

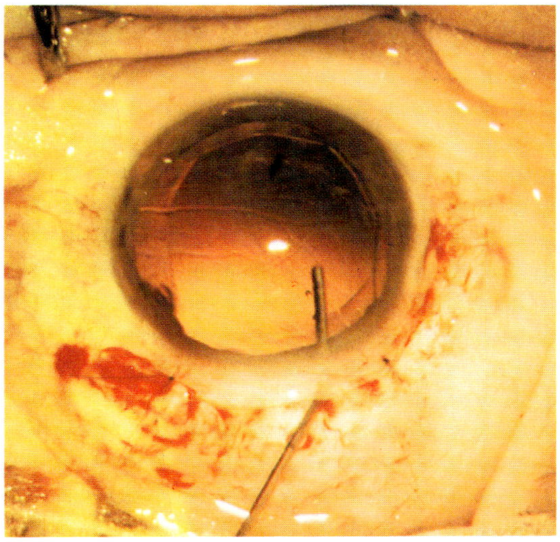

22.10 Infiltration into the fornices of the lens capsule.

22.11

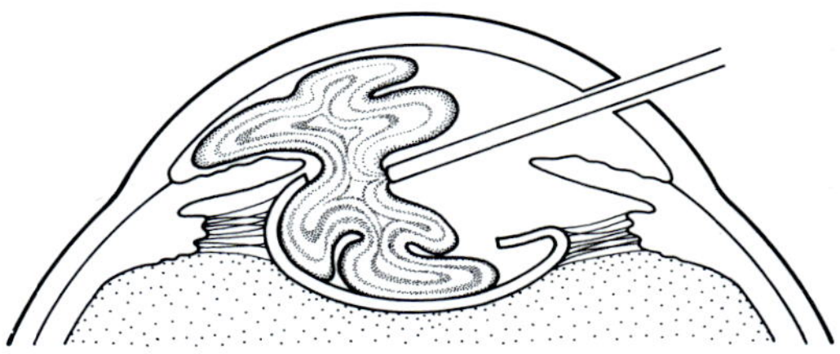

22.11 Diagram demonstrating inflation of the fornices of the lens capsule.

22.12

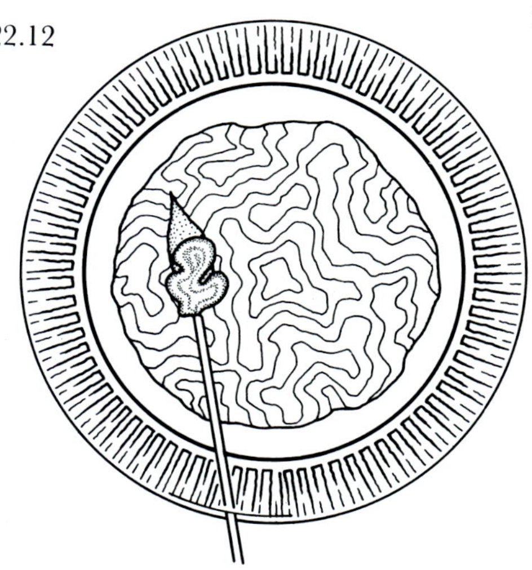

22.12 Viscoelastic covering a rent in the posterior capsule.

22.13

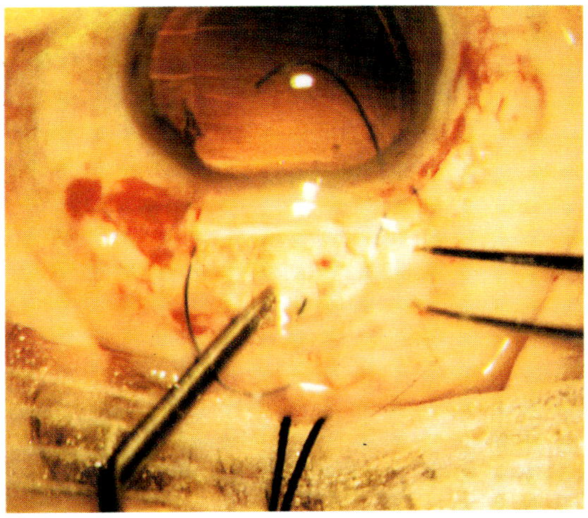

22.13 Coating of IOL prior to lens insertion.

22.14

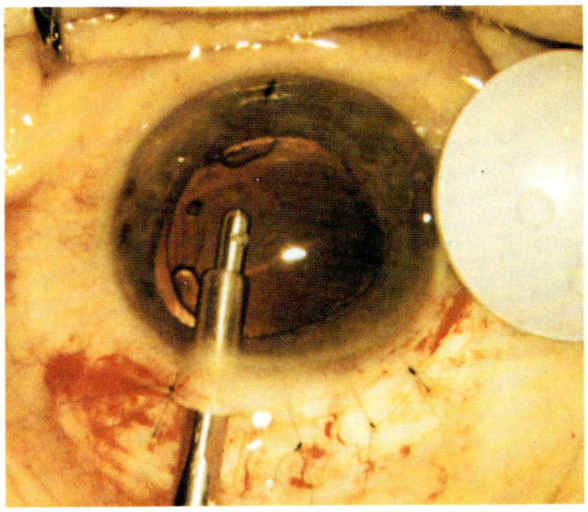

22.14 Removal of viscoelastic by I/A.

Secondary intraocular lens implantation

Viscoelastics can be used to 'seal' the limbal wound to retain air in the anterior chamber (**22.15**). The anterior chamber air is helpful in keeping the vitreous posterior to the iris plane. Additionally, viscoelastic is helpful in controlling vitreous in the anterior chamber when air is not sufficient. As before, it can be used to coat the anterior surface of the IOL prior to placement (**22.16**).

To differentiate between viscoelastic and vitreous at the wound margin, a dry cellulose sponge is used. Viscoelastic will adhere to the sponge, but will separate without causing pupillary distortion. Vitreous, however, will produce significant strands which adhere to the sponge and cause pupillary movement (**22.17, 22.18**).

22.15

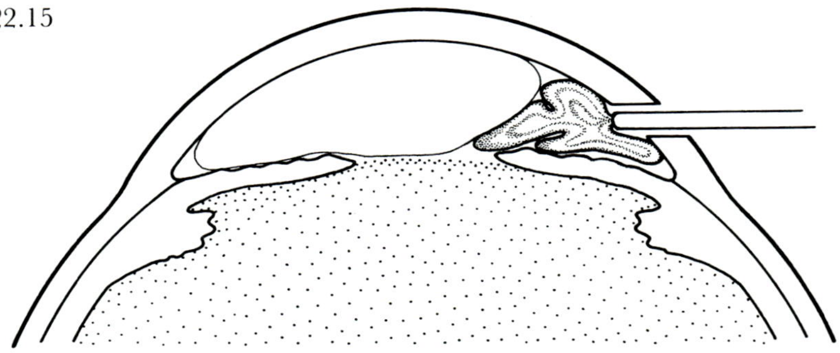

22.15 The section is sealed in order to retain air in the anterior chamber.

22.16

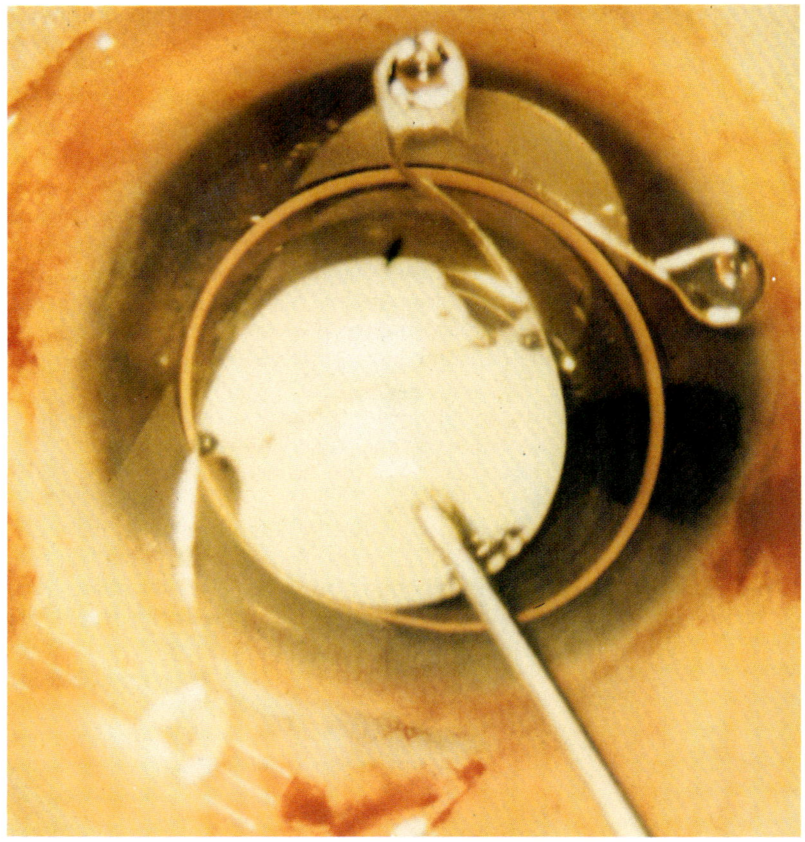

22.16 Coating of a semiflexible ACL prior to insertion. Note the use of Sheet's glide and of viscoelastic to seal air into the anterior chamber.

22.17

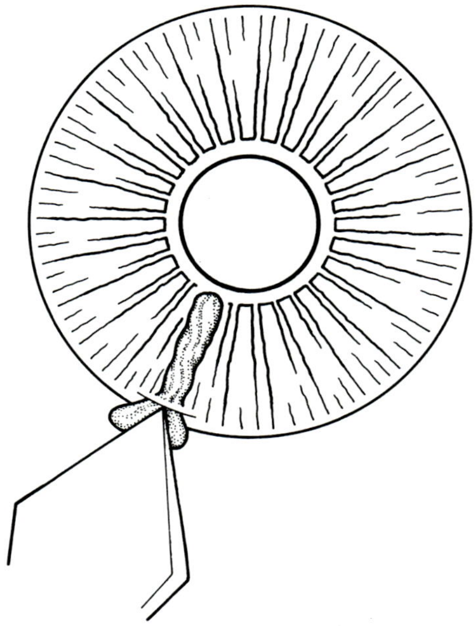

22.17 Bead of viscoelastic on the wound: when moved by a micropore sponge there is no movement of the pupil.

22.18

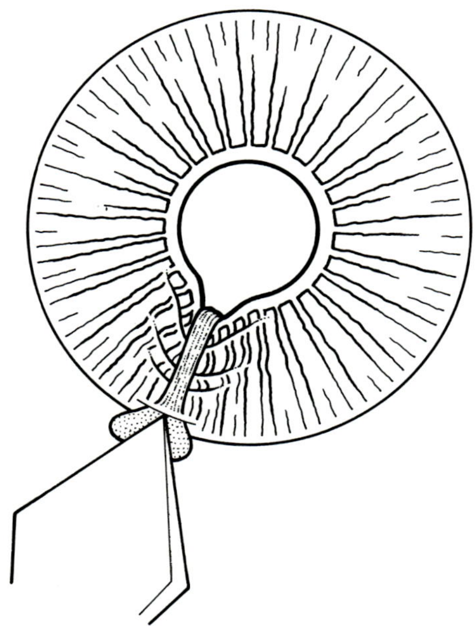

22.18 Bead of vitreous on the wound: when moved by a sponge there is pupillary distortion.

Penetrating keratoplasty

In penetrating keratoplasty and cataract extraction, viscoelastic may be used to fill the capsular bag, to coat the anterior chamber (**22.19**) prior to lens insertion (**22.20**), and to coat and protect the endothelium of the donor button (**22.21**), while suturing the button in place.

22.19

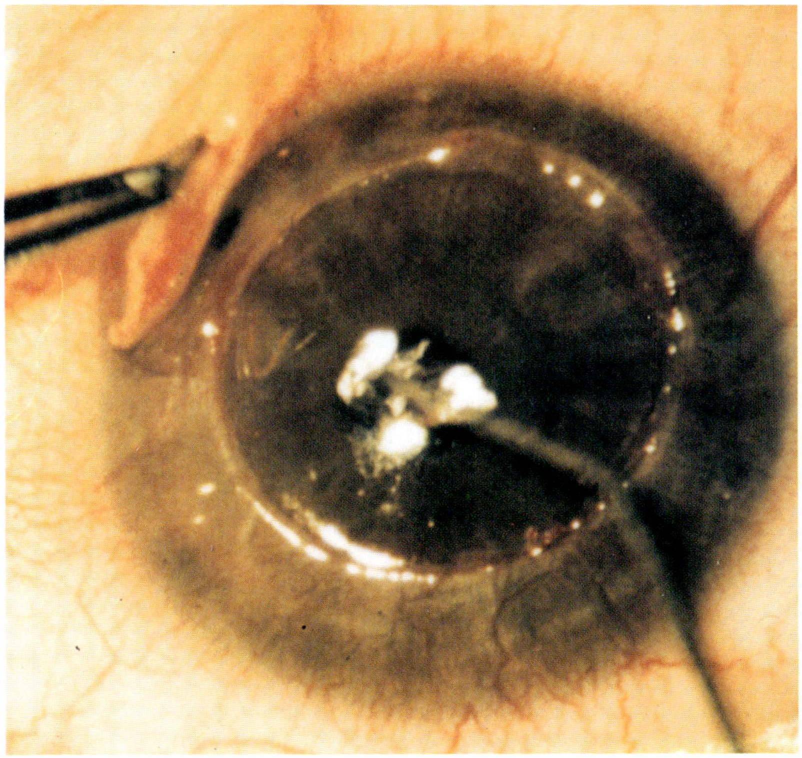

22.19 Layering of pupil and iridectomy with a viscoelastic prior to secondary lens implantation in an aphakic graft.

22.20

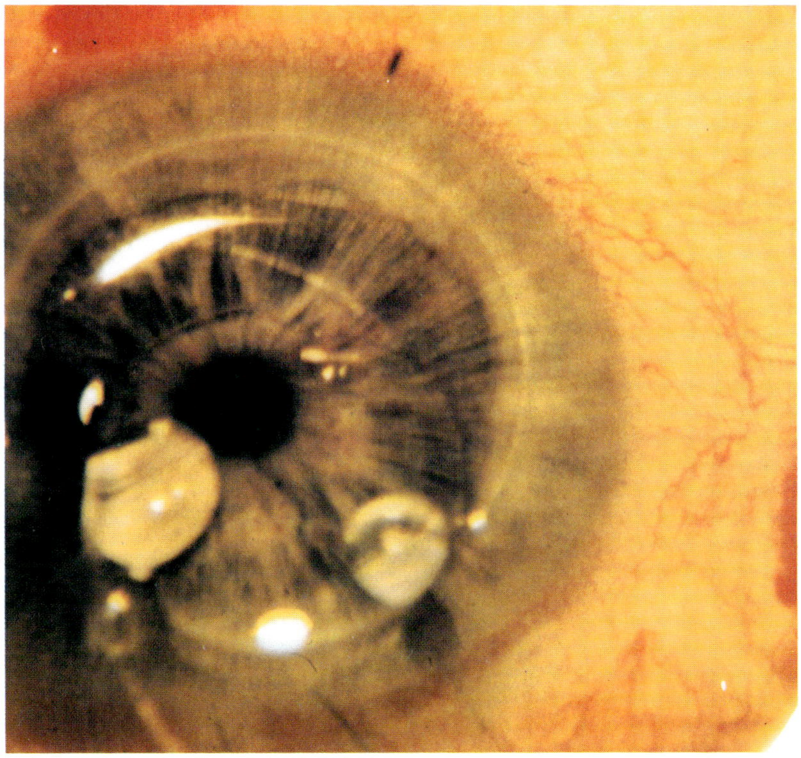

22.20 Insertion of distal loops of a Kelman ACL before graft in aphakia.

22.21

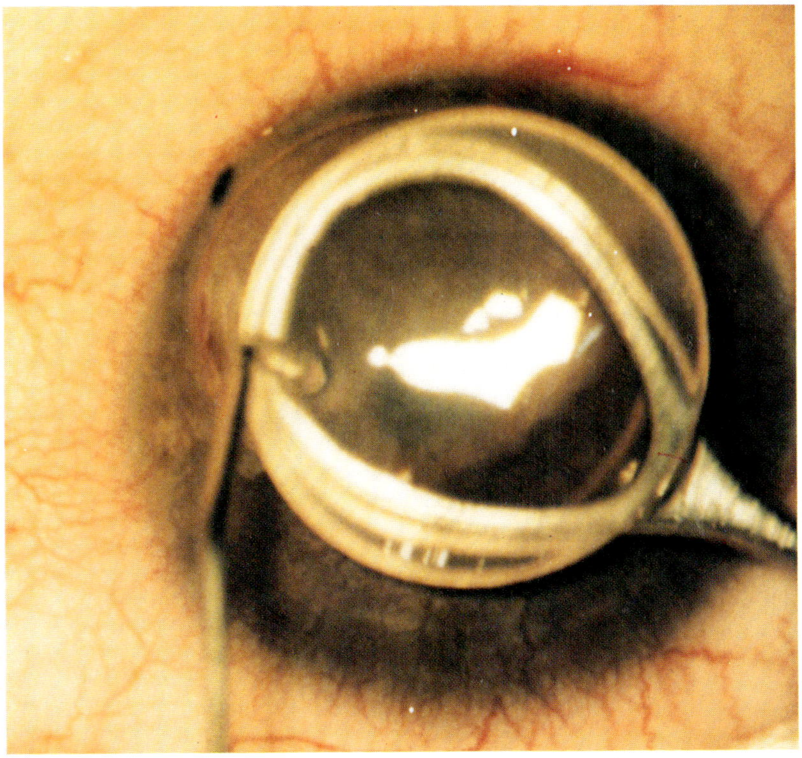

22.21 Coating the endothelium of the donor button.

Complications of viscoelastics

All viscoelastics can cause intraocular pressure elevation if left in the eye after surgery. Eyes with significant retention of viscoelastic postoperatively can demonstrate corneal edema, a deep anterior chamber, and elevated intraocular pressure. Red blood cells are seen firmly adhered to the corneal endothelium and found suspended with residual debris in the anterior chamber. The intraocular pressure peaks at approximately 14 h, and characteristically abates over the next 1–3 days. Treatment consists of ß-adrenergic antagonists and carbonic anhydrase inhibitors. Pressure elevation is less prolonged and significantly lower after anterior chamber washout and it is recommended that anterior chamber washout be performed at the close of surgery regardless of the viscoelastic type chosen.

The future of viscoelastic materials

Multiple viscoelastic agents could be developed with desired viscosities for different surgical applications. Investigators are using viscoelastics in applications such as tear film stabilizers and as vehicles for topical and intraocular drug delivery. Color-marked viscoelastics are also being investigated.

Further reading

Alpar J.J., Alpar A.J., Baca J. and Chapman D. Comparison of Healon and Viscoat in cataract extraction and intraocular lens implantation. *Ophthal. Surg.*, **19.,** 636–642, 1988.

Glasser D.B., Matsuda M., and Edelhauser H.F. A comparison of the efficacy and toxicity of an intraocular pressure response to viscous solutions in the anterior chamber. *Arch. Ophthal.*, **104,** 1819–1824, 1988.

Keates R., Waltman S. and Hoyt C. *Surgery of the Eye,* Churchill Livingstone, 57–66, 1988.

Lindstrom R.L., Larson R. and Skelnik D.L. *Viscoelastic Agents, Ophthalmology Clinics of North America,* Harcourt, Brace, Jovanovich, Inc., 173–186, 1989.

Miller D. and Stegmann R. *Healon (Sodium Hyaluronate): A Guide to Its Use in Ophthalmic Surgery.* John Wiley and Sons, 9, 1983.

Section 3:
PREOPERATIVE ASSESSMENT

23: Contraindications to intraocular lens implantation

Bruce Noble and Michael Hayward

As the use of intraocular lenses became more widespread, authoratitive lists of indications and contraindications were drawn up and published to provide guidelines for ophthalmologists beginning or contemplating intraocular lens (IOL) implantation. However, as experience with intraocular lenses increased, and with the change to extracapsular cataract surgery with posterior chamber lens implants, the indications for lens implantation have steadily widened. There are conditions that were previously regarded as relative contraindications, but that are now regarded as 'safe', and other situations in which surgery was previously absolutely contraindicated where the surgeon may now 'proceed with care' (**Table 23.1**).

As the use of lenses has increased, so too has the choice of lens styles. However, not every lens style is suitable for every clinical situation and some must be avoided altogether.

Before contemplating IOL implantation in more difficult or specialized situations, surgeons must consider their own skills, experience and the level of operating room instrumentation. The decision to implant a lens, or even to perform cataract surgery, in a complicated eye may be part of the regular experience of one ophthalmologist, but beyond the surgical skills and experience of another.

It is thus impossible to dictate rules of indications and contra-indications for lens implantation, but guidance can be given that surgeons must interpret in the light of their own limitations and skills.

Table 23.1 Considerations for IOL contraindications

IOL contraindicated	*Proceed with care*	*No contraindication*
Rubeosis iridis	Proliferative retinopathy	Other diabetic retinopathy
Uncontrolled iritis	Past history of uveitis	Heterochromic cyclitis
Ectopia lentis	Past pigment dispersion	Other forms of glaucoma
Microphthalmos	Traumatic cataract	High myopia
Buphthalmos	Corneal dystrophy	Previous retinal surgery
Flexible loop AC IOL	Vitreous loss at cataract surgery	Only eyes
Closed loop AC IOL		

Contraindications related to lens design

The use of certain lens styles has been associated with an increased risk of complications or with other difficulties in postoperative management.

Anterior chamber lenses

Rigid type: Sizing of these is absolutely critical. If the lens is too large, postoperative pain and tenderness may persist. If the lens is too small, it will be mobile within the anterior chamber, damaging both iris and corneal endothelium. Pseudophakic bullous keratopathy or glaucoma will be the end result.

With flexible polypropylene loops: These lenses are unstable and cause damage to both iris and corneal endothelium. These haptics, when exposed to ultraviolet light and resting in contact with the iris, quickly denature. The lenses are unstable on their anteroposterior axis and endothelial trauma is frequently observed.

With closed loops: These cause chronic irritation and damage to the angle with formation of peripheral anterior synechias (the angle zip-up syndrome). Intractable glaucoma is a possible sequel.

The UGH (uveitis/glaucoma/hyphema) syndrome is seen with many forms of IOLs, but is particularly associated with all these types of anterior chamber lenses.

Iris clip lenses

Whether the optic is placed in front of or behind the pupil, there is a high incidence of lens dislocation (**23.1**) and late bullous keratopathy (PBK). The risk of lens dislocation makes pupil dilatation risky and retinal examination is not easy.

23.1

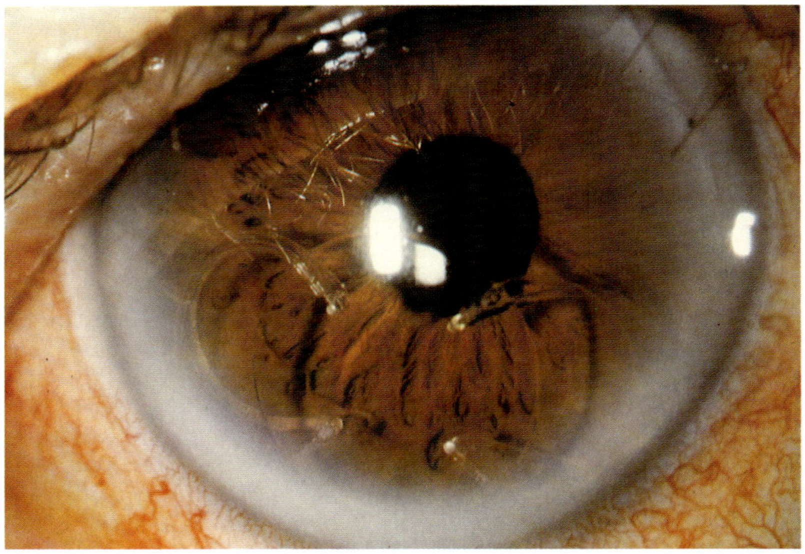

23.1 Iris clip lens dislocated into the anterior chamber.

Experimental and new designs of intraocular lens

New forms of IOL (e.g., soft hydrogel lenses, multifocal lenses and other new styles) need to be properly assessed in controlled prospective trials before being widely accepted. The design and marketing of IOLs is big business. There are many new styles with short pedigrees of assessment that are rushed onto the market by the manufacturing industry. Others are recommended to surgeons, encouraging them to gain in early experience with innovative styles, but not always in the context of a good prospective trial.

Lens implantation in the Third World

If lens implantation is to be considered in the Third World, then the surgical and intraocular lens standards should not differ from those enjoyed in the developed world. Surgeons using lenses in the Third World, designed for the Third World, must be very careful in assessing for themselves the quality of design and manufacture.

Contraindications related to eye pathology

Congenital and developmental abnormalities

Lens implantation is contraindicated in congenitally poorly developed eyes. Many of these eyes are microphthalmic (**23.2**) or abnormally large due to congenital glaucoma (**23.3**). The abnormal eye size further complicates safe lens insertion.

23.2

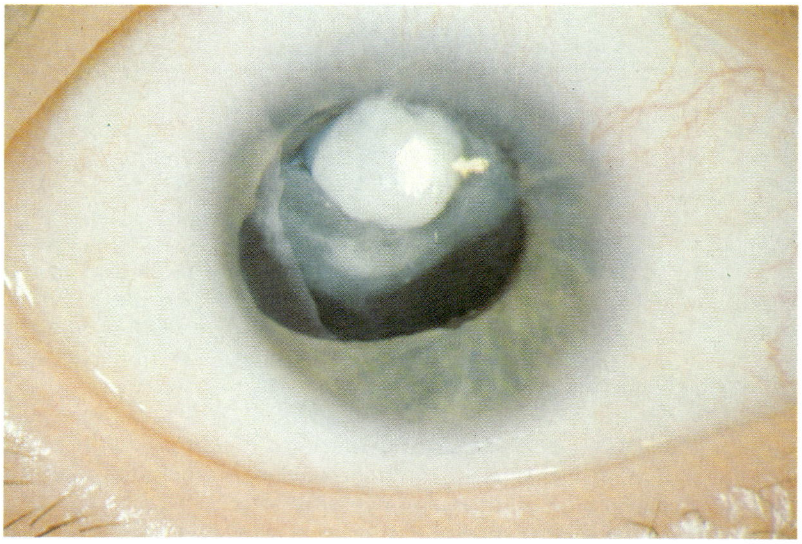

23.2 Cataract in a microphthalmic eye.

23.3

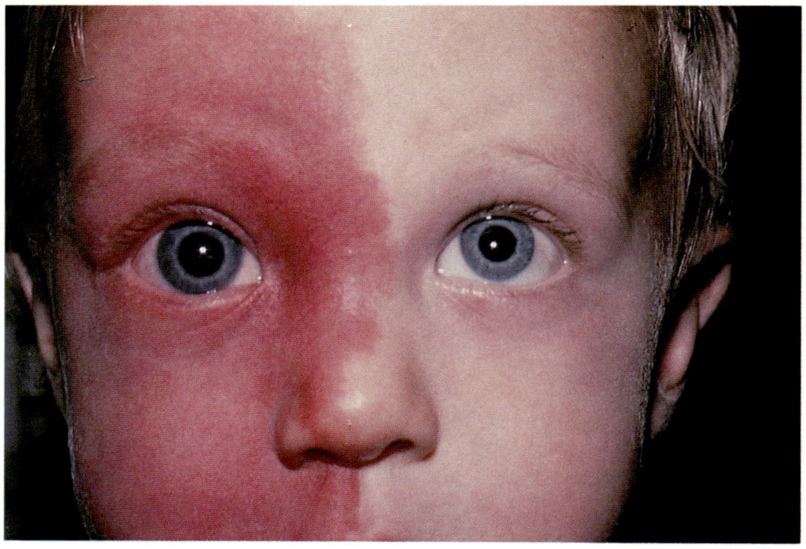

23.3 Buphthalmic eye associated with the Sturge–Weber syndrome.

Ectopia lentis (**23.4**) (e.g., associated with Marfan's syndrome or homocystinuria) is considered a relative contraindication to lens implantation. Patients presenting for surgery are often relatively young and are familiar with either contact lenses or spectacles of high power and tolerate well aphakic correction in spectacle form. Pathologically, the entire anterior segment including the drainage angle is involved and surgery on these eyes is associated with a much higher incidence of vitreous loss and retinal detachment. Special care and planning are required when contemplating any form of cataract surgery on these eyes. Posterior chamber or iris clip lenses should not be used. The use of an anterior chamber lens would be considered experimental. However, there are some congenital abnormalities, such as iris colobomata, that do not preclude lens implantation (**23.5**), although the surgery will always be more complicated.

23.4

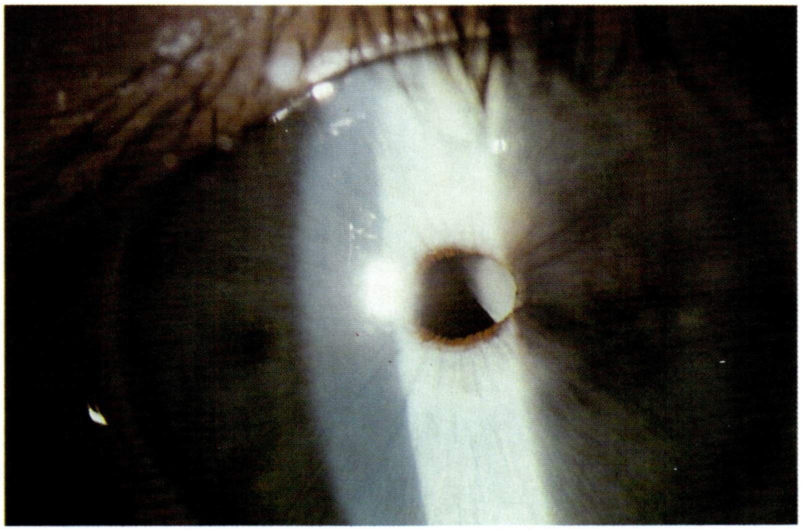

23.4 Ectopia lentis in a patient with Marfan's syndrome.

23.5

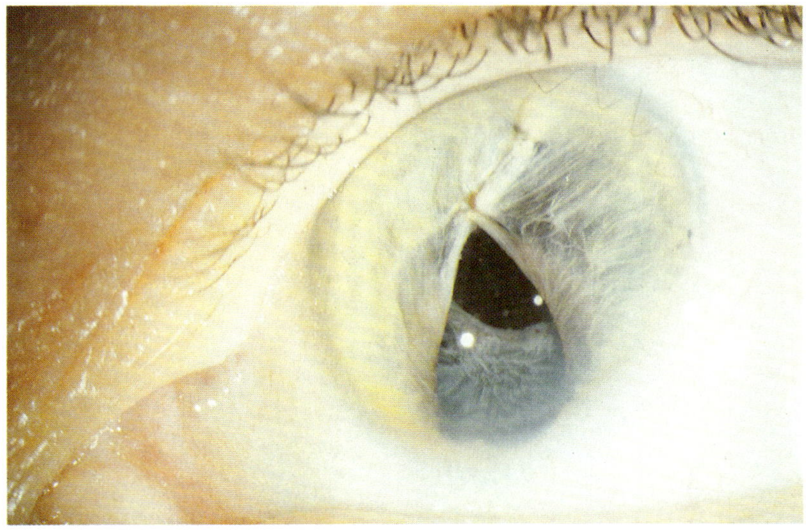

23.5 Posterior chamber IOL *in situ* behind an iris coloboma. A radial iridotomy has facilitated surgery and the anterior capsule has been used to form a 'pupil'.

Diabetes

Rubeosis iridis (**23.6**) is a contraindication to implantation. Even simple cataract surgery may lead to profound intraocular bleeding and cyclitic membrane formation, and these patients must have either simultaneous or immediate postoperative pan-retinal photocoagulation. An IOL in this situation is likely to exacerbate these postoperative problems (**23.7**).

In all other forms of diabetic eye disease an IOL may be safely implanted. Indeed, lens implantation should probably be encouraged

23.6

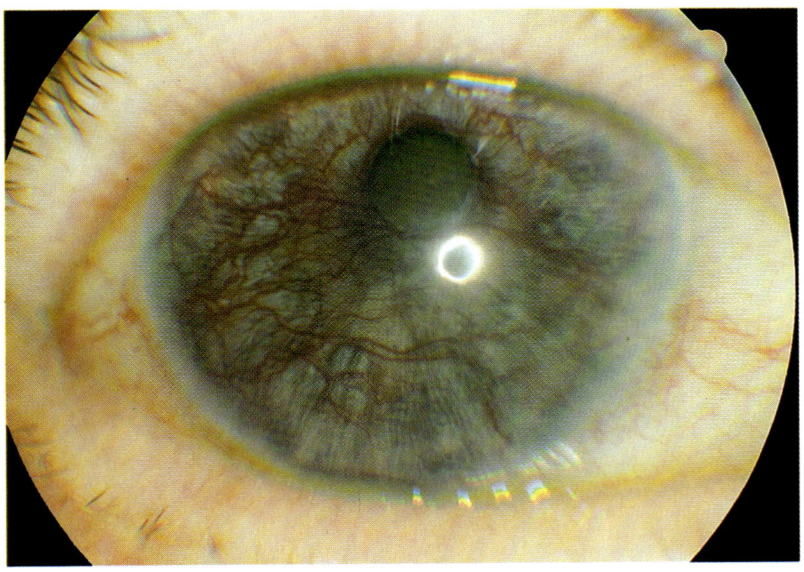

23.6 Rubeosis iridis.

23.7

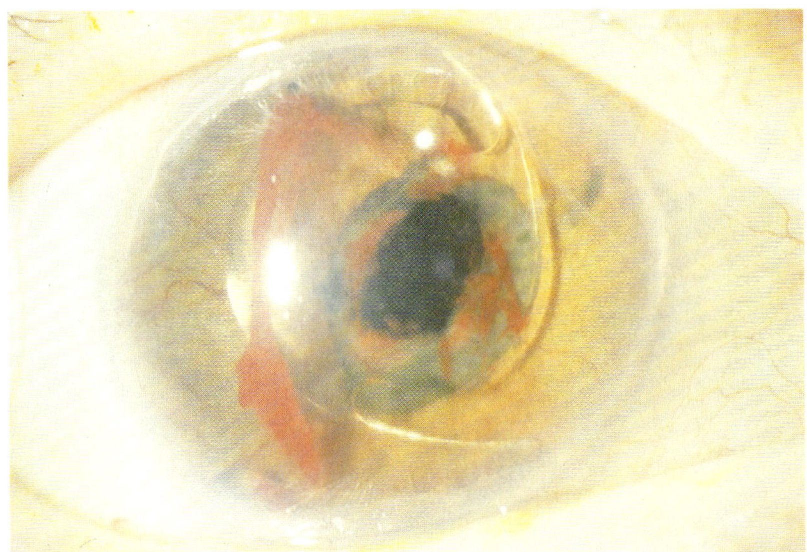

23.7 Anterior chamber lens inserted into an eye with rubeosis iridis. Notice hyphema, the small pupil despite intense efforts at mydriasis, and membrane formation.

as these patients often lose central vision due to macular disease and therefore have to rely on peripheral navigational vision. It is important in the diabetic eye that the anterior and posterior compartments are maintained (with the use of the extracapsular approach and a posterior chamber IOL) to prevent formation of rubeosis iridis in an already ischemic eye. Laser photocoagulation of the retina is possible to achieve through an IOL (**23.8**), although lasering the extreme retinal periphery may require skill and patience owing to the optical aberrations caused by the edge of the lens optic.

The diabetic eye is more liable to intense postoperative inflammation. This may take the form of a marked uveitis with fibrin clot formation (**23.9**), posterior synechias and consequent iris bombé. Some surgeons have advocated the routine use of a peripheral iridectomy, but we do not think this necessary, provided adequate monitoring and treatment are undertaken. Pigment shedding is also more common in diabetic patients and may occur dramatically during surgery.

23.8

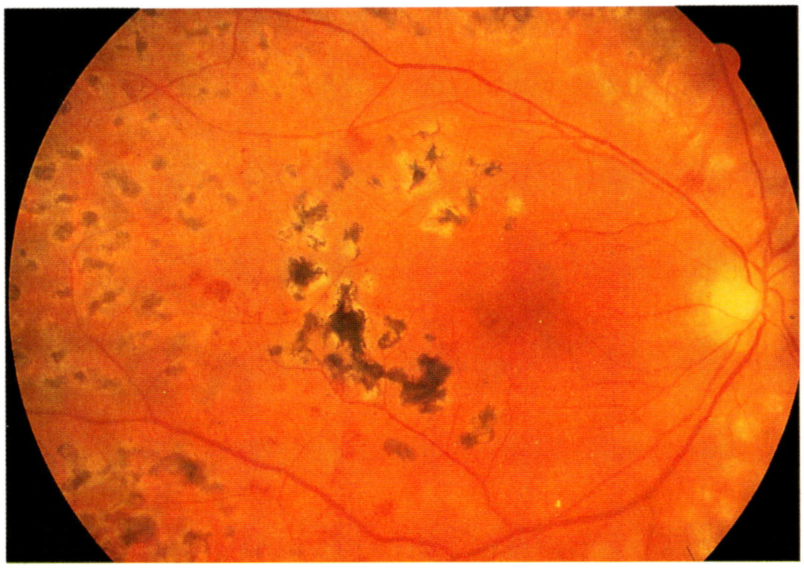

23.8 Macular and pan-retinal photocoagulation achieved through a posterior chamber IOL.

23.9

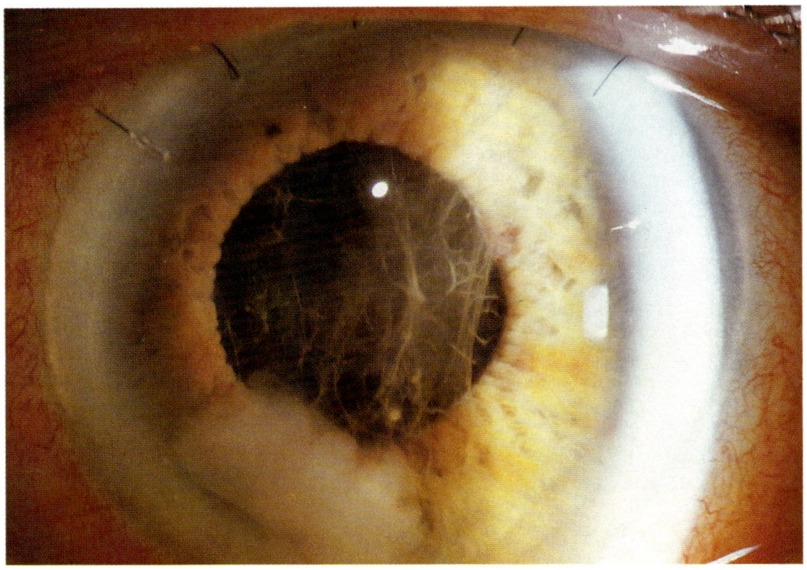

23.9 Postoperative inflammation following cataract surgery on a diabetic patient. There is also soft cortical lens material in the anterior chamber.

Uveitis

Lens implantation in the presence of aggressive anterior chamber inflammation is contraindicated. Cataract surgery should be avoided if possible, but if it is essential an intracapsular technique should be used with a broad iridectomy and possibly an anterior vitrectomy (or a formal, closed microsurgical lensectomy). The situation is more difficult when assessing a patient who has had uveitis or other forms of ocular inflammation in the past. Intraocular lens implantation may be successfully undertaken in eyes with a past history of anterior uveitis, scleritis or posterior segment inflammation secondary to sarcoid or Behçet's disease. However, the postoperative course is likely to be complicated by more active inflammation than is usual and will require more intensive and prolonged treatment. The preoperative and postoperative use of systemic steroids, either orally and/or as an IV bolus, is helpful. Intensive topical steroids are also required and some authorities advocate simultaneous systemic nonsteroidal anti-inflammatory agents. Patients may need to continue with topical treatment for a long period of time and some may need it indefinitely. There is an increased risk of aggressive uveitis, iris bombé, lens precipitates (**23.10**) and cyclitic membrane formation (**23.11**). The choice of a surface modified lens (see p. 115) may be helpful. Anterior

23.10

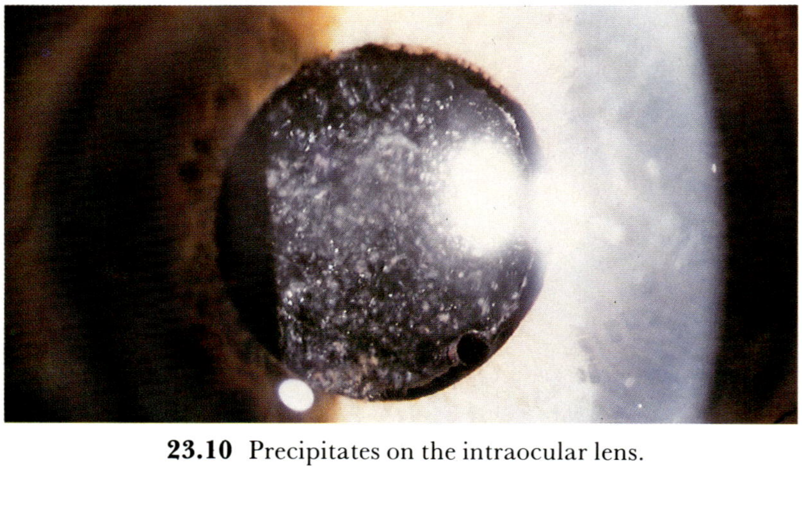

23.10 Precipitates on the intraocular lens.

23.11

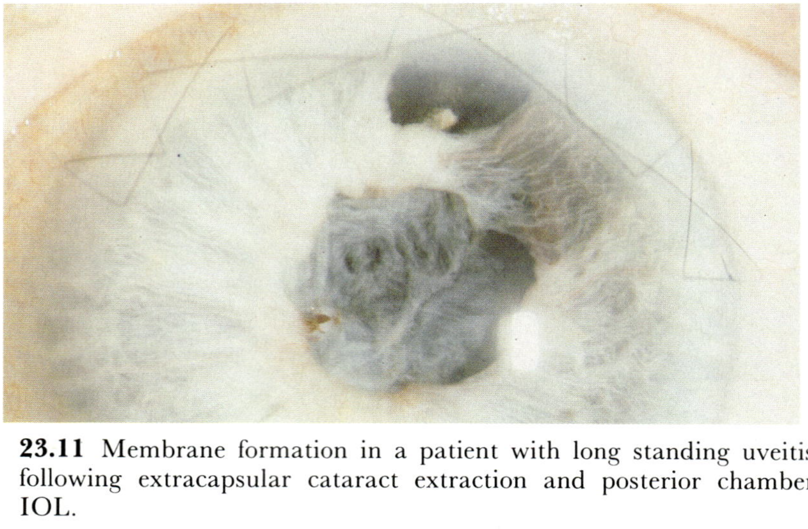

23.11 Membrane formation in a patient with long standing uveitis following extracapsular cataract extraction and posterior chamber IOL.

chamber lenses are contraindicated. A past history of posterior uveitis/choroiditis (**23.12**) is not a contraindication. Patients in whom there is a past history of scleritis should have their surgery carried out via a corneal incision to lessen the risk of postoperative scleritis.

Implantation may be safely made into patients with heterochromic cyclitis (**23.13**). Signs of increased inflammation in this condition do not usually respond to steroid treatment. However, an increase in inflammation may be seen postoperatively, which may respond normally to topical steroid treatment.

23.12

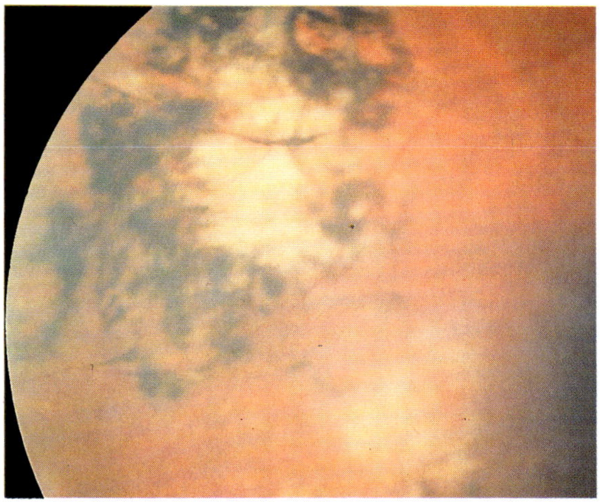

23.12 Old focus of choroiditis.

23.13

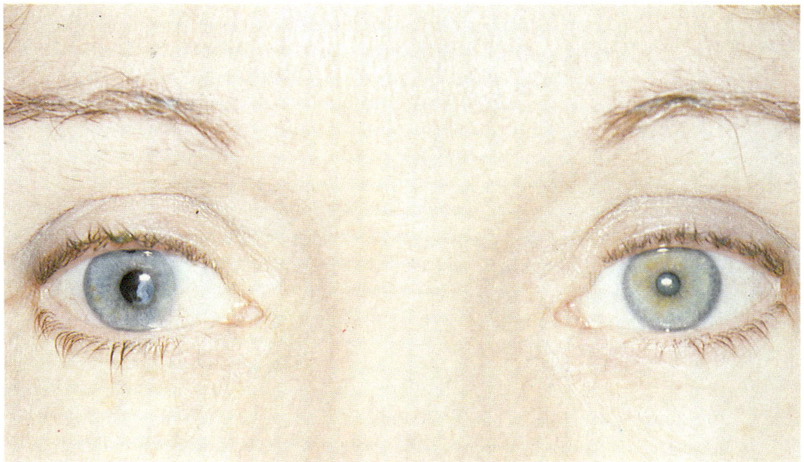

23.13 Heterochromic cyclitis.

Glaucoma

There is no contraindication to lens implantation in eyes with chronic open angle glaucoma, even if a simultaneous trabeculectomy is being performed. It is important to detect and treat early pressure rises following surgery, especially if there is evidence of gross field loss. Acetazolamide cover for the immediate postoperative period may be considered. When undertaking cataract surgery combined with trabeculectomy, or in an eye with a past history of acute closed angle glaucoma, a posterior chamber lens implant is preferred. An eye presenting acutely with phakomorphic glaucoma can also be safely implanted. We would advise the intercapsular technique as being particularly useful in this situation, as it is much easier to perform a slit-like capsulotomy in the upper part of the anterior capsule than to perform a standard can-opener capsulotomy in an anterior chamber which is either shallow or nonexistent.

A history of glaucoma caused by pigment dispersion following lens implantation in the fellow eye (**23.14, 23.15**) should warn the surgeon that a similar problem may result following surgery on the opposite eye. If possible, either a different technique or a different lens design should be used, e.g. 'in the bag' fixation rather than a sulcus fixation. There is no guarantee, however, that the condition may be avoided by these tactics as patients that have developed this condition often have evidence of pigment dispersion in the other eye prior to surgery.

23.14

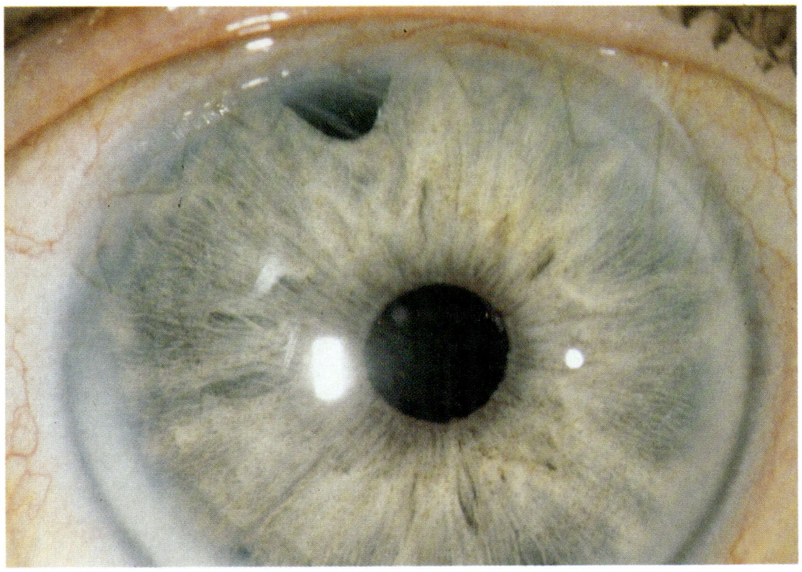

23.14 Pigment dispersion syndrome following cataract extraction and posterior chamber IOL. Note the fine pigment deposits on the anterior surface of the iris.

23.15

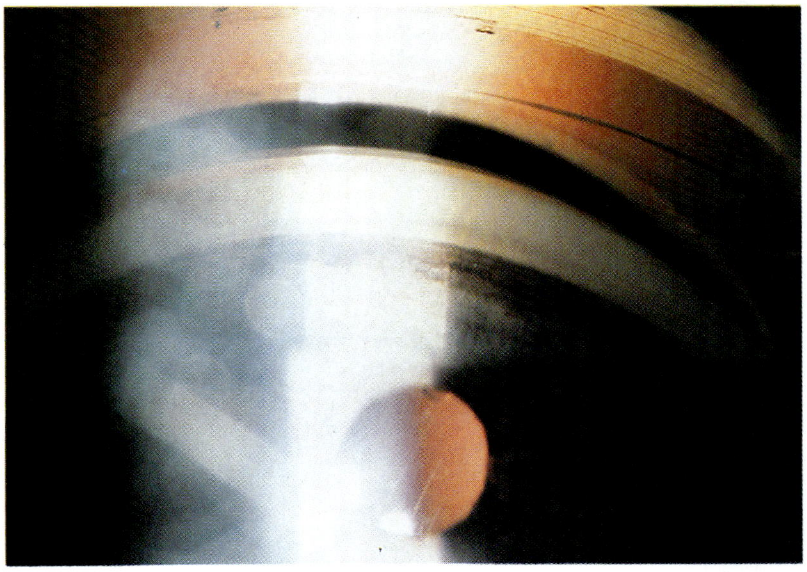

23.15 Same patient as in **23.14**, with a heavily pigmented inferior drainage angle.

High myopia

Most myopic patients benefit from the use of an IOL. Plano lenses are controversial, but the argument for inserting them is that the incidence of posterior capsular opacification may be reduced, especially if the lens is posteriorly vaulted. If a capsulotomy is required at a later date, an IOL may prevent prolapse of vitreous into the anterior chamber. However, the risk of retinal detachment remains high in these patients. For this reason, complete peripheral cortical aspiration must be achieved to enable adequate peripheral retinal examination. In patients referred for detachment surgery the peripheral retinal view is more often obscured by cortical lens remnants than by aberrations produced by the edge of the lens.

Traumatic cataract

The use of an IOL in eyes damaged by trauma is well established, but special care and planning are required, especially if there is also traumatic subluxation (**23.16**) or dislocation of the crystalline lens. Vitreous loss during cataract extraction should be anticipated under these circumstances and appropriate instrumentation used. If there is severe anterior segment disruption, one may consider performing cataract surgery followed by lens insertion at a later date, when other possible complications, such as hyphema and glaucoma, have resolved or been treated.

In children under 10 years of age many studies have shown the high incidence of amblyopia developing after unilateral surgery for traumatic cataract. This contrasts with high levels of vision achieved in children who receive primary or secondary lens implantation early in the treatment of injuries to their eye. Those children receiving contact lenses have many problems, including the large number of contact lenses required to replace ones lost or damaged. Furthermore, great persuasion is needed to encourage the child to use a contact lens in one eye whilst the fellow eye sees normally. Amblyopia is the almost inevitable outcome. Many young adults, too, abandon the use of their contact lens following surgery for unilateral traumatic cataract, with subsequent development of a divergent squint. For these reasons, either primary or secondary intraocular lens implantation should be considered for such patients (**23.17, 23.18**).

23.16

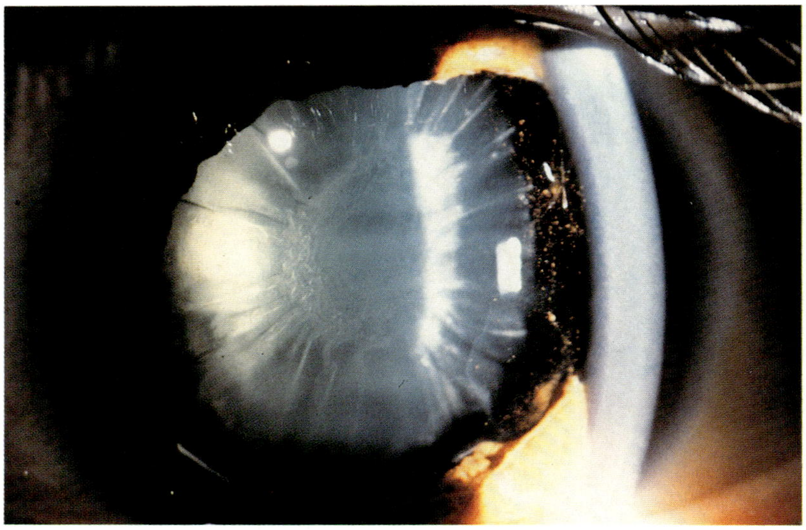

23.16 Dislocated lens following trauma. Note the rupture of zonule with vitreous presenting into the anterior chamber.

23.17

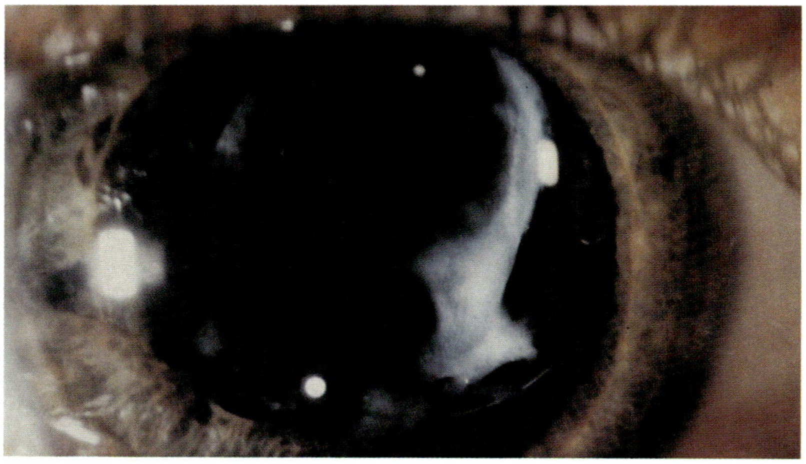

23.17 Posterior chamber IOL insertion following extraction of a traumatic cataract in a young boy.

23.18

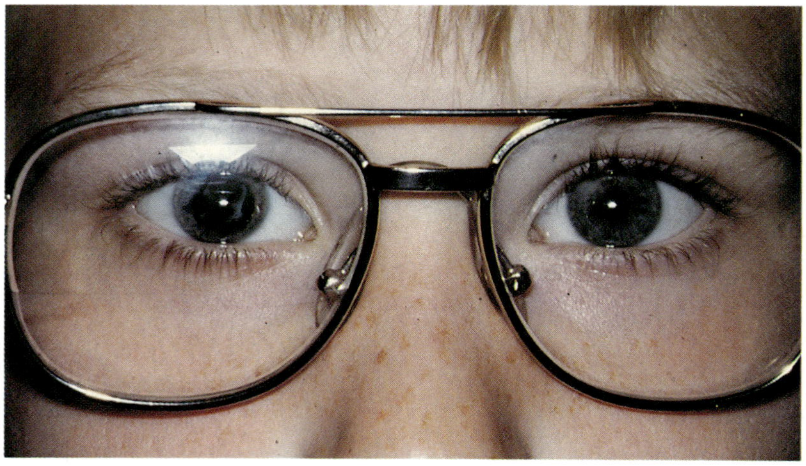

23.18 Same patient as in **23.17** three years later. Vision and fusion are both excellent. Note the bifocal spectacle lens for the right eye.

Corneal disease

In the presence of marked corneal guttata or an early Fuchs' endothelial dystrophy (**21.19**), posterior chamber lens implantation, under the cover of adequate viscoelastic agent and via a large section, is not contraindicated. A very low endothelial cell count or the presence of corneal edema (which may be present only in the morning) should indicate the need for a simultaneous corneal graft. When undertaking a corneal graft for pseudophakic bullous keratopathy, a stable anterior chamber lens or posterior chamber lens may be left *in situ*. Any iris clip lens should be removed and exchanged for a semiflexible anterior chamber lens (**23.20**). A viscoelastic agent should be used and the surgeon must ensure that the graft–host interface is watertight at the end of surgery.

23.19

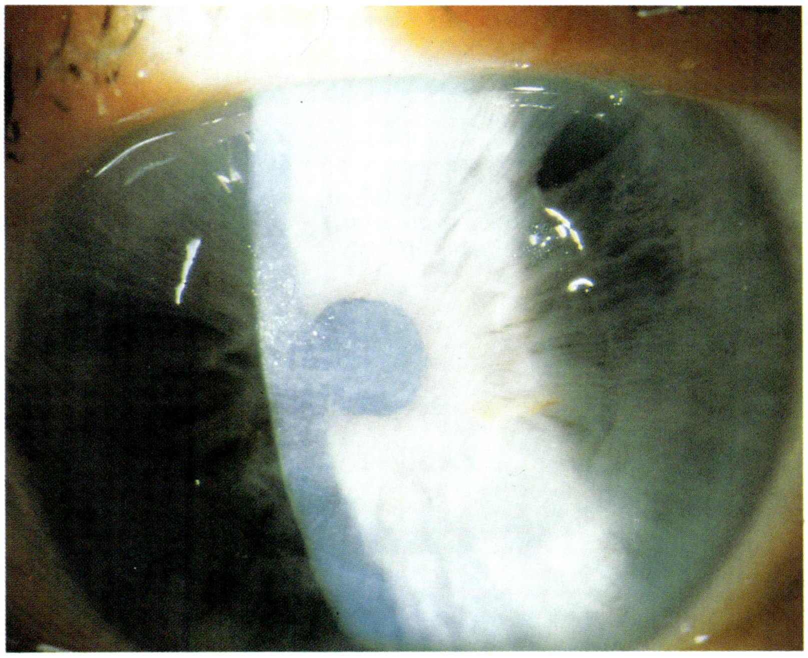

23.19 Fuchs' endothelial dystrophy.

23.20

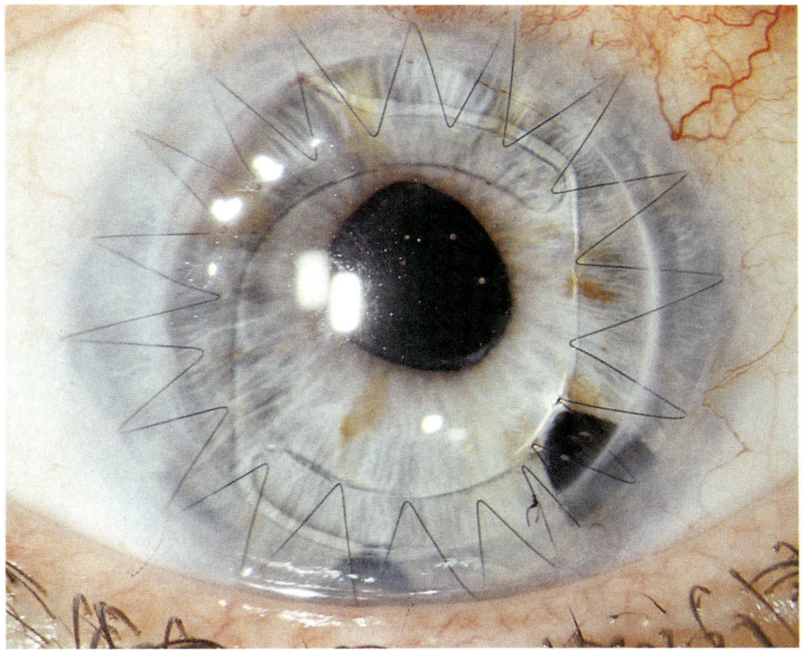

23.20 Iris clip lens exchanged for a semiflexible anterior chamber IOL during penetrating keratoplasty for bullous keratopathy.

Per-operative complications

Rupture of the posterior capsule during extracapsular surgery used to be considered a contraindication to lens implantation. However, with experience the cataract surgeon should be able to recognize a small capsule rupture as it occurs, stabilize the vitreous face with either a viscoelastic substance or air, complete the cortical toilet and proceed carefully to posterior chamber lens implantation.

However, a major disruption to the zonule or capsule makes posterior chamber lens insertion hazardous (**23.21**). This situation requires a formal anterior vitrectomy and every effort should be made to remove as much remaining cortical lens material as possible. Acetylcholine is then injected into the anterior chamber to constrict the pupil, air is introduced under a dam of viscoelastic agent and a Rycroft cannula is used to establish that the anterior chamber is completely clear of vitreous. Safe insertion of an anterior chamber lens can then be undertaken.

Vitreous loss during intracapsular surgery is not a contraindication to lens implantation, provided the vitreous is adequately cleared. In all of these situations the presence of a wick of vitreous between the section and the pupil margin is an invitation to future retinal detachment.

23.21

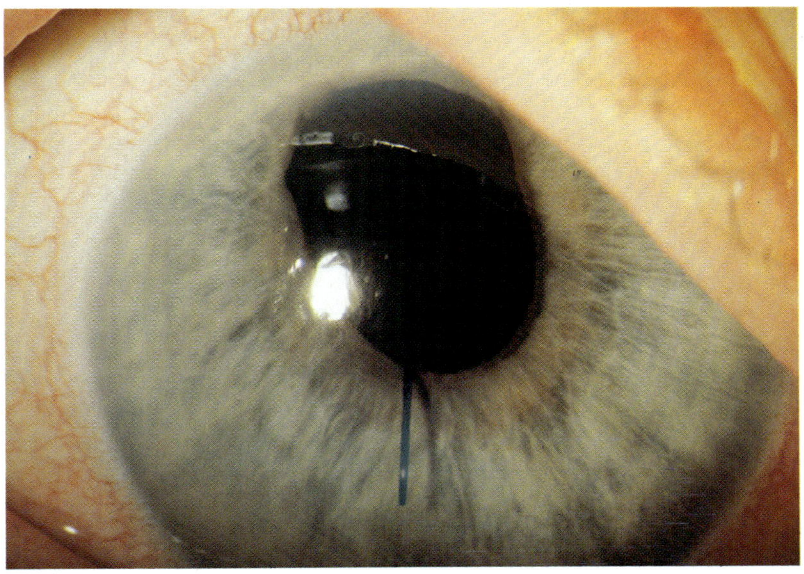

23.21 Ill-advised posterior chamber lens insertion following a major disruption of the zonule. Note the displaced PC IOL with vitreous to the wound.

Only eyes

Provided there is no ocular pathology, the risk of surgery is the same as that for a normal eye and lens implantation should proceed routinely. However, if there was pre-existing pathology in the fellow eye which led to an abnormal response during or after surgery, then the surgical technique and lens type may have to be modified.

Age of patient

Congenital cataracts: Contact lenses or spectacles are a satisfactory means of correcting vision after bilateral cataract surgery, provided the parents are well motivated. However, the birth of a child with congenital cataracts to a family of deprived or limited social and intellectual means is a management challenge to any ophthalmologist. If it seems likely that the child will not receive the benefit of close optical and parental supervision, then IOL implantation with overcorrection by spectacles is an option that can be considered. However, it must be remembered that although an IOL may be used to correct the greater part of aphakic hypermetropia, the refraction of a child's eye changes dramatically in the first few months of life whereas the IOL remains unchangeable. Spectacles and contact lenses may still be required at this early stage.

For teenage cataracts that are bilateral, contact lenses should be used to correct aphakia unless there are strong emotional or local eye reasons (e.g., marked atopy) for implantation of an IOL. Patients in the second and third decades seem to have a higher incidence of pigment dispersion following lens implantation, and an 'in the bag technique' with the use of an all PMMA lens is mandatory. In the future this problem may be overcome by the use of complete anterior capsule polishing and/or the use of lens epithelial growth inhibitors, which will enable the anterior capsule to be left *in situ* as a barrier between the lens implant and the iris pigment.

Conclusion

The surgeon must weigh up his or her own experience against the clinical challenge of the more difficult areas of ophthalmic surgery and should not be frightened to seek the advice of a colleague who may be more skilled or experienced. Since there is no universal intraocular lens the surgeon should be aware of the instrumentation and a small range of lenses that can and need to be used at different times to cope with difficult surgical problems.

Further reading

Foster C.S., Fong L.P. and Singh G. Cataract surgery and intraocular lens implantation in patients with uveitis. *Ophthalmology,* **96,** 281–288, 1989.

Lichter P.R. Intraocular lenses in uveitis patients (Editorial). *Ophthalmology,* **96,** 279–280, 1989.

McGuigan L.J.B., Gottsch J., Stanton W.J., Maumeree A.E. and Quigley H.A. Extracapsular cataract extraction and posterior chamber lens implantation in eyes with preexisting glaucoma. *Arch. Ophthalmol.,* **104,** 1301–1308, 1986.

Tasman W. Are there any retinal contraindications to cataract extraction and posterior chamber lens implants? (Editorial). *Arch. Ophthalmol.* **104,** 1767–1768 1986.

Waring G.O., III. The 50-year epidemic of pseudophakic corneal oedema (Editorial). *Arch. Ophthalmol.* **107,** 657–659, 1989.

24: Implant power calculation

Donald Sanders, John Retzlaff and Manus Kraff

The factors that affect the accuracy of implant power calculation are described below.

Axial length measurement

Accurate measurement of the axial length of the eye (the distance from the corneal vertex to the vitreoretinal interface along the visual axis) is essential for accurate implant power calculation.

There are two basic methods of ultrasonic axial length determination: the immersion, or water bath technique, and the applanation technique. With the immersion method, a small plastic eye-cup is placed on the eye of a supine patient and filled with fluid. The ultrasound probe is placed in the solution, but is never allowed to come into contact with the eye. With the applanation method, the patient is seated and an applanating cone is brought into contact with the anesthetized cornea.

In recent years, there have been several changes in applanation biometers. The ultrasound signals have been digitized and CRT tubes rather than oscilloscopes are used as a display. Algorithms have been developed to recognize the proper A-scan pattern and automatically record the axial lengths measured, rather than relying on the technician's pattern recognition ability. Water-tipped probes have often been superseded by solid-tipped probes. Power calculation software has been built into the ultrasound machines. These changes have lowered the price and increased convenience, but sometimes at the expense of the accuracy of earlier instruments (**24.1**). Conscientious measurement using good quality, well-cared for equipment is the cornerstone of accurate implant power calculation.

In an effort to offset potential errors, it is recommended that pre-operative measurements be performed always on both eyes and that a repeat measurement be carried out if:

- The difference between the two eyes is more than 0.5 mm.
- The axial length measurement seems wrong when compared with refraction.
- The patient has difficulty cooperating or fixating, in which case it is best to have another technician remeasure the A-scan without prior knowledge of previous A-scan results.

Keratometry

A potential source of serious error in manual keratometry is failure by the technician to calibrate the eyepiece to his or her eye. Readings may be in error by as much as 1 D due to this failure to calibrate; such a 1 D error translates to a 0.9 D error in calculated implant power. Autokeratometers are not subject to this error, so, in this respect, are 'technician-proof'.

Another possible source of error is the index of refraction figure used to convert the radius of curvature scale into diopters of power.

In general, we recommend remeasuring keratometry if the corneas are extremely flat or steep, if the difference in average keratometry between the two eyes is greater than 1 D, if the difference in corneal cylinder between the right and left eye is more than 1 D, or if the corneal cylinder does not correlate well with the refractive cylinder.

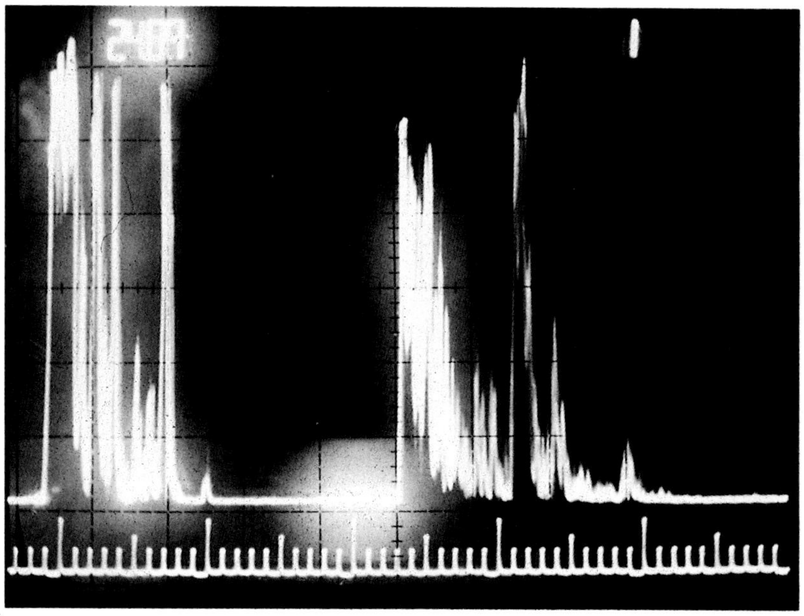

24.1

24.1 Oscillograph photographed in 1982 showing a high degree of accuracy obtained from sharp echoes. Note the high vertical echoes from the anterior surface of the cornea, the anterior and posterior surfaces of the lens and the anterior surface of the retina. The spikes that follow are orbital.

Implant power calculation formulas

The choice of implant power calculation formulas has been a major point of controversy in the past. Formulas have developed along two lines: theoretic formulas and regression-derived theoretic formulas.

Theoretic formulas

The formulas of Fyodorov, Colenbrander, Thijsen, Vand der Heijde and Binkhorst, are based on geometric optics, as applied to schematic eyes using theoretical constants. These apparently different formulas are, in fact, identical, except for the correction factors. They can all be algebraically transformed into:

$$P = \frac{n}{L - \text{ACD}} - \frac{n \times K}{n - K \times \text{ACD}}$$

where P is the implant power for emmetropia, n the aqueous and vitreous refractive index, ACD the estimated postoperative anterior chamber depth (mm), L the axial length (mm), and K the corneal curvature (D).

Regression formulas—SRK®

The general form of the regression formula used for implant power calculation is:

$$P = A + B \times K + C \times L$$

where P is the power for emmetropia, K the keratometry (D), and L the axial length (mm). A, B and C are constants.

The SRK®, or Sanders, Retzlaff, Kraff, formula has a B value of −0.9 and a C value of −2.5. The A-constant is derived separately for each lens style and manufacturer. This formula has become the most widely used formula for implant calculation.

Second generation formulas

It is generally accepted that both theoretical and regression-derived formulas perform well for eyes of axial lengths between 22 and 24.5 mm. With the dramatic shift to posterior chamber lenses, it became evident that, although the formulas continued to perform well for average eyes, the theoretic formulas tended to predict too large a value in short eyes and too small a value in long eyes, and the regression formulas had the opposite tendency.

To address this problem, a number of new formulas, described as second-generation IOL power formulas, have been developed. They are either modifications of the classic theoretical formulas, modifications of the SRK® formula or similar empirically derived approaches, or a combination of theoretical and empirical approaches. Most are aimed at convenience rather than accuracy.

Second generation theoretic formulas: Binkhorst, Hoffer, Olson, and Holladay have now incorporated estimated postoperative anterior chamber depth (ACD) correction factors; and Shammas has incorporated an axial length correction factor for long and short eyes.

Binkhorst and Hoffer both observed a correlation between measured postoperative ACD and axial length, and so adjusted expected postoperative ACD according to axial length. Hoffer's correction factor is a linear regression equation. Olson's regression formula, derived by sophisticated analysis of a group of anterior chamber IOLs, predicts postoperative ACD from corneal diameter, corneal curvature, preoperative ACD, and lens thickness.

Holladay's formula, which uses a sensory retinal thickness factor of 0.2 mm and the corneal refractive index of 1.333 recommended by Binkhorst, adjusts expected postoperative ACD with a complex equation relating ACD to both axial length and corneal curvature.

Retzlaff has recently developed the SRK/T (T for theoretic) formula. After testing many models, the Fyodorov formula was chosen as the base and the corneal height formula was chosen for ACD tailoring. The SRK/T formula gives predictions similar to the second-generation theoretic formulas and is especially similar to Holladay's formula. Furthermore, the SRK/T formula can be personalized for a specific IOL and/or surgeon in two ways. One can input either an ACD value that one desires or an SRK A-constant, and the appropriate personalized ACD value will be calculated. Alternatively, either an ACD value or an SRK A-constant can be derived from data.

Second generation empiric formulas: In 1984, Thompson *et al.* described a new intraocular lens formula designed to improve results in axial myopes. Their formula was a linear regression equation for eyes of axial length less than 24.5 mm, and it had quadratic or squared terms for both axial length and keratometry when the axial length was greater than or equal to 24.5 mm. A major problem with this formula was that it was highly specific for the data set from which it was derived, and there was no method for individually tailoring the formula to different types and manufacturers of IOLs.

Donzis *et al.* developed a 'percentage change' formula, which is a direct modification of the SRK® formula. It utilizes the SRK® A-constants, but changes the relationship between axial length and power for emmetropia to a nonlinear term whose magnitude is a function of the percentage deviation of a particular case's axial length from a mean value of 23.5 mm.

The SRK II™ formula is built upon, and is meant to replace, the SRK® formula. For eyes with axial lengths between 22 mm and 24.5 mm, the emmetropia power predictions are identical to the SRK® formula. These eyes constitute approximately 75% of cases, while 10% of cases have axial lengths less than 22 mm and 14% of cases have axial lengths greater than 24.5 mm. Thus, the SRK II™ modifications change emmetropia predictions from the standard SRK® formula for one out of every four IOL cases to be operated on.

As a help to users of SRK®, we suggest the method of modification in **Table 24.1**.

Table 24.1 Modification of SRK® to SRK II™

$$(P = A - 2.5\,L - 0.9\,K)$$

If L is < 20.0, add +3 to the A-Constant

If L is 20.0–20.99, add +2 to the A-Constant

If L is 21.0–21.99, add +1 to the A-Constant

If L is > 24.5, add −0.5 to the A-Constant

To predict postoperative refraction (R) for a given IOL power (I):

$R = P - I$ if P is *less* than 14.0

$R = \dfrac{(P - I)}{1.25}$ if P is greater than 14.0

To find the IOL power to produce a given refraction:

$$I = P - (R \times 1.25)$$

But if P (calculated power for emmetropia) is less than 14.0, $I = P - R$

Accuracy of power formulas

As a practical matter, one would like to know if there are differences in accuracy between these newer, second-generation formulas. We have looked at over 2000 cases from various sources in the United States and an even larger series provided by Dr Howard Gimbel in Canada. We compared the accuracy of the SRK II™ formula as an example of a second-generation regression formula and three second-generation theoretical formulas (Binkhorst II, Holladay, and SRK/T).

In eyes of normal axial length (22–24.5 mm), all performed equally well (**24.2**). In short eyes (less than 22 mm), again the differences in formula accuracy were insubstantial (**24.3**), as were those for moderately long eyes with axial length between 24.5–26.99 mm (**24.4**). In very long eyes (axial lengths between 27–28.99 mm), there was a slight decrease in accuracy with the SRK II™ as compared to SRK/T or Holladay formulas (**24.5**). In extremely long eyes (axial lengths greater than 29 mm), clearly the SRK II™ was less accurate than the theoretic formulas (**24.6**). However, to put this into perspective, eyes with axial lengths greater than 29 mm (**24.7**) constitute only 0.6% of the population, so approximately one case in 200 would be affected by major formula prediction differences. The data shows that of the major second-generation formulas, all perform well in all but the most extreme cases.

24.2

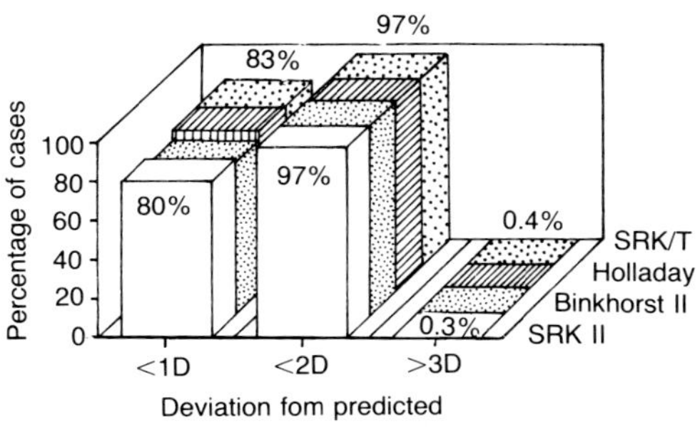

24.2 IOL power accuracy for average eyes (N = 1596), US series.

24.3

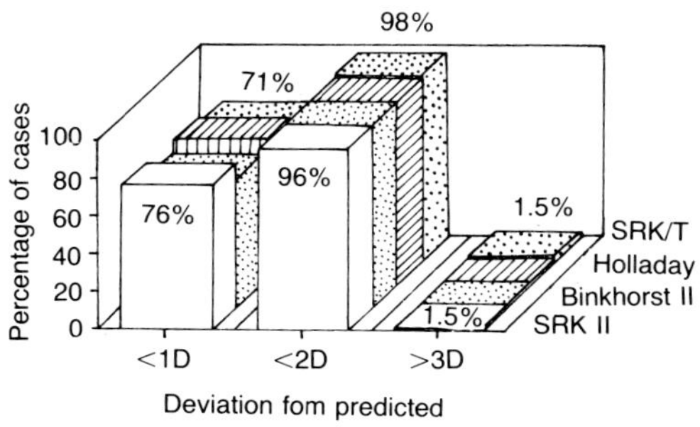

24.3 IOL power accuracy for short eyes (N = 201), US and Canadian series.

24.4

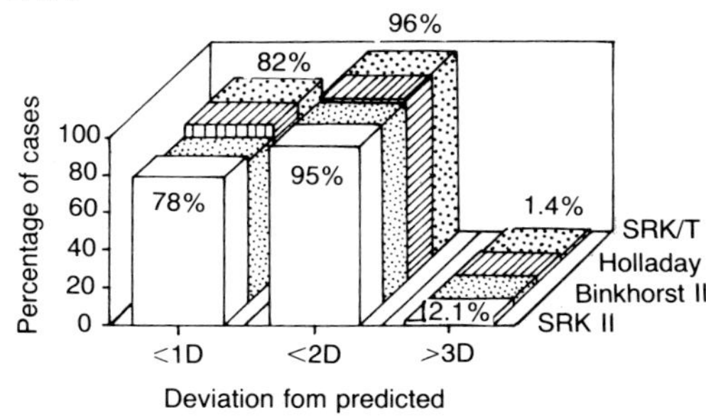

24.4 IOL power accuracy for moderately long eyes (N = 286), US and Canadian series.

24.5

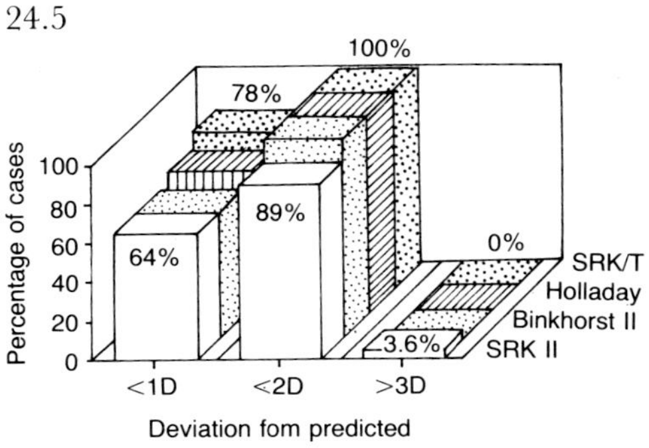

24.5 IOL power accuracy for very long eyes (N = 28).

24.6

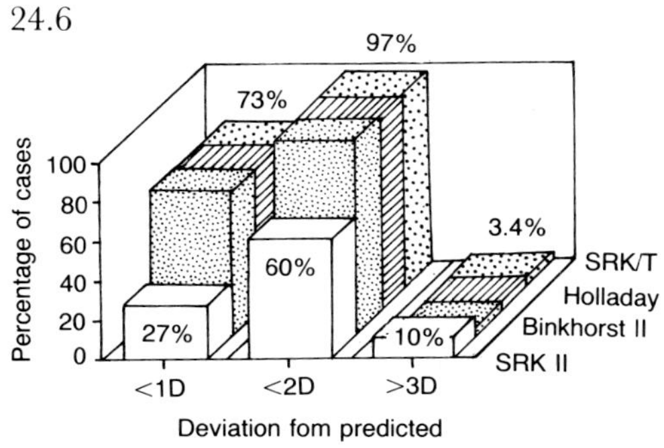

24.6 IOL power accuracy for extremely long eyes (N = 28).

24.7

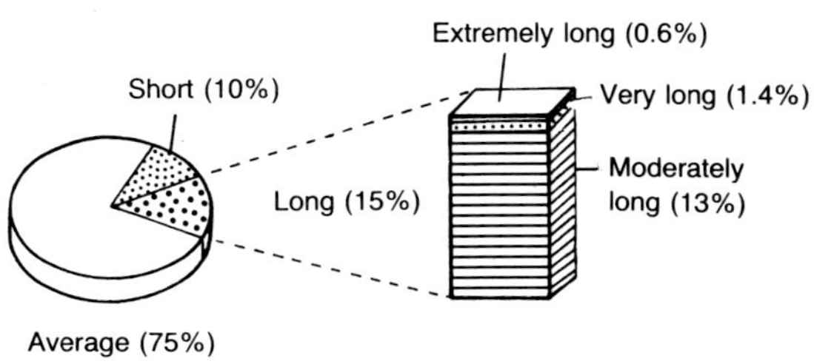

24.7 Distribution of axial length.

Surgical technique

Sulcus or bag

For capsular bag placements, the implant is further back in the eye, *decreasing the effective power of the lens*. There is usually a 0.5 D to 1.5 D loss of effectiveness by placing the implant in the capsular bag as opposed to the ciliary sulcus, and so a higher power lens should be used when the implant is placed in the capsular bag.

Orientation of the implant optic

Some surgeons implant plano convex posterior chamber lenses with the plano surface forward. This is only sensible if there is no angulation of loops or if loops are absent. Such 'flipping' of the implant decreases the effective power of the lens by at least 0.75 D, even if the position of the lens is unchanged. An additional 0.5 D loss of effectiveness occurs because the principal plane of the lens is displaced further back into the eye. Thus, a total loss of effectiveness of 1.25 D is expected by turning the lens around. In practice, if an implant power formula predicts an 18 D lens power for emmetropia using a plano convex lens with the convex-side forward, then a 19.5 D implant power will be required if the same lens is implanted plano-side forward. Flipping a meniscus optic would also displace the principal plane of the lens posteriorly and decrease the effective power. Flipping a biconvex optic would have no effect on the effective power. This is true if the anterior and posterior biconvex curves are equal. However, some manufacturers use the ratio of 1:3, mimicking the natural crystalline lens, and flipping these lenses would change their effective power.

Postoperative change in corneal curvature

Modern microsurgical techniques have a tendency to steepen the cornea postoperatively. This is especially true in corneas where the horizontal meridian is steeper preoperatively than the vertical one ('against the rule' astigmatism). Suturing of a cataract incision has a tendency to steepen the vertical meridian; with preoperative 'against the rule' astigmatism, the cornea will become more spherical and the average 'K' will be steeper after surgery.

Manufacturer variation in power labeling

Although Olson and Waters found no evidence of implant power mislabelling *per se*, there was ample evidence for industry-wide variation in methods of calculating implant power. *They found variations, due to different methods of calculating among the companies studied, to be as much as 0.95 D.* We have found differences, in certain cases, to be substantially higher than 1 D. To add to these difficulties, seemingly minor variations in manufacturing technique and lens design may change the implant power required for emmetropia.

Final selection of implant power

After the measurements have been obtained and the implant power formula chosen has been applied, the surgeon, armed with the calculated emmetropizing and ametropizing values for the patient, must make the final decision as to what strength implant to place in the patient's eye.

The following factors should be considered:

- Fellow eye refraction and cataract, if any.
- Emmetropia, isometropia, iseikonia.
- One diopter myopia, monovision.
- Lifestyle of patient: Active patients are best served by near emmetropia; sedentary patients may prefer myopia.
- Hedging: It has been found that the actual postoperative refraction varies by more than 1 D from the calculated refraction in over 10% of the cases and so it is preferable to hedge towards myopia.

The decision concerning proper implant power requires unhurried thought and planning. Effective implementation includes posting the power and style of the IOL selected beside the patient's name on the operating room wall, not using too many IOLs of different styles, and giving clear instructions to the staff for selecting an alternative IOL if this is necessary after a capsule rupture or vitreous loss.

Correction of surprises

Large, unexpected postoperative refractive errors require immediate action. If an error is identified, e.g. implantation of an 18.0 D rather than the planned 24.0 D IOL, a lens exchange must be considered, provided that further surgery is unlikely to compromise the health of the eye and that the patient is satisfied that vision can be improved by altering the refraction.

The situation is more difficult when no error can be identified: e.g., remeasurement of the axial length and corneal curvature confirm the original measurements and investigation indicates the correct power was used during surgery. In these cases, before planning a lens exchange, it may be advisable to determine the power of the IOL *in situ*, for a mislabelled implant is possible, to exclude a posterior pole staphyloma with an aberrant fovea by taking a B scan, and to recalculate the axial length and resultant new power for emmetropia.

Radial keratotomy patients

Douglas Koch *et al.* have noted a hyperopic shift that occurs after cataract surgery in patients who have previously undergone radial keratotomy. Two reasons have been suggested. The first is flattening of the cornea, which is associated with tissue swelling and is greatest in the first week after surgery. The resulting hyperopia can be alarming, but will regress with time, although a small amount of additional flattening may persist. The second is that, after radial keratotomy, the cornea, instead of being steeper in the center and flatter toward the periphery, is flatter toward the center with a steeper mid-peripheral area. Keratometry (K) readings become inaccurate because this more peripheral area, which is steeper than the central cornea, is measured. Falsely steep K readings lead to postoperative hyperopia. To compensate for this, a refraction-derived K value may be used and can be calculated by subtracting the refractive change induced by radial keratotomy from the pre-radial keratotomy K reading. Otherwise, the flattest of three K readings should be taken for lens power calculation. As further flattening may be associated with surgery, at least 0.5D should be *added* to the calculated implant power.

Further reading

Donzis P.B., Kastl P.R. and Gordon R.A. An intraocular lens formula for short, normal and long eyes. *CLAO J.*, **11,** 95–98, 1985.

Holladay J.T., Praeger T.C., Chandler T.Y. and Musgrove K.H. A three-part system for refining intraocular lens power calculations. *J. Cataract Refract. Surg.*, **14,** 17–24, 1988.

Koch D.D., Liu J.F., Hyde L.L. Rock R.L., and Emery J.M. Refractive complications of cataract surgery after radial keratotomy. *Am. J. Ophthalmol.*, **108,** 676–682, 1989.

Olsen T. Measuring the power of an *in situ* intraocular lens with the keratometer. *J. Cataract Refract. Surg.*, **14,** 64–67, 1988.

Retzlaff J., Sanders D.R. and Kraff M.C. *A Manual of Implant Power Calculation Including SRK II*, 2nd edn, Medford, Oregon, 1988.

25: Accommodation in pseudophakia

Spencer Thornton

There are three aspects of accommodation that need consideration; first is the production of an apparent or 'pseudoaccommodation' by alteration of the pupil size and the intentional refractive aim following lens implantation. Second is the use of two zone and multizone designs for bifocal IOLs. Third is the potential for movement of the IOL, which is dependent on the position, shape, haptic support and vitreous movement on accommodative effort. However, initially it is important to understand the optical principles and physical characteristics that enable the eye to focus for both distance and near.

How the eye focuses

The focal power of the eye depends on several factors: the length of the eye, the curvature and consequent refractive power of the cornea, and the effective focal power of the lens.

In order for the image to come into focus on the retina, the light must be bent so that the rays converge at the fovea. The nearer an object is to the eye, the more the light must be bent for the object to be seen in focus. The cornea, aqueous and vitreous each have a fixed refractive power, but the lens can accommodate by a steepening of the curvature of its surfaces and by a forwards movement, thereby increasing its focusing power. Frans C. Donders, in his treatise, *On the Anomalies of Accommodation and Refraction of the Eye*, 1864, credits Heinrich Mueller with the anatomical investigations of the action of the ciliary muscle in accommodation, in which he saw in the action of the most external layers of the ciliary muscle a means of augmenting the pressure of the vitreous humor, pushing the lens forwards. In addition, he noted the advance of the surface of the pupil and the retrogression of the periphery of the iris in accommodation for near objects.

Helmholtz, in his treatise on physiological optics, noted that the lens is suspended by zonular filaments (**25.1**) projecting from the ciliary muscle, which he described as nonelastic filaments holding the lens taut with the ciliary muscle in its relaxed state and relaxed when the ciliary muscle contracts. He described a slight anterior movement of the ciliary body on contraction, reducing the stress on the zonules and thereupon allowing the lens to undergo elastic recovery. He described the lens becoming thicker from front to back and its surface becoming more sharply curved as the lens focused on progressively closer objects. Thus, the lens is maximally accommodated when it is under the least stress and the ciliary muscle fully contracted. The idea of multiple factors affecting accommodation is therefore not new.

Studies of the structural organization of the lens have shown that because of their interlocking nature, cortical fibers are not stretched and cannot slide past one another, and so the only way the lens can change shape is for the fibers to alter their curvature by compression. Computer models have indicated that the forces acting on the surface of the accommodating lens body are approximately equal and are in a direction approximately perpendicular to the lens surface, providing a uniform compressive force against the entire surface of the lens. The zonules exert a force that has both a parallel (stretching) component and a perpendicular (compressive) one. The capsular fibers, however, resist stretching, and so only the perpendicular force is transmitted to the lens.

Relaxation of the zonules can account for most, but not all, of the shape change seen in the lens during elastic recovery. This suggests that the vitreous humor may take part in the focusing process by its support

25.1

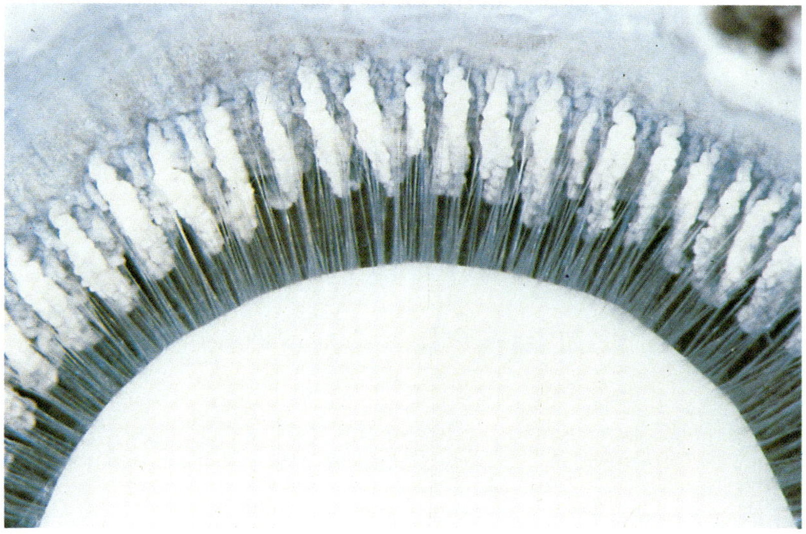

25.1 Gross photograph from behind of an autopsy globe processed using a special technique that renders the crystalline lens milky white, with excellent visibility of the zonules. This demonstrates the morphology of the zonule fibers as they pass from the lens equator on to the ciliary body (courtesy of Prof. David Apple, USA).

in the relaxed state and its possible forwards movement during ciliary contraction on accommodative effort.

The question of decreasing focal power of the lens with age is not fully understood. We know that the lens continues to grow throughout life with increasing steepness in both anterior and posterior surfaces. Despite the increased curvature of both anterior and posterior surfaces, the refractive power decreases with age producing a paradox. Why is it that an older lens has to be curved more than a younger one to focus on the same object? One possibility is that the nature of the cytoplasm in the lens fibers changes in a way that decreases the lens' refractive index with age. It is clear that a number of mechanisms are involved in age-related changes of the lens. The decrease in the refractive index of the lens is partly compensated for by the increasing steepness of curvature of the anterior and posterior surfaces, as well as by the zones of discontinuity within the lens. Zones of discontinuity detected by slit-lamp examination are found to be increased and more sharply curved with age.

The overall decrease in the index of refraction and reduced elastic recovery of the lens with age explains the phenomenon of presbyopia, and the problem of restoration of accommodation in pseudophakia becomes one of manipulation of factors exclusive of lens elasticity.

Pseudoaccommodation

With the control of postoperative refractive power and the deliberate induction of a small amount of 'with the rule' myopic astigmatism, a number of patients have a method of apparent accommodation without corrective lenses. Nakazawa and Ohtsuki measured apparent accommodation in pseudophakic eyes after implantation of a posterior chamber intraocular lens and found that the primary factor producing increased depth of focus and apparent accommodation was the ability of the pupil to constrict on accommodative effort. There appeared to be no correlation between apparent accommodation and corrected visual acuity, refractive error, corneal astigmatism or axial length. The apparent accommodation appeared to be inversely related to the anterior chamber depth and to be greater, the smaller the pupil.

Another factor contributing to an improvement in depth of focus with an IOL is that the resolving power of PMMA is no less than four times that of the noncataractous human lens seen in old age. A further factor, which appears to contribute to accommodation, is the posterior placement of the IOL. The greater the distance of the posterior IOL surface from the cornea, the greater is the focal power and the less the anterior movement necessary for increasing that focal power (Holladay *et al.* 1985).

The depth of focus of the uncorrected implanted eye may also be improved by careful planning and using a surgical technique aimed at simple myopic astigmatism (see p. 164). For this the change in corneal power must be included in the calculation of IOL power. Postoperatively, the shape of the cornea can be predicted and adjusted. Huber described a technique in which he did not adjust the amount of astigmatism during surgery, but controlled the amount of surgical ametropia by cutting the corneoscleral nylon sutures in the steeper meridian in the postoperative phase. The flatter meridian is calculated for emmetropia and the steeper meridian for simple myopic astigmatism (**25.2**). Best acuities and depth of focus have been found in subjects with between – 0.75 D and – 2.5 D of simple myopic astigmatism.

25.2

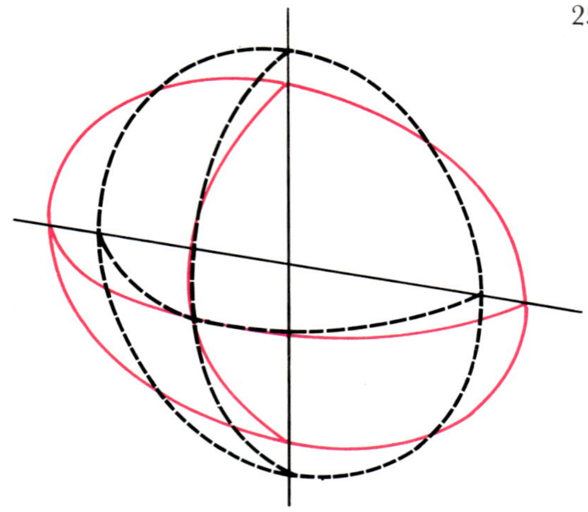

25.2 Schematic drawing of the change in corneal curvature induced by cataract surgery. The net result of surgery (red) with a slightly overtight wound at 12 o'clock will be to steepen the corneal curvature at 90° and flatten the curvature at 180°. There is little change in spheroequivalency, so for simple myopic astigmatism the flatter meridian is calculated for emmetropia.

Bifocal intraocular lenses

Bifocal IOLs have tended to follow the lead of the contact lens industry, using the same principles of optics and design. The most common type of bifocal intraocular lens uses the simultaneous vision principle and has two concentric optical zones. The central 2 mm contains the additive portion for near focus and the lens periphery is for distant focus (see p. 133). As the patient fixates on a near object, the image focused by the central portion becomes appreciated and the distance image ignored. For distant focus the image from the central part of the lens is ignored. This requires a learning process, but patients apparently adapt to it with little difficulty. The reading addition can be varied in power just as in eyeglasses. Theoretically, one can have any power at distance and near while maintaining 20/20 vision with full appreciation of the bifocal effect.

The difficulty with these designs is that deviation of the pupil size from normal or decentration of such a lens will alter the intensity balance of the two foci and may produce symptoms such as monocular diplopia, binocular diplopia, blurring of images and diminution of bifocal function.

A recent innovation is a lens that utilizes diffractive optics and provides simultaneous bifocal imaging using the effects of diffraction rather than relying on conventional refractive optics. The advantage of this diffractive design is that it provides a constant intensity of the two foci, independent of pupil size and lens centration. The diffractive microstructure of the lens is composed of 20–30 concentric optical zones, with minute steps of a few microns at the zone boundaries, and it utilizes both the conventional ray as well as the wave nature of light. With a base power calculated for emmetropia at distance and an additive power of 3.5 D for near, the diffractive lens has two powers. When focusing at distance, the higher power focuses anterior to the retina (**25.3**). The intensity of the focused light from distance overwhelms the defocused light from near, resulting in a clear image of the distant object. The brain sees one image clearly in focus with some blurred light that has no structure.

For near vision the incoming light is divergent so the two foci move posteriorly with the near focus onto the retina (**25.4**), again producing a clear single image. The chief problem with the multizone lens is that less than half the light (approximately 41%) entering the eye is in focus at any one time. This has caused some patients to note a deficit in their reading ability, particularly for very small print or in poor illumination. The two zone bifocal, when properly centered, does not have this effect because of pupillary constriction on accommodative effort.

25.3

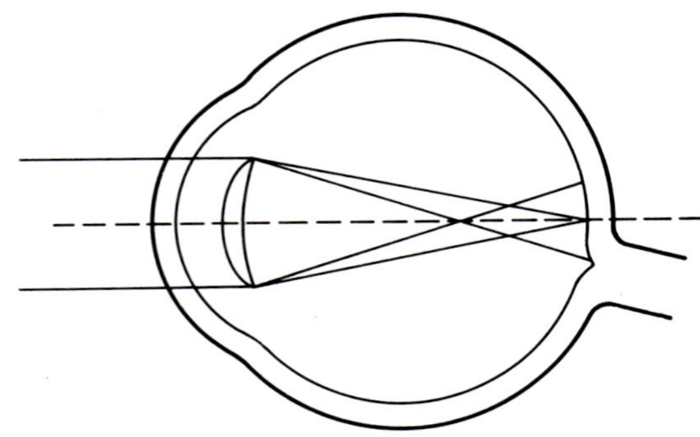

25.3 Bifocal distance vision.

25.4

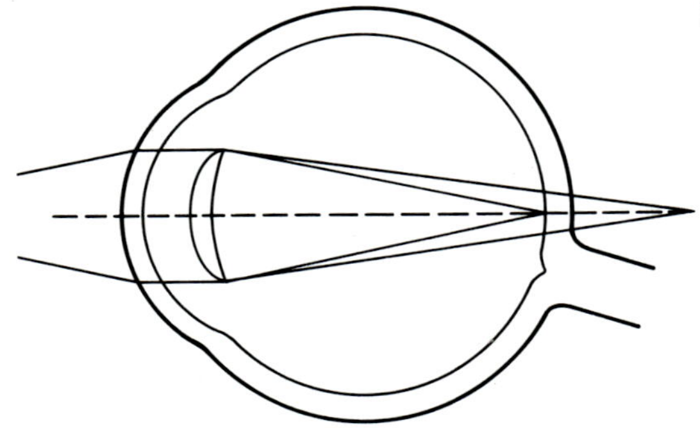

25.4 Bifocal near vision.

Potential for restored accommodation with in-the-bag implantation of a convex posterior intraocular lens

The potential for restored accommodation with a monofocal intraocular lens occurs with lenses designed with biconvex optics for implantation in-the-bag, with posterior convexity firmly held against the posterior capsule so that the capsule is slightly stretched and the lens is positioned with no pseudophakodonesis. Such a lens (**25.5**) has been designed and studied from the standpoint of the apparent accommodation produced by a change in pupil size, by posterior positioning of the lens allowing greater depth of focus, and by movement of the lens produced by anterior vitreous movement on ciliary contraction with accommodative effort (**25.6–25.9**). A-scan ultrasound measurements of changes in the anterior chamber depth in pseudophakic accommodation tended to confirm Mueller's theory of vitreous pressure pushing the lens forwards with ciliary contraction on accommodation (**25.10–25.13**).

25.5

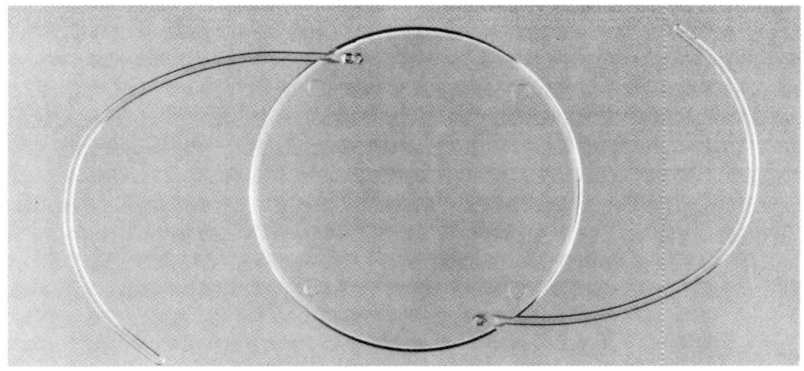

25.5 The Thornton three-piece PMMA lens for capsular fixation: 6.5 mm optic, 12.5 mm loop span with posterior convexity of the optic continuous with the curve of the anterior angulation of the haptics.

25.6

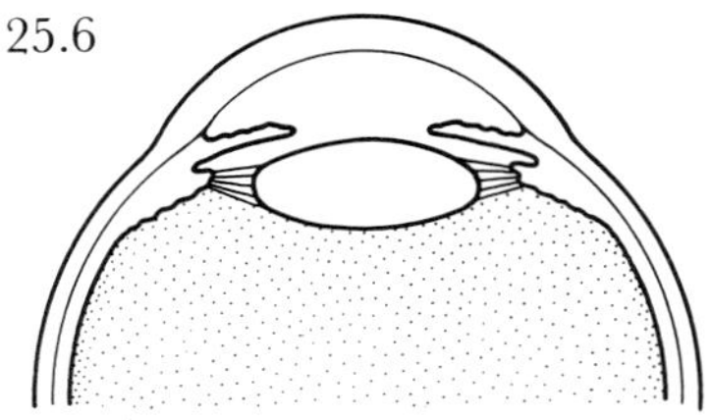

25.7

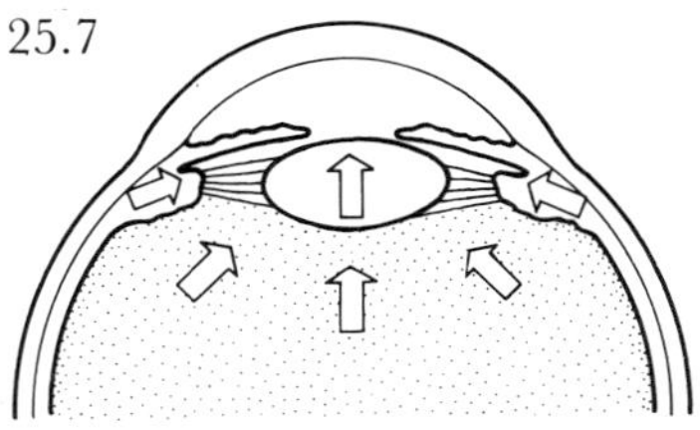

25.8

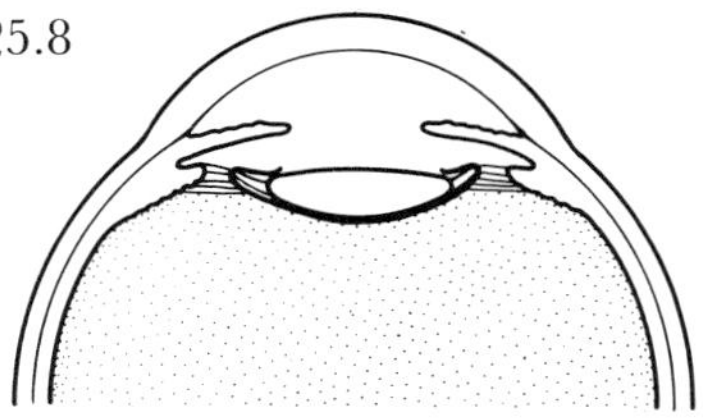

25.9

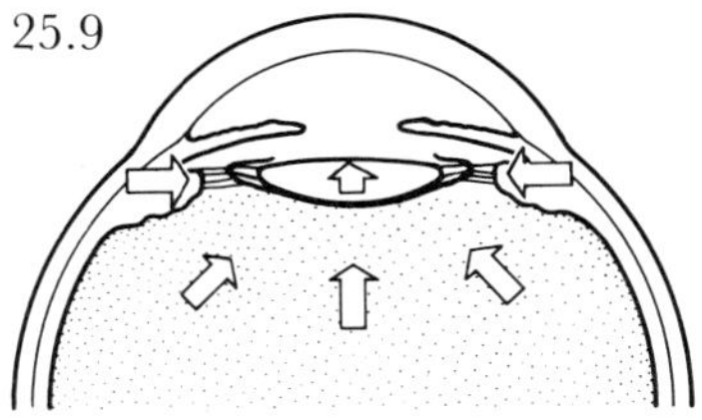

25.6 The normal eye at rest.

25.7 On accommodation, ciliary muscle contraction relaxes zonules allowing the lens to assume a more spherical shape (depending on its elasticity) and forces vitreous forwards, moving the lens forwards.

25.8 When a posteriorly convex IOL is implanted against the posterior capsule in-the-bag with haptics not long enough to press against the ciliary body, accommodation may be possible.

25.9 On accommodative effort the zonules relax and the vitreous is forced forwards, resulting in anterior movement of the IOL increasing its effective focal power.

25.10

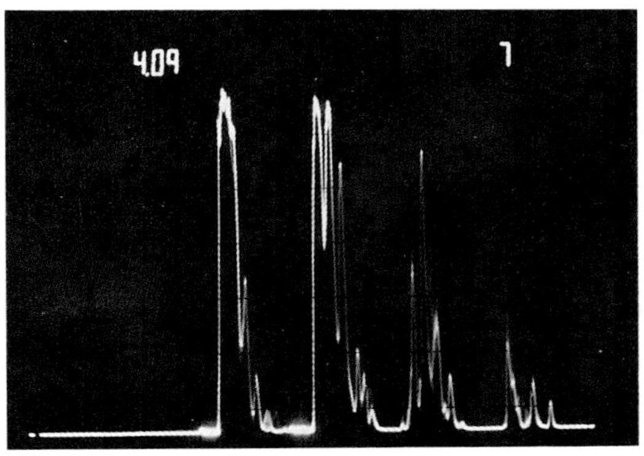

25.11

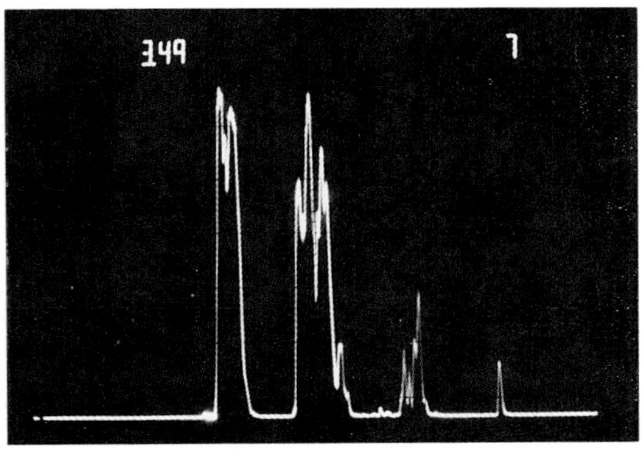

25.10 Patient A: anterior chamber depth 4.09 mm for distance fixation.

25.11 Patient A: anterior chamber depth 3.49 mm for near fixation.

5.12

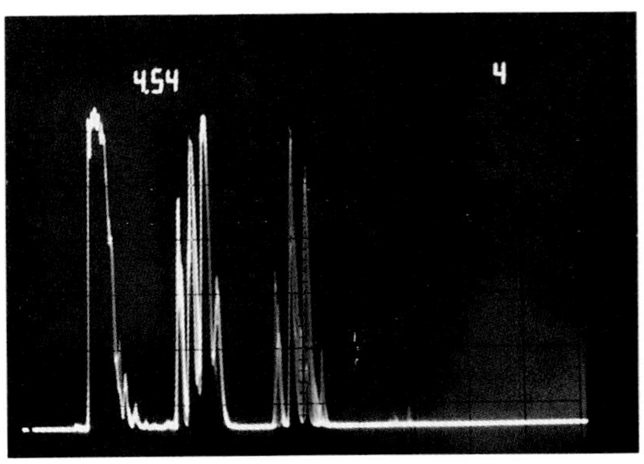

25.13

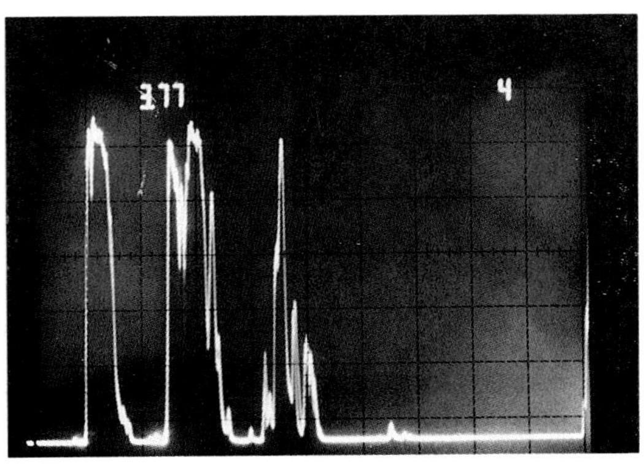

25.12 Patient B: anterior chamber depth 4.54 mm for distance fixation.

25.13 Patient B: anterior chamber depth 3.77 mm for near fixation.

Any refractive change based on movement of the lens is dependent both on the shape and position of the lens. The more posterior the lens, the more significant the change in refraction with any given anterior movement. Any movement of an intraocular lens implanted posteriorly in-the-bag will result in a significant change in refraction when compared with the movement of a lens just behind the iris plane. A lens implanted in-the-bag with the convexity against the posterior capsule will produce twice the change in near focal power compared with a lens with a convexity forwards.

It is not uncommon to see, on slit-lamp examination of aphakic patients, the vitreous face bulging forwards through the pupil, on accommodative effort. Studies have shown that following extracapsular cataract surgery and sulcus fixation of an intraocular lens the posterior capsule goes from an average of 7.6 mm from the cornea to 4.68 mm, a change of 2.92 mm. This forwards movement of the capsule appears to be due to its tendency to tighten in its zonular support. This leaves a space that is filled by forwards movements of the vitreous face or an accumulation of a fluid interface between the capsule and the vitreous face.

A solid PMMA lens with an optic size of 6.5 mm and haptic span of 12.5 or 13 mm with biconvex optics and slight anterior angulation of the haptics allows for in-the-bag placement with posterior convexity. With such a placement, accommodative effort will produce ciliary body contraction, forwards movement of vitreous and forwards movement of the lens. Thus, on accommodative effort, if the lens moves even 0.25 or 0.50 mm, there is a significant increase in the effective focal power. Clinically, this effect has been confirmed by demonstration of a reduced reading addition required for spectacles. The effect may be enhanced by planning a postoperative focal power of − 0.75 D and a surgical technique which results in a simple myopic astigmatism of about − 1.5 D.

Further reading

Hoffer K.J. The effect of axial length on posterior chamber lens and posterior capsule position. *Current Concepts in Ophthalmic Surgery,* **1,** 20–22, 1985.

Holladay J.T. *et al.* Determining intraocular lens power within the eye. *American Intraocular Implant Society Journal,* **11,** 353–363, 1985.

Huber C. Planned myopic astigmatism as a substitute for accommodation in pseudophakia. *American Intraocular Implant Society Journal,* **7,** 244–249, 1981.

Koretz J. and Handleman G. How the human eye focuses. *Scientific American,* 92–99, July, 1988.

Nakazawa M. and Ohtsuki K. Apparent accommodation in pseudophakic eyes after implantation of posterior chamber intraocular lenses. *American Journal of Ophthalmology,* **96,** 435–438, 1983.

Thornton S. Lens implantation with restored accommodation. *Current Canadian Ophthalmic Practice,* **4,** 60–82, 1986.

26: The plan for ametropia and astigmatism

Piers Percival and Spencer Thornton

Ametropia

The two surgical goals are the maintenance of binocular single vision (BSV) and the bringing of the patient near to emmetropia so that there is no longer dependence on glasses.

For hypermetropia and myopia between 3 and 8 D in the better eye follow **Flow Chart 26.1.** For ametropia in excess of 8 D the improvement in visual field and pleasure in discarding thick glasses generally outweighs the advantages of BSV so that even when the cataract is unilateral the aim, with informed consent, may be towards postoperative emmetropia.

For very high myopia, low powered or plano lenses are preferred to no lenses in order to reduce the chance of posterior segment pathology. There is an eight-fold reduction in incidence of retinal detachment in uncomplicated eyes if the posterior capsule remains intact, and in the five-year term there is a five-fold reduction in the need for opening the capsule if a posterior vaulted lens is placed in the posterior chamber in contact with the posterior capsule.

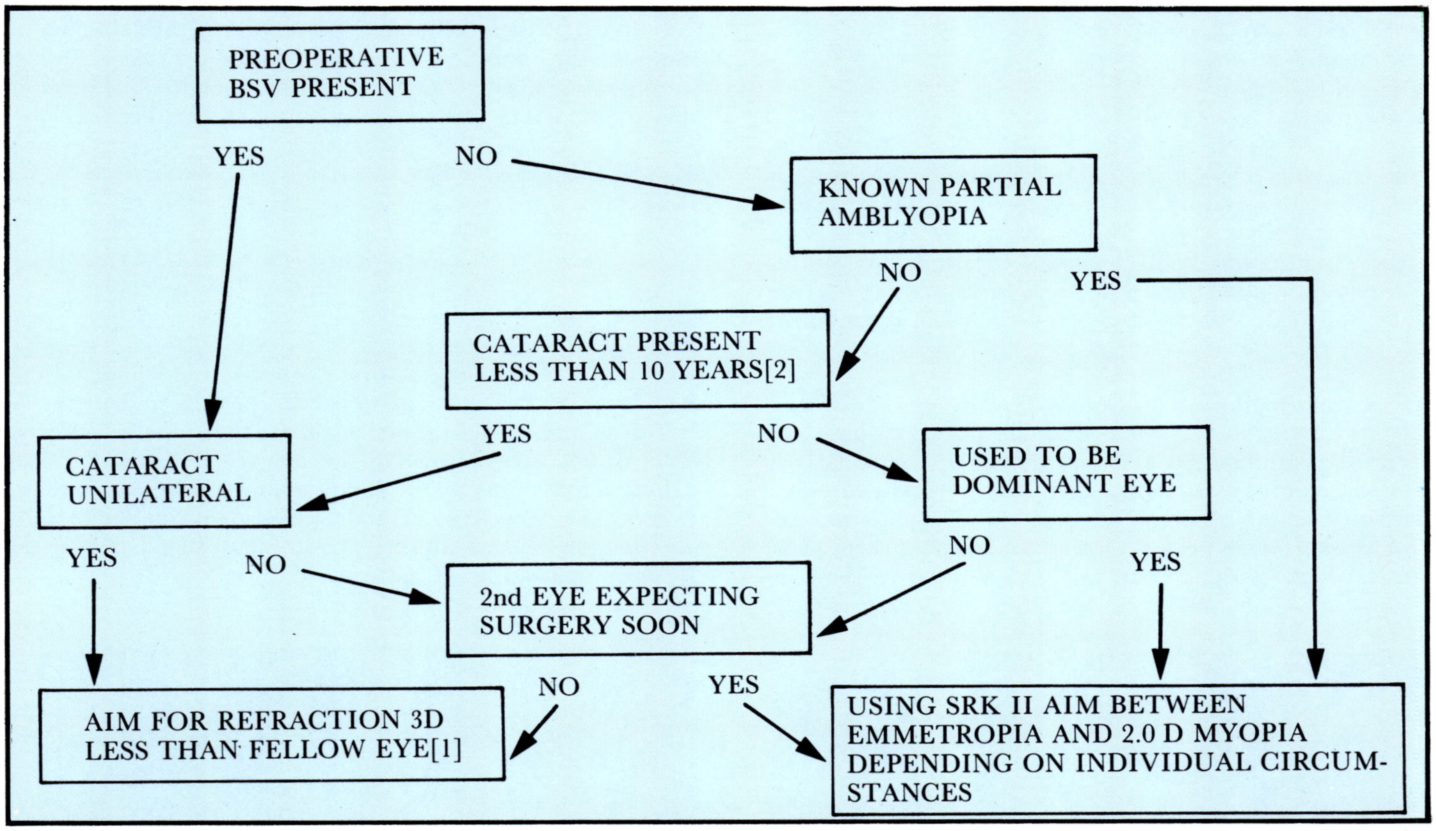

Flow Chart 26.1 For ametropia, from 3 D to 8 D. [1] BSV will normally be maintained or regained with a difference in refraction between the two eyes of up to 4 D. Hyperphoria requires a postoperative refraction that is similar in each eye. [2] If BSV has been lost for more than 15 years it is unlikely to be regained, if for less than 10 years it should be regained even in the presence of preoperative horizontal squint. If lost for between 10 and 15 years, results depend on the state of BSV before commencement of cataract.

Astigmatism

Astigmatism in excess of 2.5 D may, even when fully corrected, reduce visual acuity and produce glare, monocular diplopia, asthenopia and field distortion. It is estimated that such patients comprise 5% of the cataract population and, with the proven safety of IOL surgery, more attention may be given to intraoperative and postoperative astigmatism control. Although some of the techniques outlined in this chapter are in their infancy and are variable in effect, they are discussed to help both the patient and surgeon aim for good unaided vision. Alignment of the wound margins is an important determinant of the amount of astigmatism remaining when the eye is fully healed. Nonradial, interrupted suture bites or the shift of single running sutures produce a significant horizontal misalignment resulting in irregular steep and flat areas. On the other hand, by vertically mismatching the wound margins, one can produce a regular and predictable cylindric modification.

Postoperative aim

For monofocal lenses the aim should be about -1.5 D of cylinder, which for limbal sections is usually achieved by a slight wound compression so that the axis of the minus cylinder is at 180°. This provides a substitute for accommodation, making use of two line foci rather than a single point focus. One line offers 20/40 acuity for distance, the other offers J3 (N6) for near, and between the two the conoid of Sturm (**26.1**) offers acceptable clarity of vision without glasses, although the increase in depth of focus is achieved at the cost of a reduction in uncorrected distance acuity. Reading vision may also be enhanced (see p.161) when the implant is in the lens capsule.

26.1

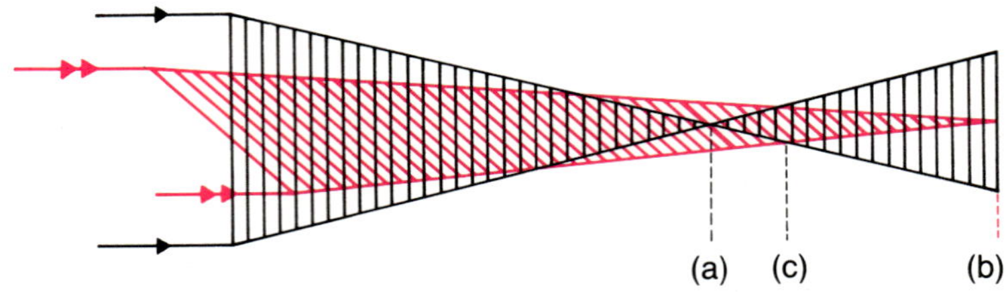

26.1 Sturm's conoid. The vertical meridian of the refracting body is more curved than the horizontal meridian. The line focus at **a** formed by vertical rays, is used for near vision. The line focus at **b** formed by horizontal rays (red), is used for distant vision. The circle of least diffusion at **c** is used for intermediate vision.

Preoperative astigmatism

The four methods that may be used surgically to modify preoperative astigmatism may be summarized:

- Wound compression or relaxation.
- Vertical mismatching of wound margins.
- A combination of the above.
- Transverse keratotomy.

Wound compression may be achieved by multiple sutures, tight sutures (especially when placed deeply) and long interrupted sutures (especially when corneal). The effect is a steeper corneal meridian. However, the treatment of the astigmatism is short lived, because if the sutures degrade or are removed (and they may have to be removed if the compression has overtreated the astigmatism), the effect is annulled. This method is not recommended for high degrees of astigmatism.

Wound relaxation is produced by too few sutures, widely spaced sutures, sutures with a short and shallow course, sclerally placed sutures and absorbable sutures or sutures that are removed early, particularly if accompanied by an excessive use of topical corticosteroids. The effect is a permanent flattening of the meridian or negation of a plus cylinder whose axis is in the direction of the suture. The method has been used to treat, for example, high 'with the rule' astigmatism where the plus cylinder has an axis at 90°, by relaxation of a 5 mm arc of wound at 12 o'clock. However, the surgeon must beware further wound decay with the passage of time and therefore should always aim to retain some degree of 'with the rule' astigmatism.

If the astigmatism is oblique, the position of the flattening technique is moved to the area of the steep axis. However, because these techniques have a variable effect and may be compounded by late wound decay, they should not be recommended alone for high degrees of astigmatism.

Vertical mismatching of the wound margins will produce a regular and predictable correction of astigmatism according to the mnemonic:

'Shallow to deep will make it steep:
The reverse of that will make it flat'

The wound is adjusted over a 50° segment of arc or a length of 5 mm at the limbus: by making the first corneal bite shallow and the opposing bite deep (**26.2**), the meridian will steepen. By making the first corneal bite deep and the scleral bite shallow (**26.3**), the meridian will flatten. This method may be relied upon for correcting between 1.5 and 3.5 D of cylinder, depending on the degree of mismatch and whether, for higher degrees, the steepening method is accompanied by slight tightening and anterior placement of the sutures or the flattening method is accompanied by early removal of the sutures.

26.2

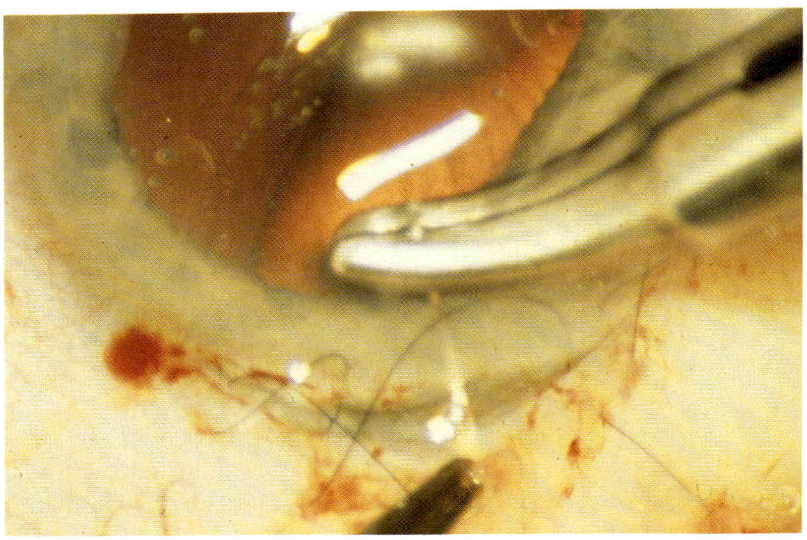

26.2 Double X suture, shallow to deep, over a 5 mm segment of wound (limbal incision).

26.3

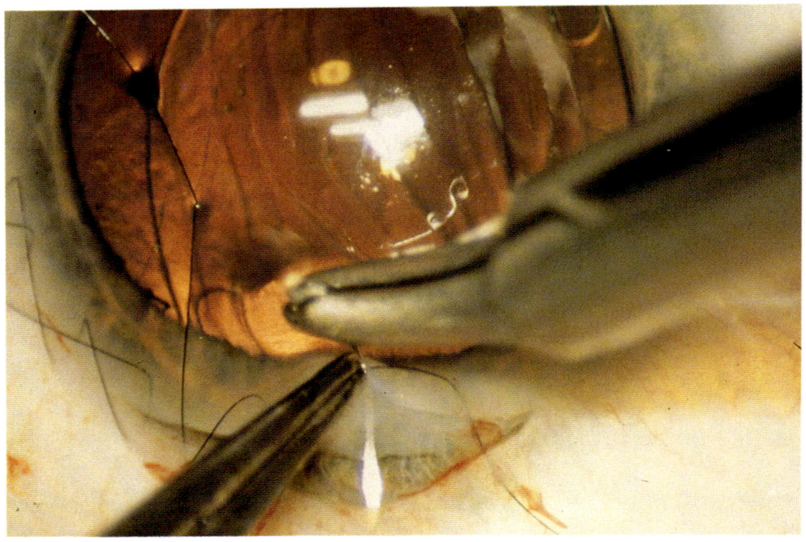

26.3 Suturing deep to shallow.

Do *not* employ long corneal sutures for steepening or absorbable sutures for flattening. Assuming that the patient may accept a residual astigmatism of up to 2.5 D, this method may be used for *treatment of up to 6 D* of preoperative astigmatism.

- Ensure the astigmatism is not recent or related to pathology, such as keratoconus.
- Ensure that your treatment, if unilateral, will be compatible with the fellow eye refraction.
- Do not depend on keratometry alone for measuring the preoperative astigmatism. Preoperative refraction is a better guide to manifest astigmatism, which is often found to be *less* than that measured by keratometry.
- Determine the axis of cylinder and relate this (plus or minus) to a segment of the wound you can adjust. For example, in **26.4** it would be appropriate to aim for correction of 3.5 D cylinder by employing **26.5** at the 12 o'clock zone. To treat a preoperative astigmatism of +4.0 D of cylinder axis 120° in a right eye it would be appropriate to employ **26.6** at the 11 o'clock zone.
- If the intention was to flatten, but the postoperative effect was not achieved, remove the appropriate sutures at one month. If the intention was to steepen but the effect overcorrected, do *not* remove the sutures for at least six months, otherwise the effect may be reversed.
- The effect of coupling (see **26.10**) is variable, depending on the type of incision, and is less exact than for transverse keratotomy. A limbal flattening procedure often increases the refractive spherical equivalent (SE) slightly towards hypermetropia. In general, one fifth of the power of the cylinder to be corrected should be added (if flattening) or subtracted (if steepening) to the power of the posterior chamber IOL. Thus, when correcting a 2.5 cylinder by flattening, 0.5 D should be added to the power of a posterior chamber lens.

Example: Preoperative astigmatism +4.5 D cylinder axis 90°
Calculated implant power for –0.7 D myopia : 21.8
Implant inserted 22.5. Flattening procedure (**26.6**)
Refraction at 1 month $-2.5/+3.0_{90°}$
Removal of sutures at 12 o'clock reduced a further 2.0 cylinder
Final refraction: $-0.25/-1.0_{180°}$

Similarly, a steepening procedure can increase the SE towards myopia and the lens power calculation should again be altered.

Example: Preoperative astigmatism +4.5 D cylinder axis 180°
Calculated implant power for –0.7 D myopia : 22.4
Implant inserted 22.0. Steepening procedure (**26.5**)
Final refraction : -1.5 cyl $_{90°}$

26.4

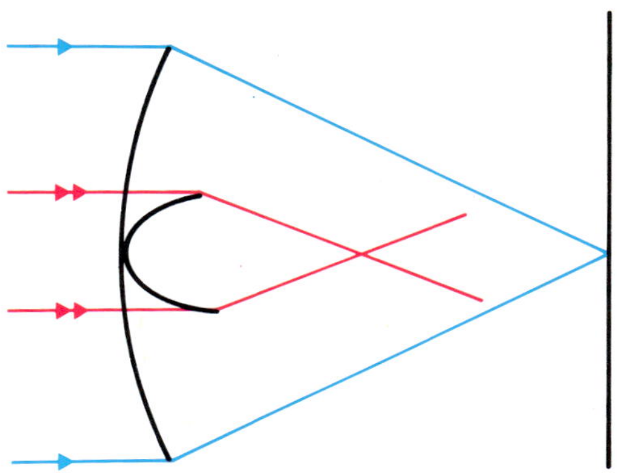

26.5

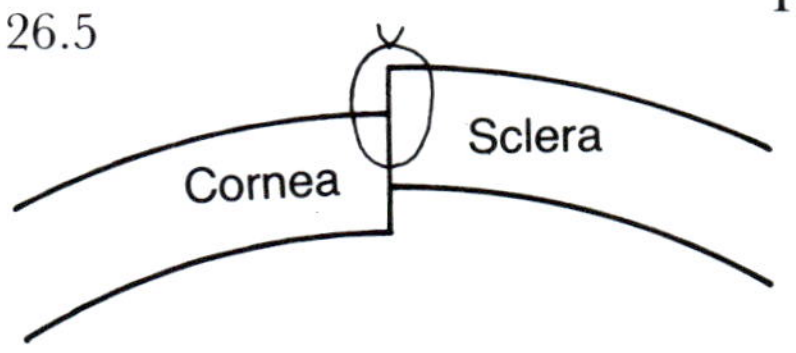

26.6

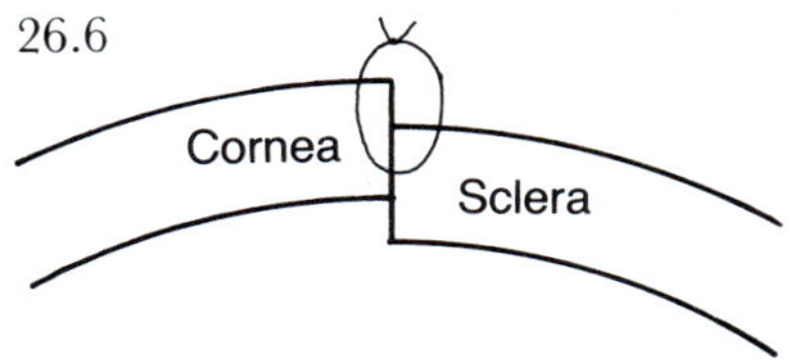

26.4 Astigmatism –5.0 D $\downarrow_{90°}$ has a cornea too steep horizontally.

26.5 Vertical mismatch for minus cylinder, axis in direction of suture. Suture shallow to deep and tighten.

26.6 Vertical mismatch for plus cylinder, axis in direction of suture. Consider early removal of suture.

Transverse keratotomy may be considered immediately before the cataract extraction for astigmatism in excess of 5 D, or for lesser amounts when the routine is for a scleral pocket incision. Informed consent should be obtained from the patient, who should understand that additional corneal incisions (which are optional) are being planned in order to enhance the unaided postoperative vision. Extension of a front cutting or square-tipped diamond blade is prepared (see text books for radial keratotomy). A Thornton Press-on Ruler (**26.7**) is used to prepare the clear optical zone and length of incision (**26.8, 26.9**).

26.7

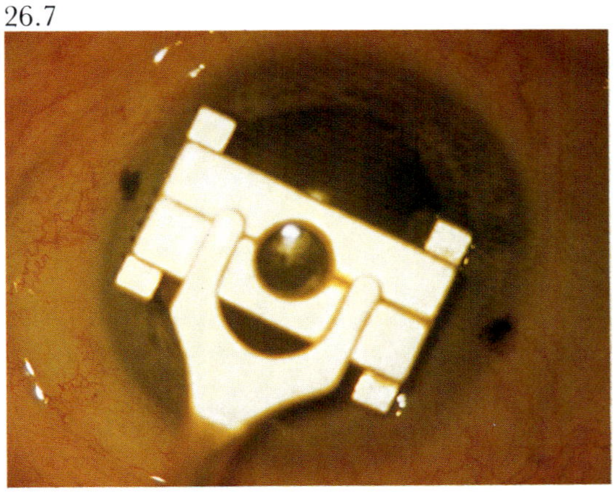

26.7 Thornton Press-on Ruler: after marking the steep axis of astigmatism to be treated with gentian violet at the limbus, the ruler, with its under surface stained, is centered on the cornea and pressed on to the eye.

26.8

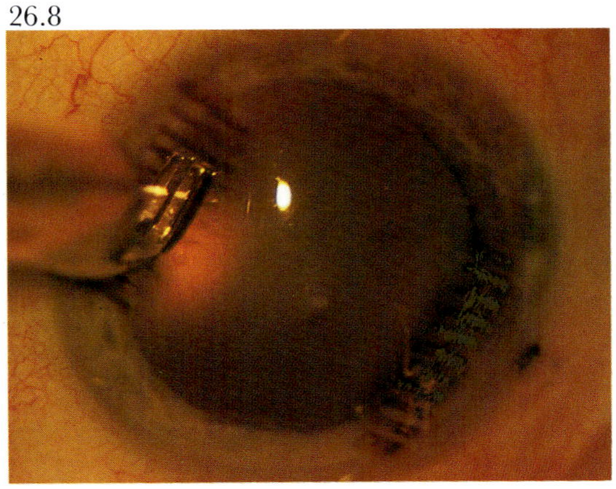

26.8 Marks from the double ruler are clearly seen. The eleven marks are each 1 mm long and spaced 0.5 mm apart. The inner edge offers a clear optical zone diameter of 6 mm and the outer edge one of 8 mm.

26.9

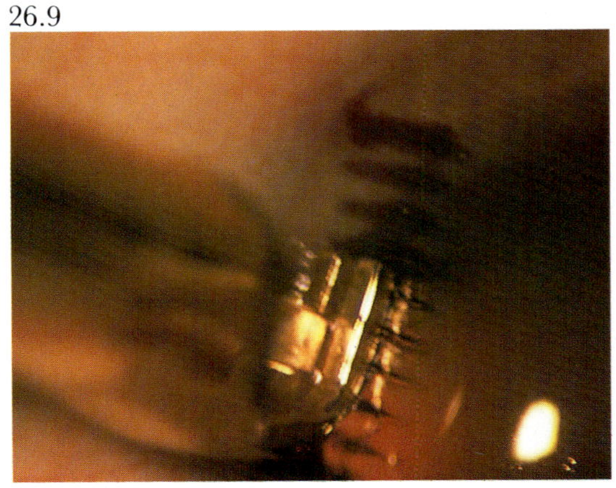

26.9 Detail of square trifaceted diamond entering at an OZ of 7 mm (midway across the marks).

Appropriate cuts are then made before commencing the cataract surgery. At an optical zone of 7 mm, paired transverse cuts 95% deep are made 1 mm long for every 0.75 D of astigmatism to be treated. The effect is variable. Two pairs at the 6.0 and 8.0 mm optical zones (OZ) should be recommended when more than 2.5 D is to be treated, but this has the danger of being more unpredictable and more likely to induce postoperative glare or irregular astigmatism. The effect of coupling should also be remembered, as for pure transverse keratotomy without radial cuts, an equal amount of steepening will occur in the meridian 90° away from the meridian that is being flattened, with no change in the spherical equivalent (**26.10**).

26.10

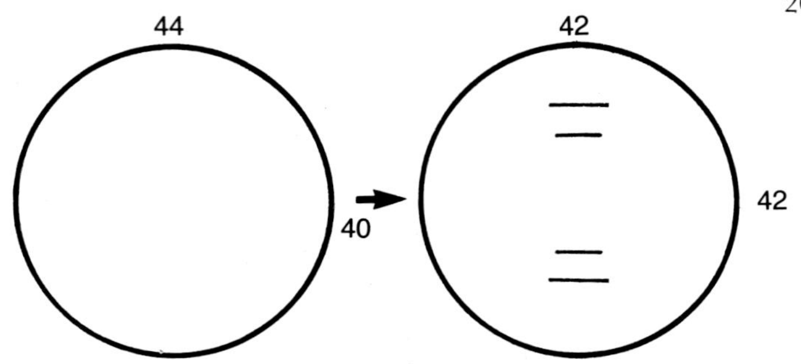

26.10 The effect of coupling: to turn a refraction of +2.0/–4.0, axis 180° into plano, a double paired transverse keratotomy is made at optical zones of 6 and 8 mm, leading to 2 D of flattening in the vertical meridian and 2 D of steepening in the horizontal meridian, with no change in the spherical equivalent.

Surgically induced astigmatism

If postoperative astigmatism occurs with a degree of frequency after cataract surgery, the surgeon should attempt to modify the technique to compensate for those factors that predispose to astigmatism. The more anterior the incision, the more likely the astigmatism. An incision 1 mm posterior to the limbus or a scleral pocket incision for phacoemulsification may be recommended to minimize astigmatism. Suture bites should be deep, not long, spaced approximately 1 mm apart and evenly tied for apposition without compression. X or double-X continuous sutures are preferred to interrupted sutures.

Consideration of treatment for postoperative astigmatism is only necessary when above 2.5 D, and then only if this is at variance with the fellow eye refraction, the patient is symptomatic, and there is a myopic component to the refraction. A flattening procedure can increase the SE towards hypermetropia, so if there is no myopic component it may be prudent to leave a hyperopic cylinder untouched (e.g., +3.0 cylinder with the rule would be preferred to a conversion to +2.0 sphere).

Treatment of overtight wound: (the axis of the plus cylinder is in the meridian of the sutures): Remove the sutures selectively or from the appropriate 5 mm arc of wound at two months if the astigmatism is over 2.5 D, remembering that wound decay may continue for six months after surgery.

Example: Postoperative refraction $-2.0/+3.5_{90°}$ (unacceptable)
Remove overtight sutures at 12 o'clock
Resulting refraction $-0.5/+1.0_{90°}$ (acceptable)

Treatment of wound slippage (the axis of the plus cylinder is at right angles to the meridian of the sutures):

- Await six months for refraction stability as the astigmatism may lessen or the patient may acquiesce with time.
- If a specific area of wound requires revision, consider wedge resection with overtightening of sutures. This prolongs further the period of convalescence.
- Consider transverse keratotomy (**26.7–26.9**) to flatten the cornea in the axis of the plus cylinder: For correction of a 2.0 D cylinder make single paired cuts with a 7 mm optical zone 3.0 mm long; for correction of a 2.5 D cylinder make double paired cuts with 6 and 8 mm optical zones 1.3 and 1.7 mm long, respectively; for correction of a 3.0 D cylinder make double paired cuts with 6 and 8 mm optical zones 1.9 and 2.6 mm long, respectively.

Example: Refraction six months after surgery: $-3.25/+4.0_{180°}$ $(+0.75/-4.0_{90°})$
Plan double paired TK tangential to 6 and 8 mm optical zones
Resulting refraction: $-0.75/-1.0_{90°}$

Further reading

Maloney W.F., Grindle L., Sanders D. and Pearcy O.D. Astigmatism control for the cataract surgeon. A comprehensive review of surgically tailored astigmatic correction. *J. Cataract Refractive Surg.*, **15,** 45–54, 1989.

Nordan L.T., Quantifiable astigmatic correction: Concepts and suggestions 1986. *J. Cataract Refractive Surg.*, **12,** 507–518, 1986.

Thornton S.P. and Sanders D.R. Graded non-intersecting transverse incisions for correction of idiopathic astigmatism. *J. Cataract Refractive Surg.*, **13,** 27–31, 1987.

Thornton S.P. Astigmatic keratotomy: a review of basic concepts, *J. Cataract Refractive Surg.*, **16**(4), 1990.

27: Hospitalization and anesthesia

Patrick Condon and John Dunphy

In-patient or ambulatory surgery

Following initial reports by Galin and Baros *et al.* (1974), and subsequently by others who demonstrated that hospitalization was not essential for successful cataract surgery, 85% of all cataract surgery in the United States converted from being carried out on hospital in-patients to ambulatory day cases in the six years between 1981 and 1987. Europe is changing more slowly to day-case cataract surgery. Davies *et al.* (1987) in the UK reported on the cost savings to hospitals involved in this change, but it must be realized that part of these savings is derived from a shifting of the cost of services from the health care industry to the family of the patients. Provided certain parameters are adhered to, it is now widely accepted that day-case surgery is not only safer for elderly patients, but that the majority prefer it.

Whereas the development of independent purpose-built facilities in the United States in the last five years has been ideal, the transition from in-patient surgery with general anesthesia (GA) to day-case ambulatory cataract surgery with local anesthesia (LA), in a hospital environment with existing staff, may be more difficult. Advantages of hospital-based ambulatory surgery include the reduced capital outlay with the use of existing equipment and staff. The disadvantages include the surgeons' lack of control over the quality of personnel in some hospitals and difficulties with the scheduling of operations due to other surgical specialty activities in the same operating room. Also, the changing role of the administration and nursing staff from admission, through preparation and actual surgery to the eventual discharge of the patients within a single day, puts a greater burden on all staff of work that would normally be spread over a three day period. A further impetus, however, to change will be the more widespread use of small incision surgery.

Preoperative selection

Tables 27.1, 27.2 and **27.3** outline the indications and contraindications to general and local anesthesia. As most patients for cataract surgery are elderly with various medical conditions, it is essential to decide the safest mode of anesthetic within one month before surgery (**Table 27.4**). Consultation with the anesthetist is helpful. A decision in favor of GA will automatically place the patient into the in-patient category. If GA is imperative yet contraindicated, it may be possible, with preoperative consultation, to optimize the patient's condition before surgery. In relation to myocardial infarction, GA should be postponed for six months. The risk of reinfarction within

Table 27.1 Ideal patient for cataract surgery

General anesthesia	*Local anesthesia*
Healthy, ASA* 1–2	Alert and cooperative
In-patient preference	Good hearing
No respiratory/CVS disorder	Short stay preference

* American Society of Anesthists classification.

Table 27.2 GA relative contraindications

CVS	Angina at rest/cresendo type Uncontrolled blood pressure Recent myocardial infarct Severe cardiovascular disease Cardiac myopathy Pericarditis Heart block
Respiratory system	Type 2 failure Severe obesity
Endocrine	Unstable diabetes Myxedema
Hematology	Severe anemia Sickle cell disease
Musculoskeletal	Cervical osteoarthritis Temporomandibular joint immobility Myotonia dystrophia Malignant hyperthermia Myasthenia gravis
Hepatic or renal failure	

Table 27.3 LA Contraindications

Uncooperative
Mental confusion
Mental psychosis
Severe deafness
Presence of severe involuntary movements
Presence of severe mechanical movements
Severe supine dyspnea
Allergy to LA drugs

Table 27.4 Preoperative assessment

Medical	Preexisting disease Current medication Hb, Hematocrit, CXR ECG, Random blood sugar
Social	Live-in relative/friend for supervising transport to/from hospital and convalescence
Decision	Suitability daycase/in-patient Suitability GA/LA Date of surgery
Explanations	Patient/relative responsibilities Fasting Preoperative drops Information leaflet concerning necessary arrangements before and after surgery

three months of a previous infarction is 37%, within three to six months 16%, and after six months 4.5%. Reinfarction is most likely to occur on the third day postoperatively. With respiratory failure, especially type 2, a combination of GA with the patient lying in the supine position decreases functional residual capacity. A simultaneous increase in closing volume results in hypoxia, compromising respiratory status and putting tissue oxygenation at risk, especially in the recovery phase. With endocrine abnormalities, it is essential that preoperative myxedema, Addison's disease and diabetes mellitus be diagnosed and appropriate stabilization with replacement therapy be instituted. Anemia of any type must be treated if GA is to be considered. Iron deficiency anemia may require preoperative oral iron, or a blood transfusion if surgery is required urgently. Changes in hemaglobin directly affect oxygen carriage to the tissues and may be critical for the elderly myocardium. In non-Caucasians, where sickle cell anemia is suspected, GA may be contraindicated, as it may also be in patients with myotonia dystrophica, myasthenia gravis and malignant hyperthermia. Where difficulties are anticipated with maintenance of the airway, such as in patients with severe cervical osteoarthritis or temporomandibular joint immobility, LA may be safer.

Only in rare situations does a combination of contraindications for both types of anesthesia preclude the patient totally from surgery.

Operative conditions

General anesthesia (GA) provides ideal operating conditions for modern microsurgical techniques. Small movements magnified by the microscope are eliminated. GA with hyperventilation can also control intraocular pressure (IOP) and reduce the complications associated with increased positive pressure within the eye. The prime requirements are secure airway control with adequate alveolar ventilation and cardiovascular stability throughout the operative and recovery period. Avoiding stimuli that increase central venous pressure and IOP is essential. **Table 27.5** compares the routines required for GA, which for cataract surgery requires in-patient stay, and for LA, which may be performed as an out-patient. GA patients on digoxin should have serum digoxin and serum electrolytes measured preoperatively to ensure an adequate dosage and to ensure that there is no relative overdosage. Patients on monoamine oxidase inhibitors should be challenged first with morphine or papaveretum and then anesthetised appropriately.

Atropine is rarely used in premedication because of tachycardia and dry mouth. It can be used intravenously in the operating room. The prevention of oculocardiac reflex is an individual matter for the surgeon and anesthetist. The newer muscle relaxants now in use generally lead to slower pulse rates. H2 antagonists should be used preoperatively in patients subject to gastrointestinal reflux. Babies less than 1 year old intended for gas induction may benefit from intramuscular atropine (15µg/kg) to protect them from bradycardia at induction before venous cannulation.

Local anesthesia can be carried out on both in- and out-patients. Whereas the preparation for LA is less rigorous than that for GA, a routine has to be observed so that scheduling of the operating list can be carried out without undue inconvenience. A repeat medical and ocular examination should be made on arrival of the patient at the hospital and, generally, no premedication is necessary.

Intraocular pressure (IOP) can be controlled and reduced by anesthesia and to a lesser extent by analgesia. IOP is raised by 2–3 mmHg in the supine position. It can be reduced by a head up tilt of 10 degrees if the blood pressure remains stable. IOP is maintained by a balance between the production of aqueous and its elimination from the eye through the outflow channels. The volume of blood in the choroidal vessels is important. The other contents of the eye remain constant throughout surgery, so that manipulation of IOP by anesthesia is through the aqueous humor and choroidal blood flow. Increased pCO_2 results in increased venous pressure (therefore less efficient drainage) and increased choroidal volume. Anesthesia aims to control pCO_2 by ventilation. Arterial pressure (also controlled by GA), plasma osmotic pressure and patient position have lesser roles in IOP control.

Table 27.5 Preoperative preparation

GA/In-patient	*LA/Day case*
Admission pm before or am of day of surgery	Breakfast at home
Preoperative fast 6 hours	Transport with relative
Recent local doctor medical report	Admission 1–2h preoperatively
Repeat medical examination, temperature, pulse, blood pressure, respiratory rate	Repeat medical examination
Adjustment of medications, e.g. insulin, steroids	Ocular preparation
Premedication with benzodiazepine	
Ocular preparation	

Drugs that may influence IOP include suxamethonium, which temporarily raises IOP by causing contraction of the extraocular muscles, and diazepam (intravenously at induction), droperidol, haloperidol, morphine, fentanyl, thiopentone, methohexitone, etomidate, propofol, and volatile anesthetic vapors, all lower IOP. Ketamine raises IOP. Inhalation agents may also raise IOP in spontaneous respiration due to increased pCO_2. Laryngoscopy and intubation raise IOP for a short period. Hypoxia will raise IOP by increasing the choroidal blood volume.

Drug therapy for glaucoma may have anesthetic consequences. Ecothiophate reduces plasma cholinesterase to such a degree that metabolism of suxamethonium and ester-type local anesthesia may be interfered with, producing apnea. Beta-blocker-type eye medication may be systemically absorbed in pharmacologically active amounts and cause bronchoconstriction and hypotension. Subconjunctival injections of mydricaine (which contains adrenaline) may lead to tachycardias and ectopic cardiac rhythms. Carbonic anhydrase inhibitors, such as acetazolamide, which lower IOP by inhibition of aqueous humor secretion by the ciliary processes, also increase choroidal blood flow by between two and three times for 30 min after administration.

Techniques and complications

General anesthesia

The patient is induced using an intubation technique and anesthesia is maintained with a combination of oxygen, nitrous oxide and an inhalation agent. The major postoperative complications are indicated in **Table 27.6**. Mortality rates have been reported of between 0.65 and 1.6 per 1000 cases, pulmonary embolism around the eleventh day being the most common cause of death.

Early studies have reported that up to 7% of those mentally normal preoperatively suffered severe dementia afterwards and up to 12% had a limited existence after their operation. Recent studies suggest that impairment of memory and reduced coordination occur for seven days after GA. Centrally acting anticholinergics and benzodiazepines have been implicated as causative factors. It has also been shown that elderly patients who became hypotensive preoperatively or hypoxic postoperatively are particularly prone to mental impairment or confusional states, so that, for the elderly, steps should be taken to avoid these situations.

Table 27.6 Major postoperative complications of GA

CVS:	Myocardial infarction. Deep vein thrombosis/pulmonary embolism.
Respiratory:	Hypoxia Atelectasis Pneumonia Aspiration
Gastrointestinal:	Nausea/vomiting (children > adults, females > males)
Urinary:	Retention (males)

Local anesthesia

Procaine was first introduced for lid akinesia by van Lint in 1914. In 1930, retrobulbar procaine became widely used and in 1943 lignocaine was introduced. In 1961, Atkinson advocated a dull needle no longer than 35 mm for retrobulbar block and suggested the use of hyaluronidase. The usefulness of orbital compression, with various devices, was shown in 1967 by Vörösmarthy and revived by Honan in 1979. From 1973 onwards, while reports of complications from retrobulbar anesthetic blocks were occurring with increasing frequency (**Tables 27.7–27.9**), the concept of posterior peribulbar extraconal anesthesia, originally introduced by Kelman, was being increasingly used by Gills, Thornton, Bloomberg and many others. For either method, surface anesthesia is required in addition to the regional block using drops of amethocaine 1% or oxybuprocaine 0.4% prior to surgery.

Table 27.7 Complications of retrobulbar anesthesia

Major retrobulbar hemorrhage	⟶	Blind from ON compression
Minor retrobulbar hemorrhage	⟶	Orbital hematoma Cancellation of surgery
Central retinal artery occlusion	⟶	Blind
Penetration of optic nerve	⟶	Optic atrophy
Globe perforation in high myopia	⟶	Retinal detachment Choroidal hemorrhage
Intradural penetration ON sheath	⟶	Brainstem infiltration Autonomic dysfunction
Levator muscle damage	⟶	Upper lid ptosis
Extraocular muscle trauma	⟶	Diplopia

Retrobulbar technique

The patient is first instructed to look upwards and to the right for the left eye and upwards and to the left for the right eye. A 3 ml mixture of 2% lignocaine with or without 150 international units of hyaluronidase is injected into the muscle cone by penetrating the skin at the junction of the lateral third and medial two thirds of the lower eyelid, just above the orbital rim. The 25 mm 22- or 25-gauge needle is then advanced upwards and medially in a direction towards the apex of the orbit (**27.1**). As the needle passes the globe it may catch in Tenon's capsule, in the expansion between the inferior and lateral rectus muscles, and cause a slight depression of the globe. Further, slight advancement of the needle tip beyond this point ensures the intraconal position of the needle tip. Aspiration prior to injection will identify and prevent inadvertent intravenous injection of the anesthetic. Approximately 3 ml of LA are used. The complications of this technique are summarized in **Tables 27.7–27.9**. In a prospective study of 6000 cases of retrobulbar block, 16 cases of CNS complications were observed, a rate of 1:380. Of these, 8 became semicomatose, two suffered convulsions and one had a cardiac arrest (Nicoll *et al.* 1987). The sequence of events after intravascular injection of LA solution is shown in **Table 27.9**. The management is with diazepam or barbiturates intravenously with ventilatory and cardiovascular support.

Table 27.8 Systemic complications of intravascular injection

TOXIC	
Cerebral cortex	Excitement, euphoria, muscle twitching, convulsion, somnolence, coma, death
Medulla	Raised blood pressure, tachycardia, tachypnea, nausea, vomiting, hypotension, apnea
CVS	Bradycardia, peripheral vasodilatation with hypotension, cardiac arrest
Respiratory system	Apnea, hypoxia
ALLERGIC	Erythema, urticaria, bronchospasm Anaphylactic shock

Table 27.9 Clinical signs of intravascular injection

Tongue and circumoral paresthesia/anesthesia
Anxiety/restlessness
Slurred speech and drop in level of consciousness
Coma with or without convulsions
Cardiovascular collapse

Peribulbar technique

First inject 4 ml of a mixture of lignocaine 4% and bupivacaine 0.5% with 150 international units of hyaluronidase in the inferior peribulbar area through the lower eyelid at the junction of the lateral third and medial two thirds, or 1.5 cm medial to the lateral canthus just above the inferior orbital rim (**27.2, 27.3**).

An aliquot of 1.0 ml of this mixture is deposited immediately beneath the orbicularis oculi muscle and then the needle is advanced along the inferior orbit to the equator of the globe. An additional 1.0 ml is injected at this point (**27.1**) and then the barrel of the syringe is angled over the malar eminence and the needle advanced in a medial and superior direction to its full depth, at which point 2.0 ml of the anesthetic are given (**27.4**). Aspiration of the barrel of the syringe is important to prevent inadvertent intravascular injection. A similar upper lid injection of 3 ml is then given transcutaneously at a point halfway between the supero-orbital notch and the medial canthus (**27.2, 27.4, 27.5**). As all orbits are shaped differently, some being shallow and others deep, it is essential while advancing the needle along the orbital floor or roof that the direction of the needle tip be redirected up or down, respectively, if it comes in contact with bone (**27.4**). Failure to appreciate this may result in an inadvertent entry of the needle and the anesthetic into the maxillary sinus inferiorly or, more seriously, into the anterior cranial fossa superiorly in cases where the bone plate is very thin.

27.1

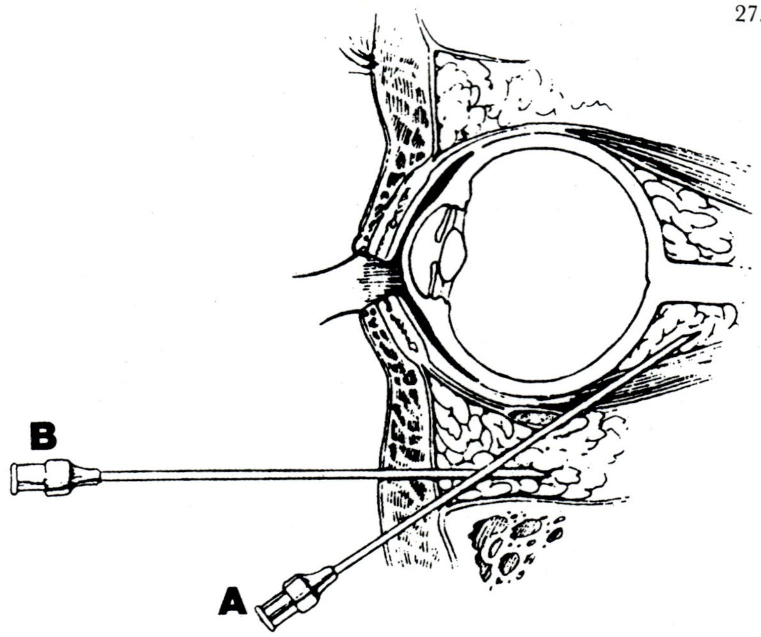

27.1 The different techniques of LA: (a) Retrobulbar injection; (b) Peribulbar injection (reproduced from *Current Therapy in Ophthalmic Surgery*, B.C. Decker, 1989).

27.2

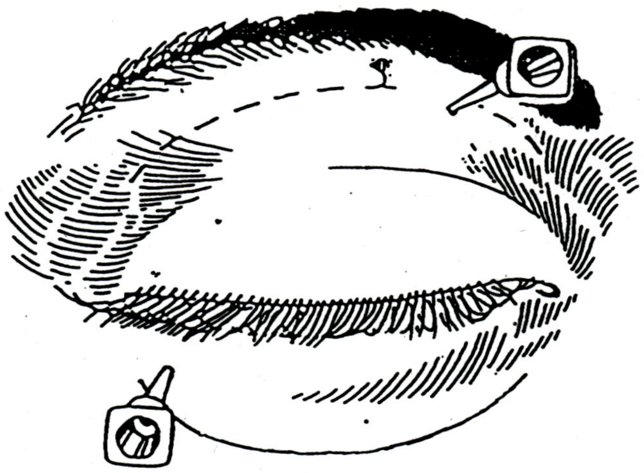

27.2 Peribulbar anesthesic injection entry sites, right eye (reproduced with permission from *Implants in Ophthalmology*, **2** (2)).

27.3

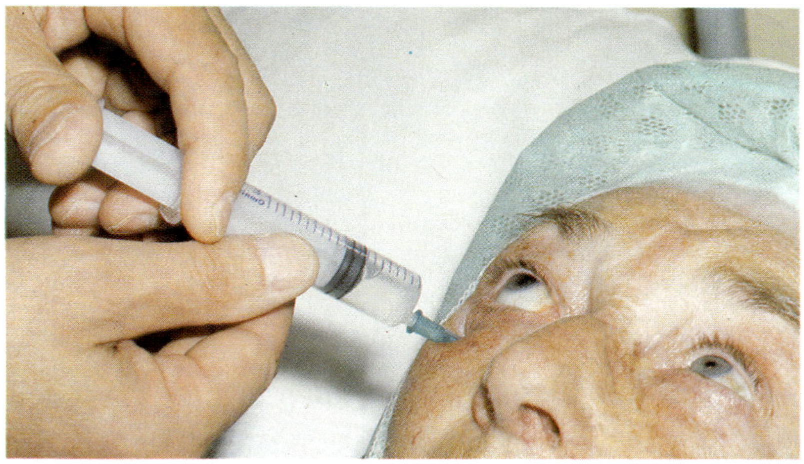

27.3 Peribulbar anesthetic – lower eyelid injection.

27.4

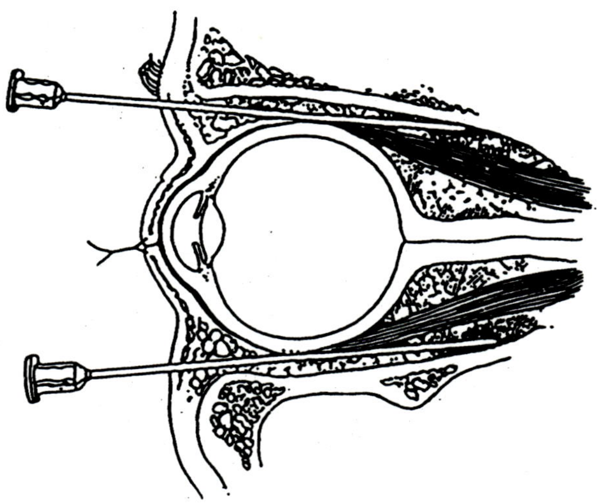

27.4 Direction of peribulbar needle within the orbit (reproduced with permission from *Implants in Ophthalmology*, **2** (2)).

27.5

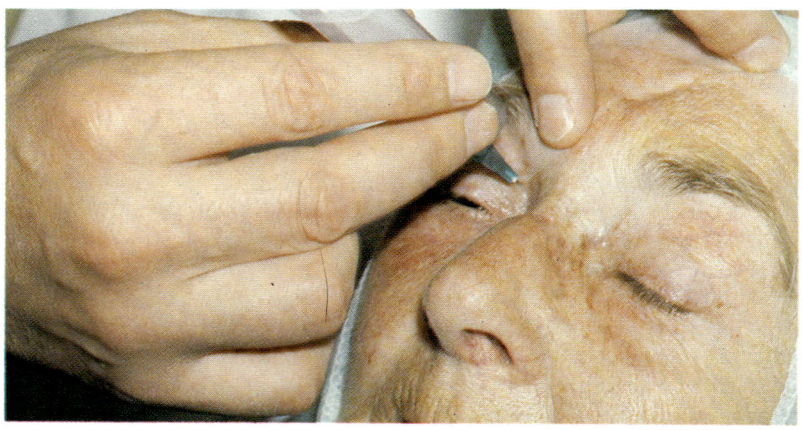

27.5 Peribulbar anaesthetic – upper eyelid injection.

The block is carefully monitored and after 10 min if eye movement is still detected, a further injection of 2–3 ml is given transcutaneously at the point between the medial one third and the lateral two thirds of the lower lid, just above the orbital rim (**27.6**). During the course of these injections, paralysis of the levator palpebrae superioris occurs with automatic closure of the upper eyelid (**27.7**). It is assumed that orbital diffusion into the extraocular muscles, as well as diffusion into the nerves controlling these muscles and the ciliary ganglion, combined with the orbicularis infiltration by the LA is the reason this method functions without the need for a facial block. Because of the relatively larger volume of anesthetic employed in this technique, ocular compression for 30 min should follow prior to surgery. Complications are rare.

27.6

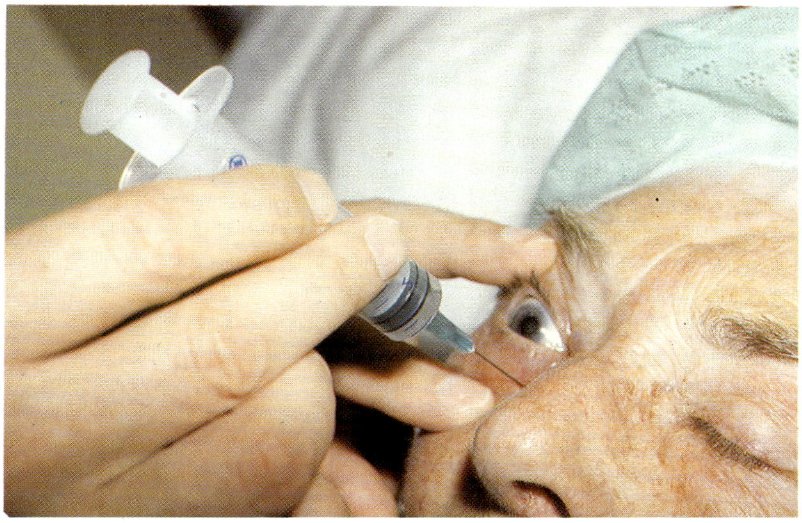

27.6 Augmentation of anesthetic with extra injection in the lower eyelid, medially.

27.7

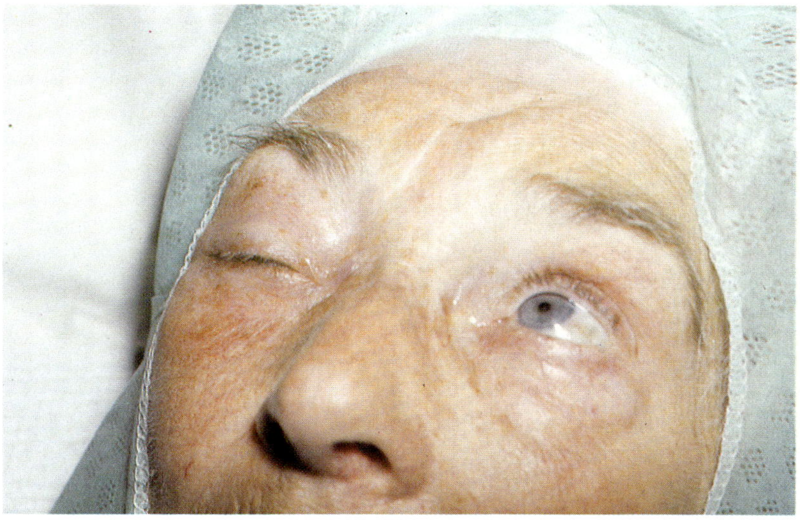

27.7 Ptosis induced with peribulbar anesthetic block.

Variations in LA techniques

Addition of adrenaline prolongs the block effectively by inducing localized vasoconstriction, but it can also cause sympathomimetic reactions of tachycardia, raised blood pressure and cardiac arrythmias in patients with cardiac problems and especially those on long-term beta-blockers, where an exaggerated response can occur. In depressive patients on monoamine oxidase inhibitors, which deplete sympathomimetic amines in the body, adrenaline can give rise to an unpredictable response resulting in hypotension and circulatory collapse. It should not be used in concentrations of more than 1:200,000.

Pain relief: Apart from the safety aspects of peribulbar anesthesia, when compared with retrobulbar techniques, the former is also less painful. **Table 27.10** lists some techniques that may be employed in order to reduce the pain of injection to a minimum.

Table 27.10 Pain relief for LA

Short-acting intravenous agents monitored by an anesthetist
Preretro/peribulbar infiltration 1% lignocaine, 27-gauge needle Skin wheal/orbicularis oculi/suborbicularis oculi
pH adjustment (a) preretro/peribulbar infiltration with a mixture of 9 ml balanced salt solution and 1 ml 1% lignocaine for skin wheal/orbicularis oculi; (b) preretro/peribulbar infiltration with 1% lignocaine and 1:100,000 adrenaline mixed with sodium bicarbonate 8.4%, 1 mg/ml, plus indomethacin trihydride 0.17 mg/ml
Warm temperature of anesthetic solution to 37°C in electric pad
N_20 and 0_2 inhalation mixture

Ocular compression

Gifford in 1948 showed that the retrobulbar LA lowers the IOP by 3–4 mmHg. However, in 1955 Kirsch and Steinman suggested that mechanical digital pressure could soften the eye more, resulting in less vitreous loss in intracapsular surgery. In 1962, Vörösmarthy introduced his oculopressor, which was followed by the Buy's mercury bag, the Gills Super Pinky and the Honan balloon. The effect of ocular compression is to express aqueous from the eye with a reduction of anterior segment and vitreous volumes. The expression of interstitial fluid and blood from the orbital tissues is also important with injections of more than 3 ml, and is particularly relevant to peribulbar anesthesia. In order to avoid the rebound phenomenon of increased production of aqueous and increased choroidal congestion during surgery, when the eye is at its most vulnerable open state, it is essential that the ocular compression device be used for at least 20–30 min prior to surgery, never exceeding 30 mmHg in order to avoid retinal vascular occlusion. If the device needs to be left on for longer periods it is advisable that the applied pressure be reduced to 10 mmHg. Whereas actual pressure monitoring by a plethysmographic dial is possible with the Honan, Nevyas and Vörösmarthy instruments, and the weight of the Buy's balloon on the eye is calculated not to exceed 30 mmHg, the manufacturers of the Gills Super Pinky and others give adequate instructions as to how to apply the devices, so that excessive pressure on the eye does not compromise the retinal circulation. Extra care should be advised for glaucomatous patients with visual field defects.

Injection needles

Since Atkinson advocated the use of a 35 mm dull needle for retrobulbar blocks in 1961, the Atkinson needle has been popular. The tip is dull, but the edges are sharp and the tip angle is 30° (**27.8**). The needles may be of 23- or 25-gauge. The dulled tip allows the operator to feel the progress of the needle by the amount of resistance of each tissue plane, thereby allowing accurate placement within the muscle cone. However, its use is painful and nerve and vessel damage remains a problem. The introduction of disposable super-sharp 27-gauge retrobulbar needles for the purpose of reducing pain resulted in a significant increase in retrobulbar hemorrhage. The Thornton needle may be 25- or 27-gauge and differs in having a thin wall of 0.08 mm with rolled (dulled) edges, although the tip is sharp (**27.9**). The tip angle is 15°. This design results in decreased resistance to insertion with less pain (without compromising the feedback of tissue plane resistance) and a reduced tendency to hemorrhage. The preferred length is 25 mm in order to obviate possible damage to the optic nerve or nerve sheath.

Monitoring of vital functions

For LA the presence of an anesthetist is optional, but monitoring must continue. Sphygnomanometer, ECG and oximeter are ideal. In practise a blood pressure cuff may be uncomfortable for the patient, but in combination with the oximeter, which has a simple clip to a finger or toe, may be all that is necessary. The oximeter passes light of two absorption spectra frequencies of saturated and desaturated hemoglobin through the skin. It therefore measures oxygen flux and indirectly indicates respiratory and cardiac function.

A sudden rise of blood pressure during the operation can be controlled by sublingual nifedipine (10 mg), which can be repeated. For tachycardia, propranolol is given intravenously in doses of 0.25 mg, which can be repeated every 10 minutes, up to four times. **Table 27.11** lists an optimal routine for LA. Premedication is not essential, but particularly apprehensive patients may be given sublingual lorazepam (1 ml), 30 min before the LA block.

Table 27.11 Avoidance of LA complications

Back up resuscitation facilities: anesthetist, laryngoscope, ambubag, endotracheal tubes, stethoscope, drugs, defibrillator
Per-operative monitoring of pulse, blood pressure, ECG, oximetry
Indwelling intravenous catheter
Thornton injection needle
Peribulbar injection

27.8

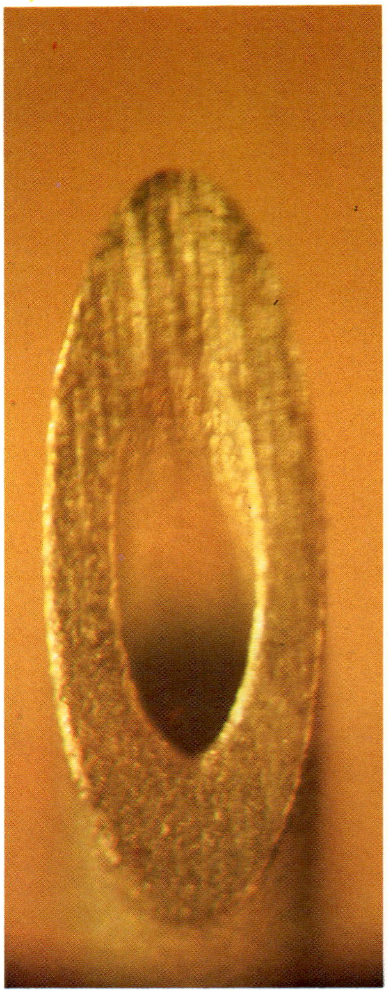

27.8 Atkinson needle tip with microscopic surface pits and dull edges (reproduced with permission from *Ocular Surgery News*, 1988).

27.9

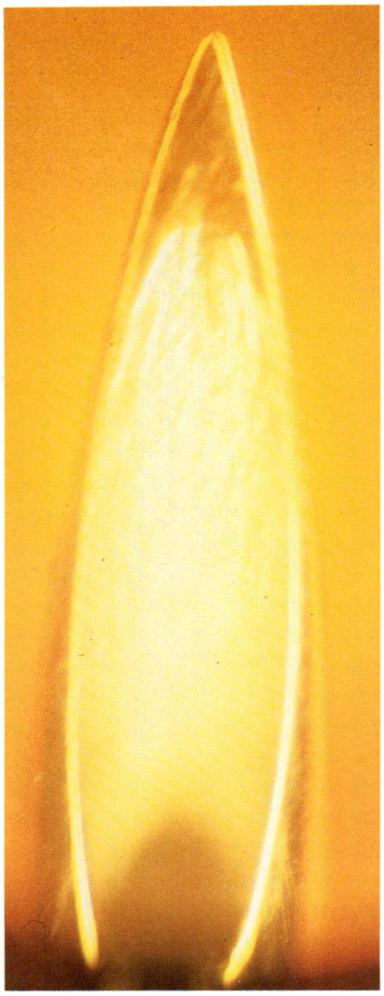

27.9 Thornton needle tip with a thin wall for reduced tissue resistance (reproduced with permission from *Ocular Surgery News*, 1988).

Further reading

Davies P.D., Limacher E. and Powell K. Out-patient cataract surgery 1982–1986. *Eye*, **1,** 728–734, 1987.

Feibel R.M. Current concepts in retrobulbar anaesthesia. *Survey of Ophthalmology*, **30,** 102–110, 1985.

Hamilton R.C., Gimbel H.V. and Strunin L. Regional anaesthesia for 12,000 cataract extractions and intraocular lens implantation procedures *Can. J. Anaesth.*, **35,** 615, 1988.

Miller R.D. (Ed.), *Anaesthesia*, 2nd Edn. Churchill/Livingstone, London, 1986.

Wong K.C.K. and Jenkins L.C. Anaesthesia for ophthalmic surgery. *Can. J. Ophthalmol.*,**20** (3), 87–92, 1985.

28: Preoperative preparation

Daniel Vörösmarthy

Preliminary examination

In assessing the patient's general health, particular attention should be paid to the mental state, pulmonary function, and the presence of cardiovascular disease. Blood pressure and urinalysis are checked routinely. A note is made of the patient's medications and any known drug sensitivities.

Next an examination is made for lesions that are a potential source of ocular infection and require postponement of surgery until resolution has occurred. These include *focal sepsis*, particularly of the teeth, paranasal sinuses and upper respiratory tract, *ocular infection*, including conjunctivitis, blepharitis and chalazia of either eye and *dacryocystitis*. Dacryocystitis must be eliminated surgically before a cataract operation can be contemplated and if this is not possible the lacrimal puncta must be temporarily closed by cautery (**28.1**).

It is not necessary to perform routine lacrimal syringing or conjunctival culture (**28.2**) preoperatively, except in suspected cases of epiphora or blepharoconjunctivitis respectively. In cases where infection is suspected these treatments and remedies must be completed at least two weeks prior to cataract surgery. After a further 48 h without treatment conjunctival cultures may be repeated and, if clear, antibiotic drops restarted five times a day prior to cataract surgery. For all other cases topical antibiotics are prescribed hourly prior to surgery but *only* during the day of admission.

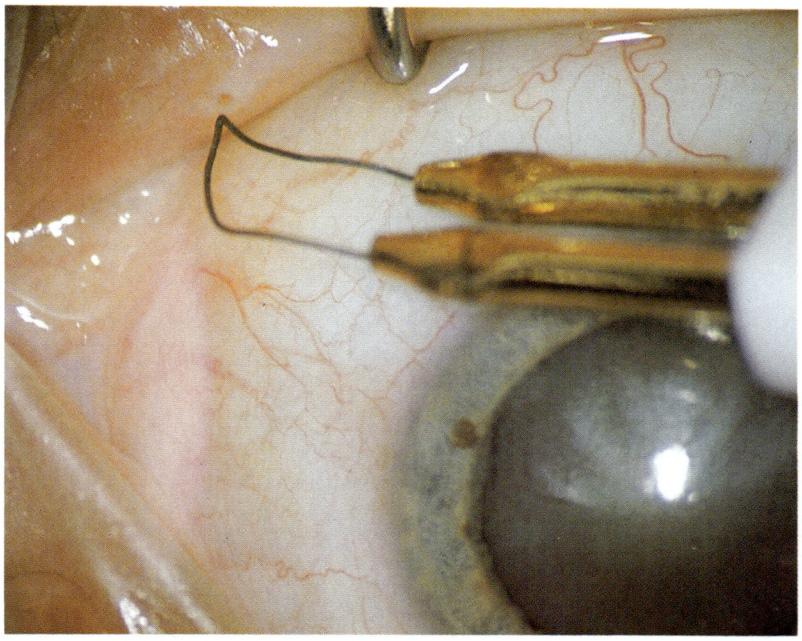
28.1

28.1 Cauterization of lacrimal punctum in a case of chronic dacryocystitis.

8.2(a)
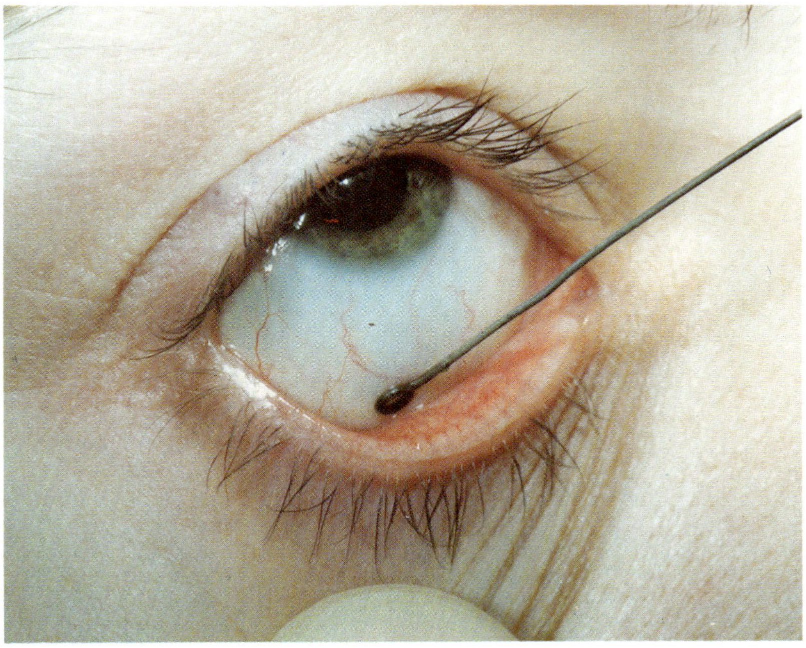

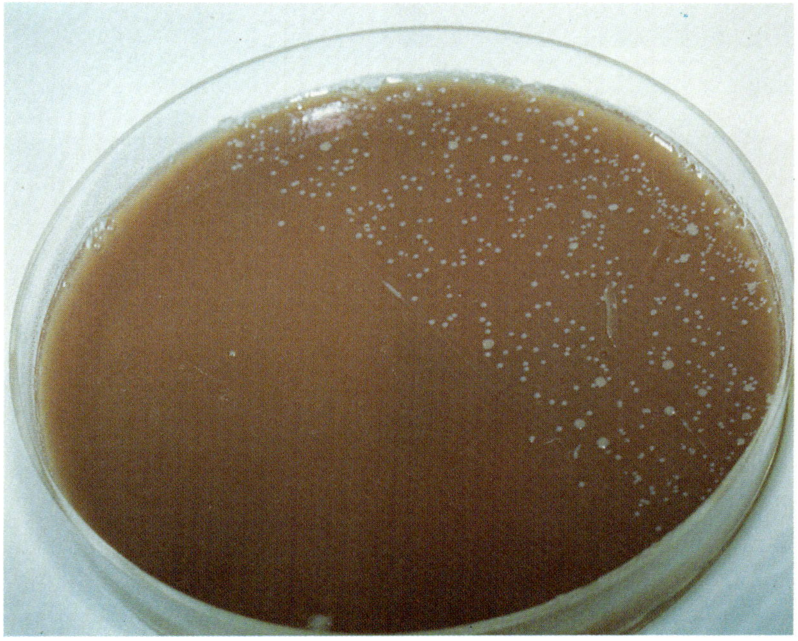
28.2(b)

28.2 Plating of a conjunctival culture (a) onto chocolate agar (b).

Preoperative tasks and the field of operation

The patient should sign, in the presence of a witness, a form of consent for the operation.

A prophylactic broad spectrum antibiotic is injected intramuscularly at the time of premedication.

The eyelashes are cut (**28.3**), as this enables better penetration of antiseptic solution to the skin and lash follicles, and easier attachment of sticky drapes to the eyelids and lid margins.

Skin preparation is carried out in two phases using an antiseptic in aqueous solution, such as povidone–iodine 10%. The first phase occurs after local anesthetic drops have been given immediately prior to retrobulbar or peribulbar anesthesia (if under local anesthetic) and ocular compression (**28.4**). The second takes place on the operating table. After towelling up, the surgical field is covered with a sterile transparent plastic drape with the lids open (**28.5**). The drape is then cut in the interpalpebral zone (**28.6**) and the cut edges of the drape are reflected underneath the lid margins by the lid speculum (**28.7**).

28.3

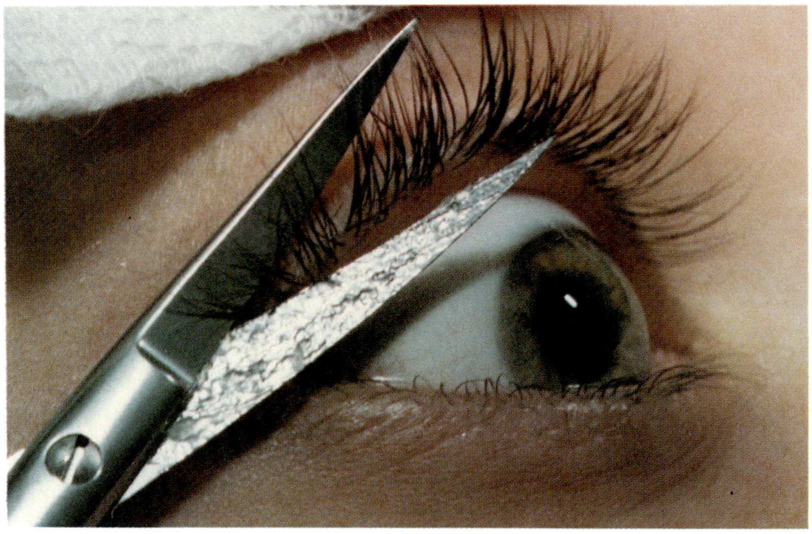

28.3 Cutting of lashes of the upper lid prior to surgery.

28.4

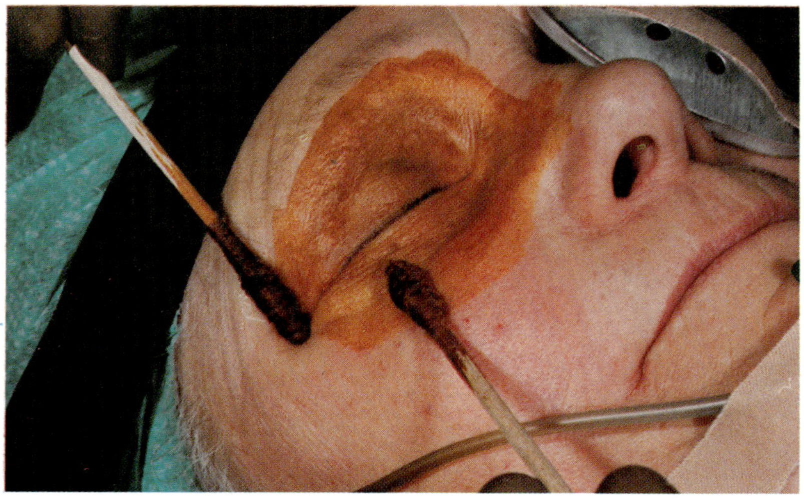

28.4 Cleansing of lid skin with 10% povidine–iodine.

28.5

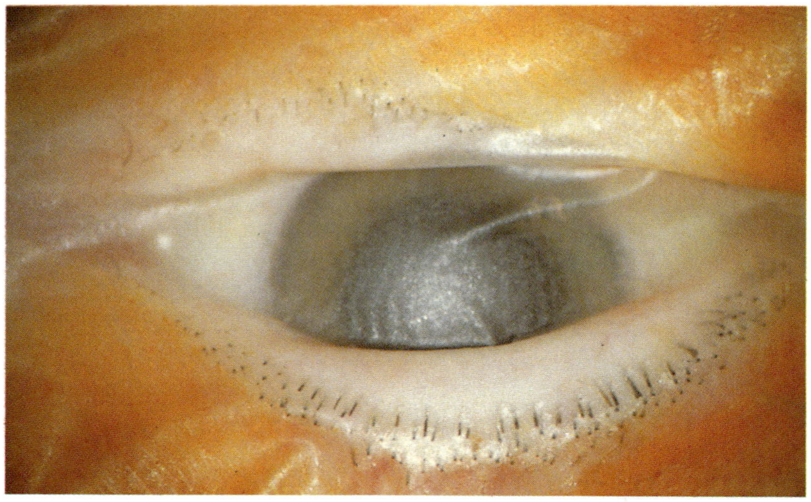

28.5 Plastic drape placed over the open lids.

28.6

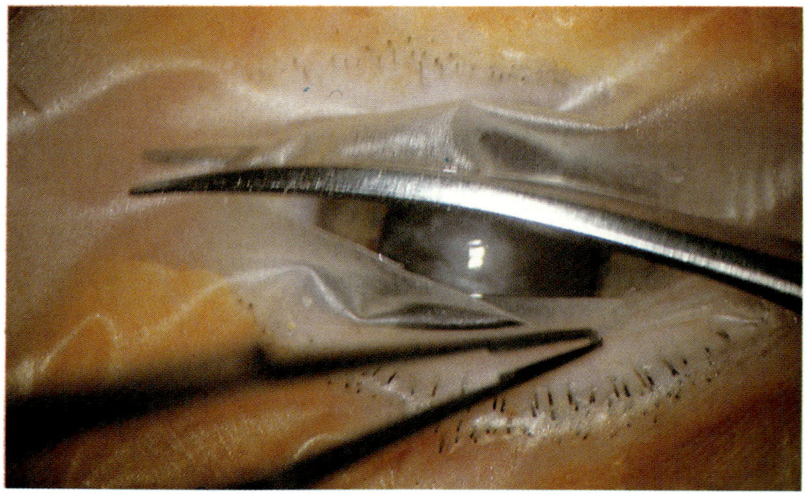

28.6 Edges of the drape are fashioned.

28.7

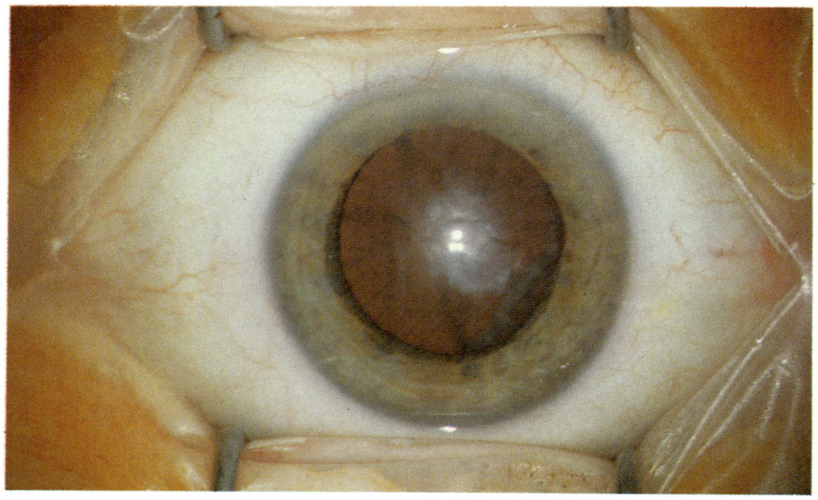

28.7 Placement of lid speculum with the edges of the drape underneath the lid margins.

The conjunctival fornices may also be cleansed with weak aqueous antiseptic (**28.8**). Continuous irrigation (**28.9**) of the surgical field is recommended, firstly to wash out the antiseptic and secondly to keep the cornea moist and clear during surgery. Excess fluid in the conjunctival fornices must be continually drained away from the chamber of the eye. This may be achieved by a wick from a gauze swab, or by a drain strip (**28.10**), or by mechanical aspiration, or by using a speculum with fine holes and a tube for mechanical aspiration (**28.11**).

28.8

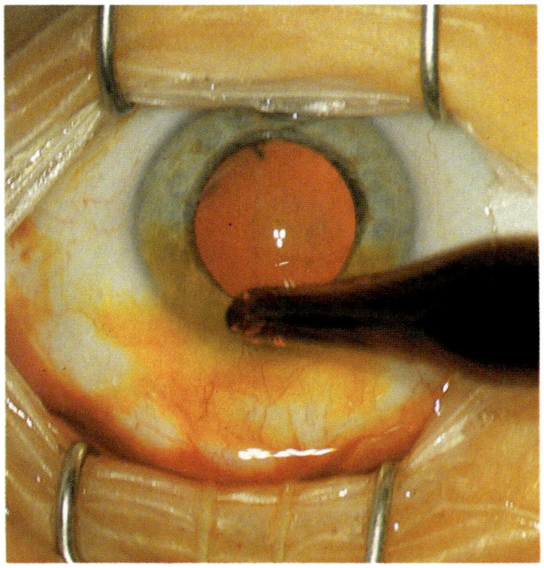

28.8 Elevation of the lids with speculum to allow a flow of antiseptic solution into the conjunctival fornices.

28.9

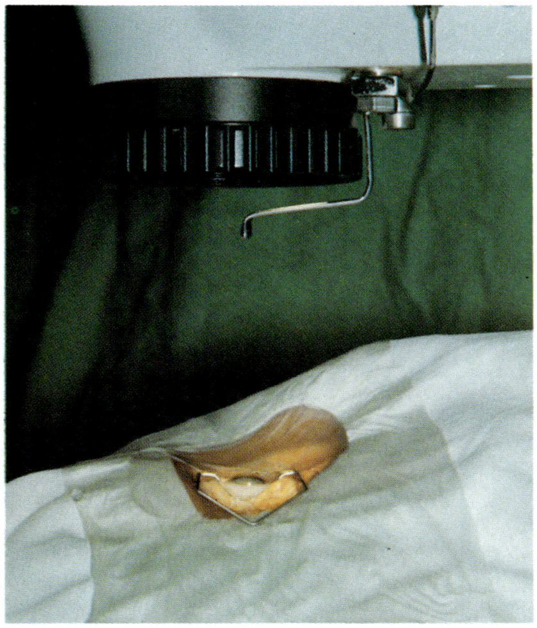

28.9 Cannula mounted on the microscope for slow irrigation drop by drop.

28.10

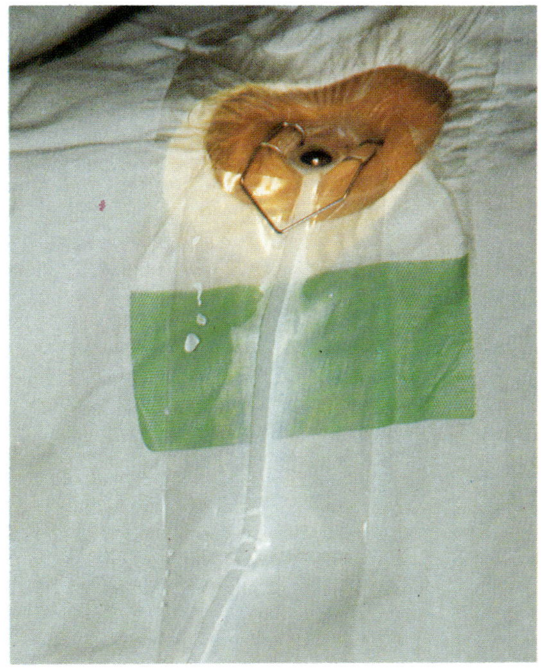

28.10 Aspiration by means of a drain strip.

28.11(a)

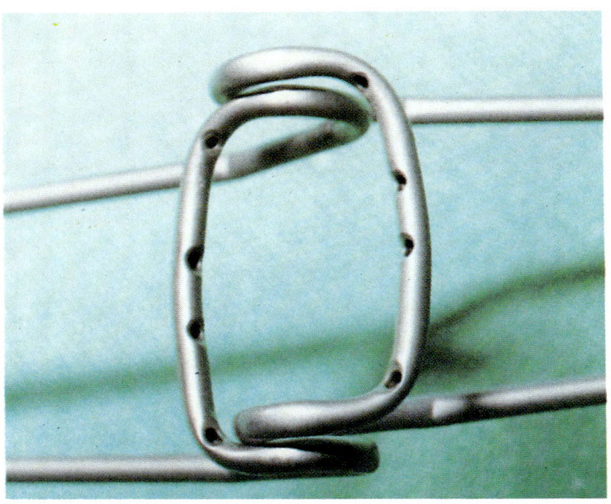

28.11(b)

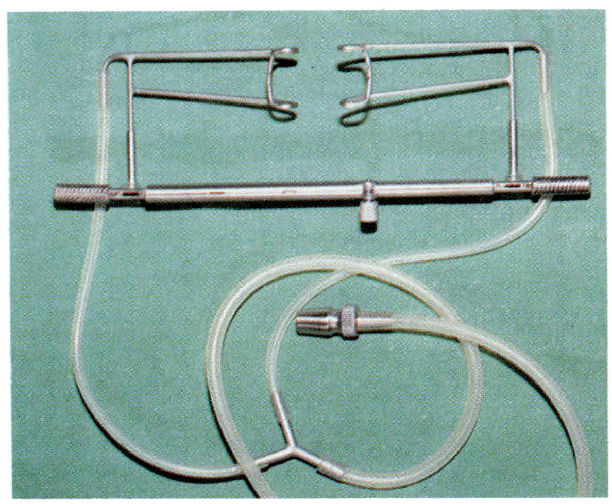

28.11 (a) Lid speculum and (b) apparatus for conjunctival drainage.

Management of the pupil

For extracapsular surgery a widely dilated pupil (mydriasis) is required to ensure adequate visibility and protection of the iris. For secondary implantation of an anterior chamber lens, a small pupil (miosis) is required in order to protect the vitreous body and open the chamber angle. Miosis is achieved by a drop of pilocarpine 2% 30 minutes before surgery. Mydriasis is more difficult because any mechanical or chemical irritation may lead to the release of prostaglandins and pupillary constriction.

The recommended treatments for full mydriasis are as follows:-

- Phenylephrine 10% and cyclopentolate 1% drops 50, 40 and 30 min prior to surgery. Other adrenaline analogues may be used if phenylephrine is not available.
- Indomethacin 1% drops 90, 60 and 30 min prior to surgery. These may also be continued postoperatively as prophylaxis against uveitis and macular edema.
- Adrenaline 1:1000 (1 ml) injected into each liter of irrigating fluid prior to surgery.
- The irrigating fluid should be warmed towards body temperature prior to surgery. Viscoelastics, if used, should also be warmed and not taken straight from a refrigerator.
- Adrenaline 1:1000 (0.1 ml) may be injected episclerally adjacent to the limbus if other methods have failed (**28.12**).
- When mydriasis appears inadequate a sector iridectomy and sphincterotomy (**28.13**) should be considered. Synechiolysis may be performed with viscoelastics (**28.14**).
- If the pupil constricts before lens implantation the use of viscoelastics in the anterior chamber will improve the mydriasis.

28.12

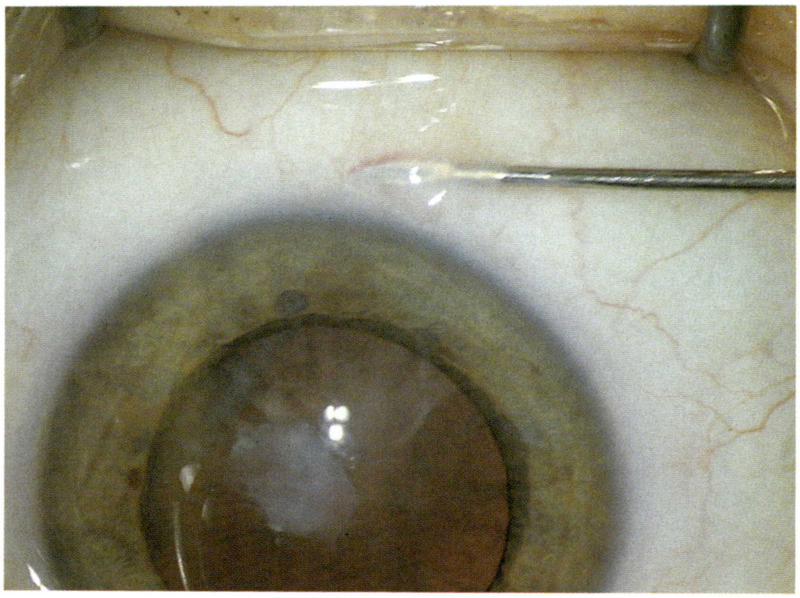

28.12 Episcleral injection of epinephrine (0.1 ml).

28.13

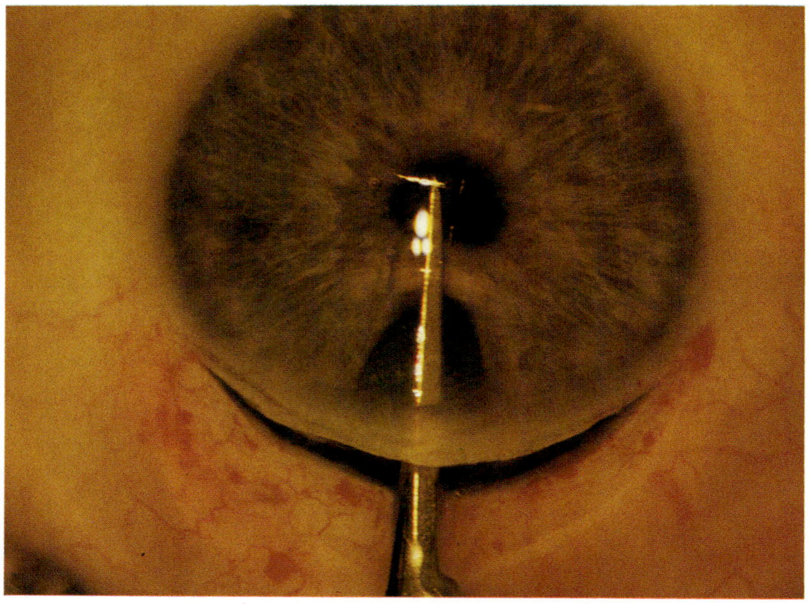

28.13 Spincterotomy to improve mydriasis.

28.14

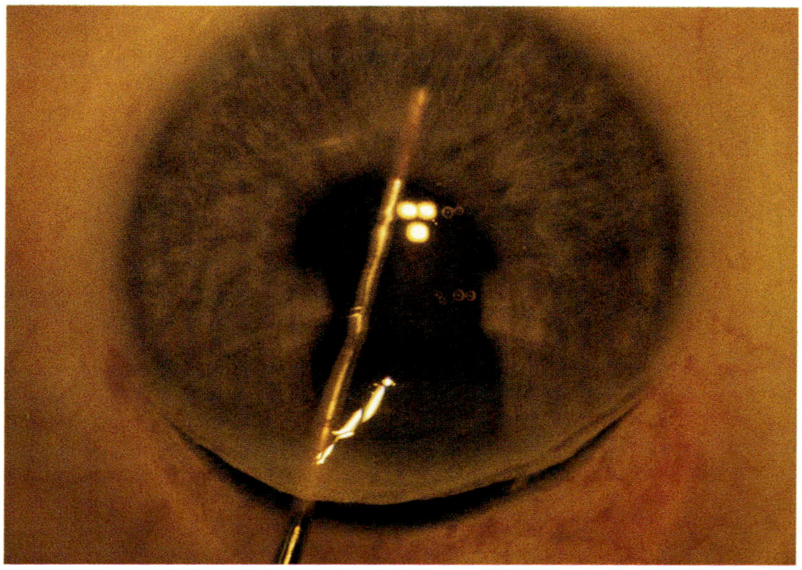

28.14 Injection of sodium hyaluronate behind the iris.

The above treatments do *not* require reversal or neutralization, for example with acetylcholine, at the end of surgery. The pupil may remain dilated for several hours, but should return to normal without additional management within two days. Atonic pupils, although sometimes caused by sphincter erosions at surgery, are also more likely after intracameral acetylcholine or the use of intensive miotics postoperatively. If it is required that the pupil be smaller at the end of surgery, a drop of the phenylephrine antagonist *thymoxamine* is recommended.

It is *not* necessary to use mydriatics on the day before surgery (e.g., atropine or cyclopentolate drops). If they are used, a lesser mydriasis may be achieved because of pupillary fatigue and there is an added risk of elevating the intraocular pressure.

Positioning the patient

A head-up tilt, so that the head is always higher than the abdomen, is recommended to avoid venous congestion being transmitted to the eye (**28.15**). If surgery is to be under local anesthesia, a pillow under the knees may improve the patient's comfort. The level of the iris should be perpendicular to the visual axis of the microscope (**28.16**). A blue light filter is recommended for the microscope light. The fellow eye should be covered and, if under local anesthesia, a tube supplying oxygen should be taped to the face underneath the drapes.

28.15

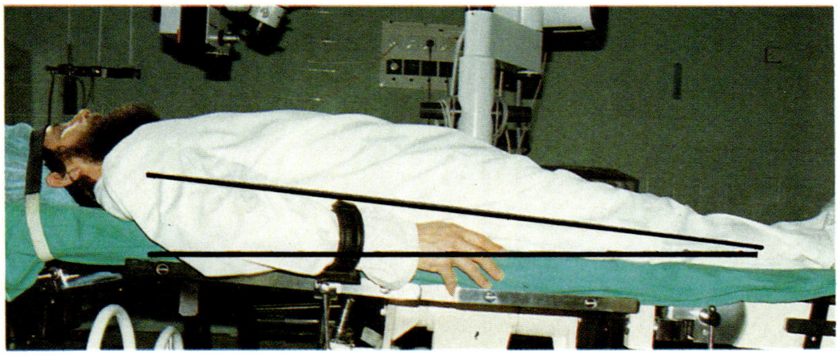

28.15 The recommended head-up tilt.

28.16

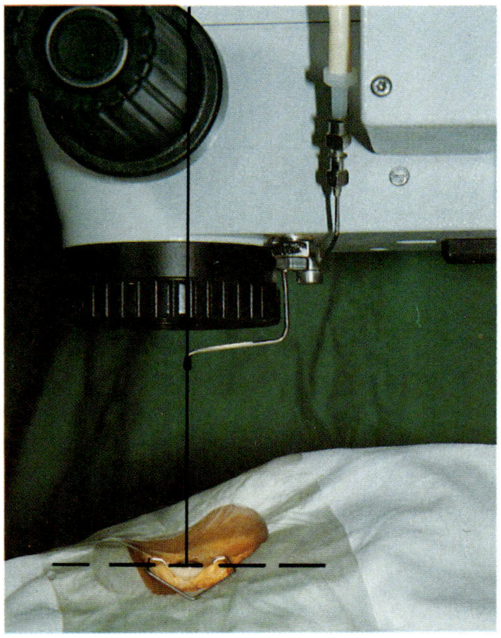

28.16 The level of the iris is perpendicular to the visual axis.

Ocular hypotony

The use of osmotic agents or carbonic anhydrase inhibitors, although useful for cases of lens-induced glaucoma, has now largely been superceded by ocular compression.

Ocular compression is an important adjunct to anesthesia and akinesia in providing the most suitable conditions for surgery. When carried out correctly it produces a controlled and sustained reduction in the volume of the vitreous body (**28.17**). After release of compression the aqueous is replaced rapidly and the vitreous slowly, creating a deeper anterior chamber and a reduction in the vitreous volume. The latter will persist for approximately 40 min and sometimes longer after surgical openings of the anterior chamber.

28.17

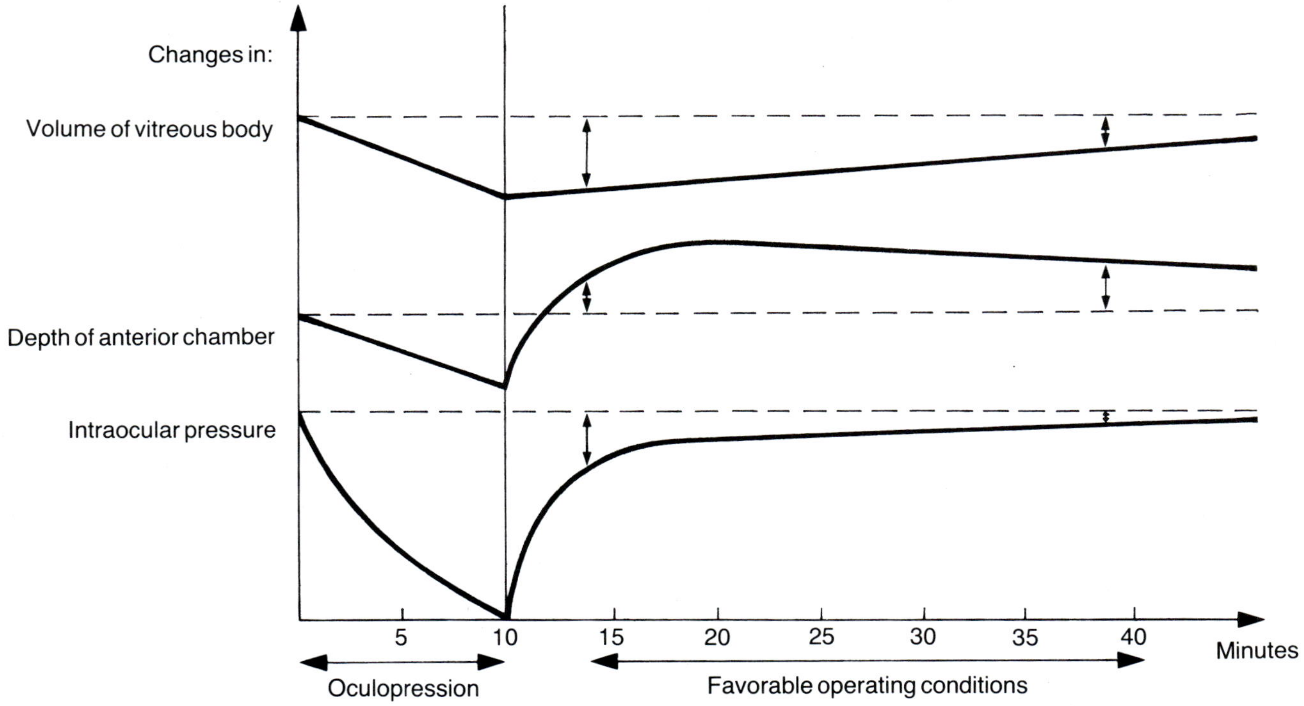

28.17 Changes in the volume of vitreous, depth of anterior chamber and intraocular pressure produced by a 10 minute application of the Vörösmarthy Oculopressor.

The oculopressor recommended (from Deutschmann's of Zittau or from Geuder's of Heidelberg) is based on the original Vörösmarthy principles and comprises three main parts (**28.18**):

- The pneumatic bellows (**28.19**) exert pressure onto the eye, and have a frame at the head that will adapt to anatomical variations and occludes the entire orbital opening. They allow an elastic compression of the eye without changing the shape of the cornea (**28.20, 28.21**). Since the orbit is sealed, the soft orbital fat allows equal pressure on the globe from every direction.
- The headrest provides support for the bellows and the possibility of transferring to either eye.
- The air pump, manometer and valves may be set for accurate control of pressure in the bellows.

28.18

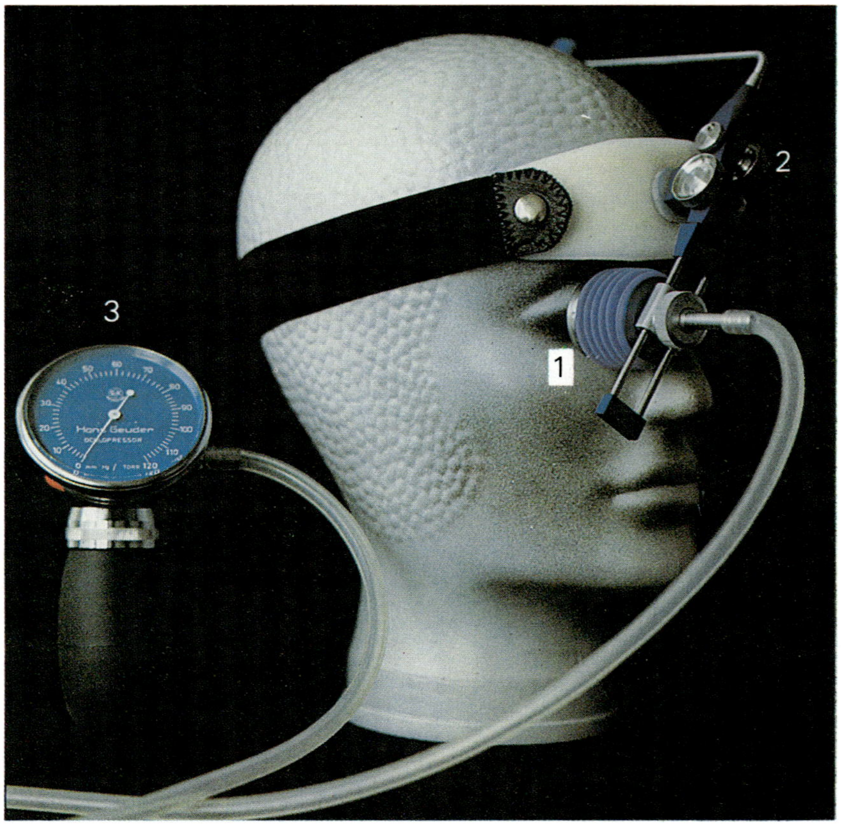

28.18 The Vörösmarthy Oculopressor: pneumatic bellows (1), headrest with support (2), airpump with manometer and valves (3).

28.19

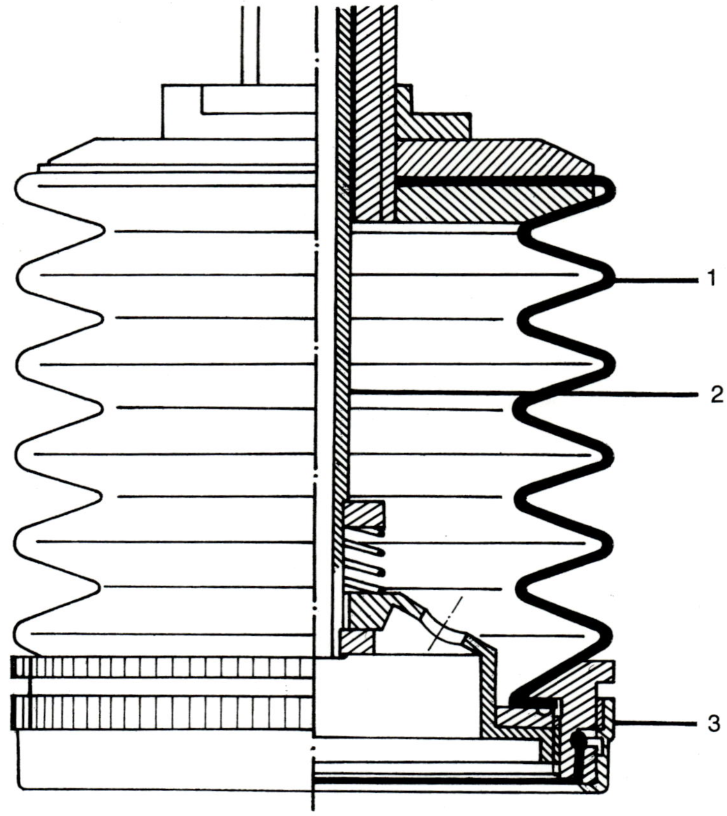

28.19 Pneumatic bellows comprising a foldable rubber cuff wall (1), a guide (2) to exert compression in the desired direction and to give expansion without friction, and a tiltable metal frame (3) fixed to the guide.

28.20

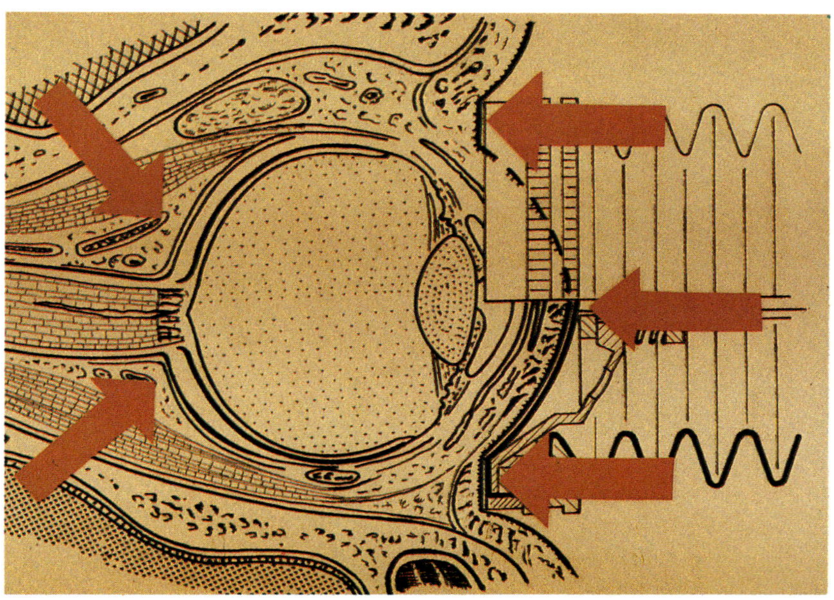

28.20 Action of the Oculopressor without a change in corneal shape. The arrows show the direction of compression (compare with **28.21**).

28.21

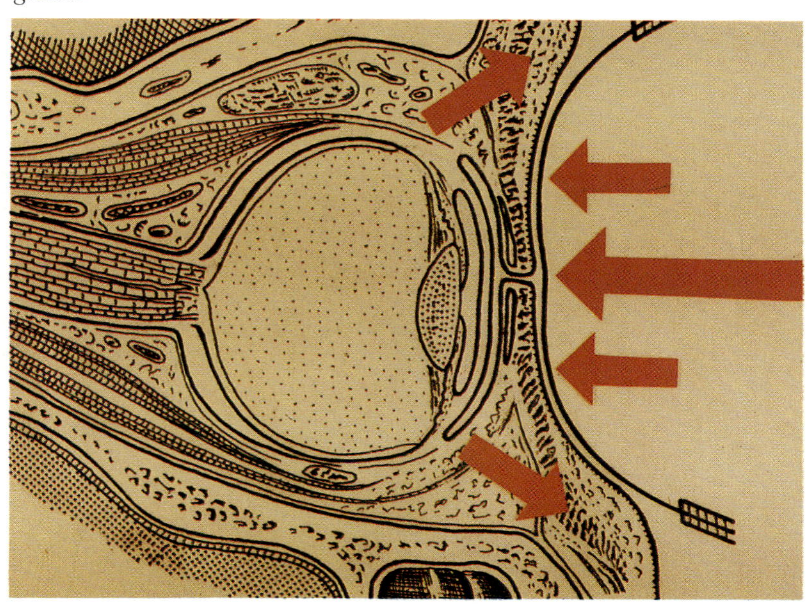

28.21 Action of a simple pneumatic balloon with a convex surface (compare with **28.20**).

Instructions for use: The oculopressor is fitted onto the patient's head in a sitting or lying position and secured with the elastic headband. The bellows are tilted back and pressed in by opening and then closing the valve. They are then tilted down to the eye (**28.22**), turned, slid and then locked into position. The oculopressor is then tilted upwards for the peribulbar or retrobulbar injection and then brought down and set in its prefixed position (**28.23**). Total akinesia prior to application is all important and a retrobulbar injection is recommended, even with general anesthesia. A higher degree of hypotony is required in young patients, especially children. Glaucoma eyes require a higher pressure and a longer period of compression.

28.22

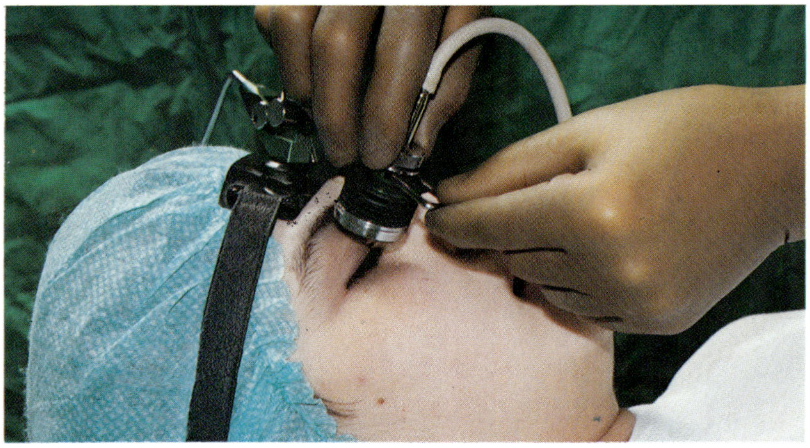

28.22 Presetting the bellows.

28.23

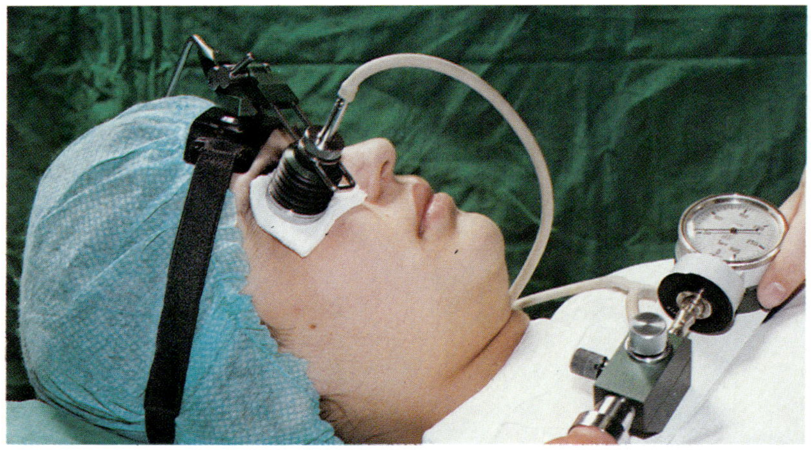

28.23 Oculopressor in action following retrobulbar anesthesia.

Coefficient of hypotonization

The change of volume (Q) is due to increased outflow, which is linearly proportional to the force (P) and duration (t) of compression:

$$Q = c \times P \times t$$

where $c = 0.281\ \text{mm}^3\ \text{mmHg}^{-1}\ \text{min}^{-1}$ and is the coefficient of outflow, which shows in mm^3 the quantity of fluid squeezed out of the eye. However, the change of volume is followed by a decrease in intraocular pressure logarithmically and not linearly.

The coefficient of hypotonization may be determined mathematically and enables a calculation of the height of compression for achieving the required hypotony if the initial intraocular pressure is known. The most frequently used compression levels, to be set for 10 min of oculopression, are given in **Table 28.1**.

Table 28.1 Determining the compression to be applied over a period of 10 min

P_1 (mmHg)	26	25	24	23	22	21	20	19	18	17	16	15	14	13	12	11	10	9	8	7
Compression level for P_2*																				
For 0 mmHg	59	58	56	55	54	52	51	49	48	47	45	43	41	40	38	37	35	34	32	31
For 1 mmHg	54	53	51	50	49	47	46	45	43	42	40	38	37	35	34	32	30	28	26	24
For 2 mmHg	48	47	45	44	43	41	40	39	37	35	34	32	31	29	28	26	24	22	20	18
For 3 mmHg	45	43	42	41	39	38	36	35	34	32	31	29	27	26	24	22	21	19	17	
For 4 mmHg	42	41	40	38	37	35	34	33	31	30	28	27	25	23	22	20	18	16		
For 5 mmHg	40	39	38	36	35	34	32	31	29	28	26	25	23	21	20	18	16			
For 6 mmHg	39	37	36	35	33	32	31	29	28	26	25	23	22	20	18	16				
For 7 mmHg	37	36	35	33	32	31	29	28	26	25	23	22	20	19	17					

* If, for example, the original intraocular pressure is 20 mmHg (P_1) and an intraocular pressure (P_2) of 4 mmHg is to be achieved, the pressure to be applied (compression level) amounts to 34 mmHg. If the original pressure is 20 mmHg (P_1) and a hypotension of 0 mmHg is desired, a compression level of 51 mmHg would be necessary. If compressions at the higher end of the scale are to be used, care must be taken not to compromise circulation to the optic nerve fibers.

Comparison with other models

The Honan balloon, Gills Super Pinky and Drews Nerf Ball are simpler instruments with features in common with the original Oculocompressor, in that they exert pneumatic compression controlled by a manometer; but there are substantial differences. Only the oculopressor has a metal guide inside the balloon which facilitates expansion in the direction desired. Further, it has a head that surrounds the eyeball and closes the whole entrance of the orbit.

Care must be taken in the design of alternative instruments that they do not simply compress the cornea (**28.21**) without protecting the eyeball from displacement and deformation. Such devices may not achieve a reliable hypotony, with the possibility of disastrous consequences during surgery.

Further reading

Alpar J. and Fechner P.U. *Intraocular Lenses*, Georg Thieme, Stuttgart, New York, 1986.

Krey H., Jacobi K.W. and Wizemann A. *Klin. Mbl. Augenheilk*, **180,** 239, 1982.

Pfandl E. *Klin. Mbl. Augenheilk*, **150,** 550, 1968.

Vörösmarthy D. *Mod. Probl. Ophthal.*, p.286, Karger, Basel/New York, 1966.

Vörösmarthy D. *Blaskovics-Kettesy Eingriffe am Auge IV*, Auflage Ferdinand Enke Verlag, Stuttgart, 1970.

Section 4:
SPECIAL CASES: PRECAUTIONS AND MODIFICATIONS TO TECHNIQUE

29: Children

David Hiles

All aphakic optical correction modalities must provide clear and accurate visual images to the eye. This is particularly necessary for children younger than six who may develop a severe form of deprivation amblyopia, often associated with strabismus. The aphakic optics must be undistorted and the visual axis free of opaque tissue in order to initiate successful occlusion therapy.

Children with unilateral complete congenital cataracts achieve the poorest visual results regardless of treatment, because of early-onset deprivation amblyopia, delay in surgery, failure of occlusion therapy, and the frequent presence of associated ocular and central nervous system developmental abnormalities. Those with unilateral partial cataracts may achieve improved visual results, because these eyes had an opportunity to develop visual responses before the cataract became dense enough to occlude the visual axis.

The visual results following surgery for traumatic cataracts are superior to those for infantile cataracts since the visual system was well developed before the trauma. The key to visual success is to remove the lens as soon as the cataract is discovered in the early sensitive period, or when the visual acuity or fixation is significantly reduced, and to apply vigorous optical rehabilitation and occlusion therapy. For unilateral congenital cataracts this should be done during the first four months of life (or during the first weeks if the cataract is complete).

Prior to surgery, all the available rehabilitative options must be discussed with the child's family. Glasses remain useful for children with bilateral aphakia (**29.1**) but are impossible for unilateral aphakes because of the associated anisometropia and aniseikonia.

Contact lenses remain the preferred option for most infants and children, whether the cataract is unilateral or bilateral (**29.2**). Keratometry and refraction may be performed under the same general anesthesia as the cataract aspiration. The lenses are fitted within the first few postoperative days or when the surgical inflammatory response has subsided. The power of the lens is increased from two to five diopters over the distance corrections to compensate for the infant's near visual world.

Small hard lenses are most easily tolerated and inserted into the infant eye. Children over one year of age may wear soft daily or extended wear lenses, which offer the advantage of minimal trauma during insertion and removal (**29.3**). Refraction is repeated every three months and lens modifications are made to compensate for the rapid myopic shift which occurs during the first three years of life in the aphakic eye. Residual refractive error and an appropriate near bifocal correction are prescribed in spectacles (**29.4**). If there is failure of contact lens wear, the surgeon should consider either an IOL or epikeratophakia.

29.1
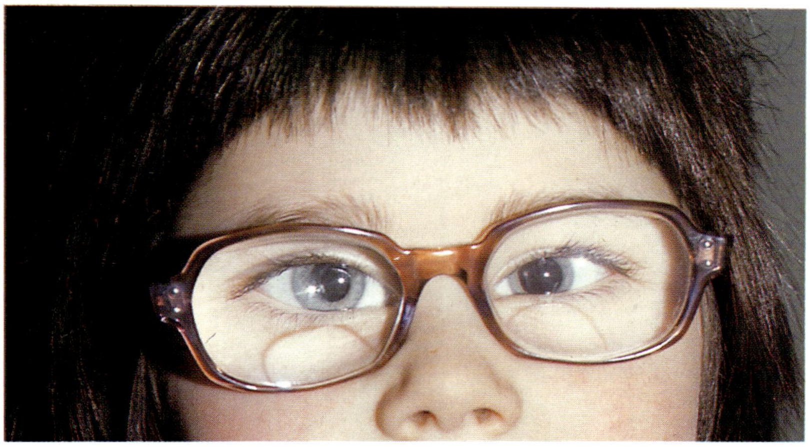

29.1 Child with bilateral aphakic spectacles with bifocal lenses for near.

29.2
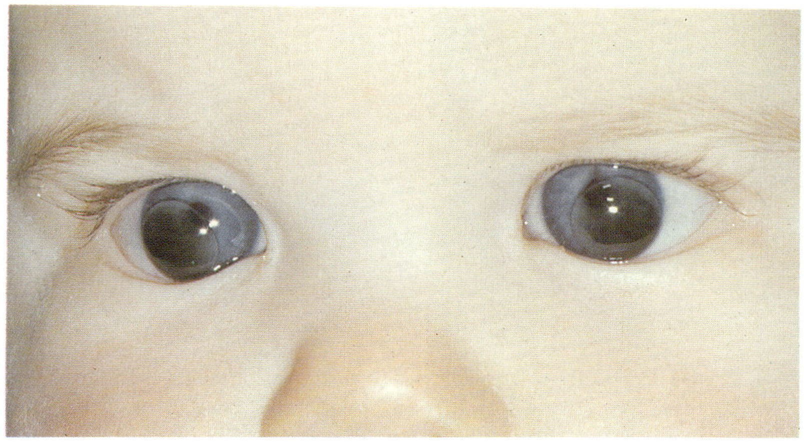

29.2 Infant with bilateral aphakic hard contact lens.

29.3
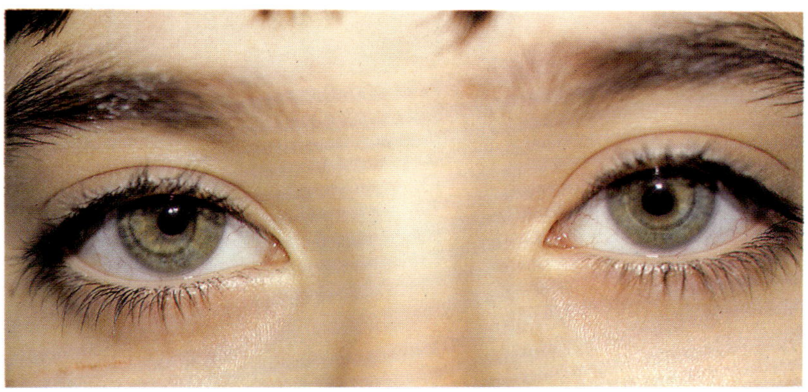

29.3 Bilateral aphakic soft contact lenses.

29.4
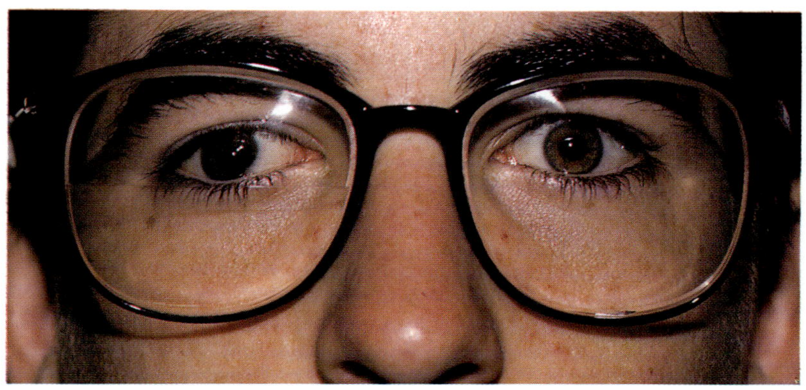

29.4 Unilateral congenital cataract showing blue-tinted contact lens and bifocal spectacle for the right eye. Note exotropia.

Indications for IOL implantation

The two advantages of IOLs over contact lenses are the likelihood of reducing the density of amblyopia and the better preservation or development of fusion. IOLs should be considered if the parent or the child refuses the concept of contact lens wear, if the surgeon deems that contact lens wear would not be successful owing to patient or parent noncompliance, or if other social or economic factors preclude adequate contact lens follow-up.

IOL implantation should be confined to unilateral aphakic children because of the unknown long-term effects of the presence of an IOL and its component materials in the human eye. In bilateral cases with asymmetric onset of visual loss, IOL implantation may be performed after contact lens failure to improve acuity. The visual results for these eyes are the same as for unilateral cataracts. If acuity fails in the fellow eye owing to increasing density of cataract, IOL implantation is not normally warranted as a primary procedure and another contact lens should be tried or an epikeratophakia graft considered.

29.5

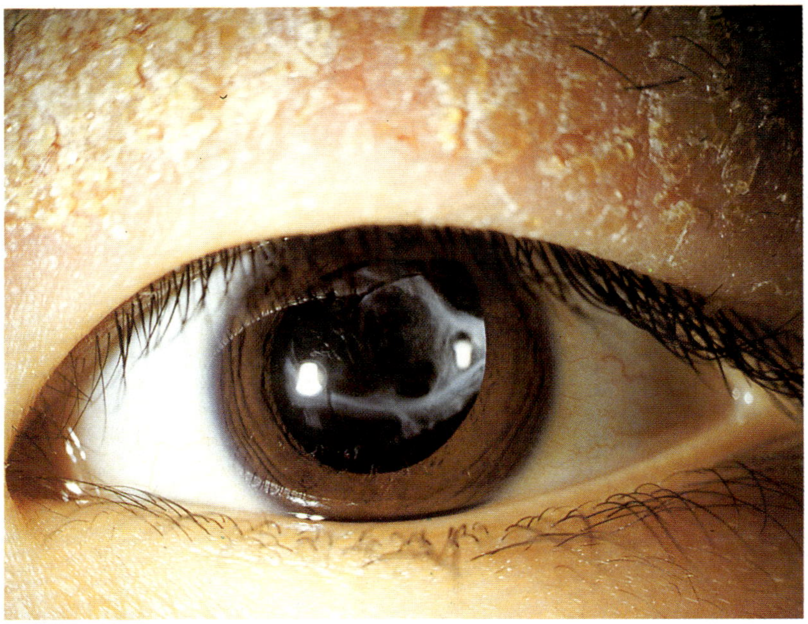

29.5 Posterior chamber implant in boy aged eight with a dermatogenic cataract. He was intolerant to contact lenses because of exfoliative dermatitis. Photographed two years after surgery.

29.7

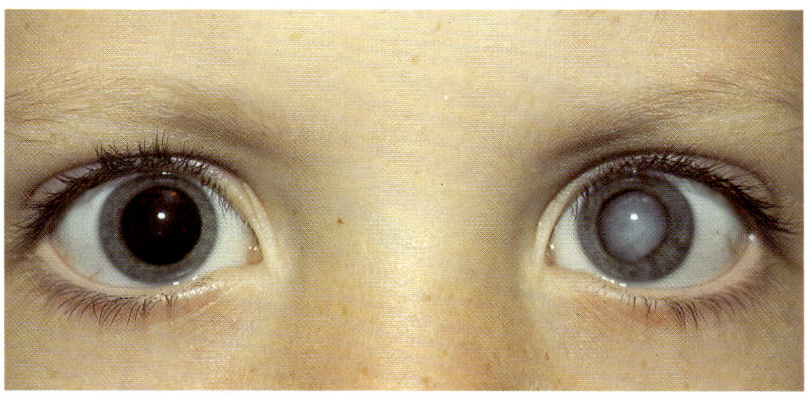

29.7 Unilateral mature cataract in a child aged three.

Infantile cataracts: These are lens opacities arising before the eighth birthday. They may be familial, metabolic, syndrome related (**29.5, 29.6**), posterior lenticonus or progressive late-onset juvenile cataracts. If unilateral and not seen at birth, in a child over the age of two and a half years, an IOL may be indicated (**29.7**). Children under eight years of age will additionally require occlusion therapy as well as a bifocal overcorrection. IOLs should not be implanted before the age of two because of the prolific production of secondary membranes and synechia formation (**29.8**) and the propensity for rapid myopic shift during the first years of life.

29.6

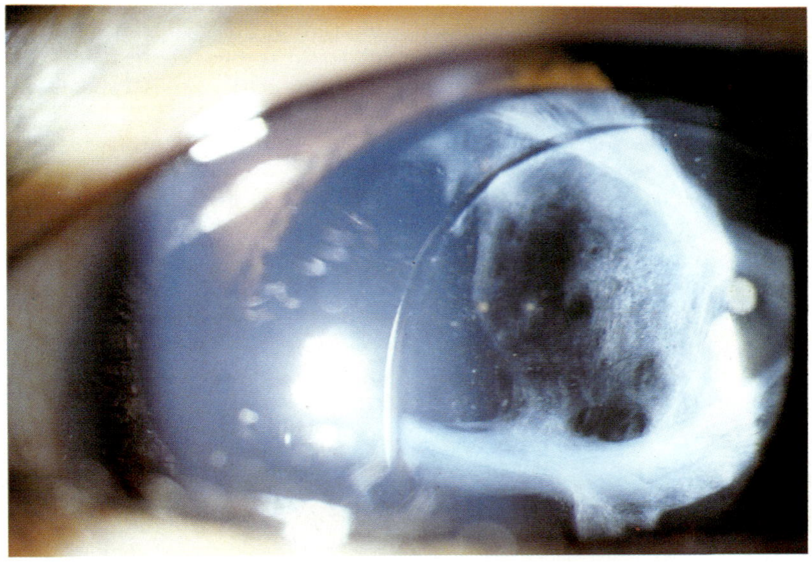

29.6 Detail of **29.5** showing lens decentration and capsular fibrosis. The posterior capsule is intact (VA 20/30 unaided).

29.8

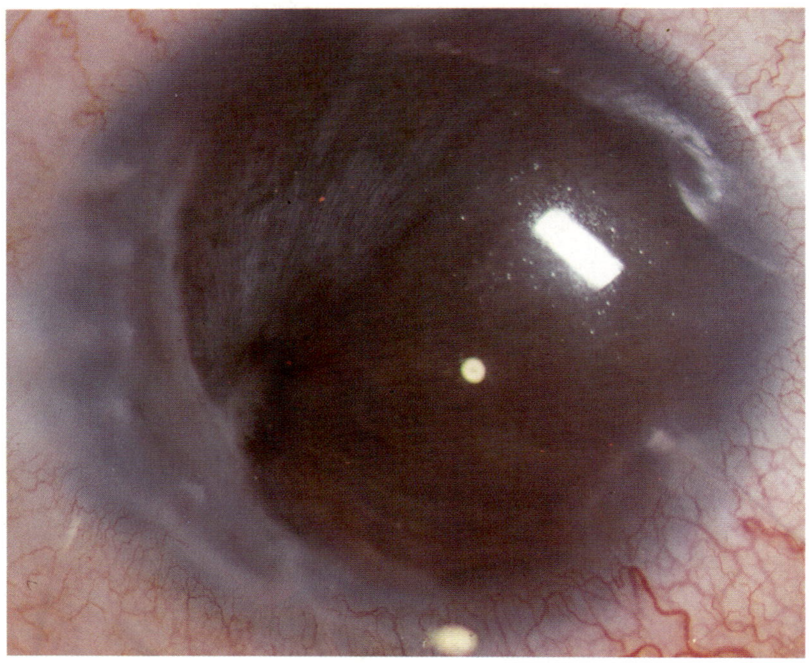

29.8 Four month old aphakic infant with posterior chamber IOL implanted through a temporal corneal incision. Note the occluded and secluded pupil with the IOL enmeshed in dense iridocapsular membrane.

Traumatic cataracts: Children with traumatic cataracts and corneal scars which preclude successful contact lens wear are IOL candidates (**29.9**). Amblyopia is related to the age of the patient at the time of occlusion of the visual axis and to the time elapsed before the eye is optically rehabilitated. The younger the age and the longer the interval before treatment, the greater is the probability of irreversible visual loss. Thus, children between the age of two and five years *who fail a contact lens trial* should receive an IOL if possible within two months of the injury. It is prudent not to implant at the time of primary repair because of inflammation and the possible elevation of intraocular pressure normally associated with trauma. The decision on primary implantation at the time of secondary lens aspiration will depend on the expected patient and parent motivation and on compliance with a contact lens. Late cataract extraction and IOL implantation is performed when the lens opacity is seen to increase, the visual fixation responses are decreased, or the corrected vision is less than 20/60. The orthoptic consequences of an IOL are superior to those of a contact lens with, in children over six years of age, a good chance of restoring full binocular single vision. However, the development of strabismus must be treated with early surgery in order to secure normal ocular alignment and peripheral, if not central, fusion.

29.9

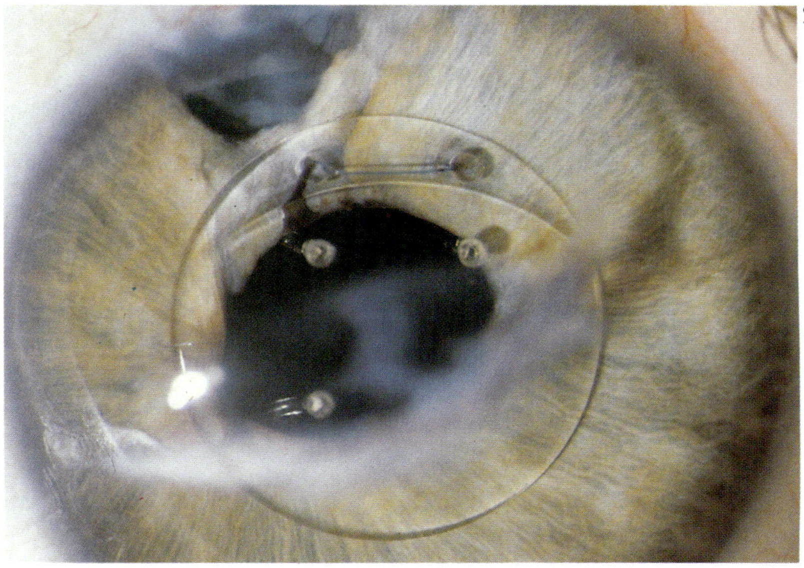

29.9 Child with traumatic corneal laceration, cataract and iris suture IOL.

IOL selection

Intimately related to IOL indications are the issues of which lens type to implant and whether to implant primarily with cataract surgery or later as a secondary procedure. The selection of the IOL depends upon the facility for fixation, the condition of the anterior segment and the age of the child.

Iris-fixated IOLs are now obsolete owing to the unacceptable risk of dislocation (**29.10**), endothelial cell loss (**29.11**), iris sphincter erosion (**29.12**), cystoid macular edema and retinal detachment. If, however, a lens is serving useful vision and is devoid of pseudophakodonesis, it should be allowed to remain *in situ* (**29.13, 29.14**).

29.10

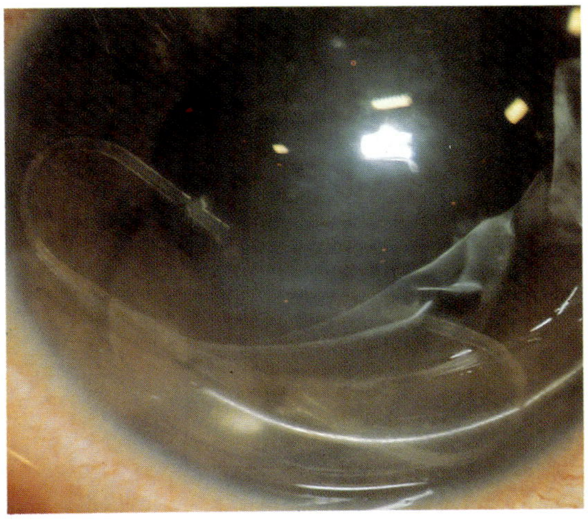

29.11

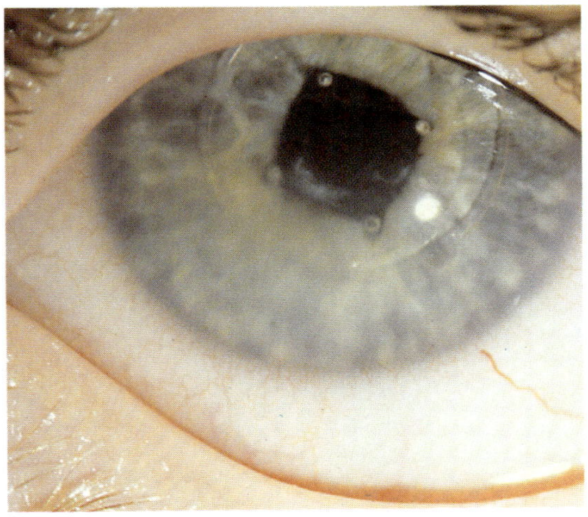

29.12

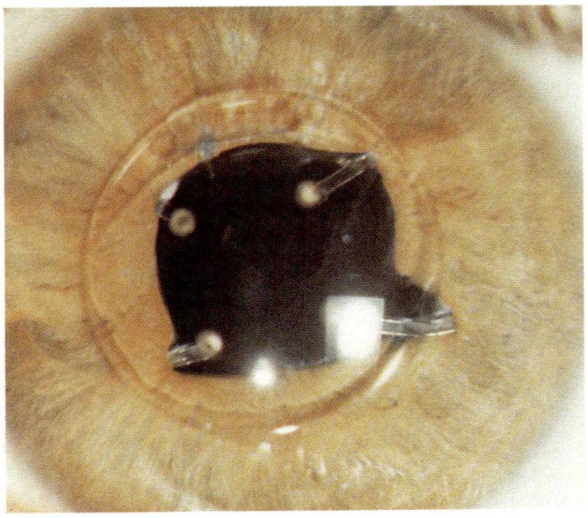

29.13

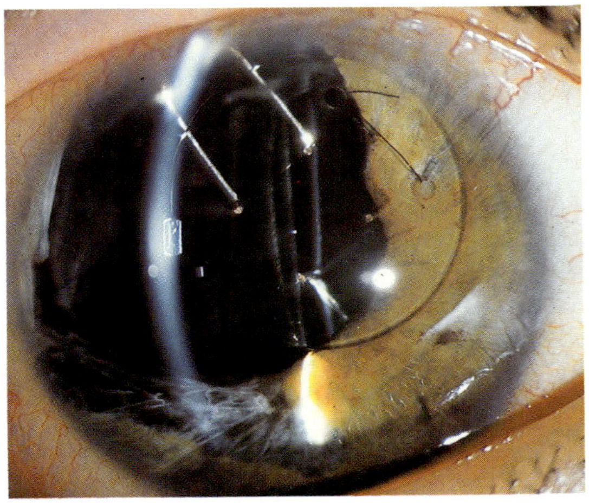

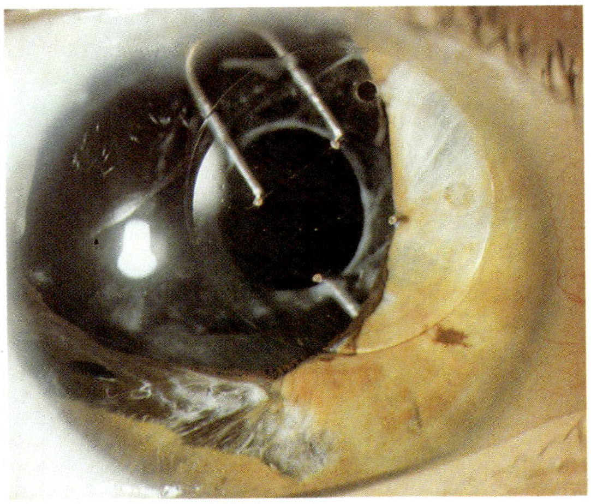

29.14

29.10 Dislocated Binkhorst two-loop iridocapsular lens into the anterior chamber.

29.11 Inferior corneal edema in patient with iris suture lens and pseudophakodonesis.

29.12 Iris suture lens with prolene loops creating an iris sphincter erosion adjacent to both inferior loops.

29.13 Twelve year old boy in 1975 with traumatic cataract, iris atrophy and a metal looped iris suture IOL.

29.14 Same patient as in **29.13** in 1985 with metal loops within the capsular bag. The prolene suture has disintegrated. Vision remained 20/25.

Anterior chamber IOLs are indicated in eyes lacking posterior capsular support sufficient for a posterior chamber lens, as occurs following lensectomy associated with anterior vitrectomy, or following trauma when the pupil is dilated or immobile because of posterior synechias. An IOL placed in front of the pupil should have minimal contact with the iris, avoid pupillary block, permit adequate secondary membranectomy, allow pupillary mydriasis and be sufficiently flexible to allow slight elongation as the anterior segment of the eye completes its growth.

The flexible one piece open-looped PMMA anterior chamber intraocular lens (**29.15**) is now recommended for all contact lens noncompliant children between three and six years of age as either a primary or secondary IOL implantation, as well as for children over six receiving secondary lens implantation.

Several specific surgical recommendations are suggested for anterior chamber implantation (**29.16–29.19**). The lens should not be placed into an eye with vitreous protruding into the anterior chamber. A vitrector should be used to clear the visual axis of vitreous and other lens remnants prior to implantation. Sodium hyaluronate is placed in the anterior chamber to protect the anterior iris surface from trauma, as well as to reduce corneal endothelial cell loss during implantation. A Sheets lens glide is used to further protect the iris when the lens passes over its surface. After the lens is in place, the wound is closed with interrupted 9-0 polygalactin sutures and 4-mirror gonioscopy is performed to ensure that the lens foot plates are in the proper position.

29.15

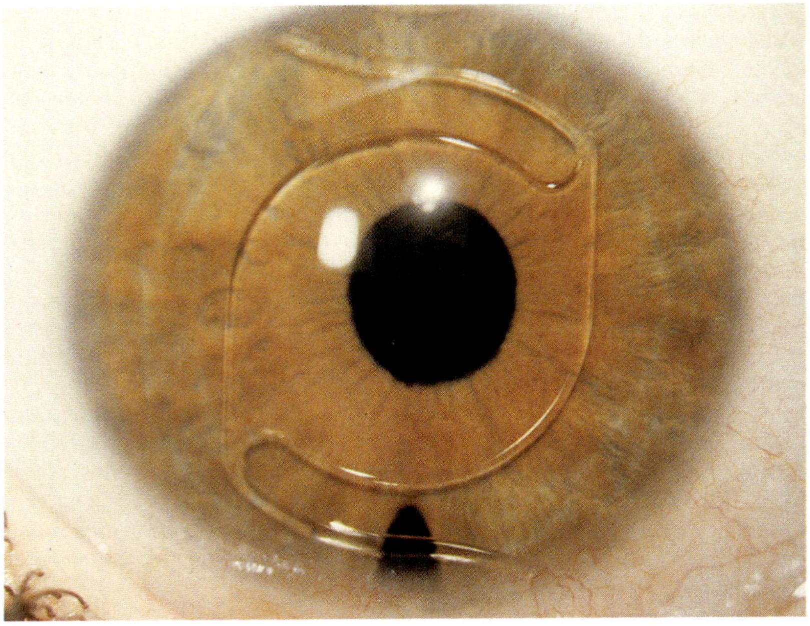

29.15 The Kelman one piece flexible open-looped PMMA anterior chamber secondary intraocular lens with four-point fixation.

29.16

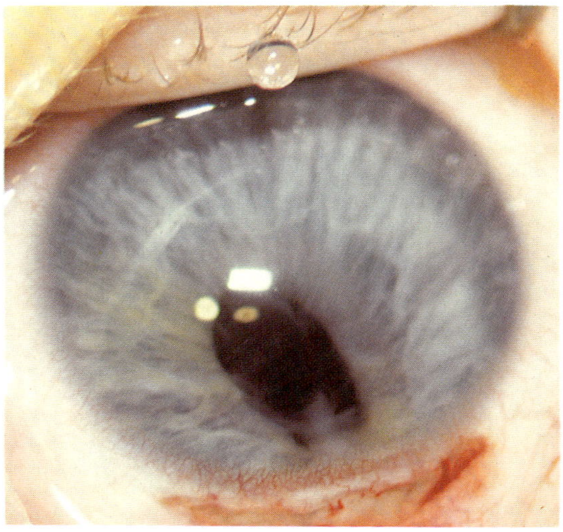

29.17

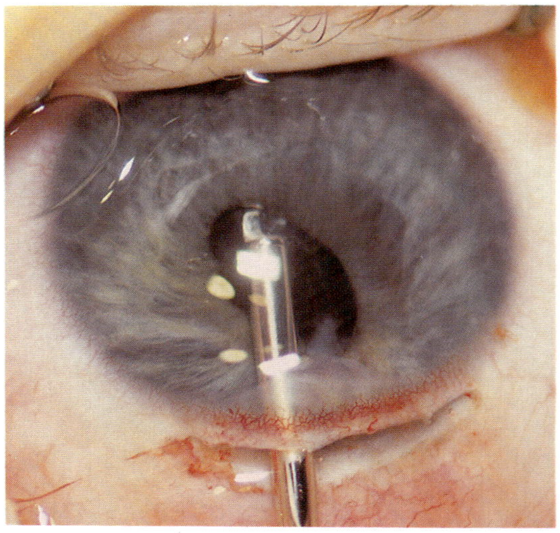

29.16 Aphakic eye with updrawn pupil and secondary membrane in a child following surgery for congenital cataract and failure of a contact lens trial.

29.17 A peritomy conjunctival incision followed by limbal corneoscleral incision. Intraocular scissors and vitrector release adhesions, remove secondary membrane, lens remnants and anterior vitreous, recreating a round pupil.

29.18

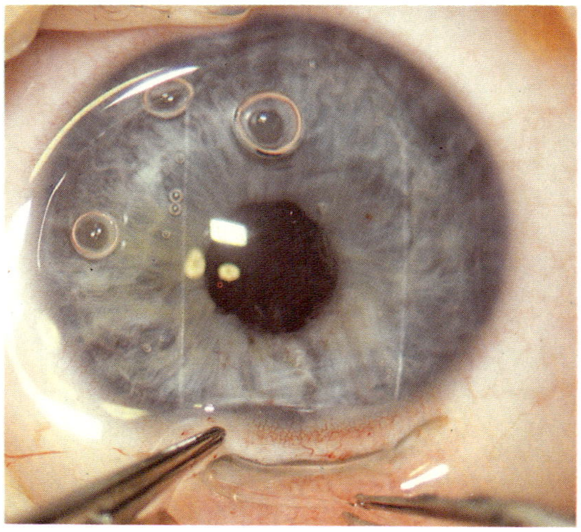

29.19

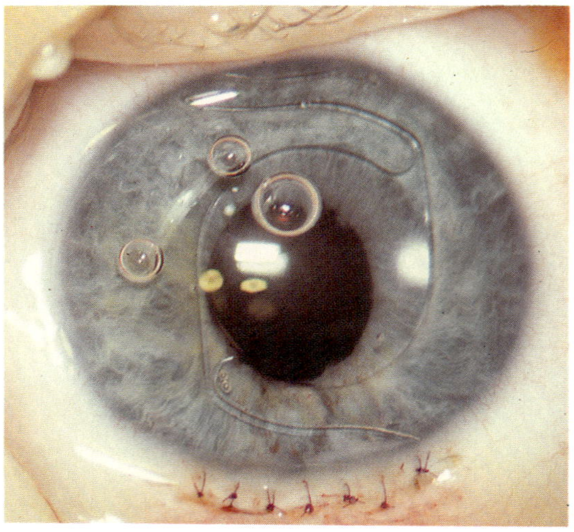

29.18 Sheets lens glide in position in the anterior chamber following the vitrectomy procedure.

29.19 A Kelman one piece flexible four pod PMMA lens vertically oriented in the final position. Closure of the corneoscleral incision is with interrupted 9-0 vicryl sutures.

Posterior chamber IOLs are recommended for eyes with otherwise normal anterior segments undergoing primary IOL implantation in children over the age of six (**29.20,** see also **29.5**).

The posterior chamber lens preferred is the Sinskey soft J loop lens design with a 10° forwards anterior angulation of the haptics, possibly incorporating the new surface modified PMMA (see p. 115). A posterior chamber lens may be implanted as a secondary procedure if the posterior capsule is intact, if vitreous is not protruding through a previously created central capsulotomy, and if the peripheral posterior capsular membrane would support and adhere to the lens haptics. Insufficient support may lead to malposition (**29.21**). A hazard of primary or secondary posterior chamber implantation is that the position of the lens haptics often cannot be determined because the space between the posterior capsule and the iris may be compressed due to scleral collapse and forwards vitreous pressure.

Meticulous attention to specific aspects of the cataract aspiration and lens implantation is necessary (**29.22–29.29**): Sodium hyaluronate, rather than continuous irrigation, is used to maintain the anterior chamber during the anterior capsulectomy. Continuous circular capsulorhexis may improve the certainty of good lens centration inside the capsular sac. Phacoemulsification may be recommended to reduce the operative time of cataract aspiration. Anterior chamber irrigation is

29.20

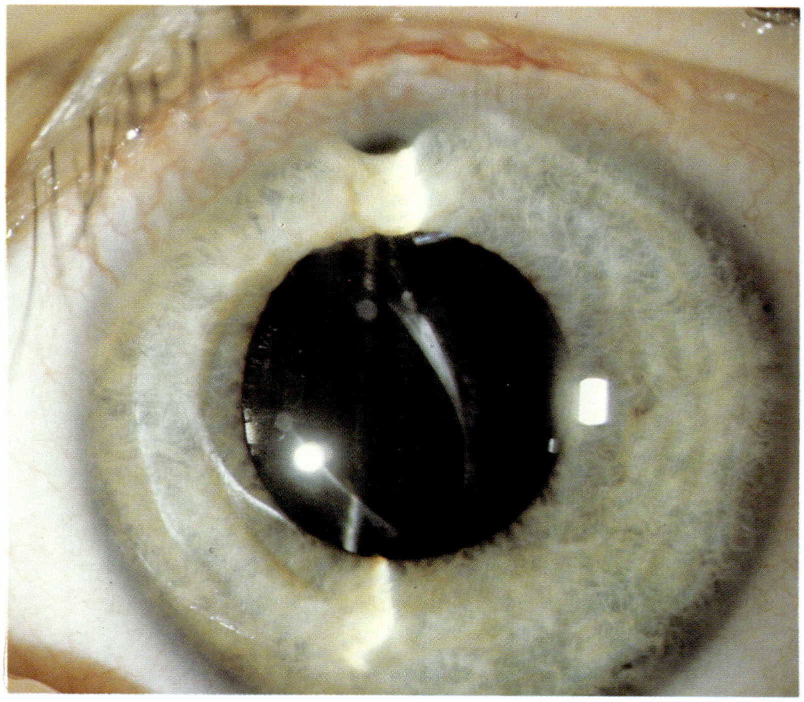

29.20 Well placed posterior chamber lens with primary posterior capsulotomy.

29.21

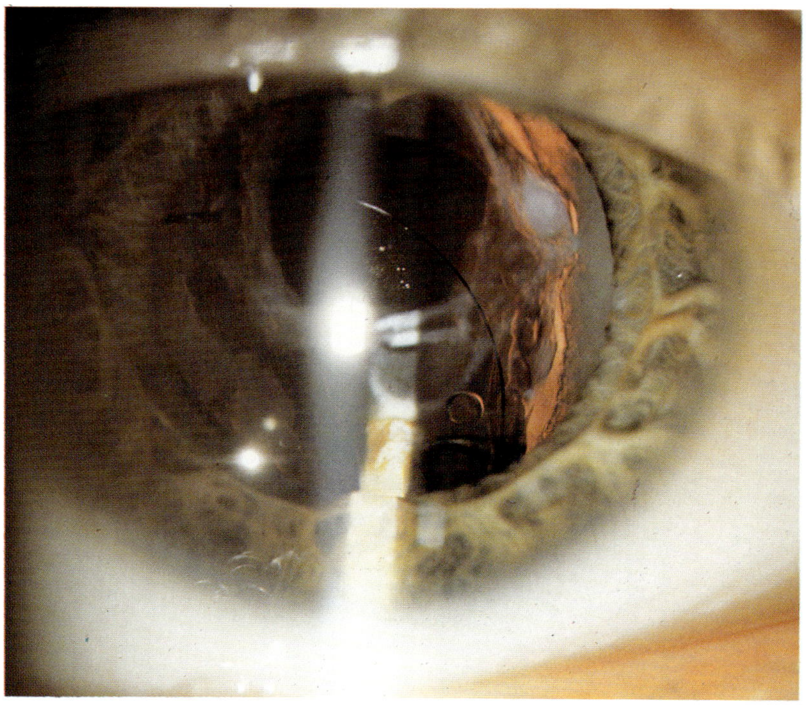

29.21 Secondary posterior chamber IOL with inferior dislocation (sunset syndrome).

9.22

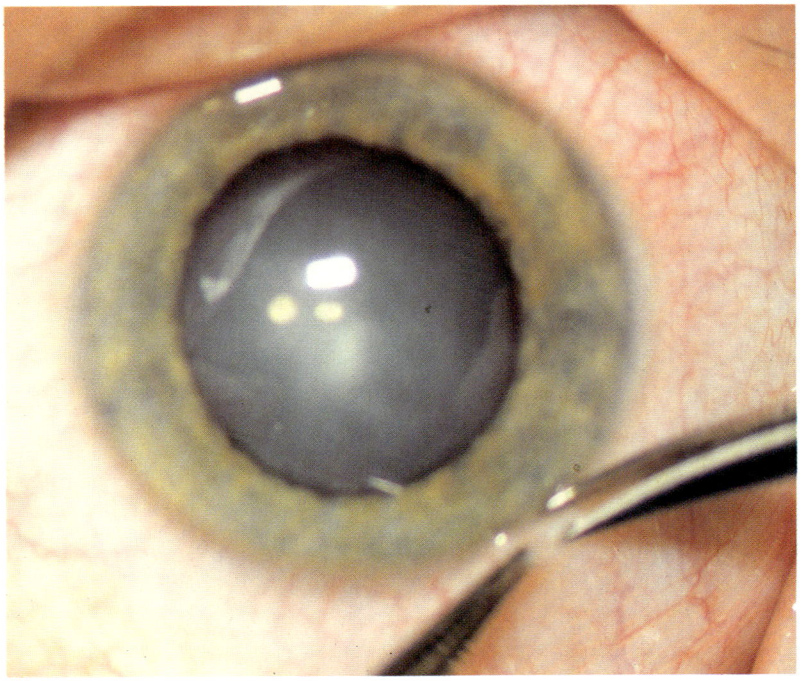

29.22 After an 8 mm cord peritomy, incision with fine scissors.

29.23

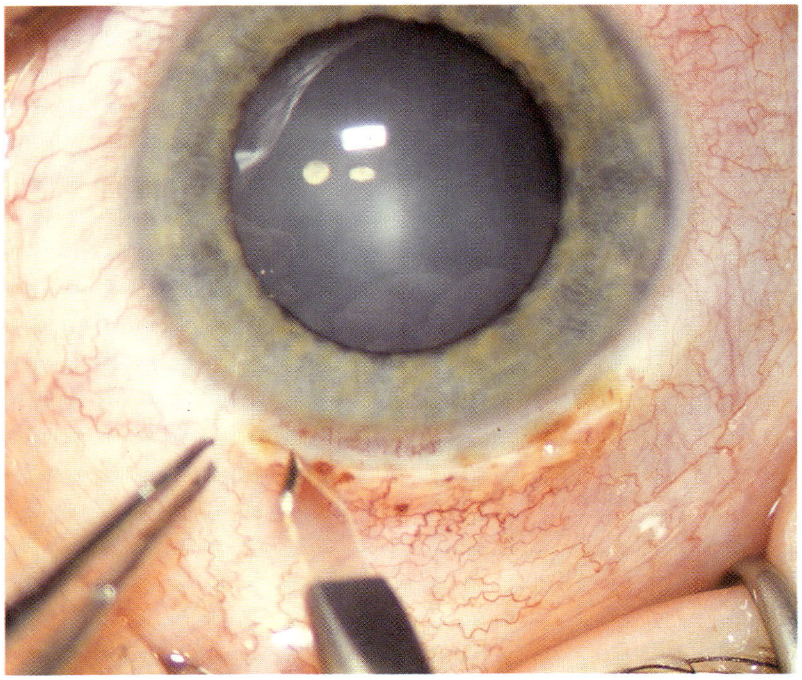

29.23 Corneoscleral limbal incision with a diamond knife.

29.24

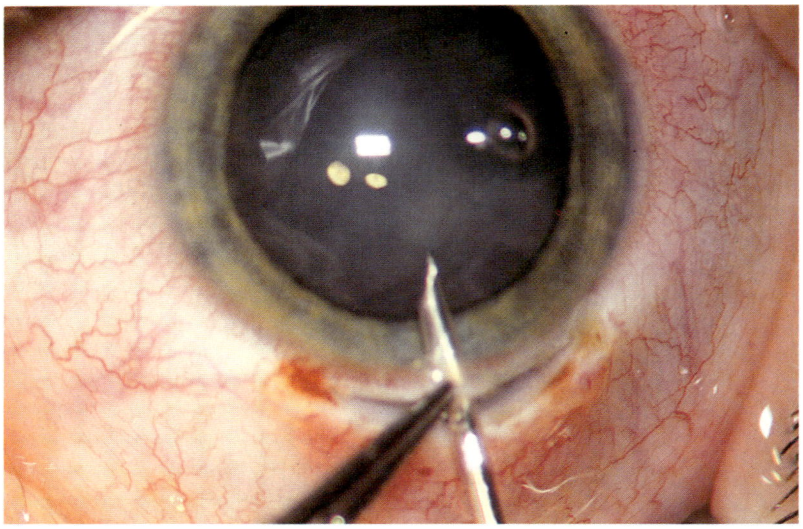

29.24 Cystitome anterior capsulotomy, with the anterior chamber filled with sodium hyaluronate.

29.25

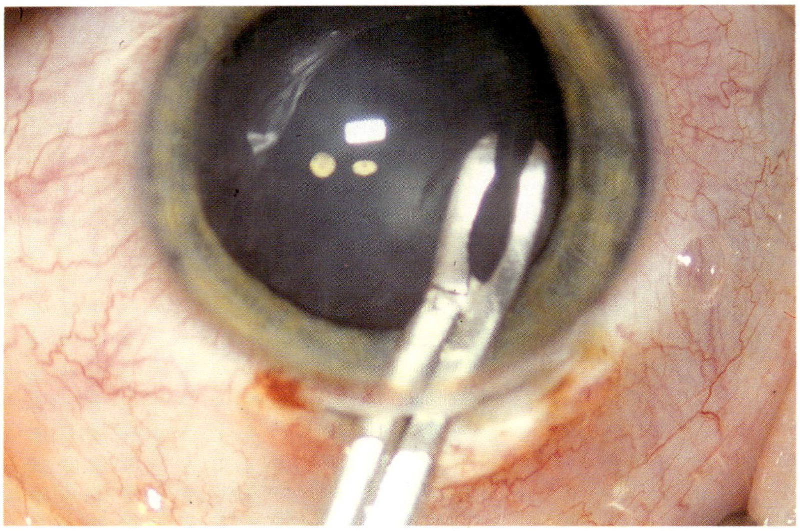

29.25 Forceps removal of the anterior capsule.

29.26

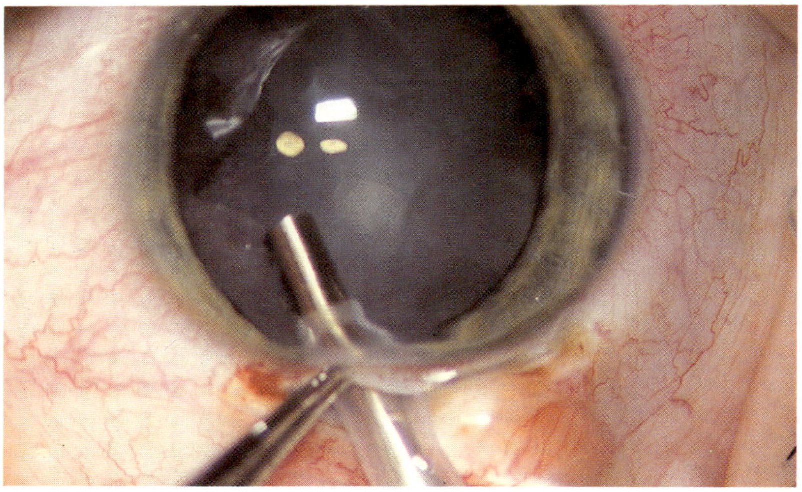

29.26 Phacoemulsification of an infantile cataractous lens. Note the bubble of sodium hyaluronate at the left-hand end of the wound.

29.27

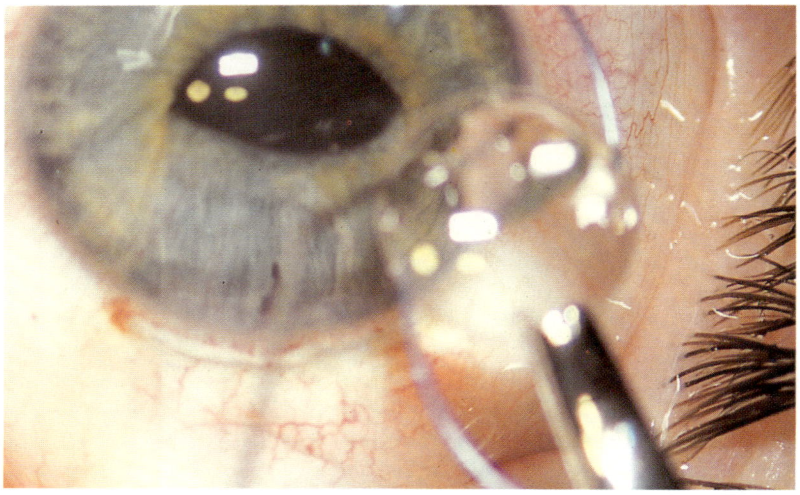

29.27 Placement of a Sheets glide into the posterior chamber under sodium hyaluronate. The Sinskey two-loop lens is grasped with lens delivery forceps.

29.28

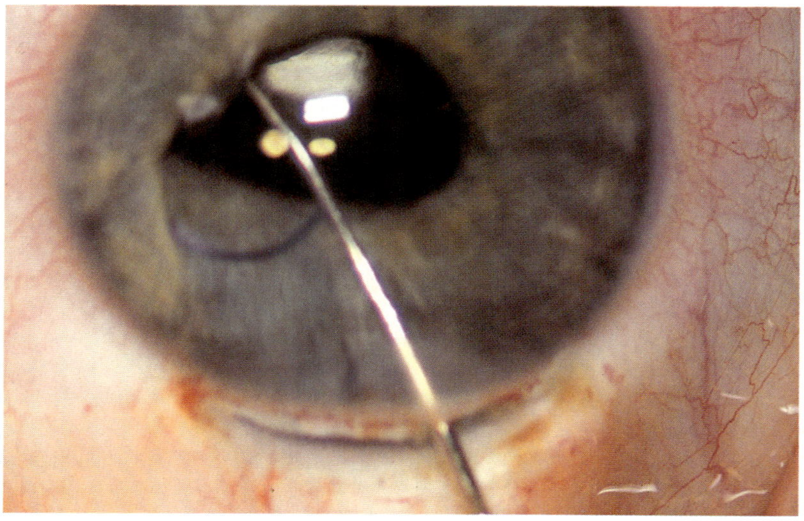

29.28 Manipulation of the lens loop with a Sinskey hook to rotate the lens to the horizontal plane and into the capsular bag.

29.29

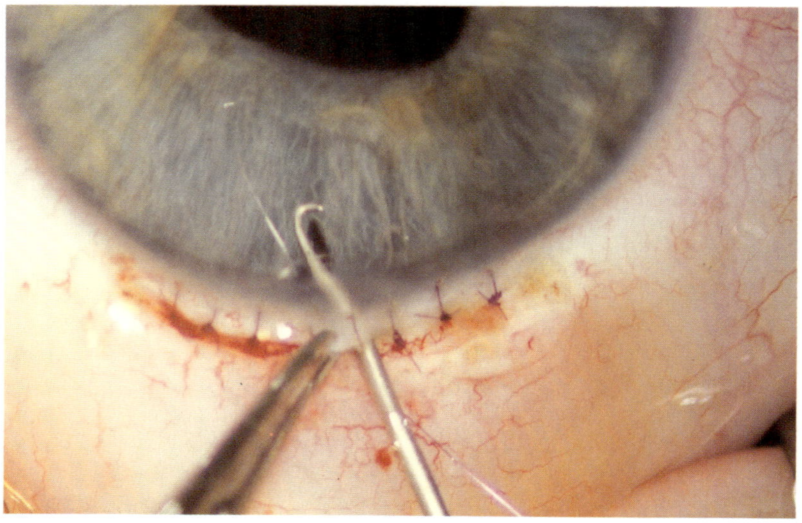

29.29 Partial closure of corneoscleral wound with 9-0 interrupted vicryl sutures. An irrigating hook passes through a peripheral iridotomy posterior to the IOL to create a primary capsulotomy.

minimized to prevent iris prolapse and pigment epithelial loss. Any iris trauma in children increases the cellular response, so predisposing to secondary membrane formation and often leading to iris capture and IOL malposition (**29.30**). Sodium hyaluronate and a Sheets lens glide facilitate atraumatic implantation. Although it is relatively easy to be certain of capsular placement of the inferior loop, there is frequently uncertainty over placement of the superior loop unless meticulous attention is paid to the preparation of capsular flaps and viscoelastic agents are liberally used to maintain the anterior chamber. Iris trauma from manipulation of the superior iris or from rotation of the implant should be avoided as this contributes to synechia formation and iris capture.

Posterior chamber IOLs require a primary posterior capsulotomy to produce a clear visual axis. To avoid iris manipulation during this procedure and the possibility of allowing vitreous to pass into the anterior chamber, a tiny peripheral iridotomy is made at the 12 o'clock position. A small irrigation hook attached to a syringe bearing sodium hyaluronate is passed through the iridotomy, under the iris and IOL haptic, to appear in the pupillary space. Sodium hyaluronate is injected ahead of the needle, as needed, to create a space between the IOL haptic and the posterior capsule. A large opening is then made by tearing the capsule without disturbing the IOL or vitreous. It should be stressed, however, that even with a primary posterior capsulotomy, in 63% of our patients, the visual axis became reoccluded by secondary membranes (**29.31**).

Unfortunately, the cellular proliferation from epithelial cell metaplasia uses the intact anterior vitreous face in children as well as the surface of the implant for scaffolding, so reoccluding the clear visual axis. The cellular response must therefore be vigorously treated with topical and possibly orbital floor corticosteroids in the early postoperative period. Topical corticosteroids must continue until anterior chamber flare and cells are absent. Systemic corticosteroids are prescribed on a decreasing daily basis over the first ten postoperative days. Since red blood cells are also a source of anterior chamber fibrosis, collections of blood must be cleared using I/A prior to wound closure.

Secondary capsulotomy by discission (**29.32**) is associated with a risk of dislodging the lens, vitreous prolapse, corneal endothelial cell loss and iris trauma. Use of the neodymium YAG laser should therefore be preferred, which is possible in most children over six years of age (**29.33**).

29.30

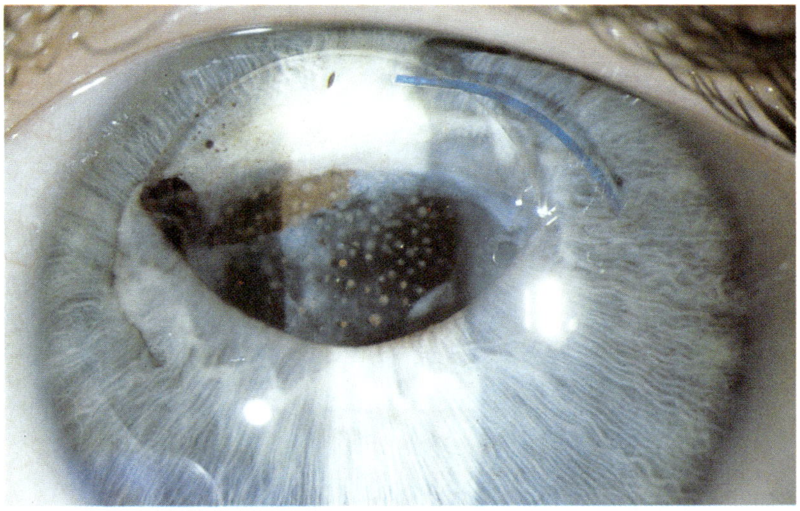

29.30 Superior iris capture with anterior dislocation of the IOL haptic and secondary membrane occluding the visual axis.

29.31

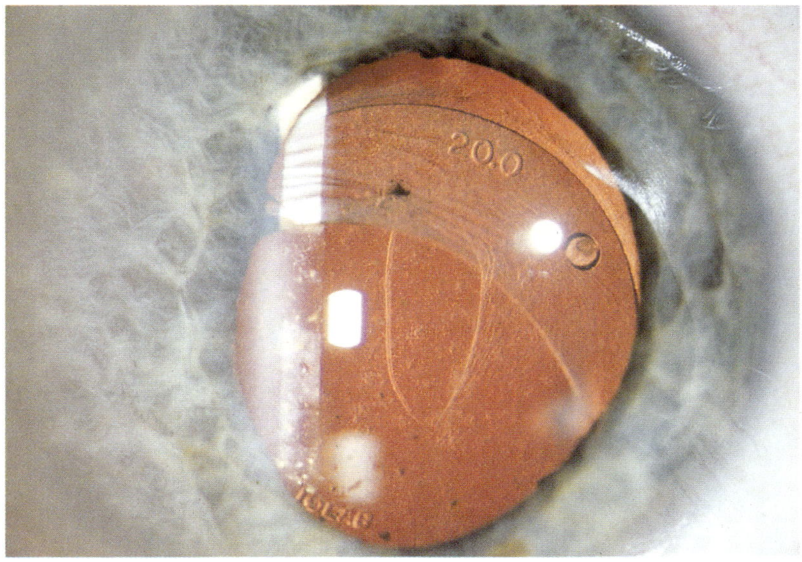

29.31 Posterior chamber lens with a dense secondary membrane occluding a primary posterior capsulotomy.

29.32

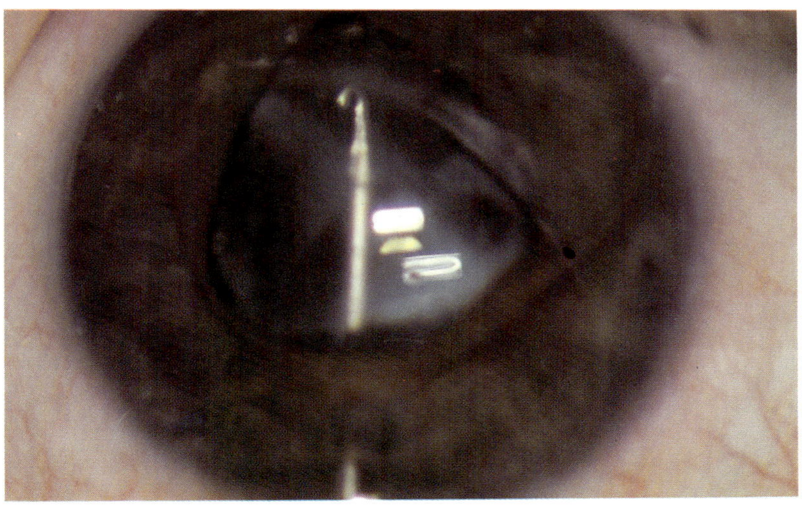

29.32 Secondary discission of posterior capsular membrane utilizing an irrigating hook attached to the syringe filled with sodium hyaluronate. Note entry through the peripheral iridectomy.

29.33

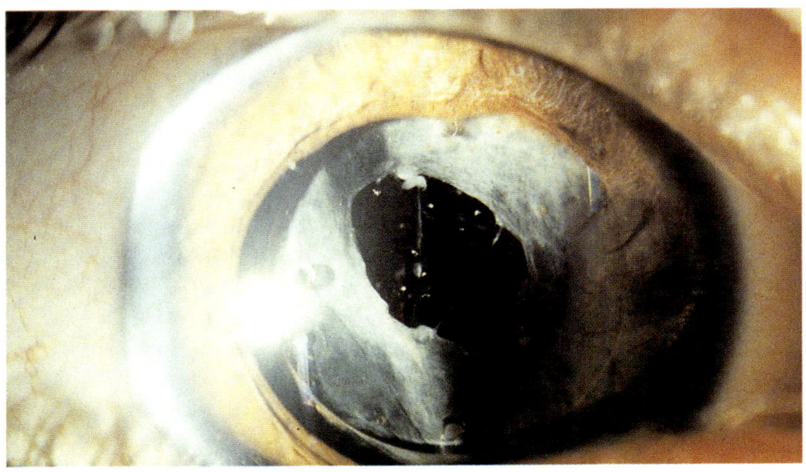

29.33 Dense secondary membrane behind posterior chamber IOL with a central aperture created with Nd:YAG laser.

Complications and results

Table 29.1 summarizes the postoperative complications of 720 eyes in children encountered in our practice, based upon the rigid selection criteria for IOL commencing in 1974, and on epikeratophakia graft commencing in 1984. Eyes with marked preexisting defects (including glaucoma) were directed towards the use of contact lenses and the high incidence of some complications in this group resulted from the original disease processes. Iris complications were mainly related to the iris-sutured lens in common use during the 1970s.

Table 29.2 summarizes the need for secondary surgery in the three groups. In many instances the technique of the original surgery predisposed to additional operations, e.g., cataract aspiration without a primary posterior capsulotomy, or the implantation of a posterior chamber IOL with subsequent reocclusion of the primary posterior capsulotomy by the regrowth of a secondary membrane. The contact lens group showed a high incidence of glaucoma surgery because of primary disease. The IOL group showed a high incidence of subluxations between 1974 and 1981 due to the use of iris-supported lenses. These lenses account for 19 of the 22 dislocation surgeries and 14 of the 16 explantations.

Table 29.3 summarizes the visual results achieved from 232 consecutive traumatic cataracts and **Table 29.4** the results from 301 unilateral infantile cataracts during the period 1977 to 1987.

Table 29.1 Postoperative complications occurring in aphakic children optically rehabilitated with contact lens, intraocular lens and epikeratophakia grafts

	CL		*IOL*		*EPI*	
	No.	(%)	No.	(%)	No.	(%)
Corneal edema/clouding	1	(1)	29	(10)	1	(1)
Cloudy graft	NA		NA		18	(17)
Iris complications	NA		43	(15)	NA	
Glaucoma	19	(6)	10	(3)	1	(1)
Endophthalmitis/infection	0		0		2	(2)
Detached retina	6	(2)	8	(3)	3	(3)
Uveitis	0		1	(1)	0	
Phthisis bulbi	4	(1)	2	(1)	0	
Dislocated IOL	NA		24	(8)	NA	
Power errors > ± 3.00 D	NA		36	(13)	18	(17)
Total eyes	328		286		106	

NA = Not Applicable

Table 29.2 Secondary surgeries performed in eyes receiving contact lens, intraocular lens and epikeratophakia grafts

	CL		*IOL*		*EPI*	
	Eyes	*Ops*	*Eyes*	*Ops*	*Eyes*	*Ops*
EUA*	28	42	2	2	13	14
Discission	129	147	129	185	12	14
Nd:YAG laser	2	2	7	7	0	0
Glaucoma	19	51	5	7	0	0
Penetrating keratoplasty	0	0	1	1	0	0
Enucleation	4	4	3	3	0	0
Detached retina	1	1	3	4	0	0
Others	8	10	4	4		
Dislocated IOL surgery	NA	NA	16	22	NA	NA
IOL explant	NA	NA	16	16	NA	NA
Graft removal	NA	NA	NA	NA	14	14
Regraft	NA	NA	NA	NA	12	12
Total eyes	328		286		112	

* Postoperative examinations under anesthesia without other surgical interventions.

Table 29.3 Best corrected visual acuities and aphakic optical modalities of consecutive traumatic cataracts in children (1977–1987)

VA	*NONE*		*GL*		*CL*		*IOL*		*EPI*		*TOTALS*	
	No.	(%)	No.	(%)	No.	(%)	No.	(%)	No.	(%)	No.	(%)
$^{20}/_{20}$ to $^{20}/_{40}$					48	(56)	67	(61)	5	(29)	120	(52)
$^{20}/_{50}$ to $^{20}/_{100}$	1	(6)	1	(25)	16	(19)	11	(10)	6	(36)	35	(15)
$^{20}/_{200}$			1	(25)	8	(9)	6	(5)	1	(6)	16	(7)
$< ^{20}/_{200}$	15	(94)	2	(50)	13	(15)	26	(24)	5	(29)	61	(26)
Total	16		4		85		110		17		232	

Table 29.4 Best corrected visual acuities and aphakic optical modalities of consecutive unilateral cataracts (age 0 to 17 years) (1977–1987)

VA	*GL*		*CL*		*IOL*		*EPI*		*TOTAL*	
	No.	(%)	No.	(%)	No.	(%)	No.	(%)	No.	(%)
$^{20}/_{20}$ to $^{20}/_{40}$			10	(11)	28	(16)	1	(3)	39	(13)
$^{20}/_{50}$ to $^{20}/_{100}$			8	(9)	52	(30)	2	(6)	62	(21)
$^{20}/_{200}$			14	(16)	21	(12)	6	(17)	41	(14)
$<^{20}/_{200}$	1	(100)	58	(64)	73	(42)	27	(75)	159	(52)
Total	1		90		174		36		301	

Further reading

Dahan E. and Salmenson B.D. Pseudophakia in children: precautions, technique, and feasibility. *J. Cataract. Refract. Surg.*, **16,** 75–82, 1990.

Hiles D.A. Indications, techniques and complications associated with intraocular lens implantation in children, pp 189–268 in *Intraocular Lens Implants in Children*, Hiles D.A. (Ed), Grune and Stratton, New York, 1980.

Hiles D.A. and Hered R.W. Modern intraocular lens implants in children with new age limitations. *J. Cat. Ref. Surg.*, **13,** 493–497, 1987.

Weidle E.G., Lisch W. and Thiel H-J. Management of the opacified posterior lens capsule: an excision technique for membranous changes. *Ophthal. Surgery*, **17,** 635–640, 1986.

30: Corneal dystrophies

Tom Casey

There are twenty well-defined dystrophies, but only a few are of special interest to the cataract surgeon. Fuchs' dystrophy is of profound importance. One of the most difficult decisions to make is the type of operation to be performed when cataract and moderately advanced dystrophy coexist. A knowledge of the natural history of the dystrophies is advisable; some of the more striking, e.g. Schnyder's, rarely need keratoplasty even when associated with cataract. Some, such as Reis-Buckler's, have a high recurrence rate in the graft. One variant of posterior polymorphous dystrophy (PPD) is associated with cataract and glaucoma and may present as simple band degeneration to the unwary. Surgeons often find difficulty in making a correct diagnosis; this is not due to a paucity of literature on the subject. The author believes that the written word is usually inadequate to describe the clinical features; diagrams and photographs are better. Once a diagnosis is made, the other features can be found in standard texts.

Reis-Buckler's dystrophy

This is by far the most common dystrophy that the corneal surgeon sees, since operations may be necessary even at the age of twenty. Indeed, such patients often bring their children with recurrent erosions, even in the first year of life. It is a dominant dystrophy. It is not known if this is a primary dystrophy of Bowman's membrane or if the condition starts in the basal epithelial cells. The pathology, which explains the honeycomb appearance of the epithelium and the recurrent erosions, shows fibrocellular connective tissue projecting in a finger-like fashion into the epithelium (**30.1**).

There is a high recurrence rate after keratoplasty, approximately 30% over a ten year period. Recurrences are more frequent after lamellar grafts, so large (7.5–8 mm) full thickness grafts are preferred and if cataract coexists, a triple procedure is ideal. Lamellar keratectomy is sometimes useful for recurrent episodes of pain but visual results are poor.

30.1

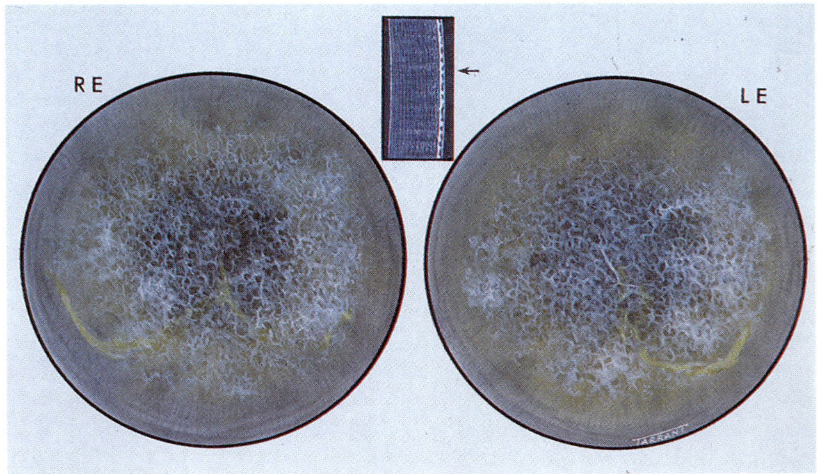

30.1 Reis-Buckler's dystrophy showing typical honeycomb superficial corneal opacities. Arrow (sagittal inset) shows the appearance of a fibrous tissue projection through basement membrane.

Granular dystrophy

This is characterized by an early onset in the axial area of the cornea, with visual symptoms from age fifteen, and often requires keratoplasty in the fourth decade. Inheritance is dominant. The early corneal opacities are approximately 1.5 mm in diameter and are situated in the anterior stroma. They later coalesce and progress deeper into the stroma (**30.2**). The epithelium is not involved and so there are no episodes of corneal erosions. Full thickness grafts carry the best prognosis, and recurrence of the dystrophy in the transplant is approximately 5% in ten years.

30.2

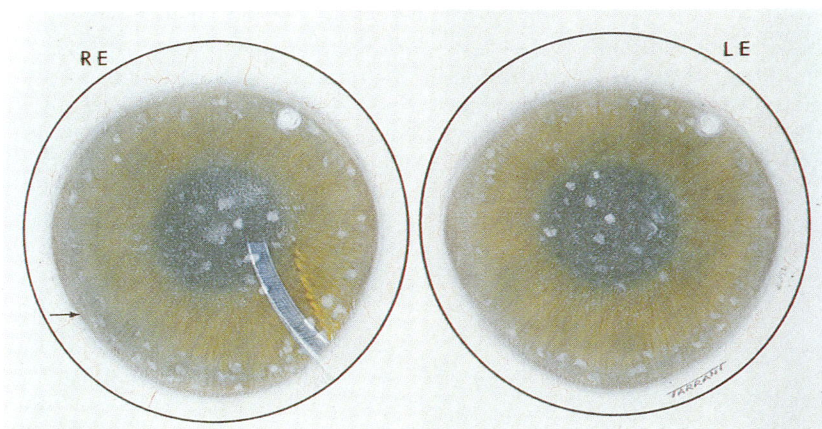

30.2 Granular dystrophy in a 40-year-old patient. Note that with time the opacities increase in size, become confluent and extend to the periphery.

Lattice dystrophy

The prognosis for grafting is excellent, except that there is a 10% recurrence rate over ten years. Inheritance is dominant. Visual symptoms appear earlier than in granular dystrophy and since the epithelium is involved, symptoms of erosions may occur. At first there are striking lines or dots in the axial region; later these progress to branching filaments and the intervening areas of the corneas have a ground glass appearance (**30.3**).

30.3

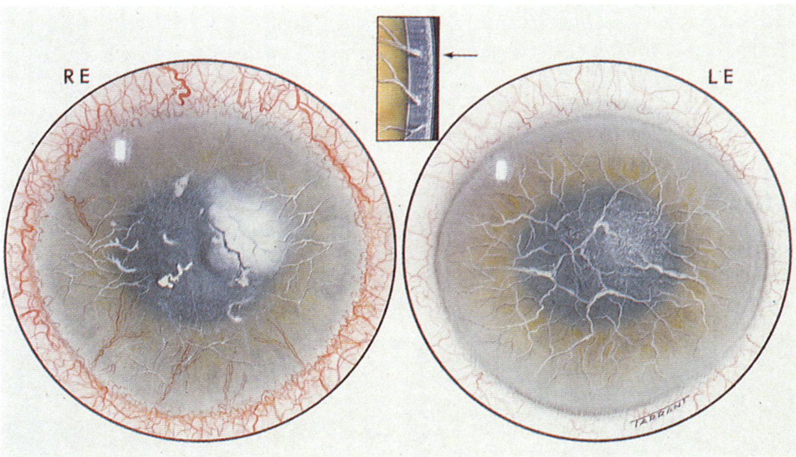

30.3 An advanced lattice dystrophy in a patient aged 70 with coexisting cataract. The right eye presented with pain and injection due to a recurrent erosion complicated by a corneal abscess. Recommended treatment was a bilateral triple procedure with a minimum interval of one year to avoid sensitization by the second graft.

Macular dystrophy

Visual symptoms may arise at the age of ten. There is a diffuse cloudiness in the superficial axial part of the cornea, which later extends to the periphery and deeper areas of the cornea (**30.4**). Within the diffuse area of the opacity there may be areas 2.5 mm in diameter which are more dense – macular opacities. Inheritance is recessive.

As in lattice and Reis-Buckler's dystrophy, symptoms of erosion are common.

30.4

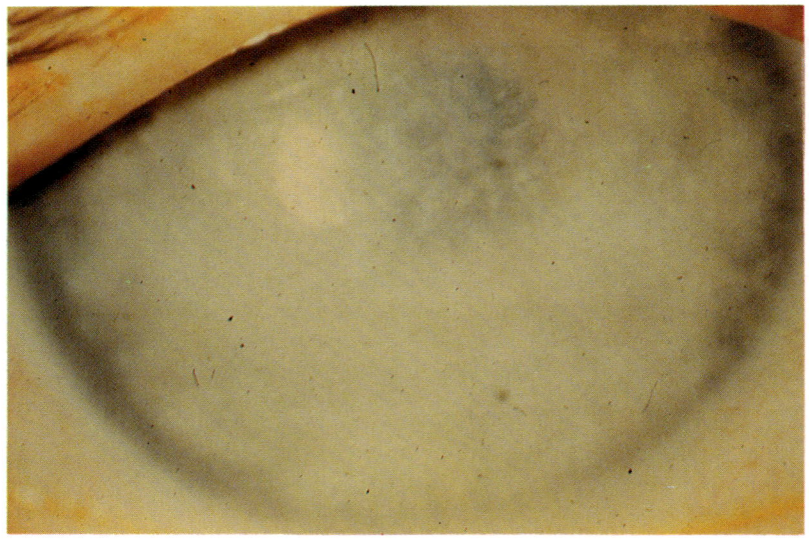

30.4 Advanced macular dystrophy requiring keratoplasty.

Posterior polymorphous dystrophy

Inheritance is dominant, but since patients have no visual symptoms, it is difficult to know when the condition commences. Blister-like lesions are noted in the endothelium from the age of twenty. The polymorphous white opacities are extremely slow in progression. Occasionally there is endothelial decompensation (**30.5**) and bullous keratopathy occurs.

30.5

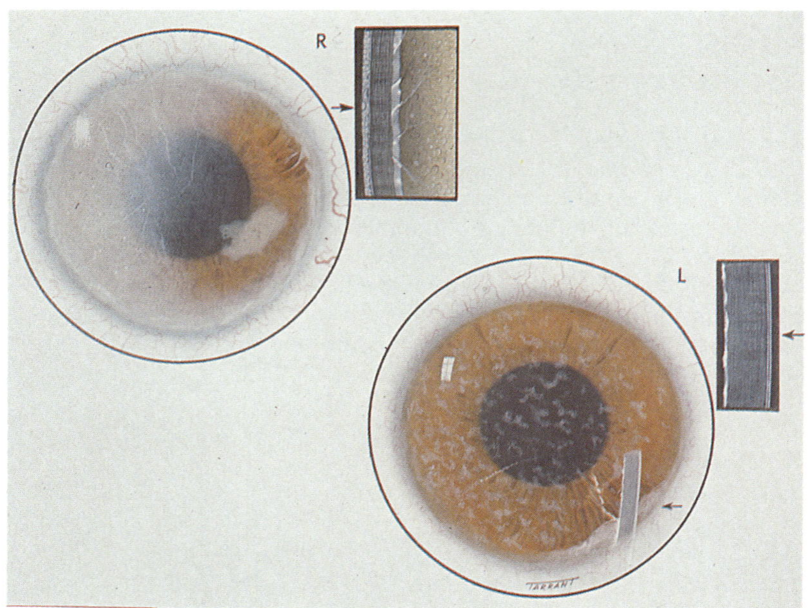

30.5 Posterior polymorphous dystrophy. The right eye showed endothelial decompensation with temporal half corneal edema. The opacities of the left eye had remained unchanged for ten years.

The prognosis for corneal grafting will depend on the presence or absence of certain associations: if a prominent ring of Schwalbe and iridocorneal adhesions are found, there is a high risk of glaucoma. Apart from cases with endothelial decompensation, when PPD and cataract coexist (**30.6**), the corneal condition can be ignored and simple cataract extraction with implantation can be carried out. Some relatives of patients with PPD present with simple band degeneration (which may recur after lamellar grafting).

30.6

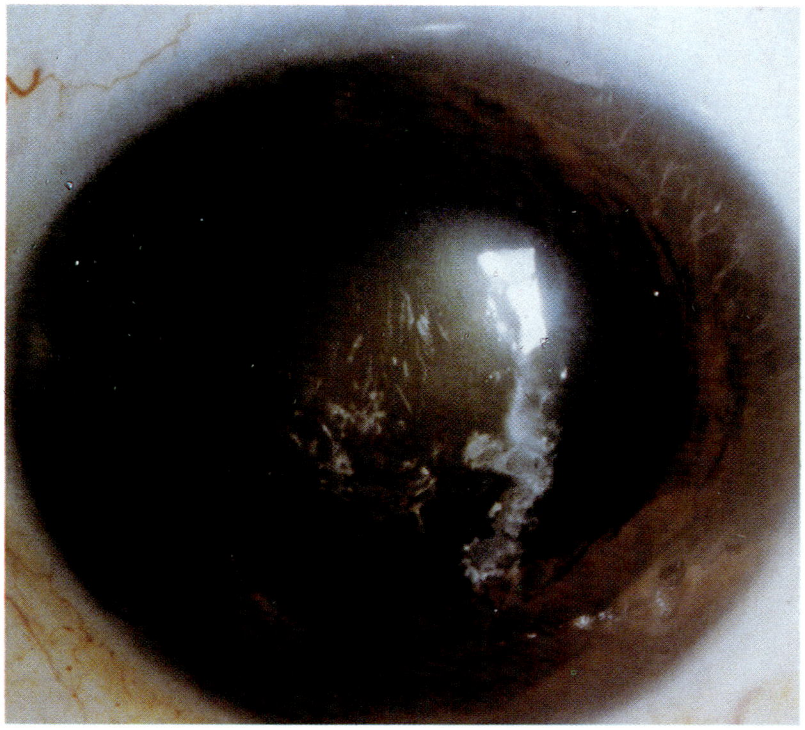

30.6 Uncomplicated posterior polymorphous dystrophy with coexisting cataract: routine ECCE with PCL implantation was planned.

Fuchs' dystrophy

The condition (**30.7**) is more common in females than males, rarely presents before the age of fifty and occasionally there is a family history (5%). It has been stated that glaucoma is a common association, but this is not so. The clinical features are excrescences on Descemet's membrane which appear on the slit lamp as tiny water droplets (guttata).

Occasionally, there is thickening of Descemet's membrane, but no excrescences. This variant may also lead to corneal edema. One of the most difficult problems for a cataract surgeon is to decide on the proper procedure when Fuchs' dystrophy and cataract coexist. If the dystrophy is widespread yet mild, extracapsular cataract extraction with posterior chamber lens implantation should be planned under the protection of sodium hyaluronate. If the dystrophy progresses postoperatively, keratoplasty presents no additional hazard, as it does in an aphakic eye after intracapsular extraction. If keratoplasty is necessary within six months of cataract surgery in the first eye, the graft triple procedure should be recommended for the second eye.

30.7

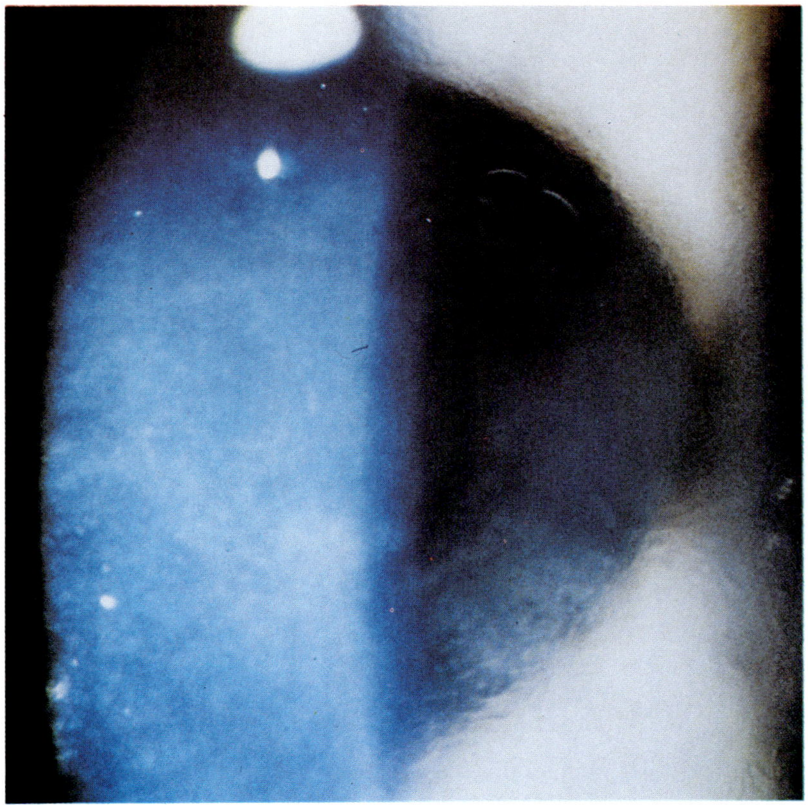

30.7 Moderately advanced Fuch's dystrophy and early cataract. Note that the cornea (right side of the slit beam) has a ground glass appearance when seen by reflected light. A triple procedure was performed because coexisting cataract tends to progress after keratoplasty.

Other findings that indicate the need for primary graft triple procedure are as follows:

- Central corneal thickness by pachymetry of 0.7 mm or more.
- The appearance of fine epithelial edema with the slit lamp. This may only be present in the early morning, and clears as the day progresses. If examination in the morning is not possible, the finding may be suggested by symptoms of greater blurring in the early morning.
- Specular microscopy (**30.8, 30.9**). If guttate spots are moderate and the intervening endothelial cells are of relatively normal density, extracapsular extraction with posterior chamber implantation may be planned. However, if intervening cells are of reduced density or there is widespread obliteration by the guttata, the graft triple procedure should be recommended.

30.8

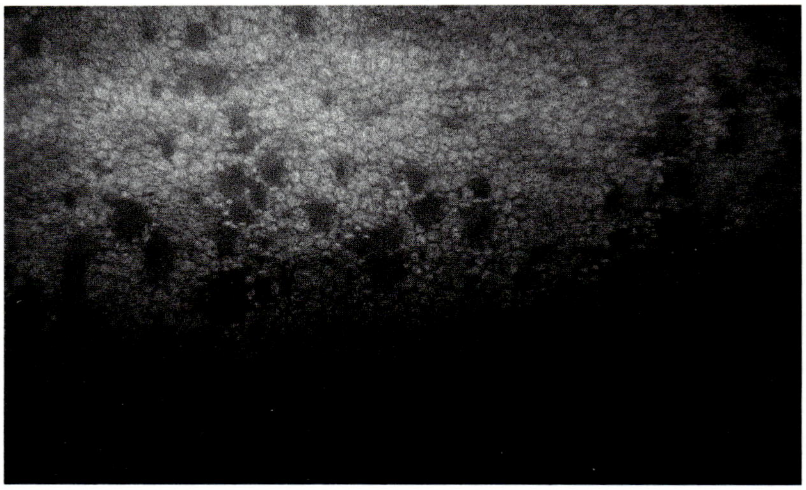

30.8 Specular microscopy of moderate guttata showing some pleomorphism, but a relatively normal density of endothelial cells. Cataract surgery was performed under the protection of sodium hyaluronate without the need for keratoplasty.

30.9

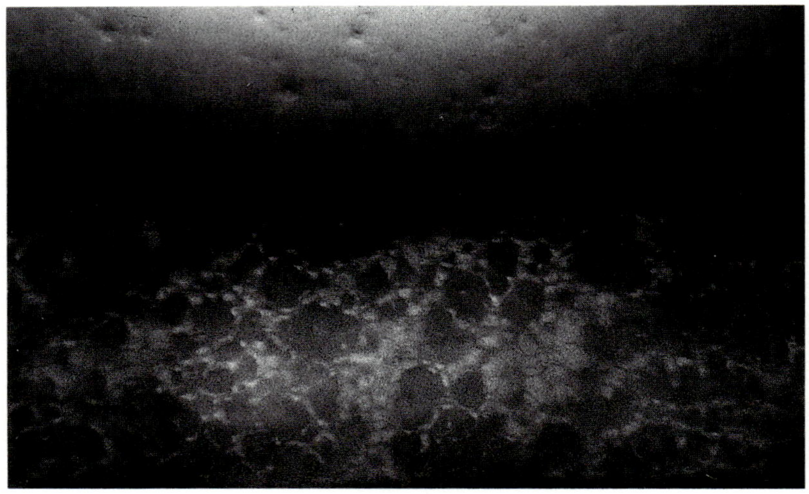

30.9 Specular microscopy in a case of 'early' Fuchs' dystrophy showing advanced guttata and endothelial cells of poor quality: a triple procedure was indicated.

Schnyder's dystrophy

The striking oval crystals (**30.10**) are present at the age of ten. They are situated in the anterior stroma and Bowman's membrane. The epithelium is not involved. There may be a faint haze in parts of the cornea unaffected by crystals. The crystals consist of cholesterol and there may be an associated arcus and problems of lipid metabolism. Corneal grafting is rarely necessary and if cataract coexists, intracapsular extraction with lens implantation is recommended without keratoplasty. Owing to the dense corneal opacification, clean phacoemulsification or extracapsular extraction would be impossible, as would later YAG laser capsulotomy. The procedure of choice for coexisting cataract would therefore be 'open sky' intracapsular extraction with careful insertion of a one piece semiflexible anterior chamber lens.

30.10

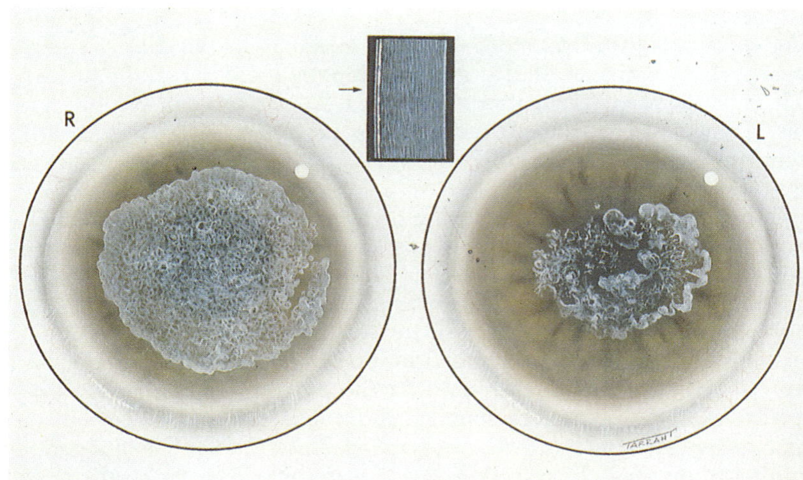

30.10 Schnyder's dystrophy showing characteristic superficial crystalline opacities. Visual acuity 20/30 in each eye.

The triple procedure

When cataract and moderately advanced Fuchs' dystrophy coexist, corneal grafting, extracapsular extraction and posterior chamber implantation is a very satisfactory triple procedure. However, the results are not as good as a routine cataract extraction because of the difficulty in predicting the final refractive power and because of the astigmatism that is commonly encountered. A two stage procedure of cataract surgery secondary to graft surgery is not now recommended because of the increased risk of graft failure, the risk of further increasing astigmatism, the increased risks from two operations and the delay in visual recovery.

Axial length measurements are made by ultrasound and the power of the implant is reduced by at least 1 D to compensate for the usual myopia after keratoplasty.

Cutting the donor disc

This is best done with a punch from the posterior surface, using either the author's or the more sophisticated, but more expensive, Hanna's punch. It is wise to bear in mind that a cornea punched from the posterior surface is approximately 0.25 mm smaller than a cornea cut from the anterior surface with the same size trephine. It is recommended that a donor disc 0.5 mm larger than the recipient opening is used, since this reduces the risk of complications from postoperative glaucoma, although surprisingly this has little effect on the refraction.

Cutting the recipient cornea

It is likely that much of the astigmatism of corneal grafting arises during this maneuver. An oval opening may be produced by uneven pressure from the speculum or the fixation forceps.

The Hessburg–Barron Vacuum Trephine, which fixates the cornea by suction during trephination, avoids some of the distortion that occurs with the Franchescetti type of trephine, but the Hanna instrument is the best.

Anterior capsulotomy

This can be either circular or square. A 5.5 mm trephine, dipped in fluorescein, marks the anterior capsule (**30.11**) and the capsulotomy may be completed with curved Vanna's scissors. Alternatively, a razor blade and straight Vanna's scissors will give a square opening (**30.12**). The nucleus may be expressed by using a lens loop in one hand and a squint hook in the other (**30.13**).

Low power irrigation/aspiration is used to remove the cortex, but greater care must be taken than in routine cataract extraction because the anterior flaps have a tendency to collapse. The aspiration hole should be placed parallel to the capsule and the irrigation ports anterior and posterior.

30.11

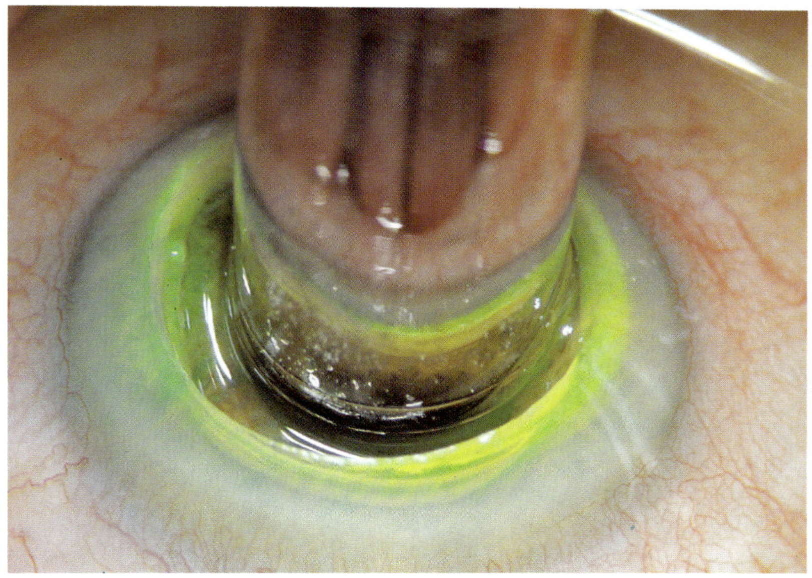

30.11 Circular capsulotomy being made with a 5.5 mm trephine.

30.12

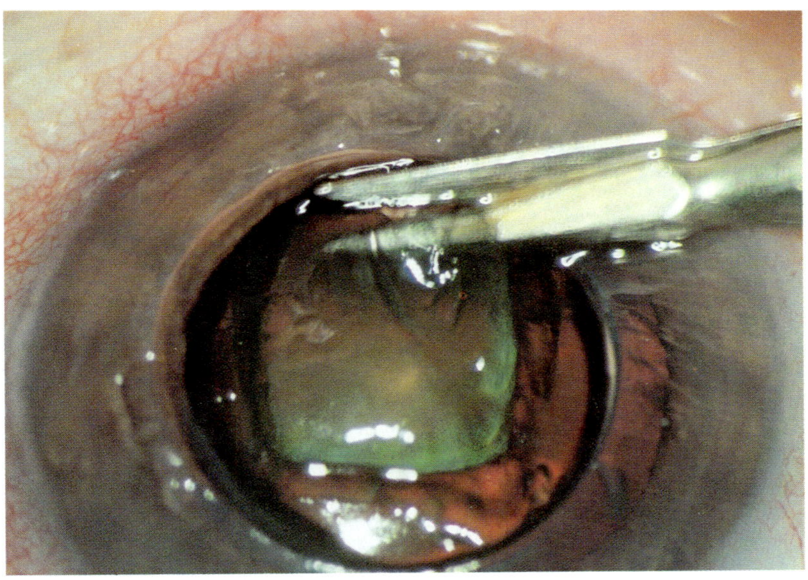

30.12 Square capsulotomy being completed with Vanna's scissors.

30.13

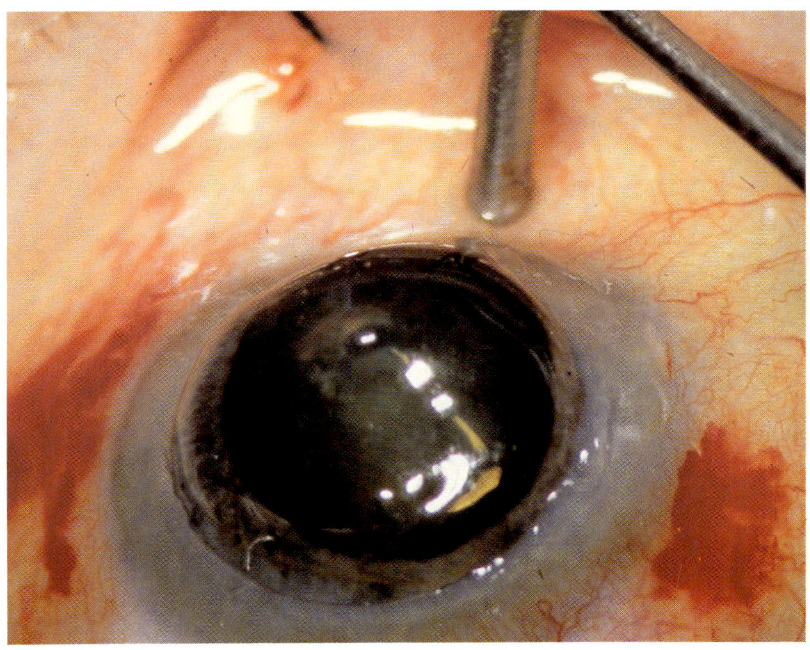

30.13 Counterpressure below the limbus with a squint hook to prolapse the nucleus.

Insertion of posterior chamber lens into capsular bag

The anterior capsular flap is separated from the posterior capsule with sodium hyaluronate. One of the haptics is inserted, and the other is flexed into position by simultaneously grasping the anterior capsular flap with the McPherson forceps.

Suturing

The primary consideration is avoidance of astigmatism. The second (**30.14**) direct suture is the most critical in determining tissue distribution. In general, direct sutures allow greater control of astigmatism. Apart from refraction and keratometry, corneoscopy is invaluable in studying corneal contours.

It must be remembered that despite tissue typing, and even in an avascular dystrophy, rejection is possible, and so patients must be kept under frequent review, even years after surgery.

30.14

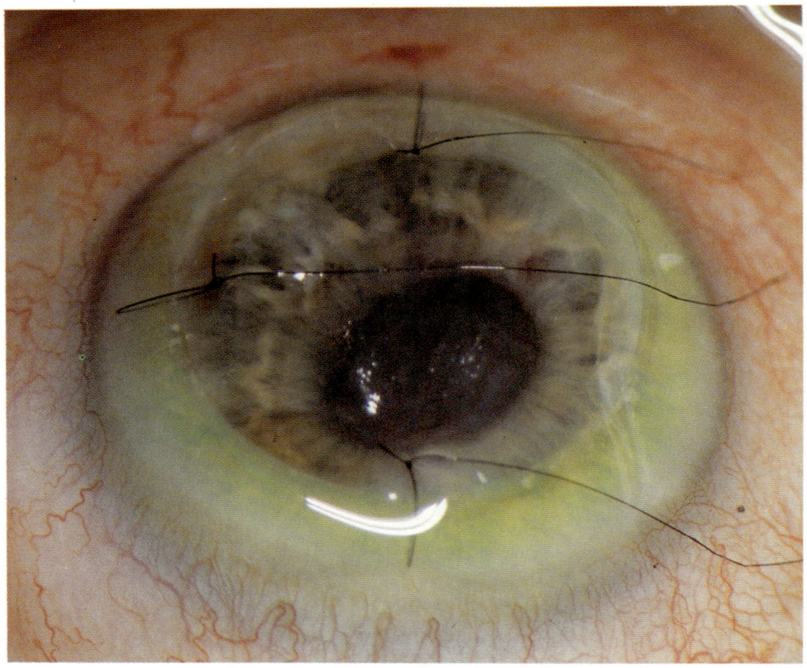

30.14 Placement of three of the four direct cardinal sutures.

31 The glaucomatous eye

Stephen Obstbaum

The incidence of cataract and open-angle glaucoma increases as the population ages. We are, therefore, witnessing an increased prevalence of the coexistence of these conditions with the increased longevity of our patients. Glaucoma is a chronic condition, potentially causing irreversible visual loss, and presenting management options that pose ongoing therapeutic challenges. Cataract formation is responsible for a reversible form of visual loss that is amenable to surgical intervention and is highly successful. Our rationale for operating on eyes with cataract and glaucoma is to improve the patient's visual function. In the past, intraocular lens (IOL) implantation was considered a relative contraindication for some eyes with glaucoma. Alternative forms of visual rehabilitation, using either aphakic spectacles or contact lenses are fraught with difficulties. In the 1970s, the major cataract operation we performed was an intracapsular cataract extraction (ICCE), and the IOLs used at that time were either pupil-supported or anterior chamber lenses. In those circumstances where an IOL was successfully implanted, vitreous migrating either around the IOL or through the pupil could obstruct the filtration angle or block a previously functioning filtering bleb. A pupil-supported lens implanted in an eye with the possibility of a shallow chamber after filtering surgery led to the potential for IOL–endothelial contact. Pupillary block occurred more frequently with pupil-supported and anterior chamber IOLs, while synechia formation and secondary angle closure were frequently observed with anterior chamber IOLs. Yet, despite the prevailing sentiment against the use of IOLs in glaucoma eyes, several studies suggested that, if the glaucoma was preoperatively controlled and the surgery was performed flawlessly, the IOL itself did little to disturb that level of control.

During the past decade, the popularity of the extracapsular cataract extraction (ECCE) and the introduction of the posterior chamber lens (PCL) have made implantation in the glaucomatous eye a safer procedure. Maintenance of an intact posterior capsule permits compartmentalization of the eye and protects the anterior segment and a pre-existing filtering bleb from the vitreous. The use of a PCL simplifies the insertion technique, and ensures placement that is distant from the trabecular meshwork and any filtration site. Capsular bag fixation, in addition, sequesters the lens from the uveal tissue.

Another adjunct for safer and more predictable surgery is the use of a viscoelastic substance, which maintains the anterior chamber during the course of the procedure, protects tissue by coating the endothelium and the iris, lyses synechias, and maintains pupil dilation during the operation. In addition, this agent facilitates capsular bag insertion of the PCL.

Miotic pupil techniques

The patient with preexisting glaucoma frequently has a pupil that does not dilate well (**31.1**). This situation may be the result of the long-term use of miotic agents, posterior synechias from preexisting inflammation or posterior synechias from prior surgery. Since visualization of the anterior capsule by mechanically widening the pupil is an essential step for safe cataract surgery, we have adopted several techniques to facilitate anterior capsule exposure.

Multiple sphincterotomies

Multiple sphincterotomies widen the pupil that dilates only moderately. This situation is generally a consequence of chronic long-term miotic therapy in a noninflamed eye, and there are usually few posterior synechias. The technique involves making small incisions through the sphincter muscle inferiorly and, at times, either temporally or nasally (**31.2**). The use of a viscoelastic material to fill the anterior chamber enhances the ease of performing this technique.

31.1

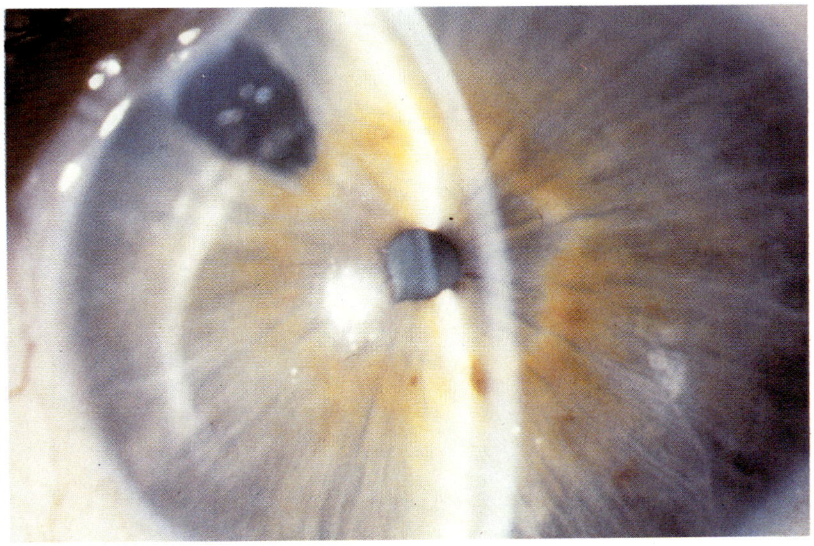

31.1 Maximal dilatation of a miotic pupil with posterior synechias resulting from glaucoma surgery.

31.2

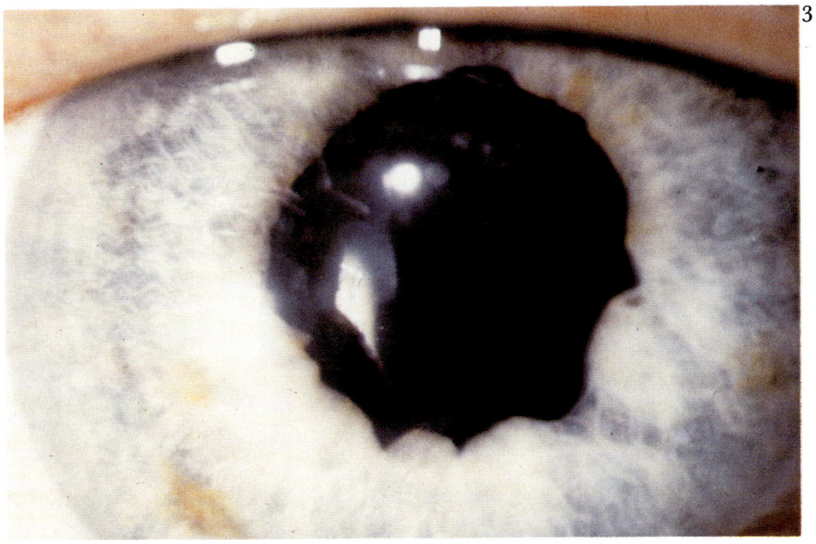

31.2 Multiple sphincterotomies adequately open the pupil for cataract extraction and IOL implantation without destroying the symmetry of the central opening.

Peripheral iridectomy with radial sphincterotomy

If the pupil does not dilate at all or dilates only minimally, some degree of posterior synechia formation is generally evident. In order to widen the pupil, a synechiolysis is performed. This procedure is readily achieved in an anterior chamber filled with a viscoelastic material. If a peripheral iridectomy already exists, a cyclodialysis spatula is introduced through it behind the iris. If an iridectomy does not exist, it is performed at this time. Synechias are swept from the peripheral portion of the iris, where the synechiae are generally absent, towards the central portion of the pupil, thereby putting less stress on the anterior capsule and the zonular apparatus. Once the synechiolysis has been performed, one can place additional viscoelastic material in the anterior chamber to assess the degree of pupil dilation. If it is adequate, one can proceed with the operation. With inadequate pupil dilation, a radial sphincterotomy is performed by placing the scissor blade through the peripheral iridectomy and extending the incision through the superior portion of the pupil (**31.3**). At times, an inferior sphincterotomy is also required to achieve a sufficiently wide exposure to the anterior capsule. Some surgeons believe that minimal lysis of adhesions should be performed, and that only a small central capsulotomy is required. However, better exposure permits more precise placement of the IOL within the capsular bag after a round capsulotomy or envelope technique (**31.4–31.6**). In eyes that have had previous angle-closure glaucoma with a peripheral iridectomy, the result may give the appearance of a keyhole (**31.7**). Once an adequate view of the capsule is achieved, the surgeon's preferred capsulotomy technique is performed. It is advantageous to create a capsulotomy that encourages capsular bag fixation of the PCL.

31.3

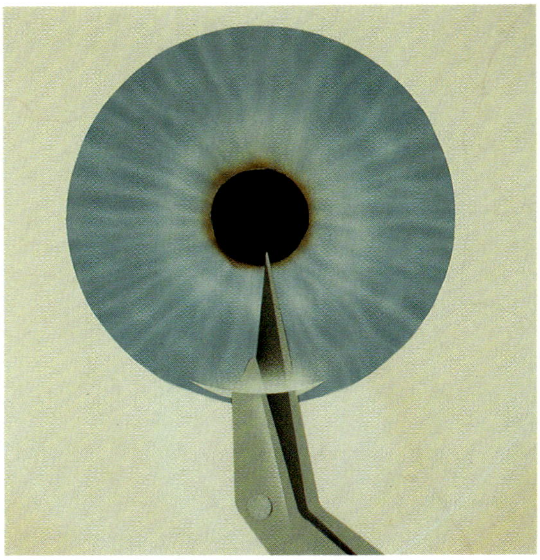

31.3 The scissor blade is placed through the iridectomy and an incision made through the superior sphincter in a chamber filled with viscoelastic material.

31.4

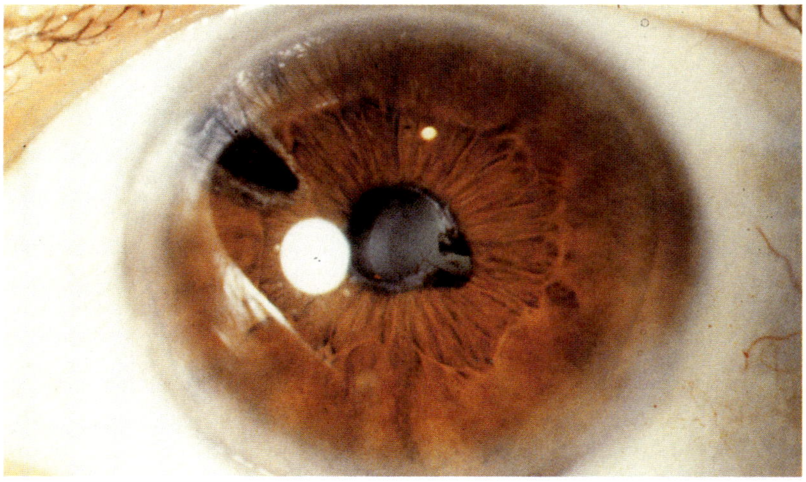

31.4 An eye with combined-mechanism glaucoma having had prior peripheral iridectomy and the development of posterior synechias (maximal dilation).

31.5

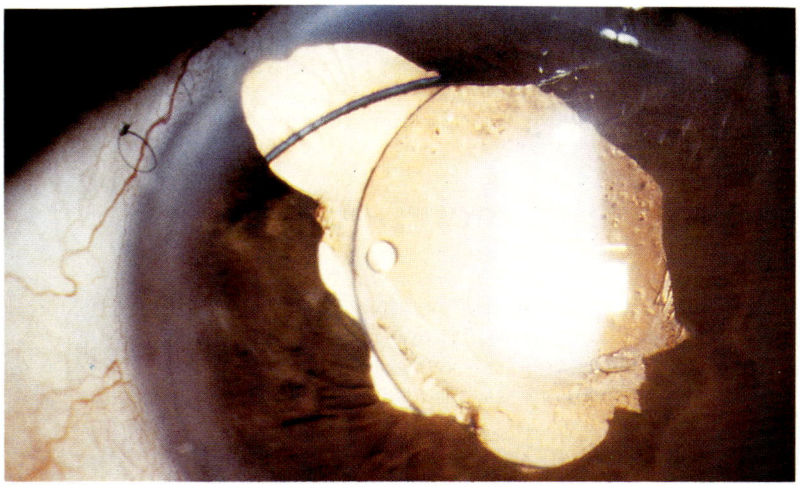

31.5 An eye shortly after surgery, which included synechiolysis, radial sphincterotomy, inferior sphincterotomies and ECCE with PCL.

31.6

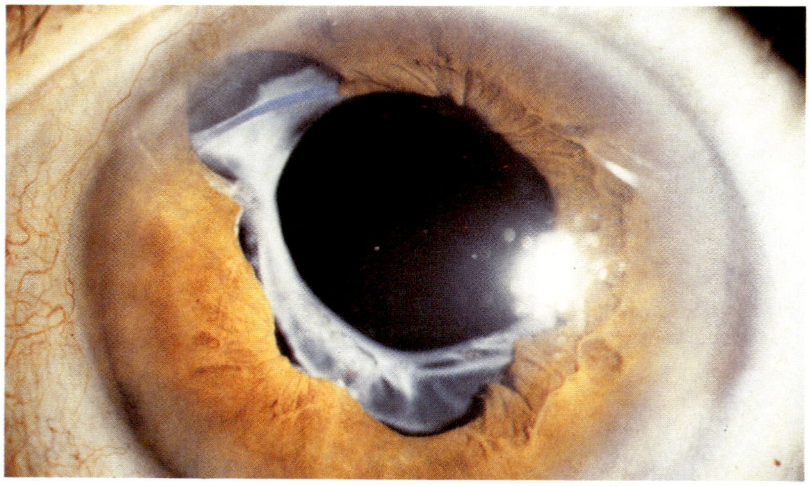

31.6 The same eye as in **31.5** photographed five years later. The IOL is within the capsular bag, and the IOP is controlled without medication.

31.7

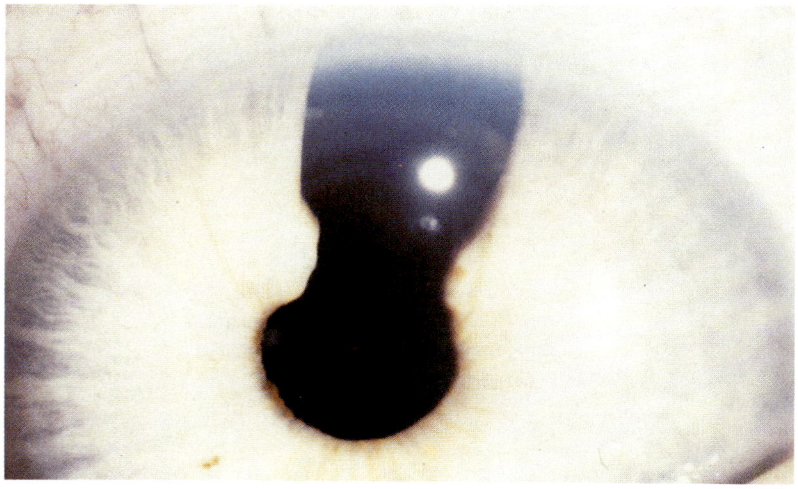

31.7 A keyhole pupil configuration of a patient with ECCE and PCL after a peripheral iridectomy for angle-closure glaucoma.

ECCE and PCL implantation in the glaucomatous eye

Patients with glaucoma have been examined in order to assess the effect of cataract surgery and PCL implantation. These groups included chronic open-angle glaucoma (COAG), angle-closure glaucoma (ACG), eyes after previous argon laser trabeculoplasty (p ALT), and eyes after previous filtering surgery (p Filtration). In each of these groups, except in pALT, there was a reduction in intraocular pressure after ECCE/PCL implantation (**Table 31.1**). Moreover, in all of these groups, almost 50% of the eyes required less medication after surgery than before, and, in 90% of the eyes, less or the same amount of medication was required after surgery (**Table 31.2**).

Of these four groups, the eyes with previous filtration imposed a specific additional consideration. This was selection of the site of the incision for cataract surgery in the presence of a preexisting filtering bleb. Several options have been proposed (**31.8**). Some surgeons make an incision either temporally or inferotemporally, others suggest using an inferior approach, and some advocate going through the filtering bleb and perhaps creating an additional filtration site at the same time. However, the recommended approach is an incision anterior to the bleb in clear cornea, because it affords the surgeon a familiar orientation to the eye while seated at the head of the patient. With only minor modifications in incision length and perpendicularity of the corneal incision, the operation is otherwise similar to the surgeon's accustomed technique (**31.9, 31.10**). In some instances, the somewhat cystic bleb can overhang the cornea (**31.11**). By simply dissecting the bleb bluntly from the corneal tissue and elevating it, an ECCE with PCL implantation can be performed satisfactorily, and minor regression of the superfluous portion of the filtration bleb will occur (**31.12**). In most instances, retention of an avascular filtering bleb is achieved.

Table 31.1 IOP in each group before and after extracapsular cataract extraction/PCL implantation.

Glaucoma condition	*Preop IOP* (mmHg)	*Postop IOP* (mmHg)
COAG	17.6 ± 2.7	16.5 ± 2.9
ACG	16.6 ± 3.7	14.3 ± 2.4
p̄ ALT	16.2 ± 2.6	17.1 ± 2.3
p̄ Filtration surgery	15.7 ± 4.8	15.3 ± 4.0

Table 31.2 The medical requirements for glaucomatous eyes after extracapsular cataract extraction/PCL implantation.

Condition	*Postop medication required*		
	Less	*Same*	*More*
COAG	11	5	1
ACG	2	6	0
p̄ ALT	8	0	1
p̄ Filtration	3	9	3
	24 (48.9%)	20 (40.8%)	5 (10.2%)

31.8

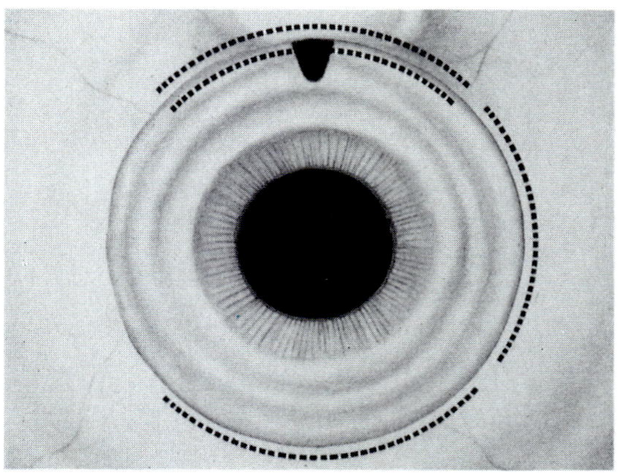

31.8 Proposed sites for the cataract incision after a filtering operation are: temporally, inferiorly, through a clear corneal incision, or through the preexisting filtering bleb.

31.9

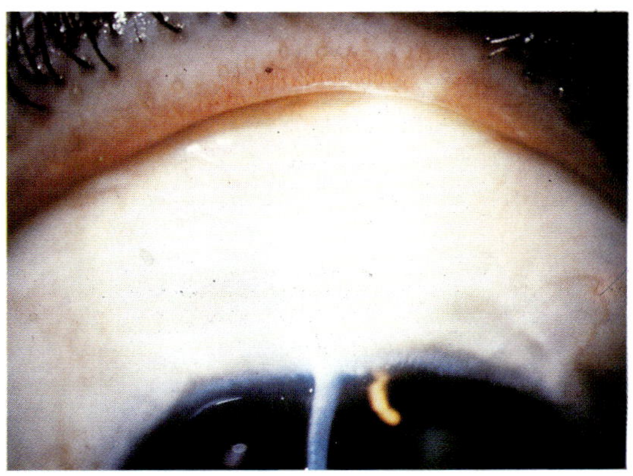

31.9 An iridencleisis procedure was performed 20 years before cataract surgery. Preoperatively there is a large, avascular bleb.

31.10

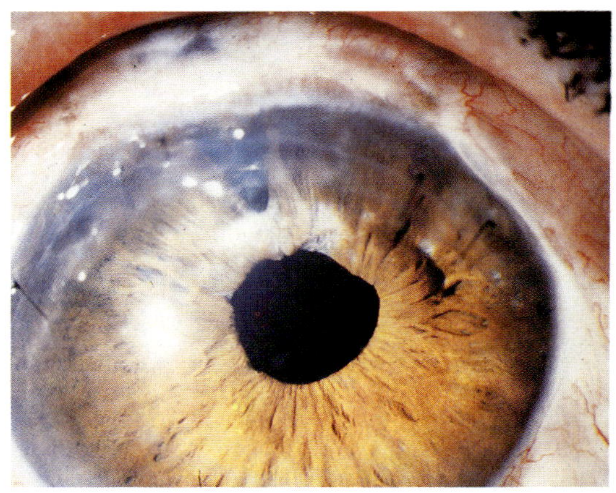

31.10 Same eye as in **31.9** following ECCE with PCL performed through a clear corneal incision anterior to the filtering bleb. The visual acuity is 20/25 and IOP is 14 mmHg. Although the bleb is smaller, it was functioning well more than three years later.

31.11

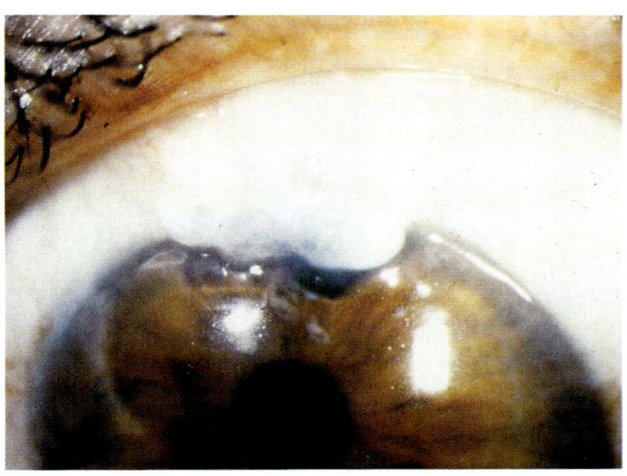

31.12

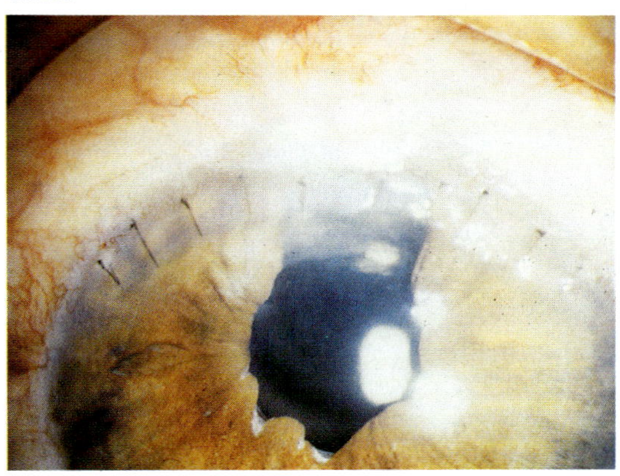

31.11 A cystic bleb extending into and overhanging the superior cornea.

31.12 After dissecting the edge of the bleb, a corneal incision was made for ECCE with PCL. The anterior-most portion of the bleb has retracted with the passage of time.

Complications

The complications that occur as a consequence of performing an ECCE/PCL implantation in an eye with glaucoma are transient pressure elevations, iritis and pigment dispersion, reduced size of the filtration bleb, posterior synechias, the so-called 'iris retraction syndrome', and cystoid macular edema.

Of these, iritis and pigment dispersion commonly occur because of the degree of iris surgery and manipulation required (**31.13, 31.14**). Proponents of a technique that does not lyse adhesions suggest that this reduces the degree of induced anterior chamber reaction. However, one must weigh the ability to perform the operation successfully and safely with the better visualization afforded by a wider pupil diameter, and the inflammation that may result. Intraocular inflammation is, to some degree, responsible for the reduction in bleb size and/or function. Frequent administration of topical steroids, as well as injecting a subconjunctival steroid on completion of surgery, is helpful in reducing the inflammatory response.

The reduction in bleb size, even when encysted with uveal tissue (**31.15, 31.16**) observed in many of the eyes with preexisting filtering operations, does not necessarily portend the demise of the filtering bleb, nor a worsening of intraocular pressure (IOP) control. The IOP control is maintained, either because of the continuation of the bleb's effect, or perhaps because of an action of the PCL *per se*.

31.13

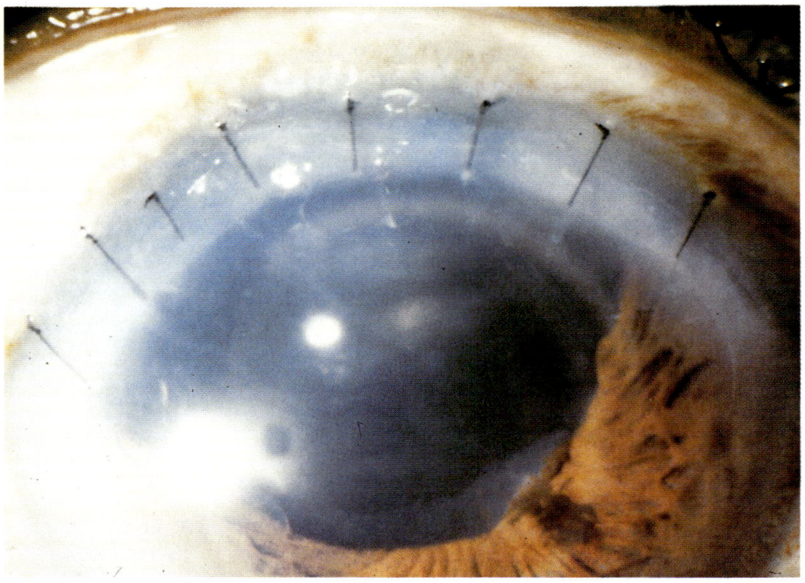

31.13 The appearance of an eye one day postoperatively that had had previous filtering surgery and a sector iridectomy. ECCE with PCL into the capsular bag through a clear corneal section was performed.

31.14

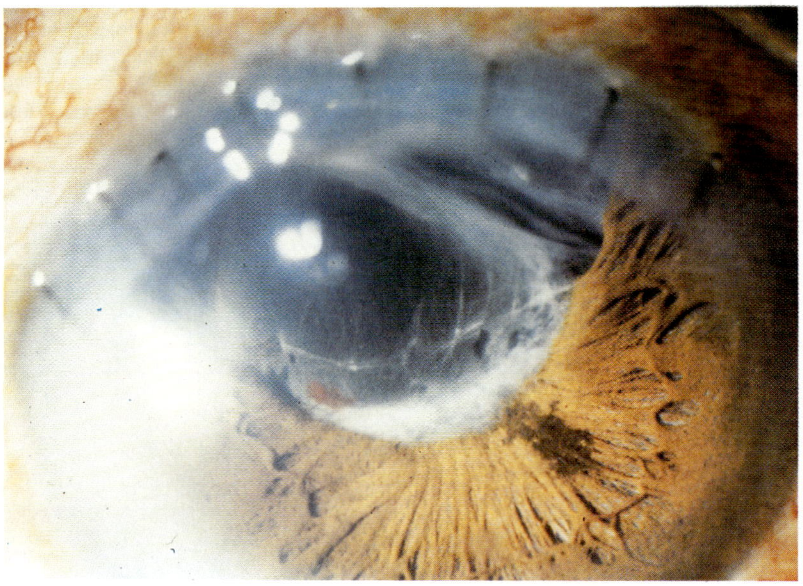

31.14 Two weeks later, the same eye as in **31.13** is inflamed, with the development of a membrane surrounding the posterior chamber IOL. Later it was necessary to open the membrane on the anterior surface of the IOL with a neodymium YAG laser.

31.15

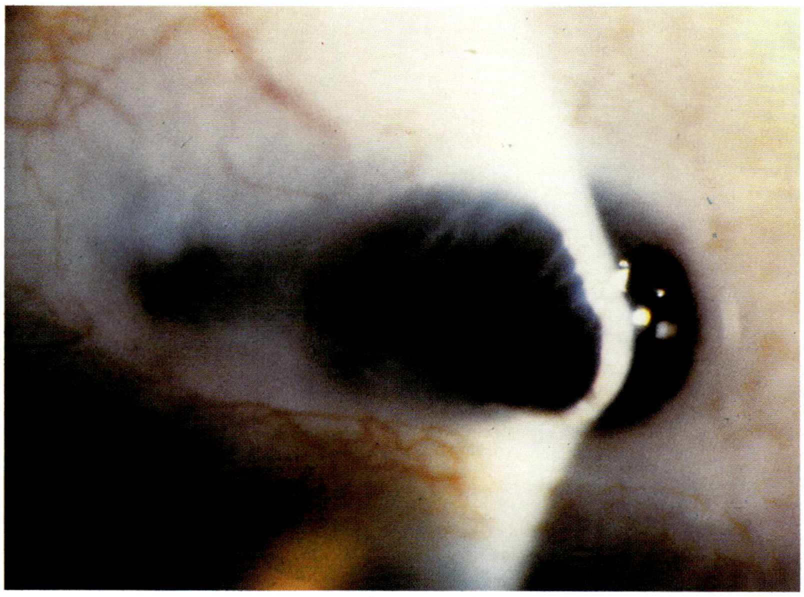

31.15 Uveal tissue present through the sclerostomy site and beneath the bleb after a Scheie procedure. The IOP was well controlled.

31.16

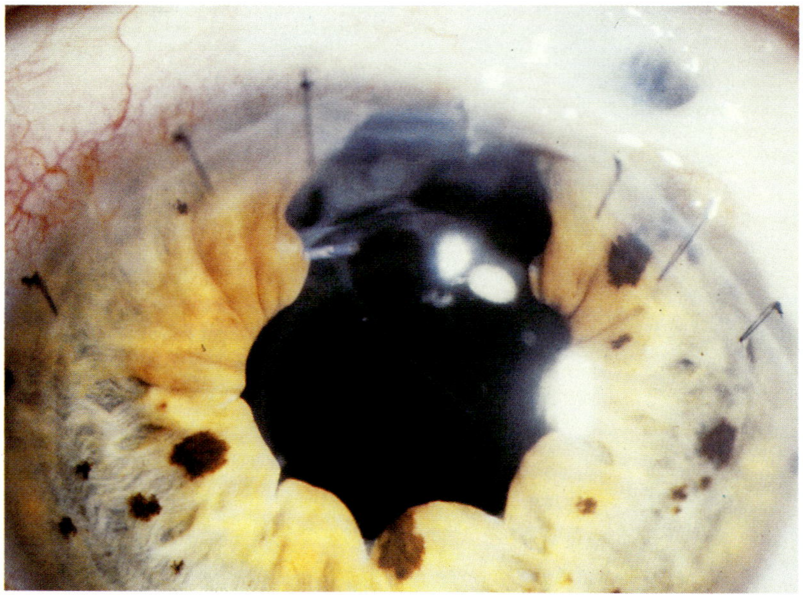

31.16 Same eye as in **31.15** after ECCE with PCL implantation: the prominence of the uveal tissue is reduced and the bleb size is smaller, yet the IOP remains controlled.

Combined surgery for glaucoma and cataract

In eyes with coexisting cataract and glaucoma, the surgical alternatives are: cataract surgery alone; filtration surgery followed by cataract surgery; or a combined surgical approach.

Cataract surgery

When the glaucoma is controlled medically and has minimal visual field loss and/or optic nerve damage, most surgeons will perform cataract/IOL surgery without adding a glaucoma procedure. In the early postoperative period, the pressure is usually controlled with little or no medication, but generally a return to medical treatment is later required.

Filtration surgery followed by cataract surgery

These eyes characteristically have intraocular pressures that require maximally tolerated medication for control and have an accompanying progressive visual field loss and optic nerve damage. In the absence of a cataract, filtering surgery would be performed to treat the glaucoma. Advocates of successive surgery recommend filtration surgery followed by cataract surgery six months later. They contend that the vision-threatening condition should be cared for first, and, once the eye has stabilized, a cataract extraction and IOL implantation can then be performed. This is an acceptable strategy if the cataract is not significantly affecting visual function. When the cataract is visually disabling, and the glaucoma is of sufficient severity to warrant surgical intervention, the proposed sequential surgery has several disadvantages: filtering surgery can produce a more rapid progression of the cataract; postoperative inflammation can cause posterior synechia formation and make the cataract surgery more difficult, and the surgeon may be forced to deviate from customary techniques if a filtering bleb is present, which may affect the competence of the functioning bleb. It also exposes the patient to two intraocular procedures. Should the filtering procedure be compromised during the cataract surgery, an immediate IOP rise could occur. While there may be some special circumstances when staged or successive surgery is warranted, for the most part, this alternative is less attractive than combined surgery, given the current state of technology.

Combined cataract and glaucoma surgery

Surgical procedures combining ECCE, PCL implantation and a form of trabeculectomy are gaining popularity.

The goal of combined surgery is to improve impaired visual function induced by the cataract, while enhancing control of the glaucoma without introducing significant morbidity. The results of combined surgery have been remarkably good. Our experience, with a follow-up of more than six years, has shown that 53% of eyes required no or less medication, 30% used the same medication, and 17% needed more medication than preoperatively. Similar results have been achieved by others. McGuigan *et al.* reported that, at one year postoperatively in their combined surgery group, 30% needed the same or more medication, compared with 75% for their nonfiltered group of patients.

Indications for a combined procedure are the presence of a visually disabling cataract, plus glaucoma recalcitrant to maximally tolerated medical treatment, or significant visual field loss and optic nerve cupping regardless of medical control, or eyes in which a transient pressure rise might cause further optic nerve damage.

The technique of a combined trabeculectomy/ECCE/IOL implantation commences with a fornix-based conjunctival flap. A rectangular superficial scleral dissection is performed and grooved incisions are made on either side for the cataract surgery (**31.17**). If the pupil is small, the trabeculectomy is completed first, the chamber is filled with viscoelastic agent, and sphincterotomies are made before the anterior capsulotomy (**31.18**). In cases with adequate mydriasis the capsulotomy

31.17

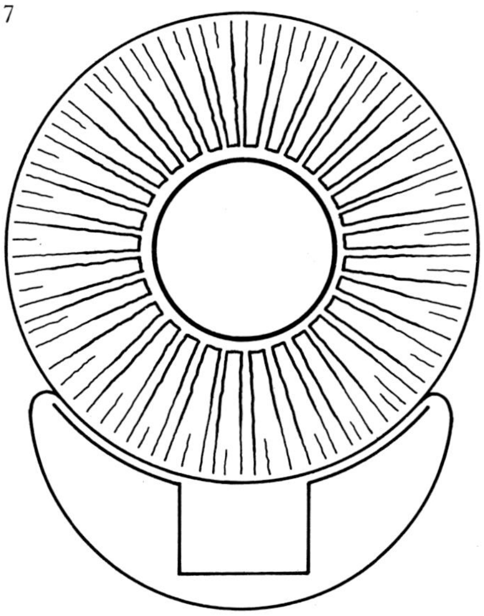

31.18

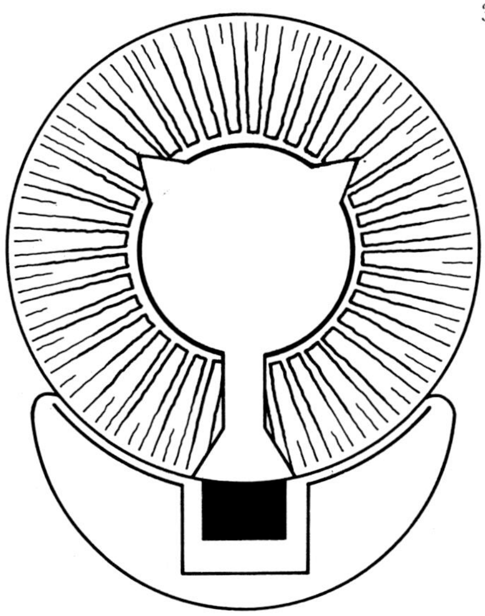

31.17 A lamellar scleral flap preparation and grooved incisions with a fornix-based conjunctival flap.

31.18 Trabeculectomy, iridectomy and sphincterotomies performed before the anterior capsulotomy in cases with poor mydriasis.

is performed before the trabeculectomy, but after the first trabeculectomy incision (**31.19**), since it is easier to do the latter when the eye is hard than when it is soft. The advantage of capsulotomy before trabeculectomy is that the chamber remains closed and cannot be complicated by hemorrhage. The limbal incision is then enlarged and the nucleus removed. A scleral punch can be utilized to remove trabecular tissue. The chamber is filled with a viscoelastic agent, and the IOL placed within the capsular bag. If the trabeculectomy is at the center of the incision (**31.17**), a peripheral iridectomy is performed on completion of the procedure and the wound is closed appropriately. If the trabeculectomy is placed at the left-hand end of the incision (**31.19**) this may be completed and closed prior to insertion of the IOL. Finally, the fornix-based flap is pulled down to cover the wound and secured with 9-0 vicryl sutures.

With bag fixation these eyes do remarkably well, without added morbidity as a consequence of the additional glaucoma procedure (**31.20**). Increasing experience suggests that IOP control in the immediate postoperative period is superior in eyes with combined surgery to operations of cataract with IOL alone.

31.19

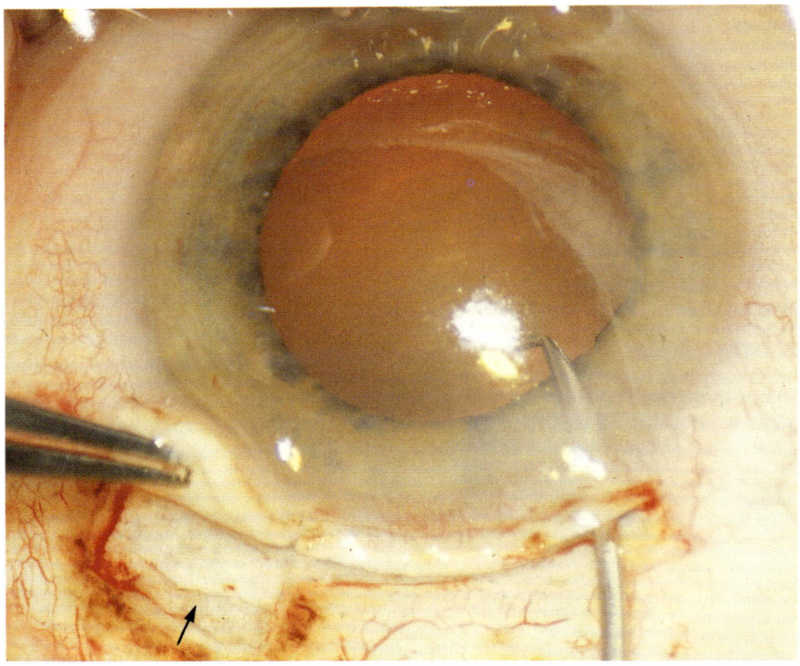

31.19 The outer flap of sclera and initial scleral incision for trabeculectomy (arrow) are made, but the capsulotomy, when the mydriasis is good, is performed under viscoelastic agent before the trabeculectomy is completed.

31.20

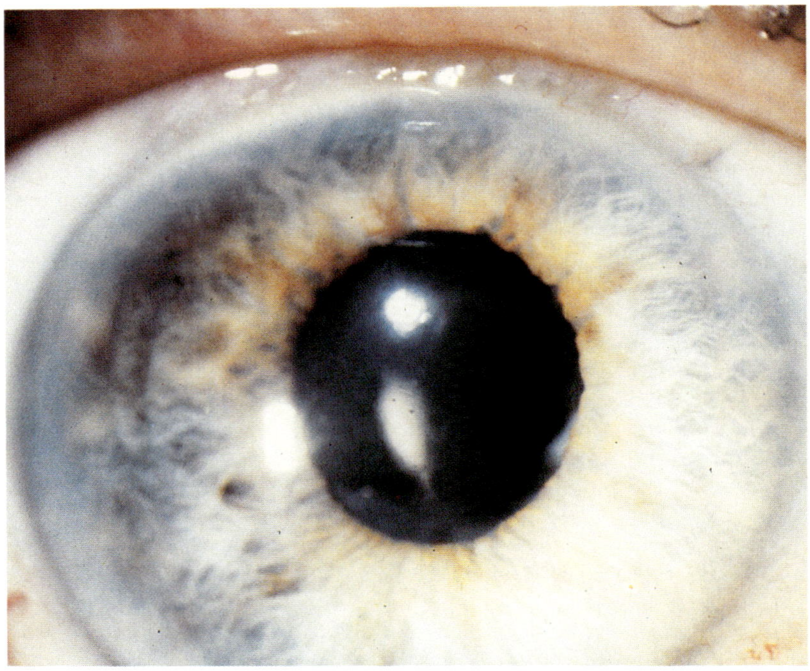

31.20 An eye with a combined ECCE/PCL/trabeculectomy without the need for a sphincterotomy about one year after surgery. The visual acuity is 20/25 and IOP is 12 mmHg.

Further reading

Fagadau W.R., Obstbaum S.A., Hermann W.K. *et al.* Glaucoma, extracapsular cataract extraction and intraocular lens. In: *Cataract Surgery*, Abrahamson, I.A. (Ed.), New York, McGraw-Hill, Inc., pp 126–131, 1986.

Krupin T., Feitl M.E. and Bishop K.I. Post-operative intraocular pressure rise in open-angle glaucoma patients after cataract or combined cataract-filtration surgery. *Ophthalmology*, **96,** 579–584, 1989.

McGuigan L.T.B., Gottsch J., Stark W.J. *et al.* Extracapsular cataract extraction and posterior chamber lens implantation in eyes with pre-existing glaucoma. *Arch. Ophthalmol.*, **104,** 1301–1306, 1986.

Murchison J.F. Jr and Shields M.B. An evaluation of three surgical approaches for co-existing cataract and glaucoma. *Ophthalmic Surg.*, **20,** 393–398, 1989.

Obstbaum S.A. Glaucoma and intraocular lens implantation. *J. Cataract Refrac. Surg.*, **12,** 257–261, 1986.

Percival S.P.B. Glaucoma triple procedure of extracapsular cataract extraction, posterior chamber lens implantation and trabeculectomy. *Br. J. Ophthalmol.*, **69,** 99–102, 1985.

Rock R.L. and Rylander H.G. Spontaneous iris retraction occurring after extracapsular cataract extraction and posterior lens implantation in patients with glaucoma. *Am. Intra-Ocular Implant Soc. J.*, **9,** 45–47, 1983.

Simmons R.J., Savage J.A. and Thomas J.V. The glaucomas and extracapsular cataract surgery with posterior chamber lens implantation. In: *New Orleans Academy of Ophthalmology: Symposium of Glaucomas, St. Louis*, The C.V. Mosby Company, pp 27–54, 1985.

Simmons S.T., Litoff D., Nichols D.A. *et al.* Extracapsular cataract extraction and posterior lens implantation combined with trabeculectomy in patients with glaucoma. *Am. J. Ophthalmol.*, **104,** 465–470, 1987.

32: Coloboma and microphthalmos

Hugh Williams and Piers Percival

Colobomata are due to a developmental disturbance in the closure of the embryonic cleft, which may be hereditary, or follow the Rubella syndrome (**32.1, 32.2**). Colobomata may involve the optic disc, retina, zonule and lens, and may be associated with scleral ectasia, which will usually be lined by gliosed layers of the retina.

Modern microsurgical techniques of lens implantation can provide good visual results (Jaffe 1987) for patients with colobomatous eyes. Previously, the difficulty of access and the poor visual prognosis owing to amblyopia in association with nystagmus, strabismus and microphthalmos, meant surgery was seldom undertaken.

32.1

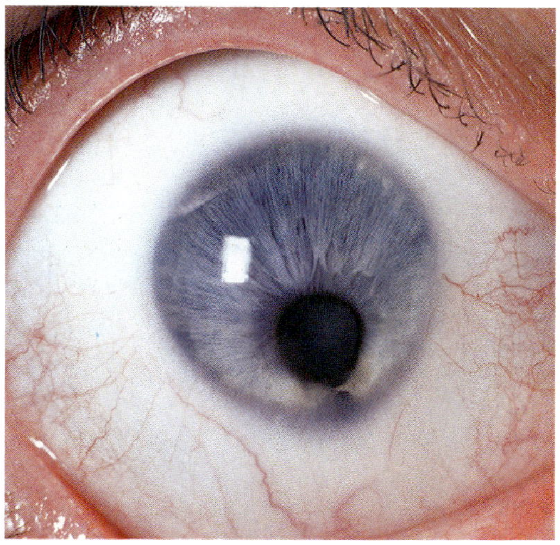

32.1 Coloboma right eye with nuclear cataract.

32.2

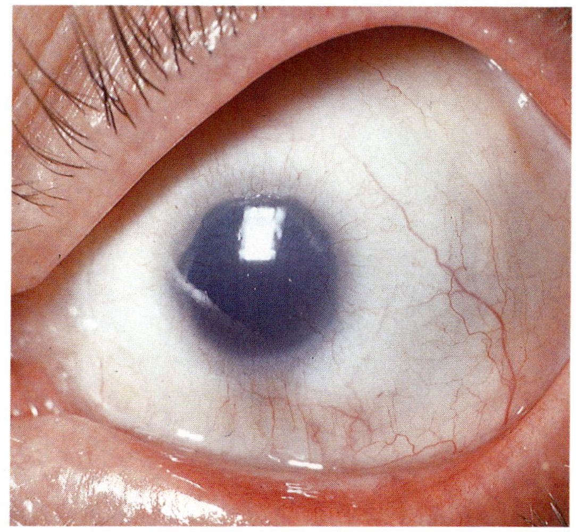

32.2 Microphthalmic left eye of the same patient as in **32.1**.

Preoperative assessment

The possible problems associated with coloboma of the iris may include any or all of the following:

- Small eye.
- Hypermetropia.
- Eccentric pupil.
- Poor mydriasis.
- Defective zonule at the site of the coloboma.
- Posterior segment deformities.

32.3

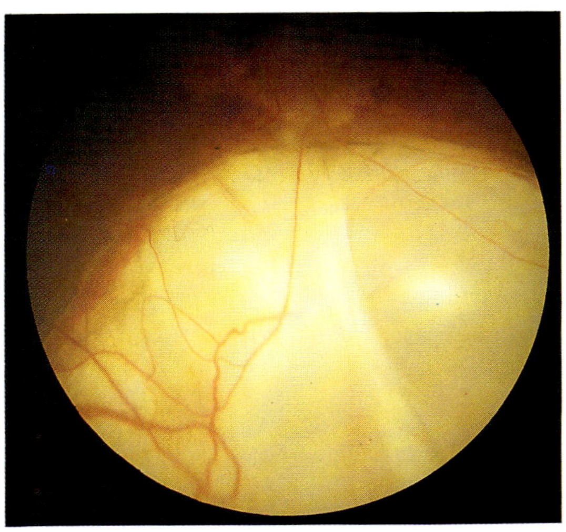

32.3 Uveal coloboma and scleral staphyloma of the same eye as in **32.1** seen through the implant after surgery.

It is of paramount importance to dilate the pupil maximally before surgery. Particular assessment will include:

- Slit-lamp examination and 3-mirror fundoscopy to reveal whether the coloboma is partial or complete. If complete, it can involve scleral ectasia, localized loss of zonular fibers and/or notching of the adjacent lens equator. Macular details, if visible, should be recorded, for poor acuity has been noted in uveal colobomata despite a normal macular appearance (**32.3**).
- Ultrasonography. An A-scan will establish colobomatous microphthalmos as well as provide axial length biometry. The latter must be taken with extreme accuracy in case a staphyloma exists below the fovea. If a posterior segment malformation is suspected, a B-scan is necessary. This may occasionally show gliosed retina to span a staphyloma (**32.4**) and be misinterpreted as retinal detachment. In such cases, the opinion of a retinal specialist may be valuable.
- Keratometry, besides providing biodata, will distinguish microphthalmos from the condition of microcornea. The corneal diameter should also be measured.

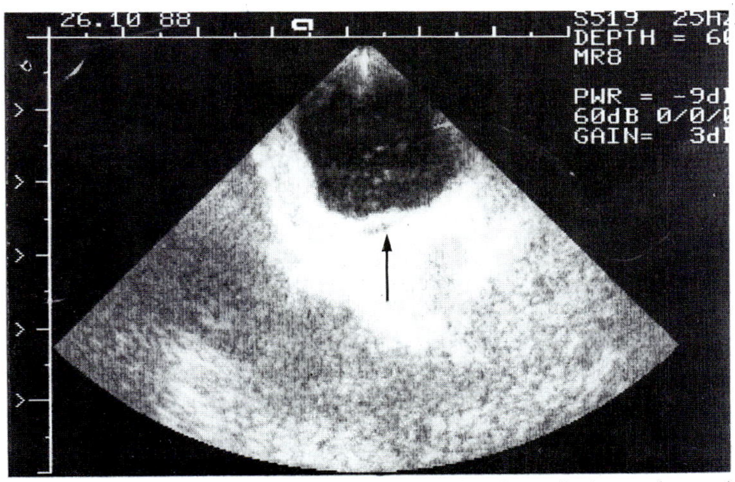

32.4

32.4 B-mode ultrasonograph showing scleral staphyloma (arrow) with overlying gliosed retina – diagnosed as retinal detachment.

The choice of intraocular lens

For a colobomatous eye of *normal* dimensions, a posterior chamber IOL of one piece PMMA with a 10° angulation of highly flexible haptics and a plano convex or biconvex 7 mm optic incorporating a u.v. filter, but no laser ridge or positioning holes, is recommended (**32.5**). The haptics should not be closed or have dialling holes (**32.6**), notches or end knobs, for these hinder explantation should it be necessary. It is prudent not to consider the use of soft lenses in abnormally developed eyes until more is learned from long-term studies in normal eyes.

For *microphthalmos* with coloboma, although most one-piece lenses have flexible loops, the overall loop spans of 13.5–14.0 mm are too large for a small eye (**32.7, 32.8**), especially since PMMA does not lose memory, so the loops retain a spring-like action, which will distort the lens capsule and adjacent structures. A PMMA lens with a 6 mm optic and a loop span of 12.0–12.5 mm may be appropriate (**32.9**).

32.5

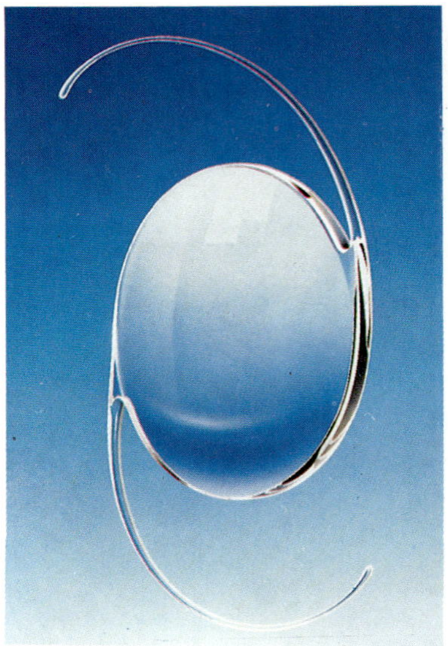

32.5 Iolab Formflex II lens 6840B, which for a 2 mm compression requires a force of 0.08 gm.

32.6

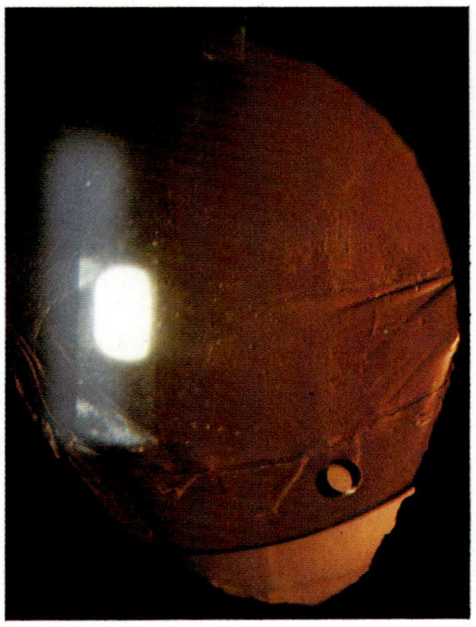

32.6 After ECCE with a wide capsulotomy the haptic has been dialled out of the colobomatous area, but a dialling hole remains, which may cause problems.

32.7

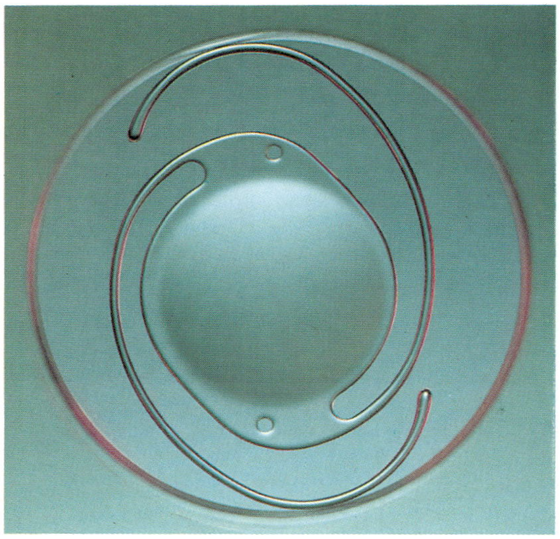

32.7 Rayner 200U encircling loop (Arnott style), with a 13.5 mm loop span, shown within a 10 mm space. The compression force required was 0.99 gm. Note that when conforming to a circle, loops do not necessarily encircle the optic and that the two-point fixation within the bag may be maintained (courtesy of Rayner Intraocular Lenses Ltd).

32.8

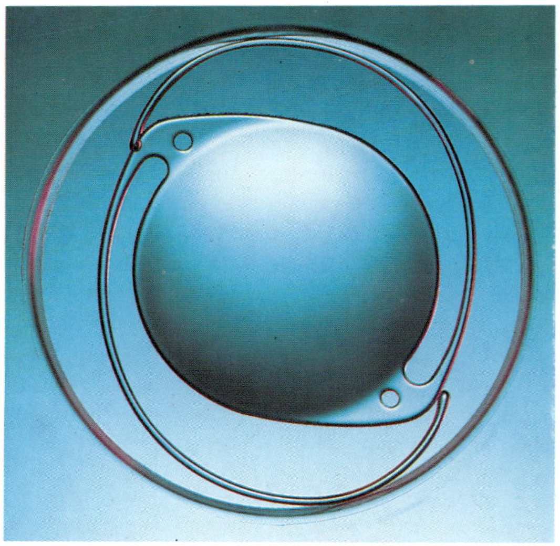

32.8 Rayner Interflex 250U, 14 mm loop span, shown within a 10 mm space. The compression force required was 0.17 gm (courtesy of Rayner Intraocular Lenses Ltd).

32.9

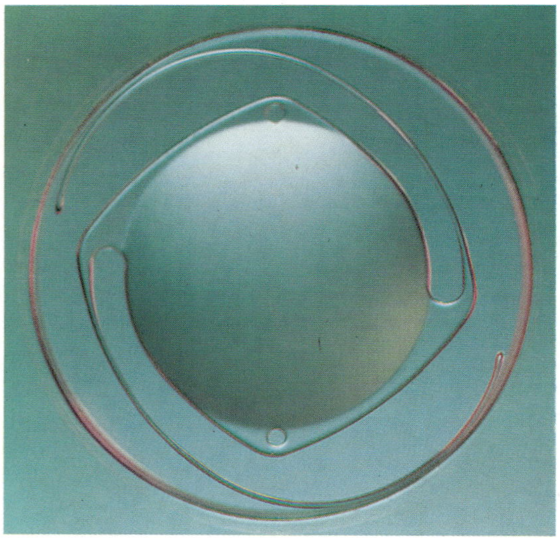

32.9 Rayner 210U, 12.5 mm loop span, shown within a 10 mm space. The compression force required was 0.14 gm. Note the even fit of loops within the circle (courtesy of Rayner Intraocular Lenses Ltd).

Force–compression ratios for some of the more flexible PMMA looped lenses now available (**32.10**) indicate the special attention required.

Galand has shown considerable variation in the dimensions of the capsular sac in cadaver eyes (p.117) and in microphthalmos the capsule diameter may be less than 9 mm. The diameter of the cornea will not necessarily be a guide to the diameter of the lens. Small corneas may be associated with lenses and axial lengths that are only slightly undersized, just as eyes as short as 16 mm may be associated with normal corneas. Therefore, the diameter of the capsular fornix should be assessed prior to lens insertion using a Sheet's glide as a dipstick. For estimated diameters greater than 8.5 mm the most suitable lens could be the 9 mm compressible disc (**32.11**).

Nanophthalmos: in the rare event of a cataract in an eye with pure microphthalmos, the resultant aphakic hypermetropia may be so great that spectacle correction will be needed in addition to the pseudophakos. These eyes may require individually made lenses or the safer option of no implantation.

32.10

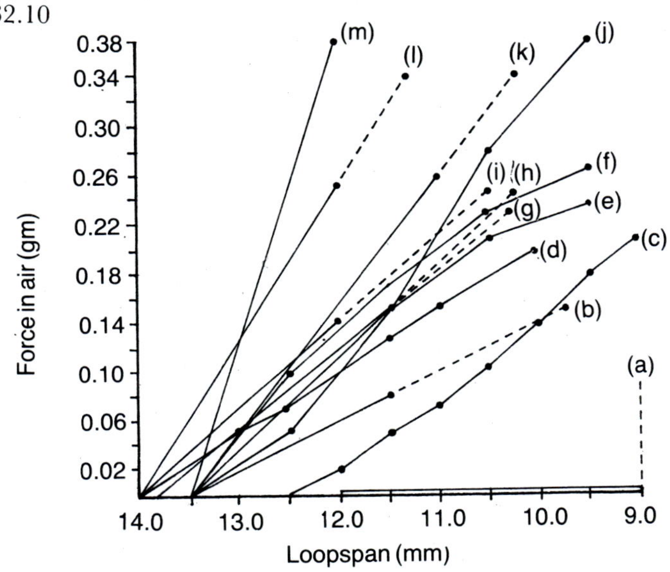

32.10 The most flexible loop lenses recommended by various companies for flexion into a 10 mm space. Solid lines represent figures released by the companies, broken lines represent the projected further flexion: (a) Pharmacia 9 mm Compressible Disc; (b) Iolab Formflex II 8640B; (c) Rayner 12.5 mm lens 210U; (d) Rayner Interflex 250U; (e) Alcon CVC IUO; (f) Alcon JF4 MUO; (g) 3M 17XE; (h) Iolab Capsulform 6440; (i) Allergan PC 24 NB; (j) Pharmacia 720; (k) 3M 190; (l) Pharmacia 725; (m) Rayner Postflex 200U.

32.11

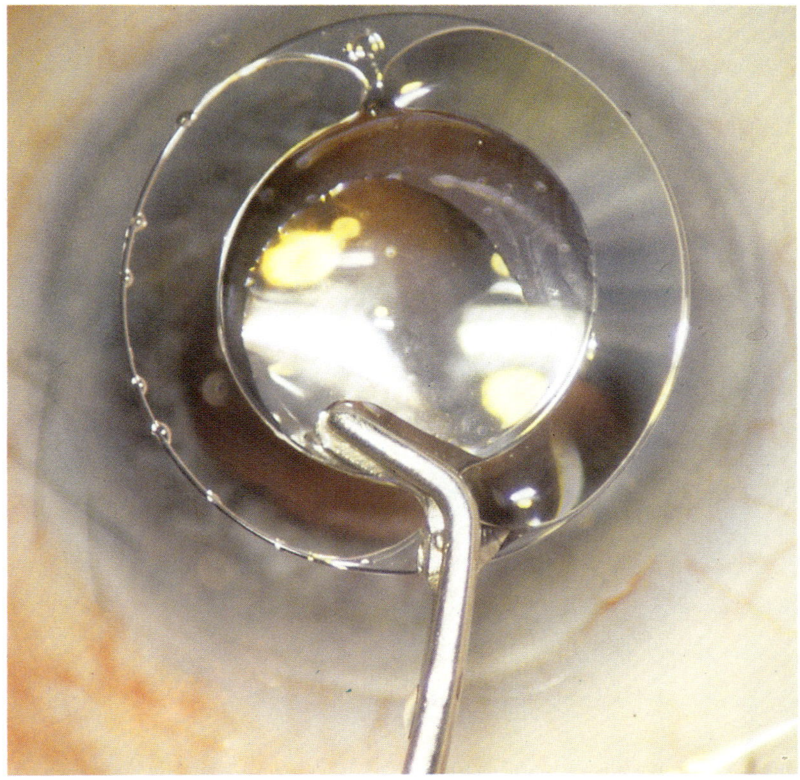

32.11 9 mm Compressible Disc lens overlying a normal sized eye.

Surgical technique

The surgeon's usual extracapsular technique may need no particular alteration (**32.12, 32.13**), but certain points merit emphasis. The entire procedure should be performed using a viscoelastic substance, which must be removed at the end of surgery.

32.12

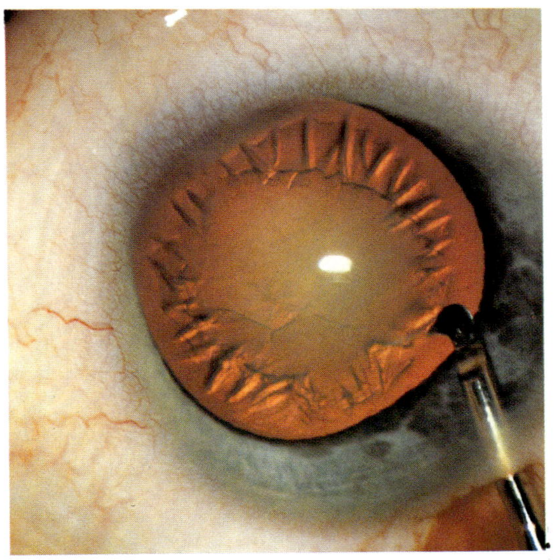

32.12 Mydriasis may be surprisingly good and allow an easy can-opener capsulotomy.

32.13

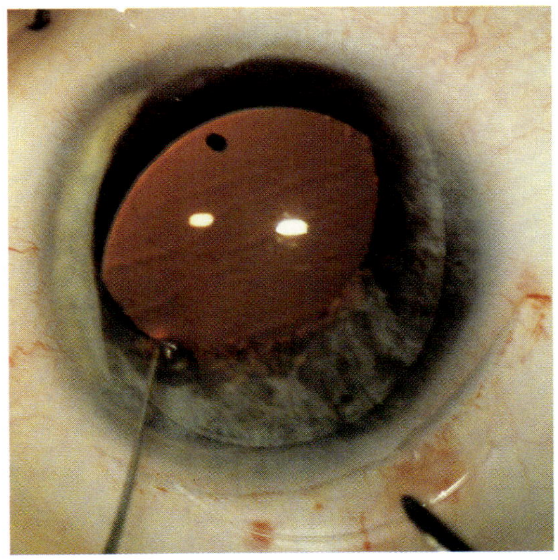

32.13 In-the-bag implantation of an Iolab Formflex II achieved by retracting the iris with the nondominant hand. Same eye as in **32.12**.

- Maximal mydriasis is essential prior to and during surgery. In cases of poor mydriasis (**32.14, 32.15**), a central iridectomy or superior sphincterotomy is performed under sodium hyaluronate (see **32.20**). This will improve pupillary centration as well as access to the lens capsule. A linear capsulotomy is the easiest approach for small pupils (**32.16**). It is unnecessary, and hazardous to the corneal endothelium, to try to close the inferior coloboma.
- If there is a coloboma of the zonule, the greatest care must be taken in performing the adjacent anterior capsulotomy. Vitreous does not usually present through the coloboma in the undisturbed state. After the nucleus is removed, the posterior lens capsule will wrinkle in the area adjacent to the zonular coloboma.
- Cataract extraction may be carried out by phacoemulsification, by standard extracapsular lens extraction or by the intercapsular technique. For nucleus extraction, it may be wise to offset the center of the section temporally (**32.16**), so that as pressure is applied to express the nucleus, it is applied well away from the area of zonular weakness. Great care must be taken with capsulorhexis adjacent to a weak area.
- In-the-bag implantation is made easier after phacoemulsification or standard ECCE by improving the visibility of the bag. This is done by using a Kuglen hook or Graether collar-button iris manipulator, held in the nondominant hand. The iris is pushed out of the way of the advancing lower haptic and subsequently the iris is retracted as the upper haptic is looped into the superior capsular bag (**32.13**). Placement of loops should avoid the area of likely zonular dehiscence. If necessary, the IOL is then dialled only so far as to move any haptic out of the iris coloboma to reduce postoperative glitter or glare.
- The intercapsular technique will ensure easy visibility of anterior capsular flaps during surgery and a small anterior capsulectomy will allow sufficient opacification of the remaining anterior capsule to avoid a halo of aphakic vision inferiorly (**32.17**). Comparison should be made with the effect of ICCE with an anterior chamber implant and the inevitable halo of aphakic vision (**32.18**). Apart from small pupils, the intercapsular technique is also recommended for small eyes when the compressible disc may be considered suitable (**32.19–32.24**).

32.14

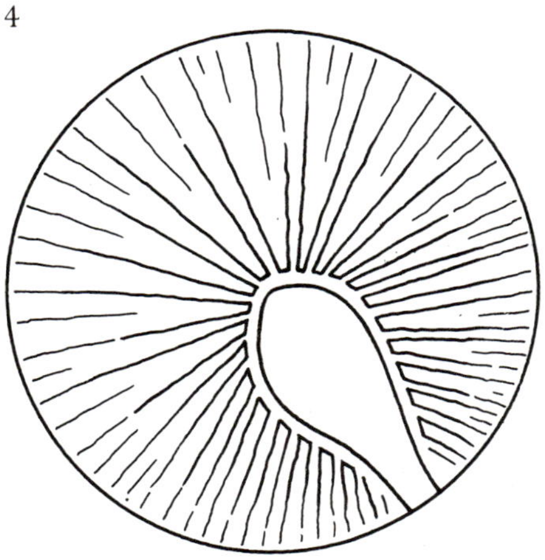

32.14 Diagramatic appearance of **32.17** before surgery, pupil undilated.

32.15

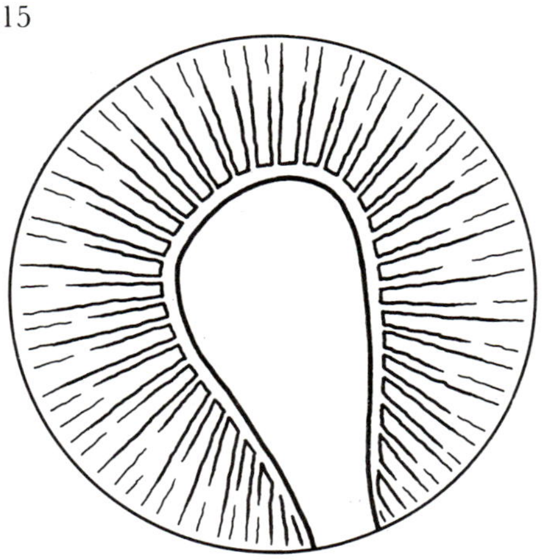

32.15 Diagramatic appearance of **32.17** before surgery, pupil dilated.

32.16

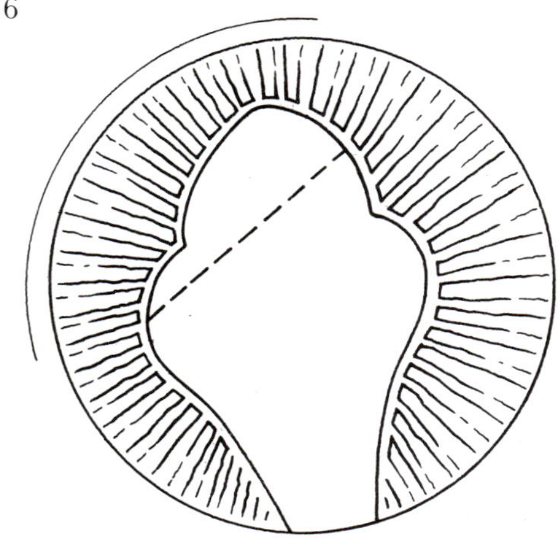

32.16 Diagram of **32.15** after sphincterotomy, showing the linear capsulotomy at a slant and temporal extension of the wound.

32.17

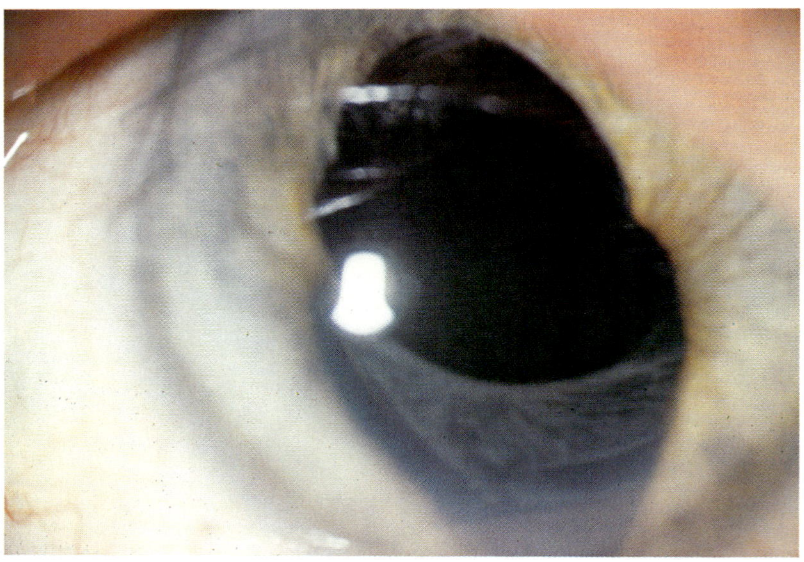

32.17 Posterior chamber lens in a colobomatous eye showing the improved centration of the pupil by performing a superior sphincterotomy and a capsulotomy small enough to allow fibrosis to cover the coloboma inferiorly.

32.18

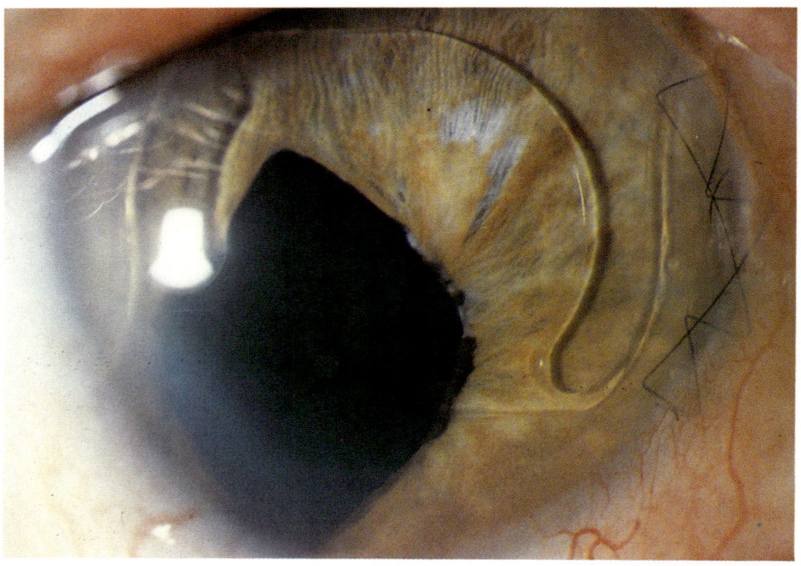

32.18 Fellow eye of that in **32.17**. After ICCE and a failed contact lens trial, a secondary ACL was implanted, with a superior sphincterotomy to improve centration of the pupil. Note halo of aphakic vision.

32.19

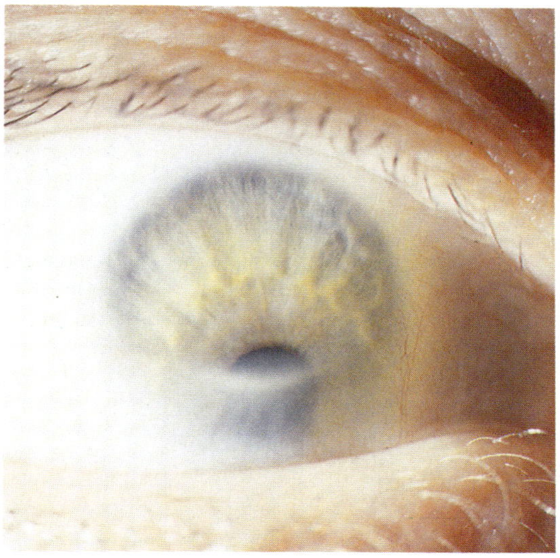

32.19 Severe developmental abnormality: corneal diameter 7 mm, complete coloboma, nystagmus and inferior corneal opacity. The fellow eye was amblyopic and had a corneal diameter of 5 mm.

32.20

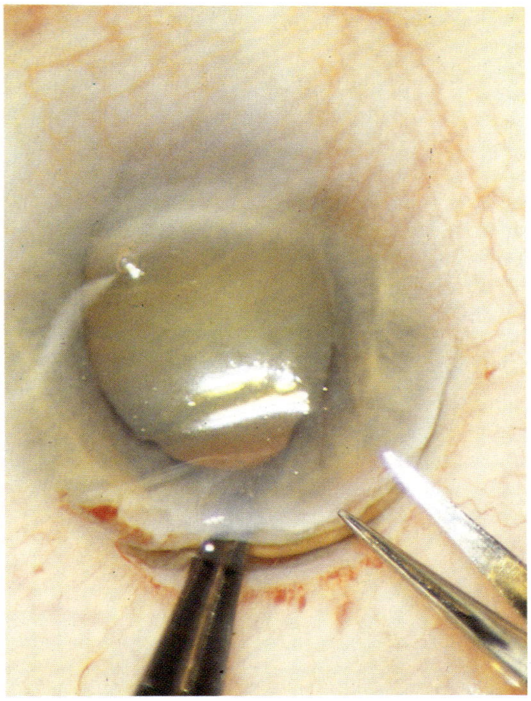

32.20 Superior central iridectomy after maximal mydriasis, same eye as in **32.19**.

32.21

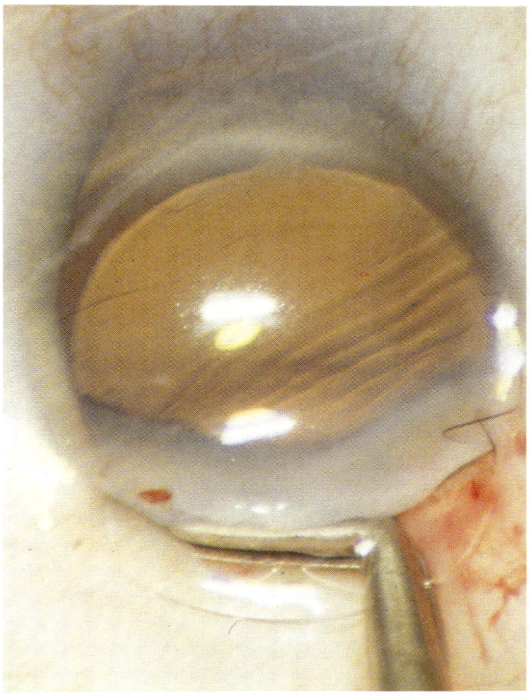

32.21 Implantation of a Compressible Disc into the capsular sac under sodium hyaluronate. Note the 9 mm disc can be compressed through a 6 mm wound. The optic diameter is 6 mm, the corneal diameter 7 mm. Compare with **32.11**.

32.22

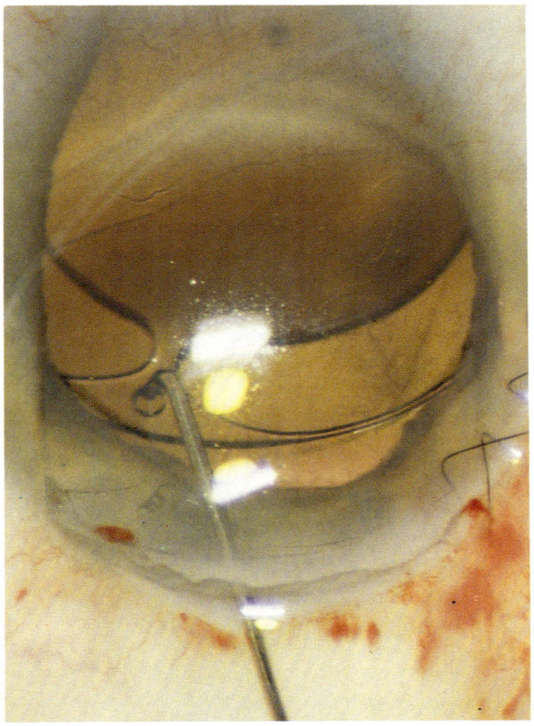

32.22 The dialling hole is now rotated through 90° with a Sinskey hook. Note that in this eye the superior position of the wound has been chosen for insertion of the implant. A temporal approach is preferred.

32.23

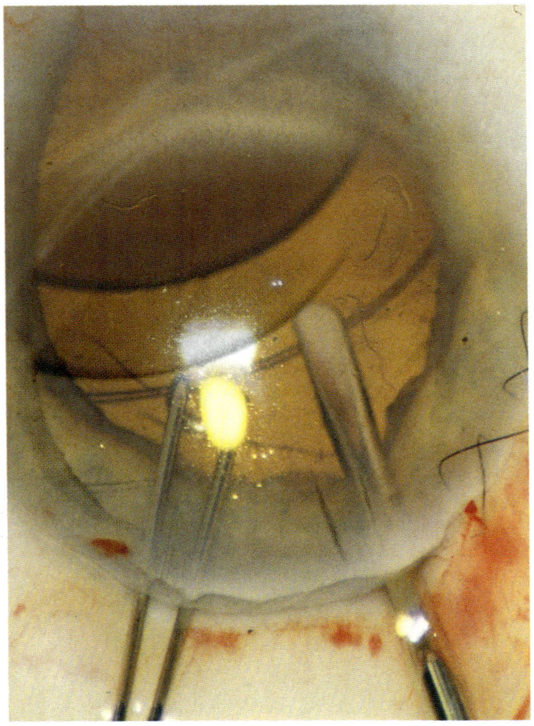

32.23 The upper rim of the capsule is now retracted with one hand, while the upper rim of the lens is flexed behind with a notched hook. Minimal downward pressure should be exerted on the lens.

32.24

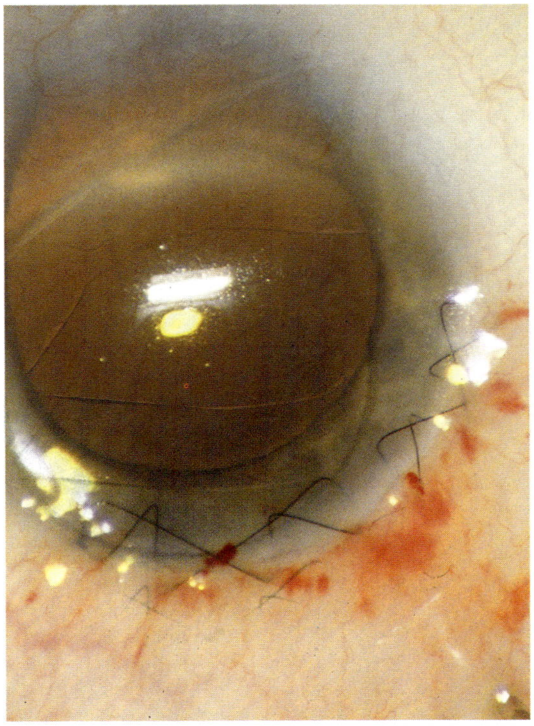

32.24 After a small capsulorhexis the wound is closed and the lens remains totally within the capsular sac.

Complications

Specific operative complications may be anticipated with congenital defects unless due care is taken as described above. If the posterior lens capsule is ruptured without incurring vitreous loss and sufficient capsule remains to provide a safe support, a posterior chamber IOL may be placed with the haptics directed into the ciliary sulcus away from the area of zonular weakness. If vitreous is lost, automated anterior vitrectomy should be performed. If there is insufficient posterior lens capsule to support an IOL, a secondary anterior chamber IOL should be implanted horizontally with the haptics lying to either side of the coloboma (**32.18**). Sunset syndrome may arise postoperatively if an area of zonular dehiscence has been extended at surgery. This may require explantation within the lens capsule and, if the eye is of normal size, be replaced by an anterior chamber lens. Microphthalmic eyes should not receive anterior chamber lenses.

Further reading

Davison, J.A. A short haptic diameter modified J-loop intraocular lens for improved capsular bag performance. *J. Cataract Refract. Surg.*, **14,** 161–166, 1988.

Duke-Elder, W.S. *System of Ophthalmology*, Vol 3, 456–481, H.Kimpton, London, 1964.

Jaffe, N.S. and Clayman, H.M. Cataract extraction in eyes with congenital colobomata. *J. Cataract Refract. Surg.* **13,** 54–58, 1987.

33: High myopia

Piers Percival and Georges Baikoff

Persons with axial high myopia (HM), even when phakic, are predisposed to choroidoretinal atrophy, macular hemorrhage, lattice degeneration, retinal breaks, vitreous traction and retinal detachment (RD). Custin has suggested that the life time risk of RD with myopia greater than –5.0D is approximately 2.4%, 40 times higher than that for emmetropes (0.06%).

Definition of high myopia

Preoperative refraction is no exact index since it does not exclude myopia of a lenticular origin. Postoperative refraction excludes myopias of a lenticular nature, but does not exclude those myopias that are caused by high corneal curvature. Likewise, the implanted IOL power is not a precise parameter, as lenses have different *A* constants of calculation. This method also is unable to exclude myopias due to high corneal curvature. The most exact method is that based on axial length. On consideration of mean values for emmetropic eyes, the mean keratometry approximates to 43.6D and the mean axial length to 23.2 mm. If the keratometric value is kept unchanged and an attempt is made to equate data for a myopia with spectacles of –6.00D, the axial length must be increased by approximately 3.3 mm (equivalent to approximately 9D of implant power). Thus, the deriving value of an axial length of 26.50 mm or greater is recommended for standardizing the definition of high myopia.

Incidence of retinal detachment following cataract surgery

In the absence of HM the incidence of RD following ECCE may be as low as 0.2%, provided the posterior capsule remains intact, but rises substantially if complications occur at surgery or the capsule is later opened. Difficulty in computing the exact statistics on the incidence of RD arises from a variance in reporting of the definition of myopia (by refraction or axial length), length of follow up of the groups studied, whether surgical complications are included, breakdown of patients with primary or secondary capsulotomy, and decimation of numbers by inadequate follow up.

High incidences may be weighted by high risk cases, e.g. family history of RD, fellow eye RD, or vitreous loss at surgery. From a review of the literature and personal observation, an attempt to indicate the expected chance of RD in cases without such risks is shown in **Table 33.1**. The higher the axial length, the higher the chance of RD. Males are more predisposed to RD than females. Some protection is afforded by an intact posterior capsule and it is reasonable to recommend an IOL for all high myopes who have cataract, *even if the requirement is for a plano power*. The reasons for this are that the patient may be offered near to emmetropic vision without glasses and that the need for secondary capsulotomy will be substantially reduced by capsule fixation of a posterior vaulted lens.

Table 33.1 Approximate incidence of retinal detachment to be expected within 3 years of uncomplicated surgery.

	Axial length		
	< 25 mm	25–26.5 mm	> 26.5 mm
ICCE	1%	6%	11%
ECCE open capsule	0.7%	3.5%	8%
ECCE closed capsule	0.2%	0.8%	4%

Note: incidence should be raised by a multiple of 6 if vitreous loss occurs at surgery.

Prophylaxis for retinal detachment

Prophylactic cryocoagulation or photocoagulation for high risk cases not only fails to eliminate later RD, but may also contribute to other pathologies, such as macular pucker. The recommended routine is not for preoperative treatment, but for a regular examination of the peripheral fundus postoperatively. Treatment is recommended if a retinal break is discovered, or if equatorial or peripheral retinal pathology is discovered in association with a past RD in either eye, a family history of RD or recent symptoms.

Choice of IOL

One-piece PMMA looped posterior chamber lenses are recommended for HM, with wide-diameter optics for improving the visibility of the fundus periphery. For capsular bag fixation the loop span should be 13.0–13.5 mm, and for ciliary sulcus fixation it should be 13.5–14.0 mm. The loops should be angulated forwards 20° and the optic should be biconvex or convex posterior in order to lessen the migration of epithelial cells over the posterior capsule. Power calculation should aim for low myopia (–1.0D ± 1D).

Clear lens extraction

The case for clear lens extraction, although recommended by some for patients with myopia over 2D yet intolerant to both contact lenses and spectacles, has been refuted by Goldberg and by many others. The surgery is not without an increased risk of RD (**Table 33.1**). This risk may be increased by between six and ten times if vitreous loss occurs, which although rare is an unpredictable event. Accommodation is lost and visual results are far from spectacular even in younger patients. Alternative treatments for those requiring spectacle power in excess of –12.0D and who are failed contact lens wearers include epikeratophakia, keratomilieusis, intracorneal inlays and anterior chamber lenses.

AC lenses in phakic eyes

Lens design

In the 1960s, in parallel with the development of implants for aphakia, Barraquer and Strampelli attempted the correction of high myopia by the introduction of a negative lens in the anterior chamber. However, shortly after their debut, the lenses were roundly criticized and ultimately rejected. Today the implants in the anterior chamber derived from the Kelman multiflex are those that are the best tolerated. Three models of AC implants for the correction of myopia have now appeared: the implants of J. Worst and P. Fechner of the iris claw type (see p. 86), composite implants of the angle support type (Praeger, Momose) and the Baikoff design (**33.1**).

The mode of fixation for a phakic eye merits some discussion. The Worst and Fechner iris claw lens has no contact with ocular structures except for the iris. It presupposes the introduction of a needle under the iris to bring it to the lens claw and carries a risk of damage to the crystalline lens. Fyodorov proposed the introduction into the posterior chamber of silicone lenses that lie on the anterior face of the crystalline lens. Results are not yet known, but one drawback is that the contact of silicone on the crystalline lens may encourage cataract formation. Also, the thick peripheral borders might be expected to cause significant iris chafing.

The anatomy of the anterior segment is different in phakia from that in aphakia, and the anterior chamber implant for high myopia must have a different profile from that used in aphakia. Vaulting is pronounced (**33.2**), so that the optic is 1 mm in front of the pupil and 2 mm behind the central corneal endothelium. Contact with intraocular structures is limited to four points on the scleral spur and there is no risk of contact with the lens, which is suspended by the zonule. Since the optic edge is necessarily thick, the optic diameter has to be limited to 4.5 mm. The power has no limit. These implants are designed to correct from –9 to –30D.

33.1

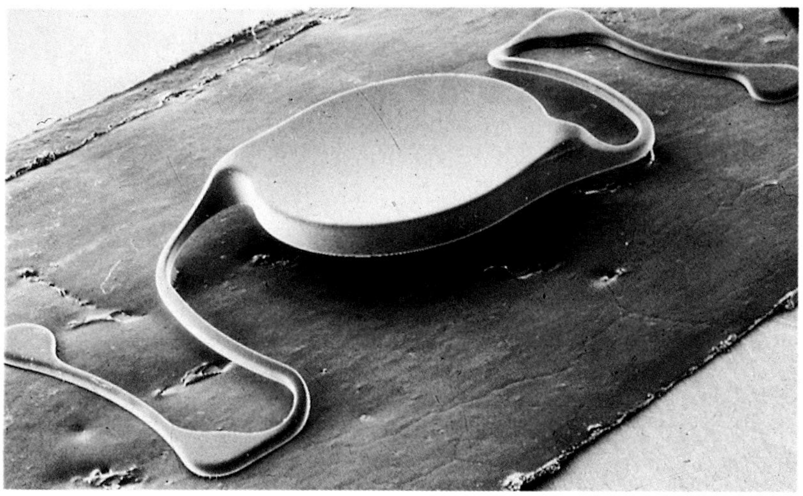

33.1 Appearance of the Baikoff implant by scanning microscopy. Note that the precise vaulting of the loops permits the lens to be in front of the iris surface and the natural crystalline lens.

33.2

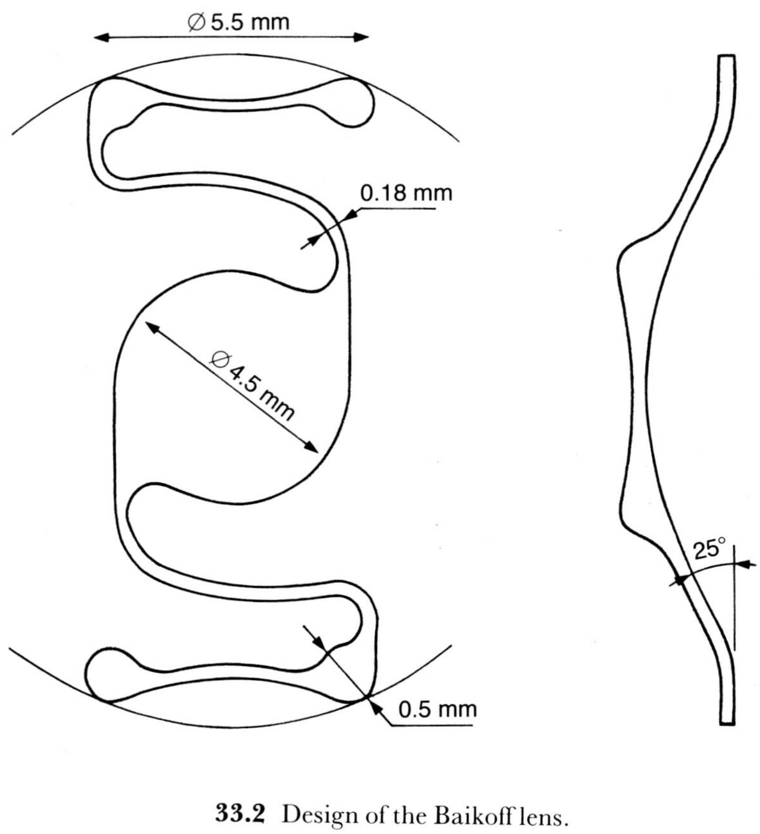

33.2 Design of the Baikoff lens.

Technique

Implantation is similar to that of secondary implantation in aphakia. The particular vaulting of the lens and the absence of contact with the structures of the iris make an iridectomy unnecessary (**33.3**). There is no risk of mechanical pupillary block. If inflammatory pupillary block arises, mydriasis must be instituted.

As we have not observed alteration of the crystalline lens, or persistent inflammatory reaction, or the development of goniosynechias, we believe there to be little risk of iatrogenic cataract or glaucoma. Accommodation is preserved. The pupil reacts normally (**33.4**) and may be dilated if necessary (**33.5**). There is no stress on the posterior segment, which rests intact after the procedure. These points are particularly advantageous if one compares the procedure to clear lens extraction, where there is a risk of inducing capsular opacification, retinal detachment and macular edema.

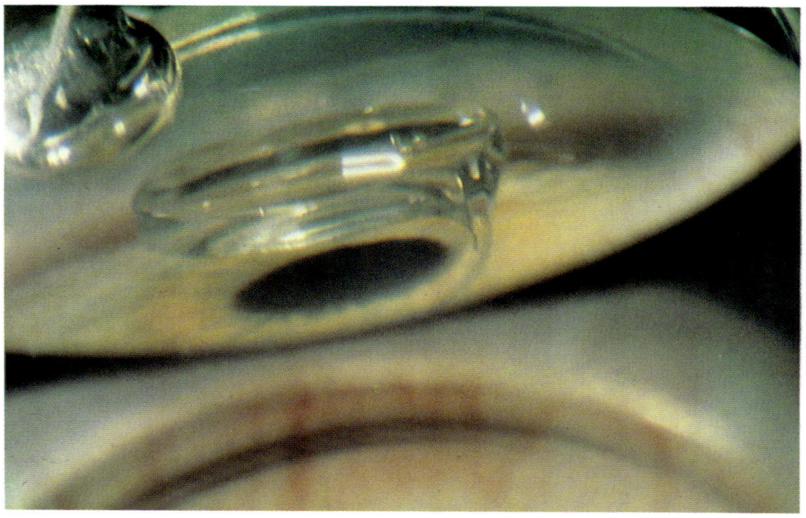
33.3

33.3 Gonioscopy of the lens *in situ*. The posterior face of the implant is 1 mm in front of the pupil. The anterior face is 2 mm behind the cornea.

33.4
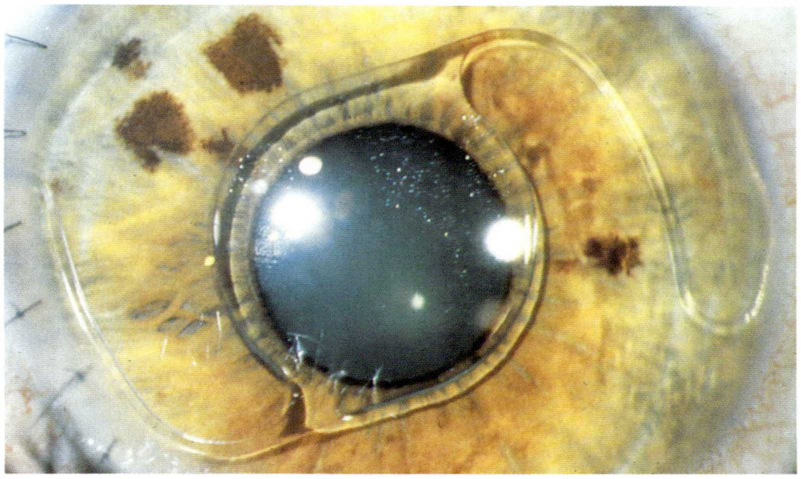

33.4 Negative implant in the phakic eye several months after surgery.

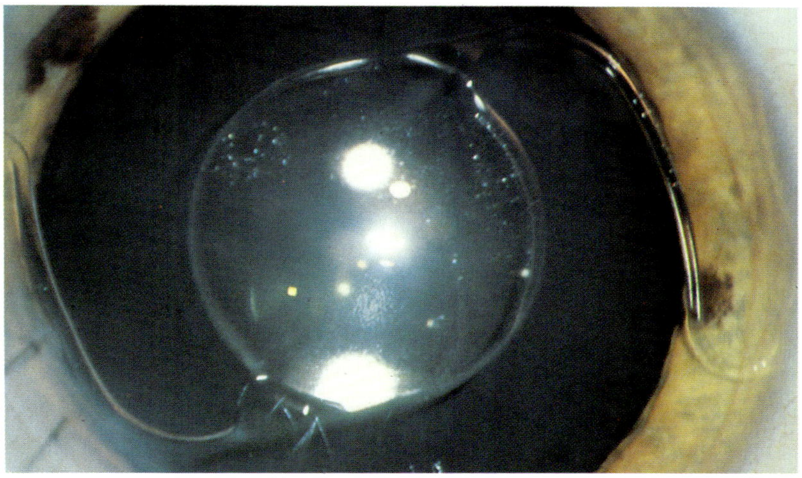
33.5

33.5 Same eye as in **33.4** with the pupil dilated. Visual access to the fundus of the eye is obtained without difficulty.

Results

A study conducted by five independent groups in France between October 1987 and February 1989 encompassed 103 operated eyes. Seventy-four patients underwent surgery: the mean age was 35 (with a range of 20–55 years). The mean myopia was –15.26 D (with a range of –8 to –25 D).

On day one, the mean visual acuity was 0.37, and at the end of six months 0.45. Following refraction, the mean distant acuity was increased to 0.7 (20/30), representing a gain comparable to that obtained preoperatively with contact lenses. There was no case of a decrease in corrected visual acuity, as may be found after epikeratophakia. The mean refractive error (spherical equivalent), was less than 1 D (a range of –4 to +2 D). Complications included a 5% incidence of uveitis, necessitating intensive local treatment with corticosteroids, and a 4% incidence of later lens rotation within the anterior chamber. One hypopyon was noted, which resolved without sequel. In no case did the uveitis incur visual damage. There were no cases of glaucoma, secondary cataract or any posterior segment complications. The mean endothelial cell loss after two months was approximately 4%, but further studies are required to determine whether this could be progressive.

Further reading

Custin B.J. *The Myopias: Basic Science and Clinical Management.* Philadelphia, Harper & Row, 1985.

Dardenne M.U., Gerten G.J., Kokkas K. and Kermani O. Retrospective study of retinal detachment following neodymium:YAG laser posterior capsulotomy. *J. Cat. Refr. Surgery,* **15,** 676–680, 1989.

Davison J.A. Retinal tears and detachments after extracapsular cataract surgery. *J. Cat. Refractive Surg.*, **14,** 624–632, 1988.

Goldberg M.F. Clear lens extraction for axial myopia. *Ophthalmology,* **94,** 571–582, 1987.

Percival S.P.B. High myopia: new definitions and significance of IOL implantation. *European J. Implant Refractive Surg.*, **4,** 137–140, 1986.

Van der Heije G.L. Some optical aspects of implantation of an IOL in a myopic eye. *European J. Implant Refractive Surg.*, **1,** 245–248, 1989.

34: Exfoliation syndrome (pseudoexfoliation of the lens capsule)

Ahti Tarkkanen

Clinical features

Exfoliation syndrome (ES) is characterized by grayish flecks that coat the surfaces of the anterior of the eye (**34.1**). The deposits can be found on the lens capsule, the ciliary processes, the zonules and the pupillary margin. The pathological deposits produce three different zones on the anterior lens capsule: a translucent central disc; a granular girdle around the periphery, called a peripheral band; and a clear zone separating these two areas. The central disc in the pupillary area may be quite faint and is easily missed without the dilatation of the pupil. Its border, however, is then exposed and is more clearly outlined by a few dandruff-like deposits and a grayish white ring at the edge. The central disc is not a constant feature of exfoliation. The peripheral band, however, is always present, and shows the characteristic granular appearance. The clear intermediate zone contains no deposits. Occasionally, however, one may see some loose flakes and a bridge extending from the peripheral band to the central disc. In addition, the flakes have been observed as precipitates on the posterior surface of the cornea, floating freely in the anterior chamber, on the anterior surface of the iris, in the pupillary border, and in aphakic eyes on the hyaloid. The pupillary border may appear atrophic with a characteristic 'moth-eaten' appearance. Transillumination of the iris in the midperiphery is often seen. On gonioscopy, the pigmentation of the trabecular meshwork may be seen to extend anterior to Schwalbe's line (Sampaolesi's line).

ES is known to be age-dependent. There is a clear increase with advancing age. The prevalence is low in populations aged less than 60 years while there is an increase from 1% in the age group 60–69 years to 4.8% in the group 70–79 years. In populations aged 80 years or more, the prevalence has been found to be over 8%. There are exceptional populations, though, in which the appearance of ES seems to take place about 10 years earlier. Familial occurrence of exfoliation syndrome has been described by several authors. ES has now been described in practically all populations of the world, but recent data support the opinion that ES is not uniformally distributed in different countries.

About 20% of patients with ES show abnormalities of intraocular pressure. This data can lead to the conclusion that glaucoma capsulare results from an overload of an already impaired drainage system by exfoliation material and by pigment granules. This combination is often followed by high intraocular pressures and a rapid loss of visual field. Corticosteroid testing has indicated that primary open-angle glaucoma and glaucoma capsulare are separate disease processes.

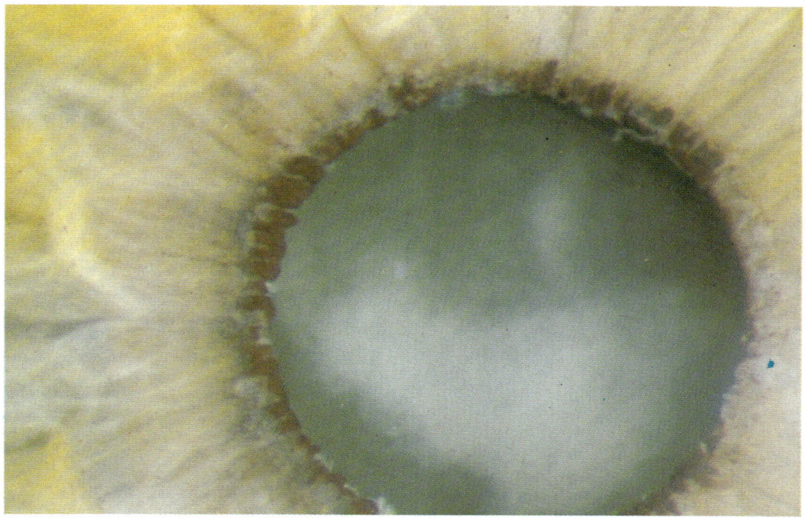

34.1

34.1 Dandruff-like flakes of exfoliation at the pupillary border in a cataractous eye.

Pathology

Exfoliation material shows a fibrillar structure. The fibrils are 20–30 nm thick with 10 nm subunits and may be 800–900 nm long. Sometimes they may show a banding periodicity of 50 nm. The material arises probably from the ciliary body, perhaps as the result of an unknown metabolic disorder. From these areas, the material enters the aqueous humor and is deposited on the anterior lens capsule, zonules, vitreous face, iris, trabecular meshwork and corneal endothelium. Histochemical studies have demonstrated the presence of glycosaminoglycans. Our recent results on lectin binding to the exfoliative material show that glycoconjugates present in the superficial zonular lamella, the zonular fibers and the nonpigmented epithelium of the ciliary body, have a rather similar lectin-binding profile as compared with those of the exfoliation material. Of interest is that the lens capsule was essentially unreactive with all the lectins used.

Cataract surgery

Cataract surgery (**Flowchart 34.1**) in ES may be linked with several problems. Eyes with ES may show spontaneous subluxation of the lens in 2% of cases, which may go unnoticed owing to the absence of iridodonesis. This may be explained by an increased iris rigidity through infiltration of the iris stroma by exfoliation material. There may be a strong bonding of the posterior surface of the iris to the pre-equatorial lens capsule, preventing good pupillary dilatation. The zonular fibers are known to be weak in ES and the central posterior lens capsule very thin. The ciliary epithelium may show marked degenerative changes (**34.2**). These features make ES a major risk factor in extracapsular cataract surgery. In one series of unselected cataract operations the incidence of vitreous loss was 1.8% in cataracts without ES, and 9% in those with ES. When in doubt, sector iridotomy is preferred and the haptics of the intraocular lens should be placed into the ciliary sulcus. Anterior chamber intraocular lenses are not recommended in ES, because the haptics in the chamber angle may further compromise aqueous outflow. In our studies on autopsy eyes the sulcus–sulcus distance was found to be 14 mm. Therefore, the IOL of choice would be that with a 14 mm overall haptic diameter.

Elevated intraocular pressures in eyes with ES are commonly found. Hence, it is essential to measure intraocular pressure on the first morning after surgery. If the pressure is elevated, topical beta-blocking agents and/or oral acetazolamide have to be administered. Furthermore, the blood–aqueous barrier may break down during ECCE due to degenerative changes in the ciliary epithelium, as well as to pathological fenestrations of the iris capillaries. This in turn may lead to massive fibrinous exudation into the aqueous humor. At the end of the operation, a paraocular injection of steroids is recommended, as well as hourly topical corticosteroids if signs of fibrinous exudate appear (see p. 249).

34.2

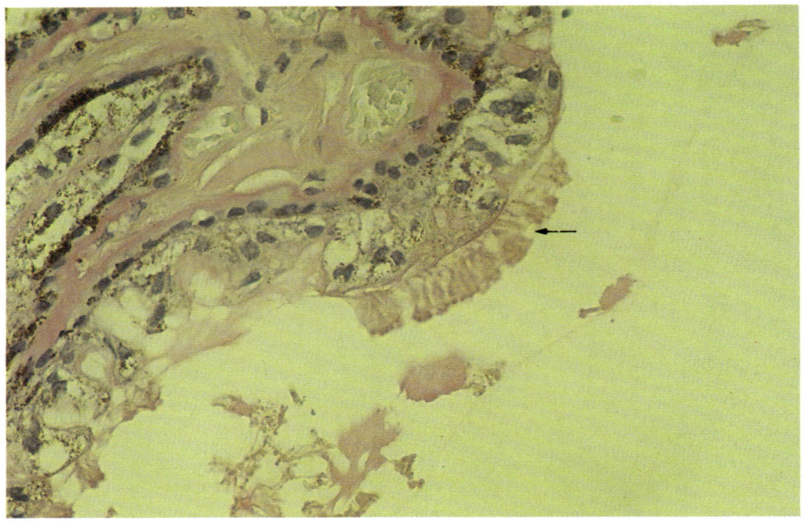

34.2 Brush-like depositions (arrow) of exfoliation on the ciliary epithelium. Both epithelial layers show marked degenerative changes.

Flow chart 34.1 Cataract surgery and IOL implantation in exfoliation syndrome (ES)

Preoperative	Full dilatation of the pupil,	If ES presents: • Rule out spontaneous subluxation • Check intraocular pressure carefully	If ocular hypertension or capsular glaucoma present: • Lower intraocular pressure by medication If capsular glaucoma is treatment resistant: • Consider glaucoma triple procedure
Intraoperative	Problems	• Poor pupillary dilatation • Weak zonules • Thin posterior capsule • Weak blood–aqueous barrier	Solutions • Phacoemulsification not recommended • Sector iridotomy may become necessary • Choice of IOL: 14 mm haptic diameter • Sulcus fixation preferred • Paraocular corticosteroids recommended
Postoperative	Measure intraocular pressure on the first morning		If elevated: • Lower by topical beta-blocking agents and oral acetazolamide
	Check the aqueous for fibrinous exudate		If present: • Hourly topical corticosteroids

Further reading

Naumann G.O.H. Exfoliation syndrome as a risk factor for vitreous loss in extracapsular cataract surgery. *Acta Ophthalmol.*, **66,** Suppl.184, 129–131, 1988.

Ruotsalainen J. and Tarkkanen A. Capsule thickness of cataractous lenses with and without exfoliation syndrome. *Acta Ophthalmol.*, **65,** 444–449, 1987.

Tarkkanen A. and Forsius H. (Eds). Exfoliation syndrome. *Acta Ophthalmol.*, **66,** Suppl.184, 1988.

Section 5: HISTOPATHOLOGY

35: Biocompatibility

Akio Yamanaka

What are the characteristics of a good IOL material? There are many points to consider, but the material should at least have good biocompatibility and not biodegrade in the eye. The polymers should have suitable refractive characteristics for the optic part of the lens, and compatible tensile strength and elasticity with the haptics. Biocompatibility consists of mechanical compatibility and interfacial compatibility.

Mechanical compatibility

Factors that influence biocompatibility at the macro level are shape, size, ease of manipulation during surgery, suitable fixation and softness of the IOL. In this regard, major advances have been made in recent years. For example, corneal dystrophy after using an iris clip lens with ICCE (**35.1**) is now avoided by switching the operation method to the use of the posterior chamber lens (PCL) with ECCE. In-the-bag fixation in ECCE with the use of viscoelastic material during surgery is expected to be safer still (**35.2**).

Compared with hard IOLs, soft IOLs are mechanically more physiological in terms of the softness of the living eye tissues from the biomimetic standpoint.

35.1

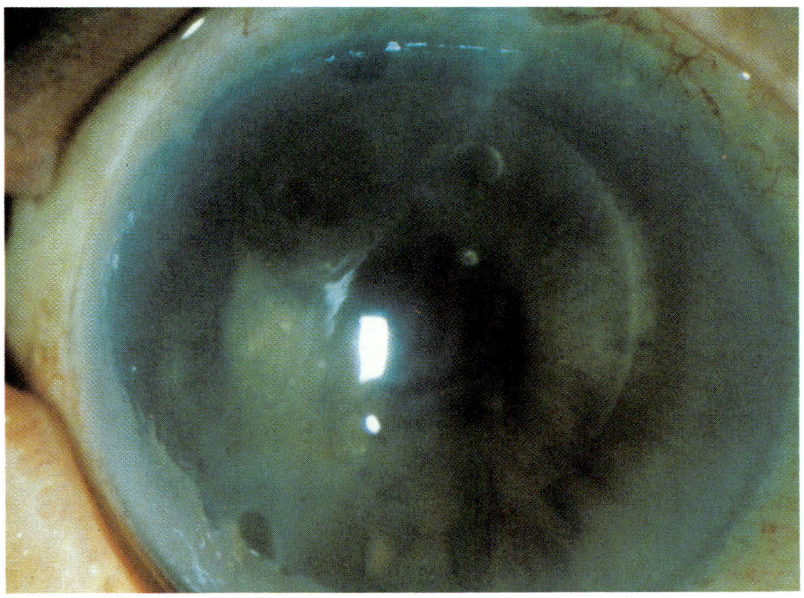

35.1 Endothelial corneal dystrophy caused by subluxation of the Medallion Lens.

35.2

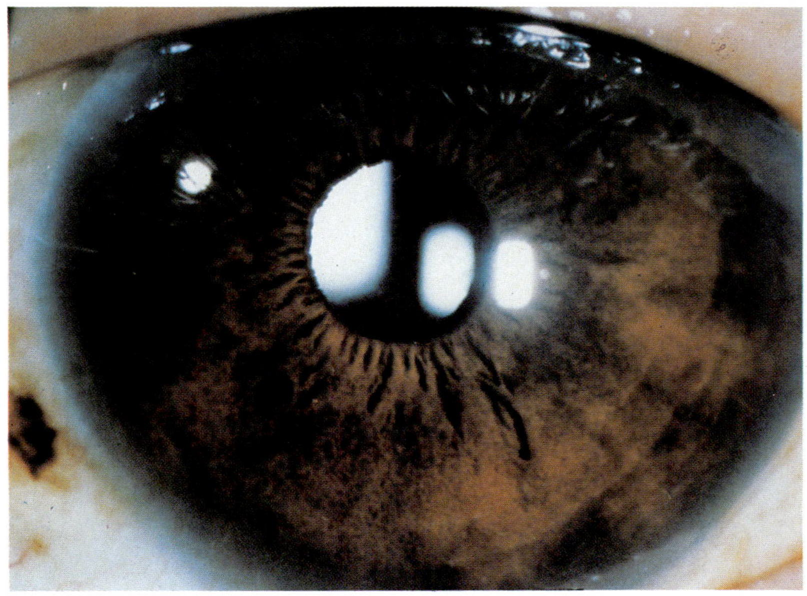

35.2 PMMA PCL *in situ*.

Interfacial compatibility

Factors that influence biocompatibility at the molecular level (**Table 35.1**) are measured by the contact angle of water to the plastic (wettability), the electric potential of the plastic surface, the rate of protein adsorption, the complement activation by the plastic, and the oil repellency.

Glow discharge, sputter etching, and grafting of the molecules onto the polymer surface are techniques for surface modification, which alter the surface character and can improve biocompatibility. However, for clinical use, especially in cases of molecular grafting, it is also essential to know the biocompatibility of the altered surfaces after biodegradation.

Table 35.1 Molecular factors for IOL biocompatibility

- Surface character
- Contact angle (wettability)
- Electric potential
- Water repellency
- Oil repellency
- Surface modification
- Complement activation for immunological reaction

The contact angle of water on the plastic surface is explained in **35.3**. A low contact angle shows good wettability; the higher the contact angle, the more hydrophobic is the material.

The relationship between cell culture and various kinds of plastic that have different surface contact angles is shown in **35.4** Polymethylmethacrylate (PMMA), 6-nylon, polyvinylidene fluoride (PVDF), polypropylene (PP) and polyethylene terephthalate (PET) were compared. From this cell culture experiment, it can be seen that biocompatibility at the cellular level, as judged by fibroblast cell growth on the surface, improves with moderate increases in wettability of the plastics. Surface treatment by glow discharge or sputter etching also decreases the contact angle and improves cell growth. However, not all plastics behave in the same way: for each there may be an optimum wettability beyond which the biocompatibility may decrease.

35.5 shows the cell growth on polymers used for IOLs, including silicone, polyhydroxyethylmethacrylate (PHEMA) and the new polyfluorocarbons. In this series it is clear that the roughness of the surface is one of the factors that influences cell growth on the plastics. If the surface is smooth, cells do not grow.

Although the role of the surface electric potential is not well known, it changes in proportion to the change of the contact angle and therefore may influence biocompatibility.

In conditions of an extremely high (very hydrophobic) or low (hydrophilic) contact angle, cells do not grow on the plastic **35.6**. The rate of adsorption of serum protein by each polymer is almost proportional to the contact angle and influences the complement activation.

35.3

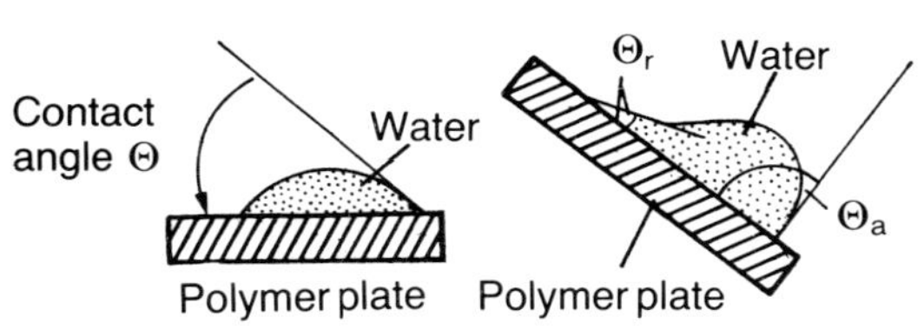

35.3 Contact angle of water droplet on polymer plate. $\cos\theta = (\cos\theta_a + \cos\theta_r)/2$, where θ_a is the advancing contact angle and θ_r is the receding contact angle.

35.4

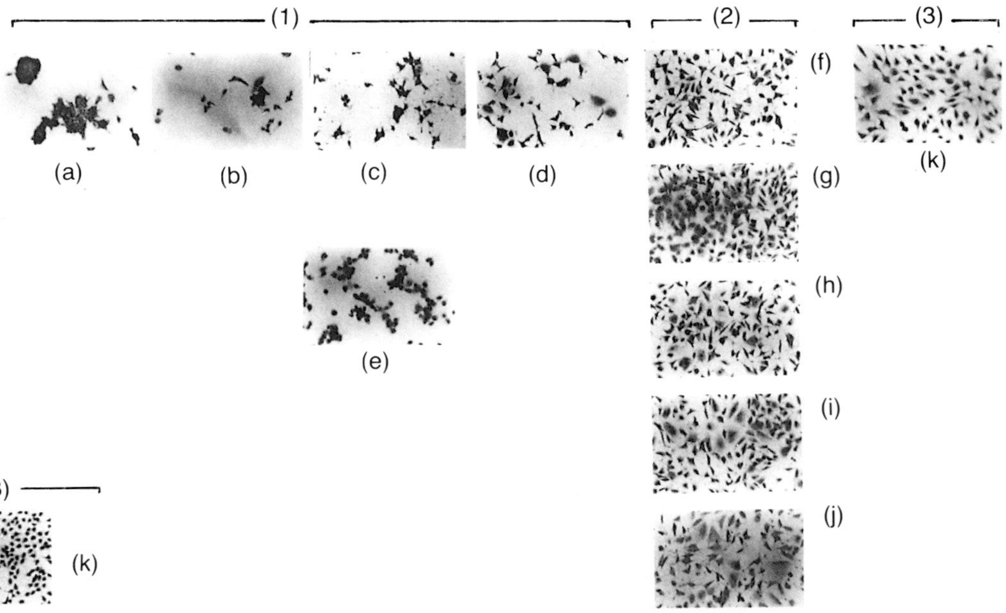

35.4 Relationship between contact angle (in brackets in list below) and biocompatibility of plastics judged by cell culture method. The surfaces of the plastics were treated by glow discharge under vacuum (0.17–0.19 mmHg). Fibroblasts of 3T3 mouse were seeded on the disinfected plastics and cultured for 24h in a 6 cm Falcon dish in MEM (Eagl's) +10% fetal calf serum, at 37°C, 5% CO_2 in air, then fixed with 100% ethanol and stained with Giemsa solution. An increase in wettability caused an increase in cell growth on the plastic surface. (1) *Not plasma irradiated*: (a) PP (94°); (b) PVDF (82°); (c) PMMA (68°); (d) 6-Nylon (57°); (e) PET (67°). (2) *Plasma irradiated*: (f) PMMA (47°); (g) PVDF (46°), (h) 6-Nylon (45°), (i) PET (44°), (j) PP (40°). (3) *Control*: (k) Falcon plastic dish (31°).

35.5

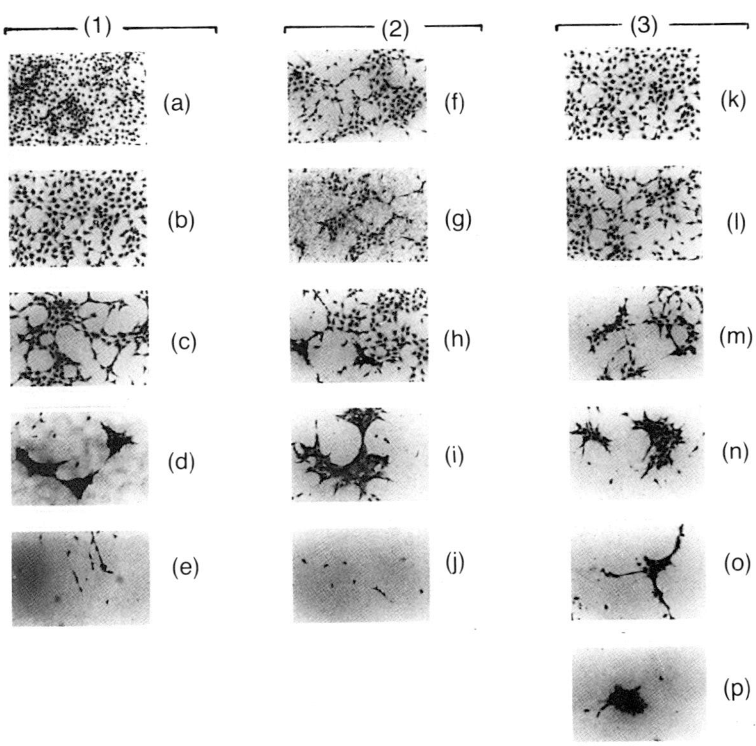

35.5 Biocompatibility of plastics judged by 3T3 cell culture (contact angle in brackets in list below). (1) *Polymers used for IOLs available on the market*: (a) Nylon (51°), (b) PVDF (82°), (c) PMMA (68°), (d) Isot. pp (94°), (e) PHEMA (56°). (2) *Silicone rubber*: (f) Sample 1, (g) Sample 1 (rough surface), (h) Sample 2 (surface treated by glow discharge, (i) Sample 2, (j) Sample 3 (95.5°). (3) *Fluorocarbon compound*: (k) PVDF (82°), (l) T 530 (89.2°), (m) α-F–CH_3 (51.6°), (n) 5FM (93.9°), (o) α-F–4F, (p) 4FM (87.2°).

35.6

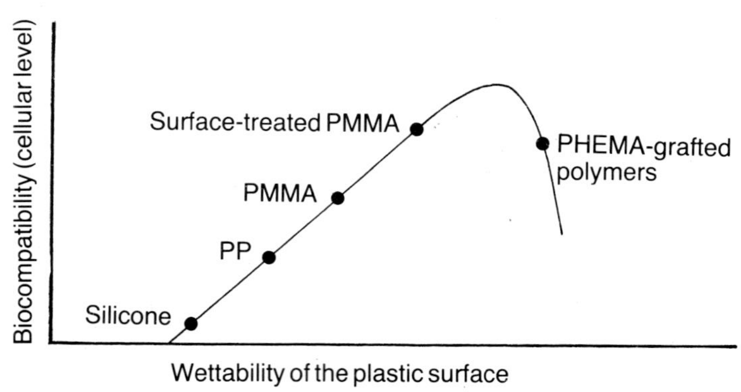

35.6 Relationship between biocompatibility at cellular level judged by cell growth and wettability.

Recently, Ikada proposed the theory that materials with extremely hydrophobic or extremely hydrophilic surfaces both show excellent antithrombin-formation characteristics, because of their low interfacial free energy with respect to water. This phenomenon may explain why IOLs of differing surface wettability (i.e., the hydrophobic silicone and the hydrophilic PHEMA) both give good clinical results. In this respect, poor cell growth may be a parameter of good biocompatibility.

Thus, the cell culture results (**35.4, 35.5**) are comparable with the clinical results (**35.7**).

Cell growth on the surface of an IOL can be observed clinically by the use of a specular microscope (**35.8–35.10**), or by the histological study of explanted IOLs (**35.11**), or by the study of postmortem eyes. The cells are of three types: large foreign-body giant cells, fibroblast-like cells and small round cells.

35.7

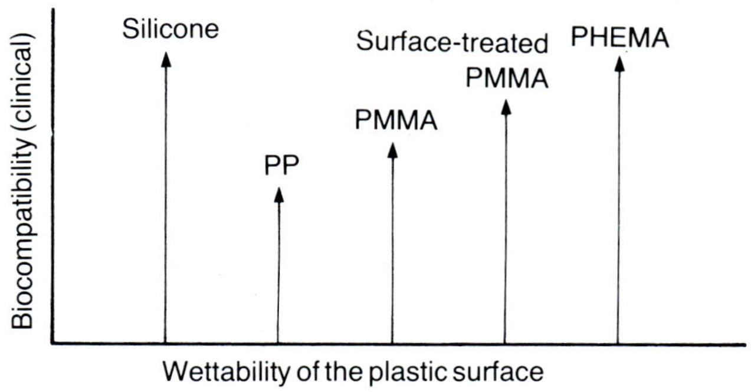

35.7 Relationship between clinical biocompatibility judged by the cellular reaction caused and wettability.

35.8

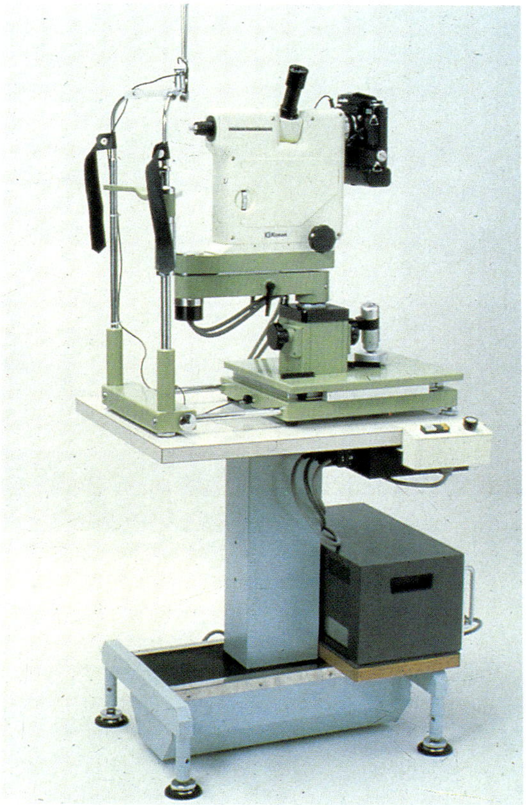

35.8 Pocklington wide field specular microscope (courtesy of Keeler's Ltd).

35.9

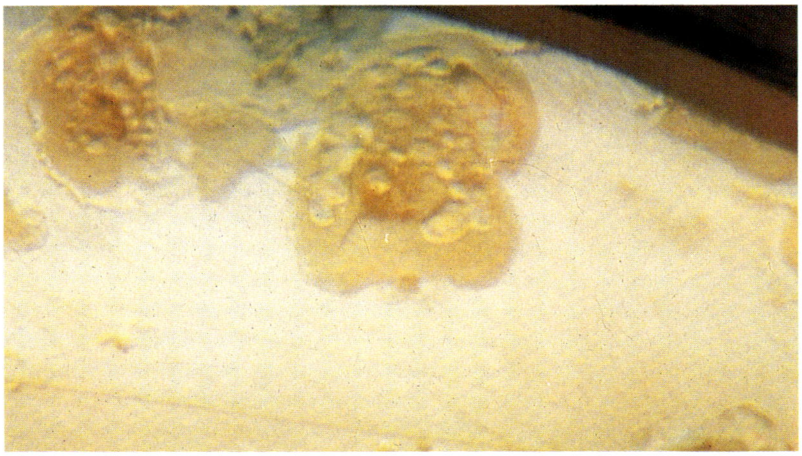

35.9 Specular microscopy showing giant cells on a PMMA PCL surface (× 75).

35.10

35.10 Specular microscopy showing cells on the surface of a silicone IOL (× 75).

35.11

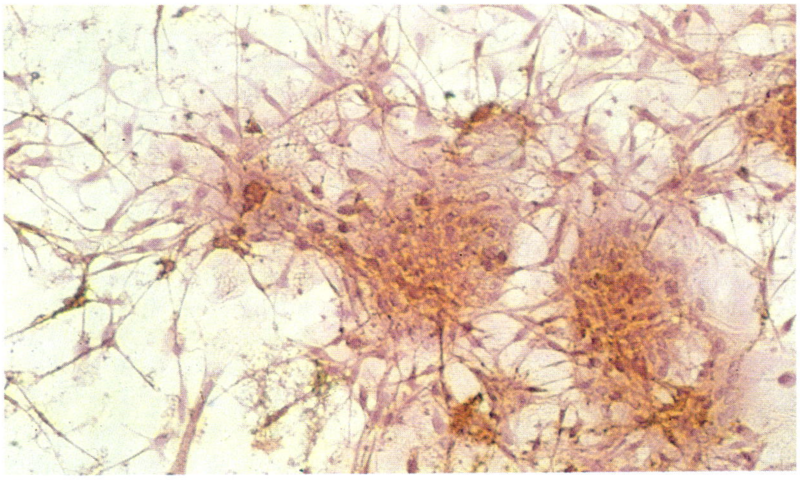

35.11 The spindle-shaped cells and conglomerated foreign-body giant cells detected by Walter's lens-implant cytology technique on a post-operative lens-induced uveitis, two years after implantation (× 50).

The three cell types may also be shown by scanning electron microscopy (**35.12–35.14**). The cells decrease in number in the long term but the IOL may become encapsulated by a collagenous membrane (**35.15**). Walter and Apple have noted this also in a human eye. The membrane shields the IOL from its surroundings, protects it from biological attack by enzymes, and ensures fixation. This kind of encapsulation is a normal reaction to a foreign body in living tissue.

Extremely hydrophobic IOLs (silicone, **35.16**) or hydrophilic IOLs (PHEMA) both show poor cell growth and good biocompatibility, with little cellular reaction clinically. A quantitative estimate of biocompatibility in quiet eyes can be achieved using a laser flare cell meter and fluorophotometry.

35.12

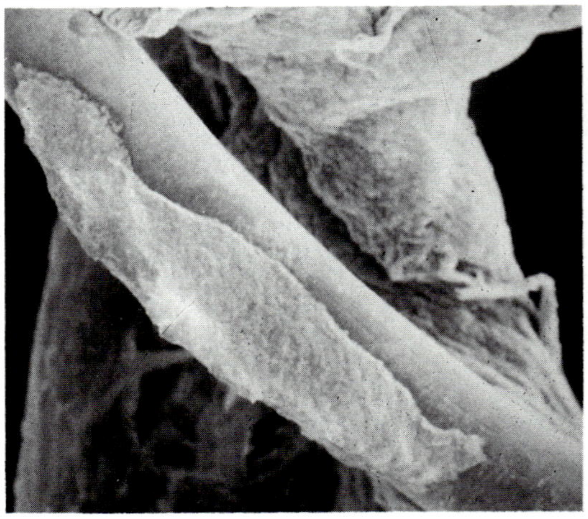

35.12 Giant cell on an explanted IOL(SEM, × 100).

35.13

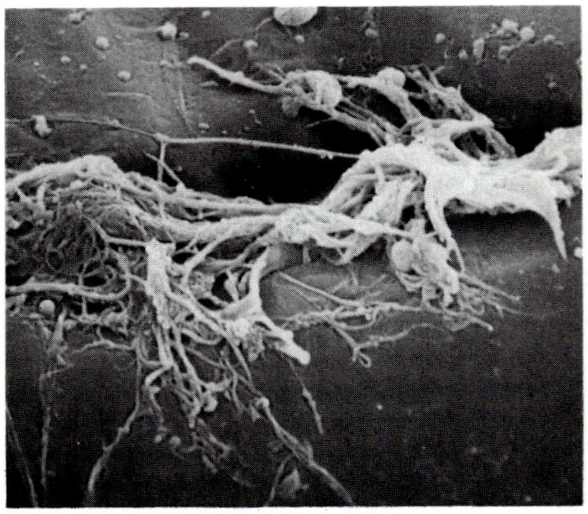

35.13 Fibroblast-like cells on an explanted IOL(SEM, × 600).

35.14

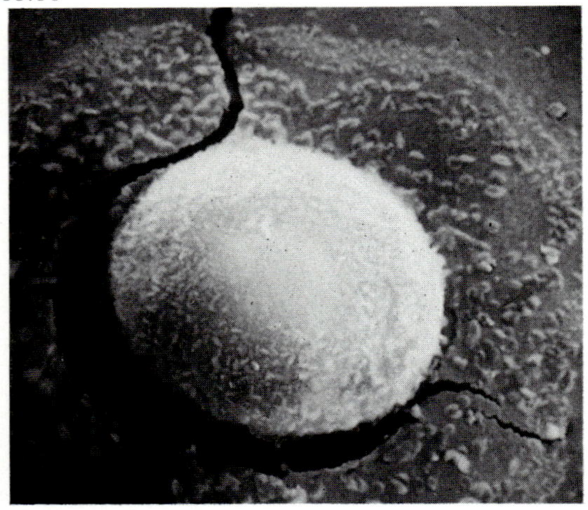

35.14 Small round cell on an explanted IOL(SEM, × 2000).

35.15

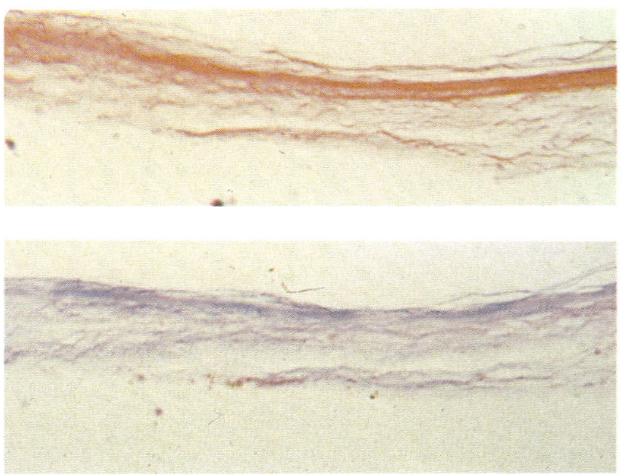

35.16

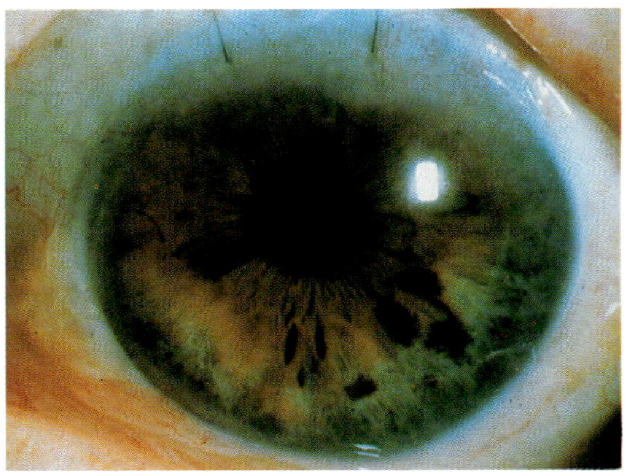

35.15 Collagen membrane on an IOL implanted in a rabbit eye (× 80). Above: Phosphotungstic acid–hematoxylin stain of membrane showing collagen as red and fibrin as blue. Below: Masson trichrome stain of membrane showing collagen, reticular fiber and hyaline material as blue, and fibrin as red.

35.16 Silicone PCL *in situ*.

Future developments

The effects of IOL materials on complement activation and macrophage function were studied by Kiyosawa *et al.* It is interesting that the extent of complement activation measured by C5a and macrophage function was found to vary with each material, its shape and the residual amount of ethylene oxide gas in the IOL material. According to Kiyosawa *et al.*, fluorocarbon polymers do not activate complement and in this respect could possibly prove to be a preferred IOL material for the future. These materials have water- and oil-repellent natures and so are quite different from other new materials, such as the hydrophilic polymer PHEMA or the hydrophobic and lipophilic polymer silicone.

Further reading

Ikada. *Biomaterials*, Nikkankogyo Shinbunnsha, 1988.

Kazusa R., Yamanaka A., *et al.*, Cellular reaction against implanted intra ocular lenses in lens-induced uveitis, *Folia. Ophthalmol. Jpn.*, **39,** 2151-2154, 1988.

Kiyosawa T. *et al.*, Effects of intraocular lens materials on complement activation and macrophage function, *Acta Soc. Ophthalmol. Jpn.*, **92,** 603–610, 1988.

Oshima K., Yamanaka A. *et al.*, Proliferation of fibroblast-like cells on plastic lens implant with or without glow discharge treatment, *Transactions, Eleventh the Annual Meeting of the Society for Biomaterials*, April 24–28, **7,** 204, 1985.

Yamanaka A. *et al.*, General consideration on plastics used for IOL implantation Part 1. Materials of the lens, *Afro-Asian J. Ophthalmology*, **1,** 13–16, 1982.

36: Posterior chamber fixation

David Apple, Robin Morgan and Julie Tsai

One advantage a posterior chamber IOL has over an anterior chamber IOL is its position behind the iris, away from the delicate structure of the anterior segment, including the cornea, the aqueous outflow channels, the iris, and the ciliary body (**36.1**). The only type of IOL that has no direct contact with uveal tissues is a posterior chamber IOL implanted entirely within the lens capsular sac.

As posterior chamber lens implantation evolved, the type of fixation achieved in the early years depended largely on chance or on the surgeon's individual preference. In general, the loops were anchored in one of three ways:

- Both loops in the ciliary region (**36.2–36.4**). We now know from autopsy studies that true ciliary sulcus fixation of both loops was, and still is, achieved much less often than had been previously assumed.

36.1

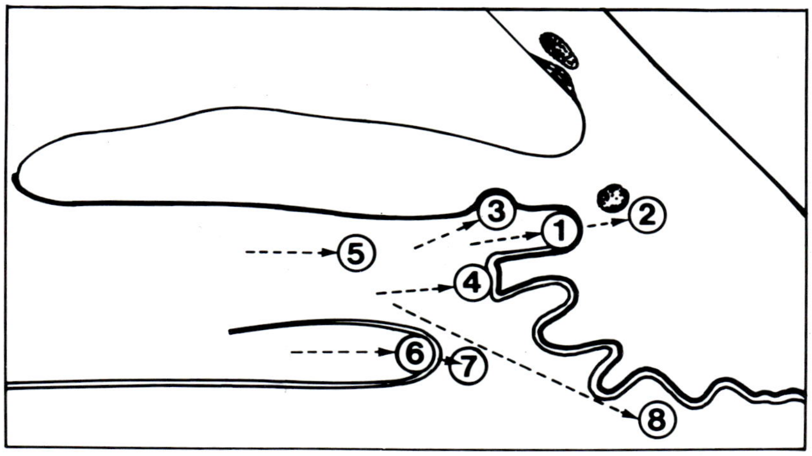

36.1 Schematic illustration showing possible placement sites of posterior chamber lens loops: (1) Loop in the ciliary sulcus. (2) Loop after erosion into the ciliary body stroma in the region of the major iris arterial circle. (3) Loop in contact with the iris root. (4) Loop attached to a ciliary process. (5) Loop in aqueous without tissue contact (can cause 'windshield wiper' syndrome because of inadequate fixation). (6) Loop in the lens capsular sac. (7) Loop ruptured through the lens capsular sac (a rare occurrence). (8) Loop in the zonular region between the ciliary sulcus and the lens capsular sac. The loop may penetrate the zonules (zonular fixation) or extend as far posteriorly as the pars plana (pars plana fixation).

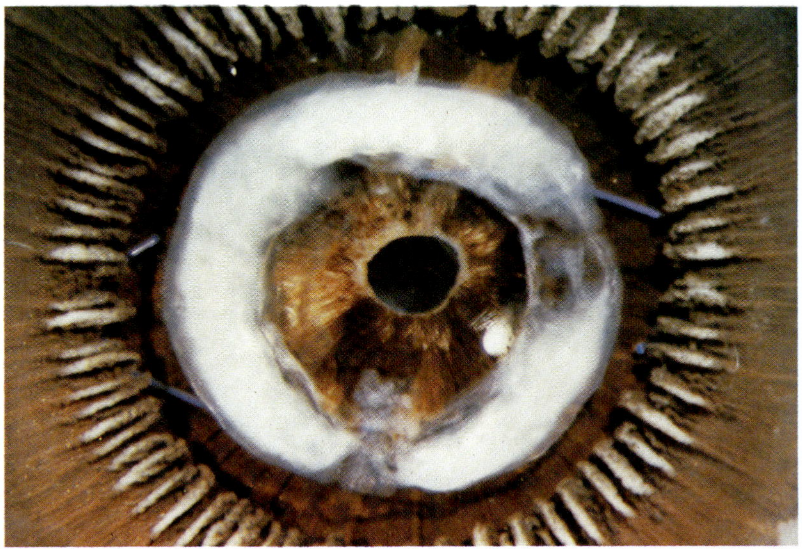

36.2

36.2 Gross photograph from behind of an autopsied eye showing placement of a modified J-loop Sinskey-style IOL with both loops in the ciliary sulcus. Centration is excellent. A complete Soemmering's ring is present, and the central visual axis remains clear.

36.3

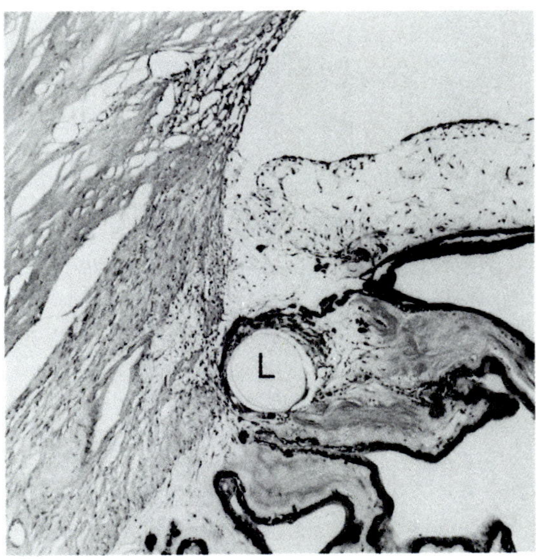

36.3 Photomicrograph of an eye showing a loop (L) situated in the ciliary sulcus. The loop has migrated into the substance of the ciliary body stroma. (Hematoxylin and eosin stain; magnification x20.)

36.4 Photomicrograph of a sagittally sectioned postmortem eye with a loop fixated at the junction of the iris root (top) and ciliary body (bottom). The loop biomaterial dissolved during tissue processing and the loop site is seen as an empty, circular space behind the iris. Note the dense fibrous encapsulation around the loop and the close proximity of the iris dilator muscle (pink horizontal band of tissue) within the iris stroma, immediately above the iris pigment epithelium. (Hematoxylin and eosin stain; magnification x150.)

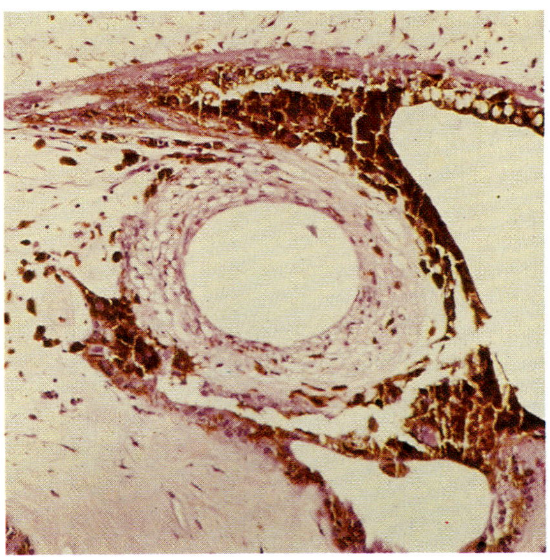

36.4

- Both loops within the lens capsular sac. Capsular fixation evolved from the original work of Cornelius Binkhorst, who popularized the use of extracapsular cataract extraction in conjunction with his two-loop iridocapsular IOL (**36.5**). In the early years of posterior chamber implantation, capsular or in-the-bag fixation (**36.6–36.10**) was intentionally performed by only a handful of surgeons; widespread use did not occur until the mid-1980s.

36.5

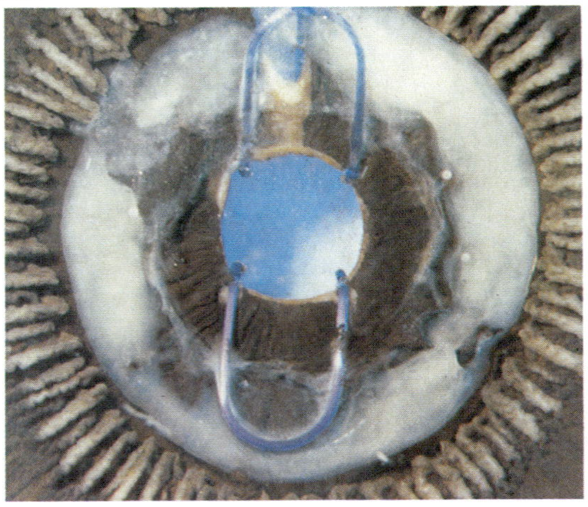

36.5 Gross photograph from behind of an autopsy eye showing placement of an iridocapsular-type IOL. Note the staking rod within the iridectomy above. The visual axis is clear, the lens is well centered, and the retained cortex forms a Soemmering's ring peripherally.

36.6

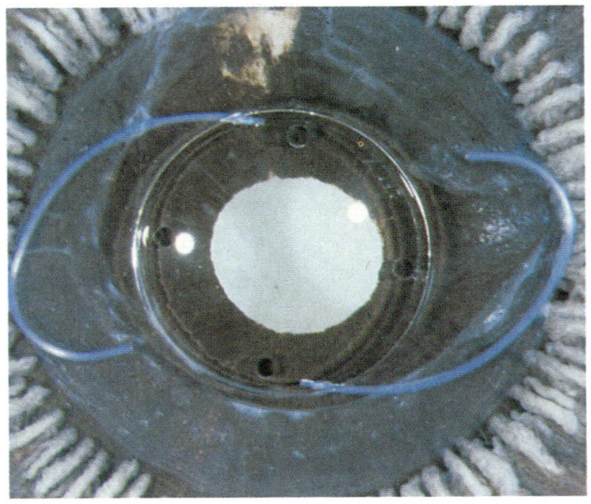

36.6 Gross photograph from behind of an autopsy eye showing a perfectly centered, modified J-loop posterior chamber lens implanted in the lens capsular sac. An iridectomy is present at 12 o'clock. Note the C-shaped bend of the loops. The lens capsule shows only a faint gray Soemmering's ring.

36.7

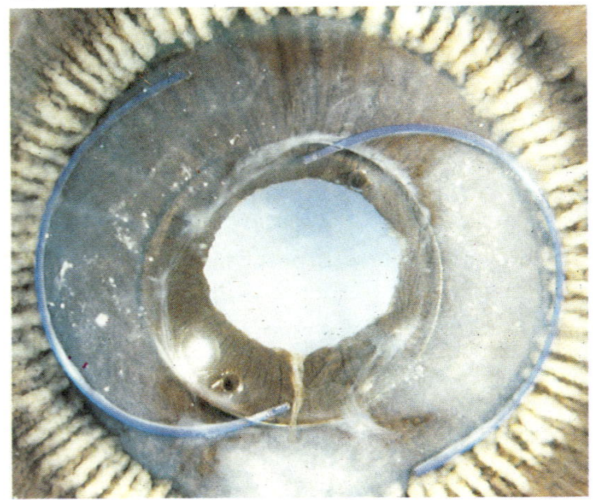

36.7 Gross photograph from behind of an autopsy eye showing in-the-bag placement of a Simcoe C-loop-style posterior chamber IOL. The optic is well centered and the loops conform to the circumference of the lens capsular bag. There is moderate retention of cortical material in the periphery, but the central visual axis remains clear.

36.8

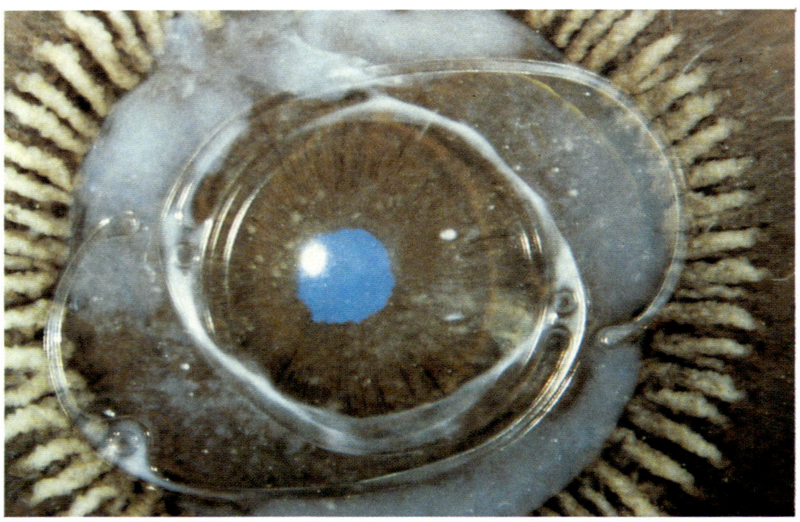

36.8 Gross photograph from behind of an autopsy eye showing a one-piece all-PMMA-style posterior chamber IOL (Arnott–Jaffe style), with both loops implanted in the capsular bag. The loops show moderate compression in order to conform to the diameter and shape of the capsular bag. The central visual axis shows a few scattered opacities. The optic is well centered and is surrounded by a ring of cortical material, which represents retained and regenerate cortex.

36.9

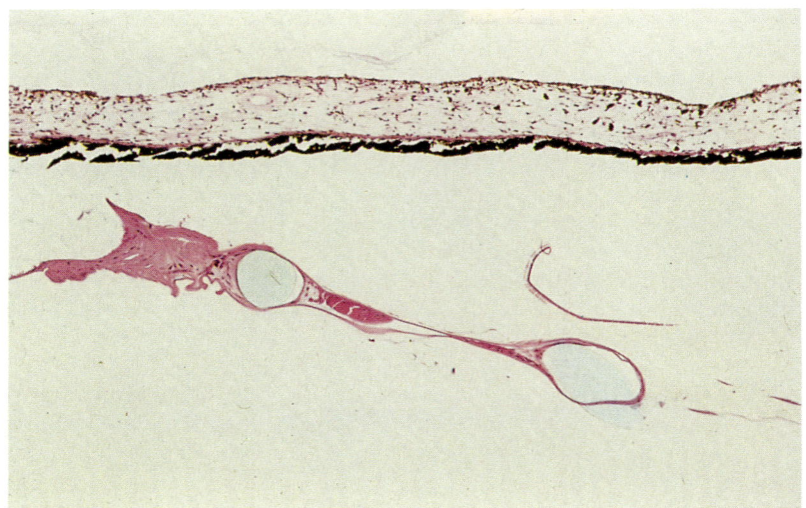

36.9 Photomicrograph of the fixation site of a closed-loop posterior chamber lens designed specifically for in-the-bag implantation (Sheets-style IOL). The proximal and distal portions of one of the blue, closed, polypropylene loops are visible posterior to the iris. Cross sections of the blue loop are surrounded by remnants of the lens capsular sac. (Hematoxylin and eosin stain; magnification x30.)

36.10 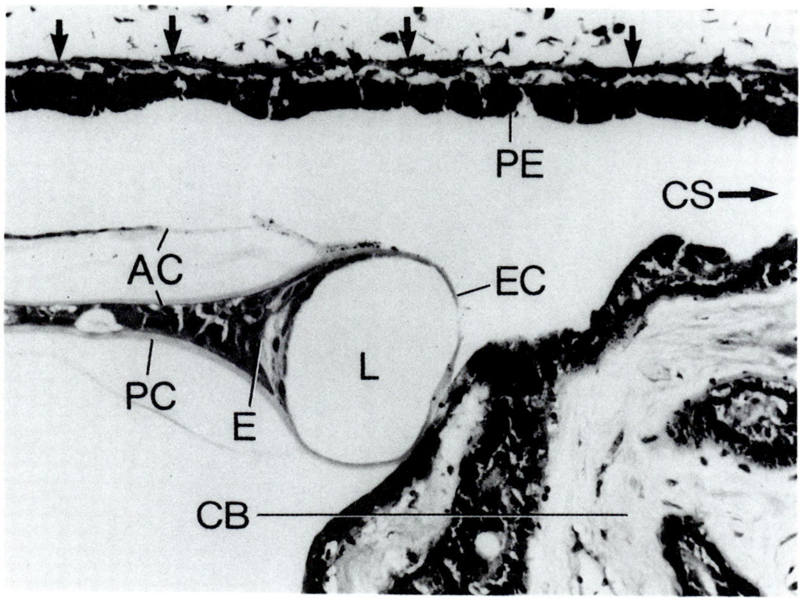

36.10 Photomicrograph of a capsule-fixated posterior chamber lens loop (L) in an autopsy eye. The IOL was well tolerated and the patient had good visual acuity until the time of death. The loop (L) is firmly secured between the equatorial capsule (EC) and posterior capsule (PC) and an abundant flap or rim of anterior capsule (AC). Note the artifactual lamellar splitting of the anterior capsule that occurred during tissue processing. The ciliary sulcus (CS) is situated to the right and above the ciliary body (CB). The dilator muscle of the iris (small arrows) is particularly clear, just above the iris pigment epithelium (PE). This muscle and the sphincter muscle are responsible for the constant movements of the pupil, one of the major factors in the pathogenesis of chafing defects. Note the residual lens epithelial (E) cells adjacent to the lens loop. (Hematoxylin and eosin stain; magnification x20.)

- One loop (usually the leading or inferior loop) in the capsular sac and the other loop (usually the trailing or superior loop) in a variety of locations anterior to the anterior capsular flap (**36.11, 36.12**). This has been the most common type of fixation since the late 1970s, when the flexible posterior chamber IOLs were introduced. Retrospective analysis of clinical cases, autopsy studies, and experience with animal implantations have shown that this asymmetric fixation occurs in *most* implantations when a lens is inserted behind the iris, without any specific intention as to where the loops should be placed. The direction of the lens as it enters the posterior chamber is usually the deciding factor in determining where the loop is fixated. The IOL passes through the pupil in an oblique fashion during the insertion process. Typically, the inferior loop passes into the equatorial fornix of the capsular sac at 6 o'clock. Then, as the superior loop is inserted, often without good visibility, the loop springs into a site behind the iris, but anterior to the anterior capsular flap at 12 o'clock.

Another cause of asymmetric fixation is the 'pea pod' effect in which a loop exits from the capsular sac, either during intraoperative manipulations, such as dialing, or postoperatively. The major causes of 'pea podding' are the pressure of a radial tear in the anterior capsule or too scanty an anterior capsular flap after a large capsulotomy. An abundant anterior flap is necessary to secure the loop in the equatorial fornix (**36.10**).

Since the introduction of viscoelastic agents, and with the trend towards smaller anterior capsulotomies with smooth rims that do not damage the capsular zonule apparatus, atraumatic removal of the lens substance has become possible. An adequate rim of anterior capsule will provide equatorial support for the loops and easier, more consistent and more permanent in-the-bag IOL placement. (**36.6–36.8**).

There are several possible loop-fixation sites and these have been confirmed histologically by analyses of postmortem globes implanted

36.11 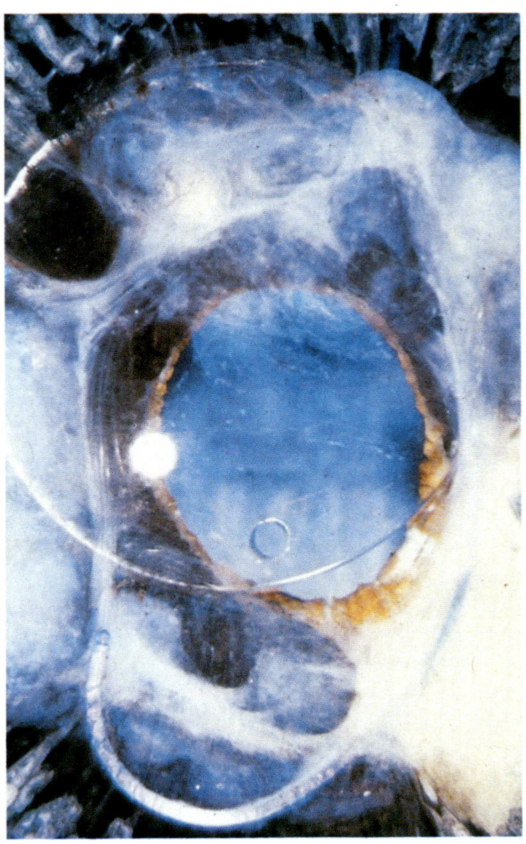

36.11 Gross photograph from behind of an asymmetrically implanted posterior chamber IOL. The inferior loop was fixated within the capsular sac, and the superior loop, positioned in the ciliary region, eroded superiorly causing upward decentration of the optic. A portion of the lens edge and a positioning hole are visible within the pupillary aperture. Note the presence of Soemmering's ring composed of large amounts of retained cortical remnants and fibrous tissue, indicative of incomplete cortical cleanup.

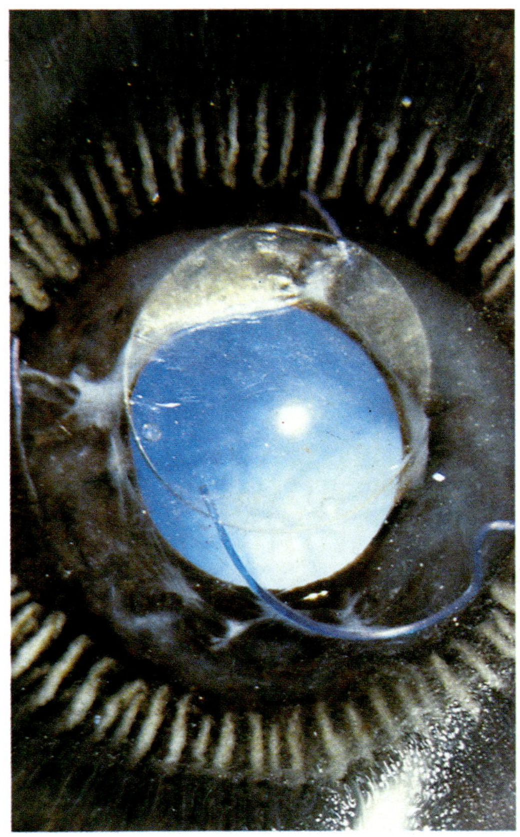 36.12

36.12 Gross photograph from behind of an autopsy eye showing a C-loop posterior chamber IOL implanted asymmetrically, with one loop in the ciliary sulcus (upper left) and the opposite loop (with the Lester notch) in the capsular bag. Notice the extensive upward decentration of the lens optic, so that the optic edge and a positioning hole are within the pupillary aperture.

with posterior chamber IOLs. When the loops fixate directly onto the surface of the ciliary sulcus, they are secured in the angle formed by the junction of the posterior iris root and the anterior margin of the ciliary processes or pars plicata. This site is theoretically the ideal placement area for uveal fixation, because a fibrous encapsulation around the loop often develops, enhancing fixation and preventing deep loop erosion into the ciliary body. However, fixation of both IOL loops at this site (**36.2**) is achieved in fewer than one in five cases.

The loops may migrate or erode through the ciliary epithelium and into the stromal tissues of the ciliary body. This is the most common form of uveal fixation. The loops may encroach upon or compress the major iris circle and other vessels in the ciliary vascular plexus. At times a loop may migrate through the ciliary body stroma and become embedded in the ciliary muscle, or may even come to rest on or near the supraciliary space adjacent to the sclera. Such a migration may play a role in the pathogenesis of lens malposition (**36.13–36.21**), particularly after asymmetric implantation (**36.13, 36.17, 36.19, 36.21**).

36.13

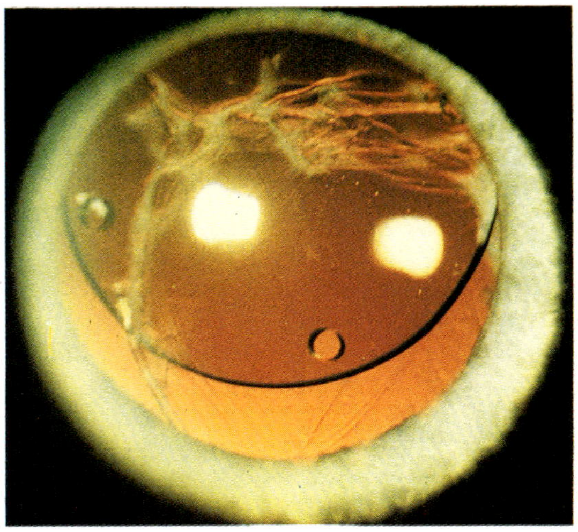

36.13 Clinical photograph of a sunrise syndrome. The inferior loop was implanted in the capsular sac and the superior loop in the ciliary sulcus. The unequal pressures exerted on the loops caused an upward decentration (courtesy of Douglas Koch, Houston, USA).

36.14

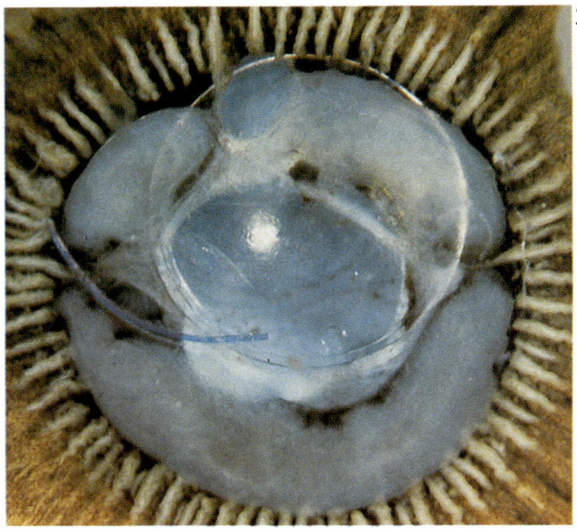

36.14 Gross photograph from behind of an autopsy eye showing a Sinskey-style posterior chamber lens with both loops in the ciliary sulcus. Note the marked decentration of the IOL, primarily in an axis perpendicular to the longitudinal direction of the loops. Note also the extensive posterior capsular opacification and epithelial pearl formation.

36.15

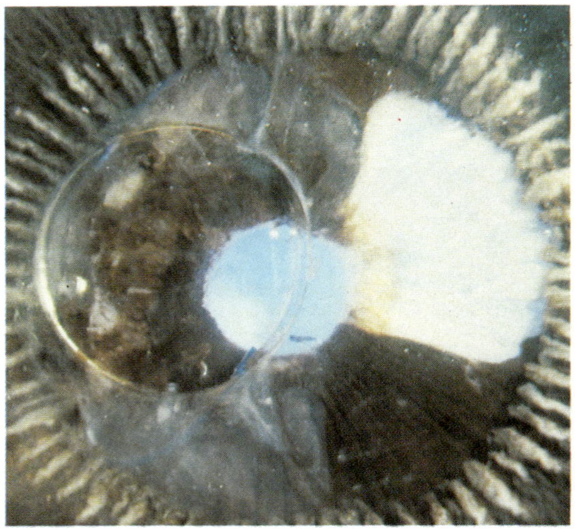

36.15 Gross photograph from behind of an autopsy eye containing a modified J-loop posterior chamber IOL, with both loops implanted in the ciliary sulcus. Note the extreme decentration of the lens optic, so that one edge is in the center of the pupil and one of the positioning holes is near the upper edge of the pupil. The decentration is to the left, perpendicular to the long axis of the lens loops. The large iris transillumination defect was surgically induced.

36.16

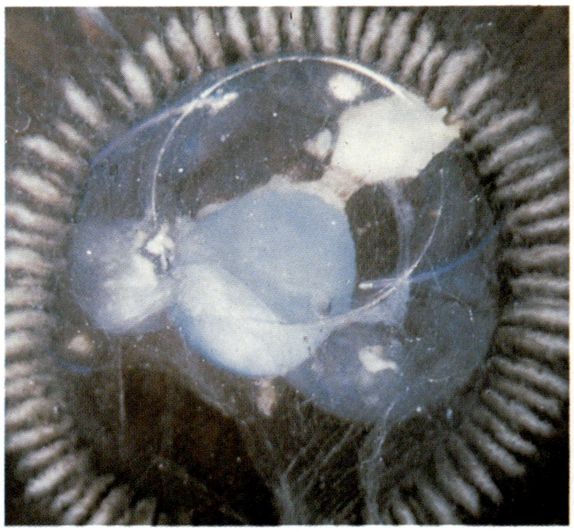

36.16 Gross photograph from behind of a globe with a posterior chamber lens that is displaced upward (sunrise syndrome). The loops were implanted symmetrically in the ciliary sulcus. The decentration was caused by an inferior zonular disinsertion, which displaced the capsular sac and optic superiorly, so that the optic edges are seen within the visual axis. Note the arcuate defect in the capsular sac at 7 o'clock and the iridectomy at 1 o'clock.

36.17

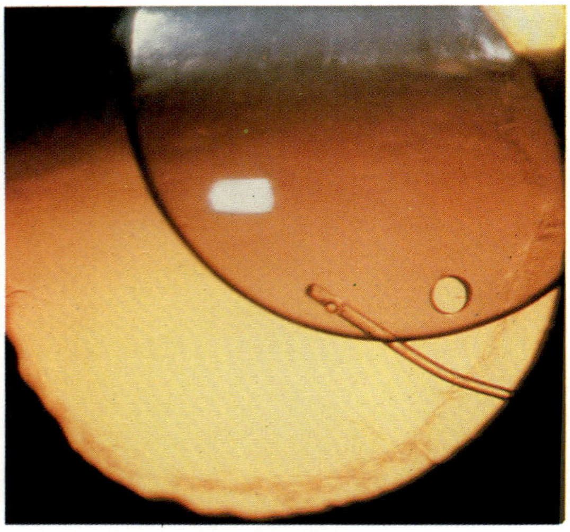

36.17 Clinical retroillumination photograph of a malpositioned posterior chamber lens. During implantation a wide, 8 mm anterior capsulotomy was performed, seen below through the dilated pupil. It is possible that the surgeon was unable to see the edges of the capsular flaps during the lens insertion and so could not achieve symmetrical loop fixation. Alternatively, because the large capsulotomy left an extremely small anterior flap, one of the loops could have slipped from the capsular bag during dialing of the IOL or during the immediate postoperative period.

36.18

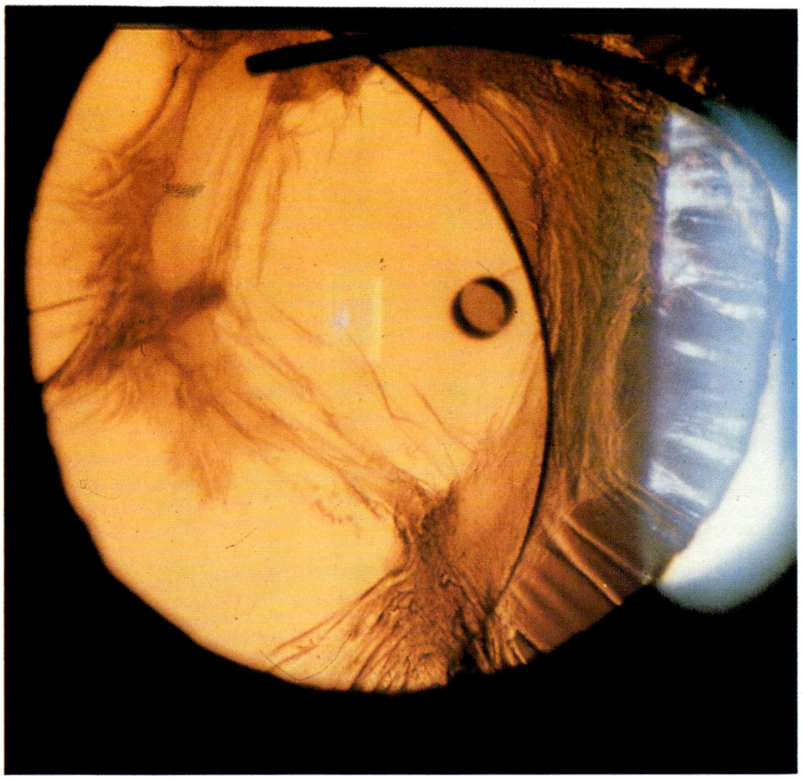

36.18 Clinical photograph showing a posterior chamber IOL that is horizontally displaced to the left, so that the edge of the lens, a positioning hole, and one of the loops are within the visual axis. Ruptured and stretched zonular fibers are seen on the right. This is an unusual case of horizontal displacement, which is more frequently caused by asymmetric loop fixation, rather than the zonular rupture seen here.

36.19

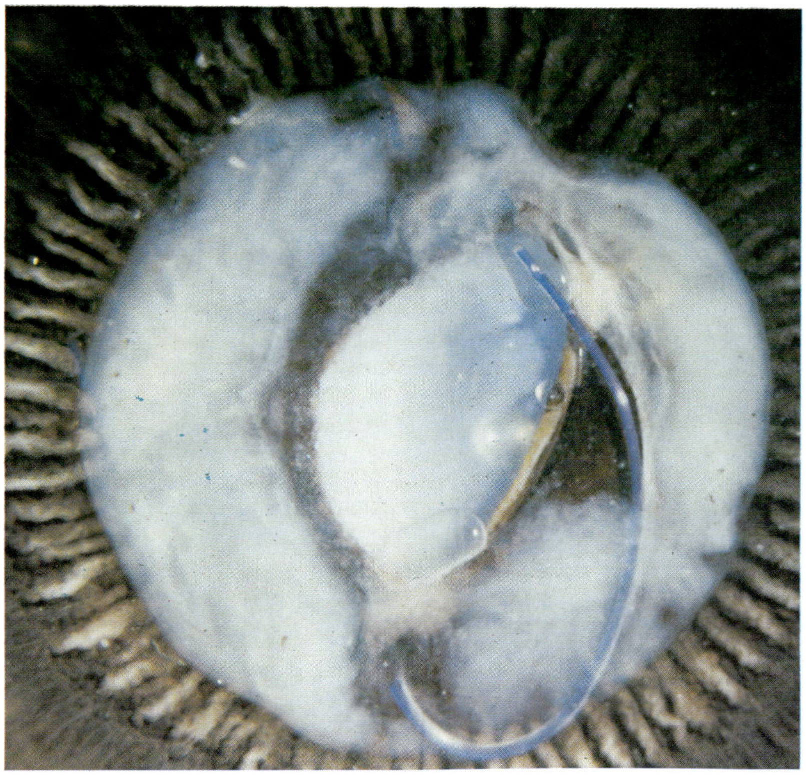

36.19 Gross photograph from behind of an autopsy eye showing a modified J-loop posterior chamber IOL implanted with the inferior loop in the capsular bag and the superior loop in the ciliary sulcus. A small iris transillumination defect is seen under the superior loop behind the dense Soemmering's ring. Note the upward decentration of the optic and the pupillary capture of the superior optic, which protrudes anterior to the iris.

36.20

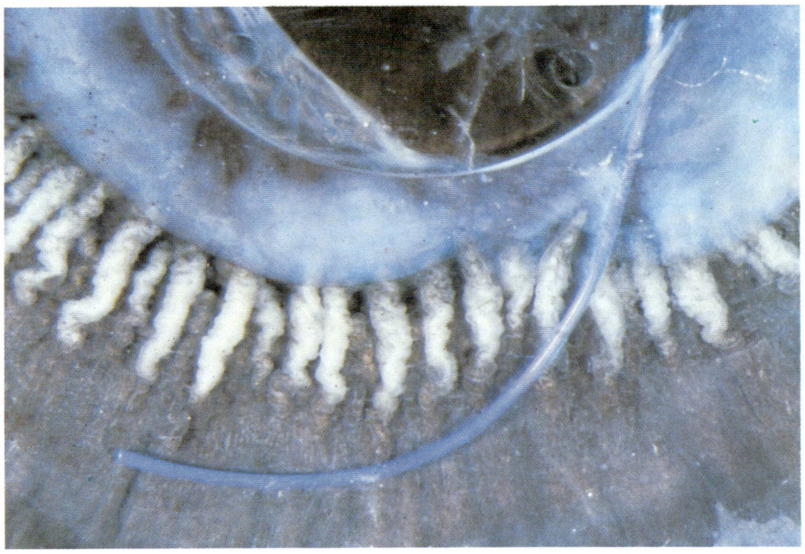

36.20 Gross photograph from behind of a postmortem eye showing one loop that has penetrated the zonules and is situated in the pars plana. This phenomenon, in which neither sulcus nor bag fixation was achieved, was seen in as many as 8% of autopsy specimens, and is associated with a high incidence of decentration.

36.21

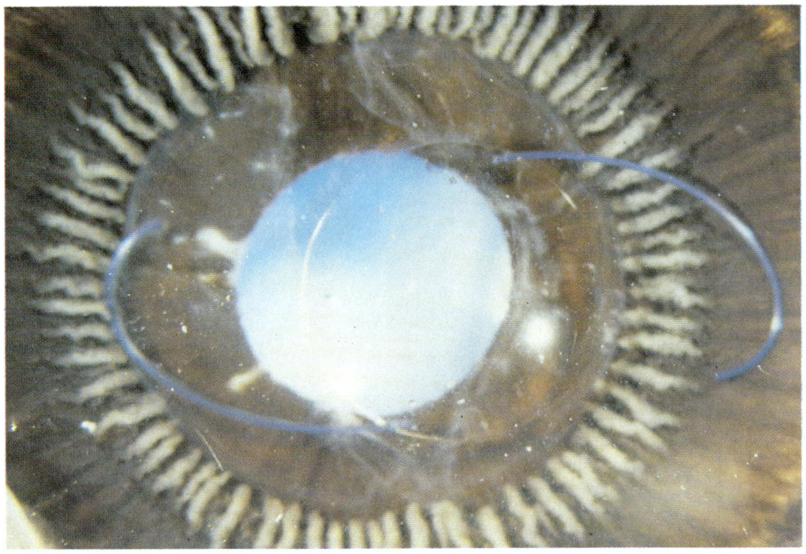

36.21 Gross photograph from behind of an autopsy globe containing a modified J-loop posterior chamber IOL in which the loop on the left was implanted in the capsular bag and the loop on the right extended through the zonules and landed in the pars plana. This caused an extreme amount of decentration to the right, so that the left edge of the optic and the positioning holes are in the pupil. Note the apparent tear of the posterior capsule, seen superiorly.

When both loops are secured in the lens capsular sac, one achieves the only type of fixation in which IOL contact with uveal tissues is avoided. Fixation of iris support, iridocapsular, anterior chamber, or uvea-fixated posterior chamber IOLs, by definition, implies direct contact of the loop or haptic with delicate ocular tissues.

If IOL loops are either intentionally or inadvertently placed in front of the capsular sac, as occurs in as many as 8% of cases, the loop may be positioned so that it is neither in the ciliary sulcus nor in the lens capsular sac. The loop may slide between these structures and become entangled in the zonules (**36.23**) or it may pass through the zonules to settle as far posteriorly as the pars plana (**36.20, 36.21**).

The fixation sites shown in **36.1**, which designate a loop that is placed anterior to the anterior capsular flap, have led the authors to use not only the term 'sulcus fixation', but also the terms 'uveal, ciliary or ciliary-region, zonular, or pars plana fixation' to designate the placement site of any IOL placed in front of the anterior capsule. The more frequently used clinical term 'ciliary-sulcus fixation' is too often used in a general sense, when the loops may be fixated behind the iris, anywhere in front of the anterior capsular flap. Simply placing the loops behind the iris and allowing them to land or settle where they may, may lead to needless decentration.

The excellent success rate now achieved with posterior chamber IOL implantation is associated with improved IOL designs and improved surgical techniques, including the meticulous placement of loops. Explantation of posterior chamber IOLs owing to a complication is now rarely required after correctly implanted capsule fixation.

Two measurable factors that can be analyzed are decentration and posterior capsule opacification (**36.13–36.26**). At present we have had access to approximately 1,300 eyes obtained postmortem with all types of IOLs. Approximately two-thirds of these globes contained posterior chamber IOLs and by reviewing the clinicopathologic data on these cases we have verified to our satisfaction the efficacy and advantages of capsular fixation, particularly in terms of achieving optimal centration.

36.22

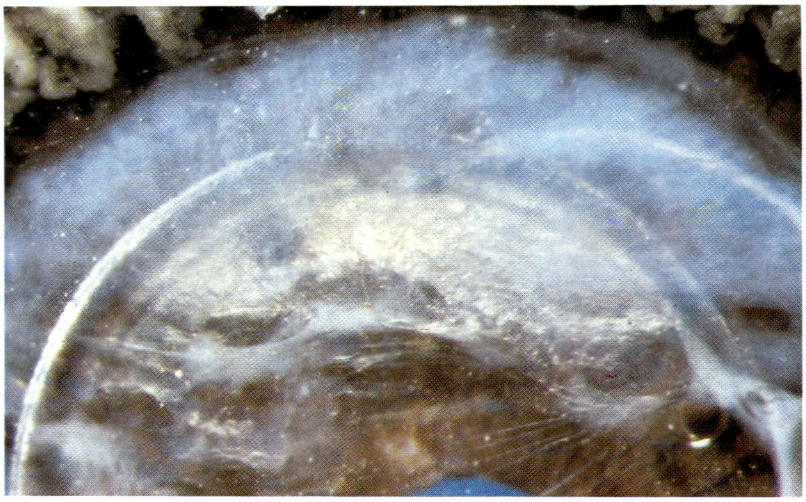

36.22 Gross photograph from behind of an autopsy globe showing the presence of a moderately dense layer of epithelial cells. Note the folds in the capsule, which are caused by a fibromuscular metaplasia of residual lens epithelial cells.

36.23

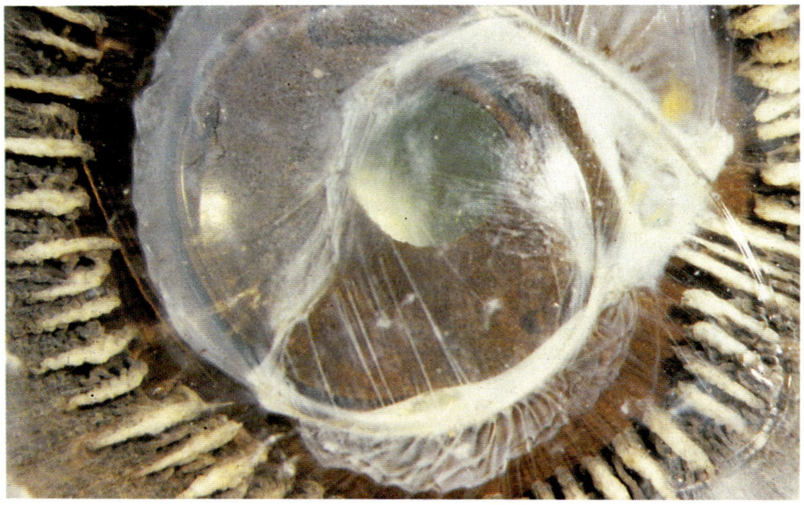

36.23 Gross photograph from behind of an autopsy globe showing a one-piece posterior chamber IOL implanted with the loop on the left in the ciliary sulcus, and the loop on the right implanted at the junction of the pars plicata and pars plana. Note the marked distortion of the capsular bag with numerous irregular folds and foci of fibrosis. Note also the focal stretching of the zonules in several quadrants. Although the optic is fairly well centered, this position of the loops leads to a higher incidence of fibrosis.

36.24

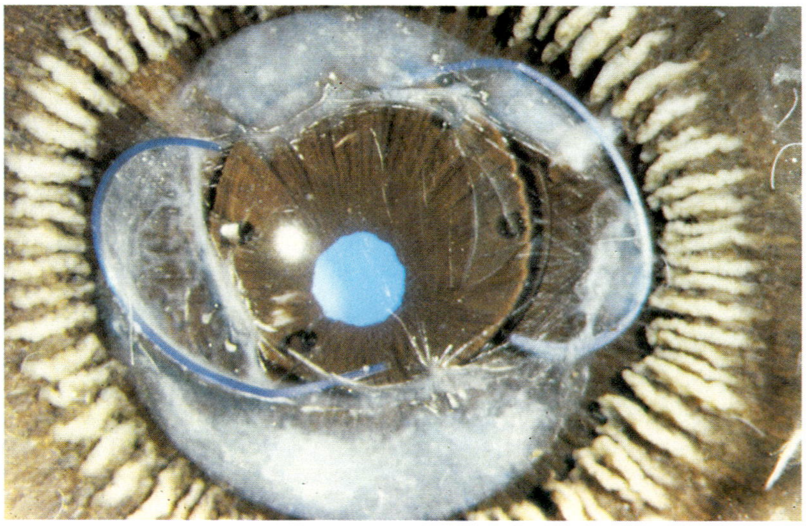

36.24 Gross photograph from behind of a modified J-loop posterior chamber IOL that is symmetrically implanted in the capsular bag. Note that the most extensive proliferation of peripheral cortical material is in the quadrants that are distal from the location of the two loops. The equator is stretched at the site of the two loops (3 and 9 o'clock), whereas no stretching of the bag is present at 12 and 6 o'clock, where the most abundant cortical proliferation has occurred.

36.25 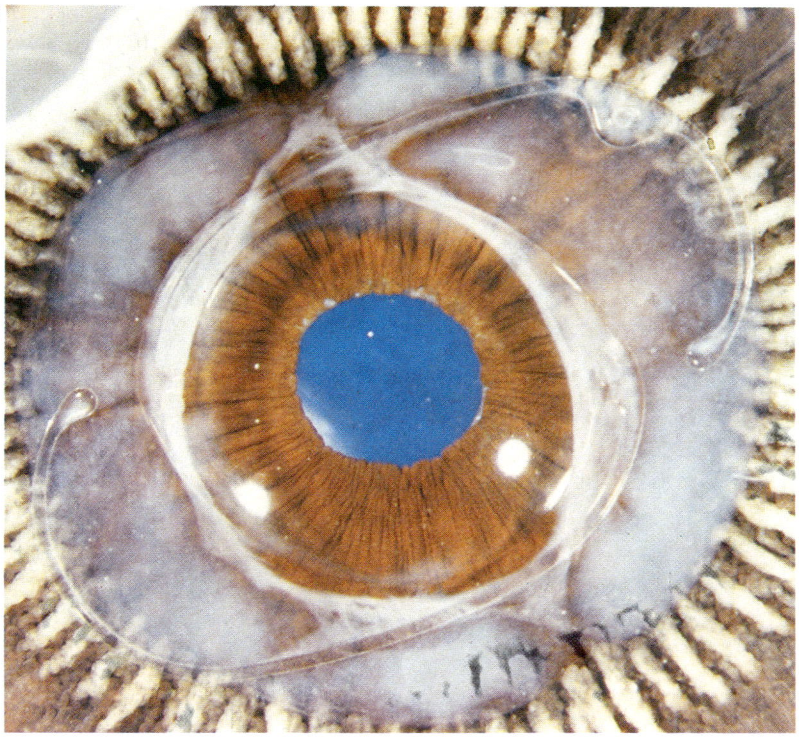

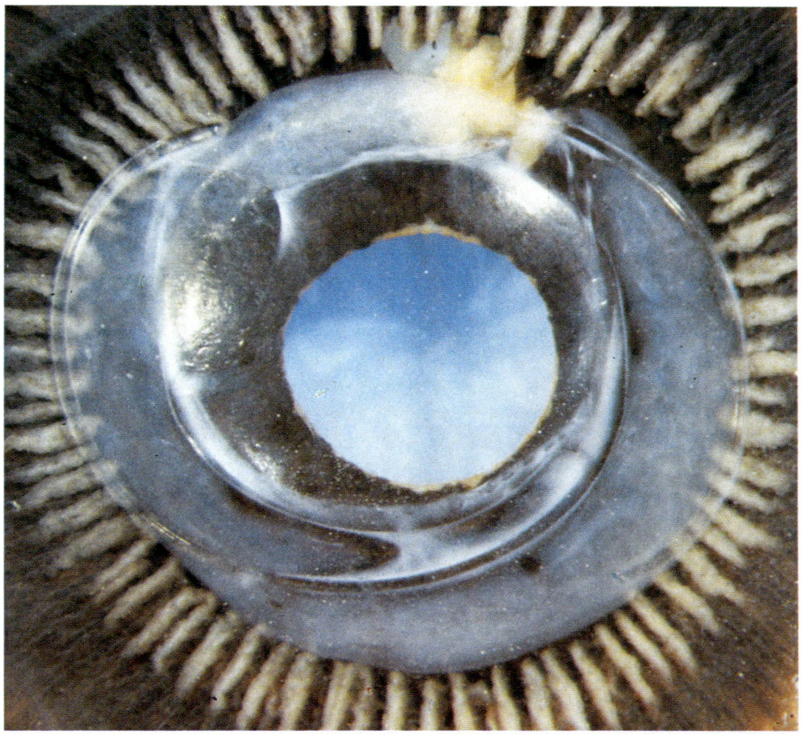 36.26

36.25 Gross photograph from behind of an autopsy globe containing a one-piece all-PMMA modified C-loop posterior chamber IOL implanted within the lens capsular bag. The loops create a significant stretch on the capsular bag. It is believed that this causes the posterior capsule to adhere tightly to the posterior aspect of the optic, providing a cell-free zone. Note the clarity of the visual axis behind the lens optic.

36.26 Gross photograph from behind of an Arnott–Jaffe-style one-piece posterior chamber IOL with both loops implanted in the lens capsular bag. The loops are compressed to conform to the capsular bag and the optic is well centered. The visual axis remains clear. The retained or regenerate cortical material is confined to the area peripheral to the lens optic.

Advantages of placing both loops in the capsular sac

- Positions the IOL in the proper anatomical site.
- It is as easy to place both loops symmetrically in the capsular sac as in the ciliary sulcus.
- Intraoperative stretching or tearing of zonules by loop manipulations in front of the anterior capsular leaflet is avoided.
- Low incidence of lens decentration and dislocation.
- No evidence of spontaneous lens dislocation into the vitreous cavity.
- IOL is positioned a maximal distance from the posterior iris pigment epithelium, iris root, and ciliary processes.
- IOL is positioned a maximal distance behind the cornea.
- No direct contact by or erosion of IOL loops or haptics into ciliary body tissues.
- Avoids chronic uveal tissue chafing and reduces the blood–aqueous barrier breakdown and/or pigment dispersion into the anterior chamber.
- Surface alteration of loop material is less likely.
- May reduce posterior capsular opacification.
- Easy to explant, if necessary.

Causes of posterior chamber IOL decentration

- Asymmetric loop insertion, one loop in the lens capsular sac, one loop in the ciliary region (**36.11, 36.12, 36.13, 36.19–36.21**).
- Escape of a loop initially placed in the lens capsular sac, either intraoperatively (during rotation or dialing of the IOL) or postoperatively because of too large an anterior capsulotomy that does not leave enough anterior capsular flap to hold the lens in place (**36.17**).
- Sliding or slippage of a loop that is sandwiched between the iris and anterior capsular flap, but not securely fixated in the ciliary sulcus (**36.14, 36.15**).
- Perforation of a loop through the iris or displacement through an iridectomy.
- Optic migration during pupillary capture (**36.19**).
- Distortion or bending of a loop during insertion, usually during excessive flexion or pronation of the superior loop, causing a difference in loop length and subsequent asymmetric fixation. Permanent loop distortion is most likely to occur in three-piece IOLs with polypropylene loops that do not have memory retention qualities.
- Intraoperative tearing of zonules, especially by manipulation or dialing of loops in front of the anterior capsule.
- Pressure or traction exerted on the loop and/or optical component of the IOL by proliferating residual lens epithelial cells and their derivatives. A fibrous or myoepithelial metaplasia of these cells

produces a cicatricial contraction of the capsular sac (**36.22**). This phenomenon may be exacerbated by an asymmetric anterior capsulotomy.

- Asymmetric contracture of capsular flaps, which may cause a peapodding effect of the lens optic, likened to the squeezing of a toothpaste tube (**36.14, 36.19**).
- Zonular disinsertion, whether the loops are in the bag or out (**36.16**).
- Loop disinsertion at the site where the loop is staked into the loop–optic junction.
- Loop fracture.

Symptoms from decentration may include glare, halo, monocular diplopia, and other visual aberrations. These may occur because of the presence of optic edges or other lens elements, such as positioning holes within the pupillary aperture (**36.13–36.19**), and may be clinically significant despite the normality of Snellen visual acuity tests. The symptoms may be exacerbated in conditions such as dim light when pupillary dilatation occurs.

Visual aberrations caused by optic components in the pupil may be reduced by increasing the diameter of the optic, or eliminating the positioning holes. However, the best way of avoiding these symptoms is to reduce the chance of decentration by ensuring symmetric loop placement.

Correct design of the IOL

Published studies have reported the diameter of the evacuated and crushed capsular sac to be approximately 10.3–10.8 mm. These measurements of crushed or flattened capsular bags are not totally relevant to in-the-bag IOL implantation. In most cases, the bag does not completely collapse and flatten to a larger diameter after ECCE. In general, a lens opened with a relatively small capsulotomy, especially with continuous circular capsulorhexis, retains its original shape and diameter. Shunsaku Ohmi analyzed a large series of autopsy eyes with posterior chamber IOLs and found the mean capsular bag diameter to be 9.6 mm (standard deviation, 0.4 mm). The diameter of the ciliary sulcus was 11 mm (standard deviation, 0.5 mm).

The original Shearing posterior chamber IOL measured 12.5 mm in diameter, and was not as flexible as today's modified J-loop and C-loop designs. If the lens was too small for the eye or if a loop eroded into the ciliary body, the IOL became decentered and 'windshield wiper' syndrome and other undesirable IOL movements occurred. These problems prompted most lens designers to increase the loop span and most flexible, looped IOLs in current use measure from 13.75–14.5 mm in diameter. These IOLs were sized to ensure consistent ciliary region fixation, to provide a snug fit and thus prevent the IOL from dislocating. In general, when such IOLs are used with capsular fixation, the flexible loops must bend or crimp to conform to the much smaller diameter of the capsular sac. The loop tip may even extend to the edge of or over the optic.

Most lenses designed specifically for in-the-bag placement have a smaller total diameter (10.0–12.5 mm). As more surgeons now prefer capsular bag implantation, use of these smaller diameter IOLs has increased. It is likely that this trend will help reduce the incidence of problems associated with severe bending and crimping of lens loops, capsular distortion, and the spring effect that can occur when the loop is exposed to contractile forces within the capsular bag.

In general, the final configuration of the loops of all IOL styles should preferably assume a C-shape that conforms to the circular capsule (**36.26, 36.27**). However, there is significant compression and bending of J-loop or modified J-loop loops (**36.6, 36.24**). The distal portion of J-loop or modified J-loop IOLs frequently exerts a unidirectional force that causes stretching and ovalling of the capsular sac. This results in the formation of folds or striae parallel to the long axis of the lens, which may occasionally cause symptoms.

36.27

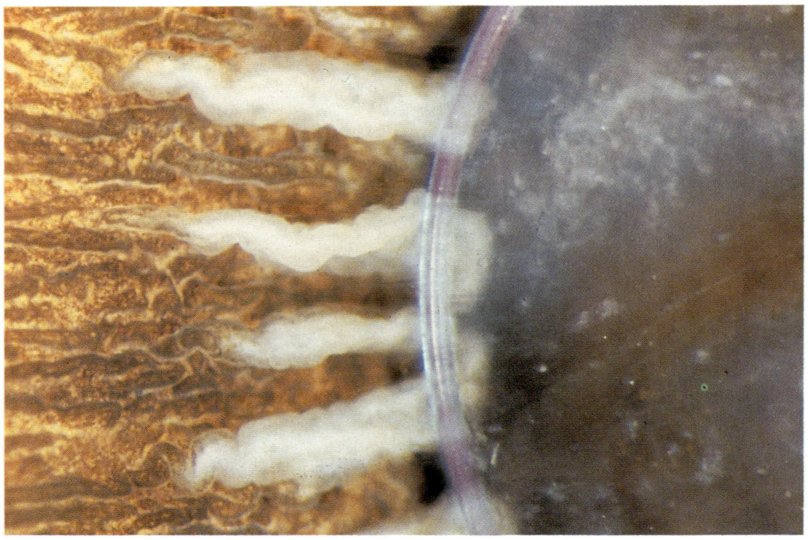

36.27 High-power gross photograph from behind of an autopsy eye containing a modified C-loop all-PMMA posterior chamber IOL. A segment of the PMMA loop implanted in the capsular bag is present, situated in the physiologic position adjacent to the ciliary processes. The loop exerts a gentle radial pressure on the capsular equator, rendering the posterior capsule taut.

There is now a definite trend among manufacturers to produce lenses with more C-shaped or rounded loops (**36.25–36.27**). These subtle modifications are adaptations of the original Simcoe C-loop and variations of the original Sinskey and Kratz designs. Modified or short C-loop lenses are now widely used because surgeons find these IOLs easy to insert and the loops conform to the circular shape of the capsular sac (**36.27**).

Posterior capsular opacification is a significant postoperative complication. Evidence is accumulating that placement of a well-designed posterior chamber lens in the lens capsular sac provides a gentle but taut radial stretch on the posterior capsule (**36.26, 36.27**), which reduces opacification. The original Anis IOL (**36.28, 36.29**) was designed to create such a symmetrical radial stretch on the capsule. A similar prototype IOL (**36.30, 36.31**) has been tested, and is also designed to achieve this goal. Of the present open-loop flexible IOLs, the one-piece all-PMMA posterior chamber designs appear to be especially effective in providing a symmetrical stretch. This may aid in minimizing posterior capsular opacification by reducing the folds in the capsular sac and holding the posterior capsule firmly against the posterior surface of the IOL optic. If IOL loops are placed in front of the anterior capsule, there is no mechanical means to prevent shrinkage and/or corrugation of the capsule (**36.23**). In such cases, as the bag shrinks, traction on the zonules with stretching or rupture may occur.

36.28

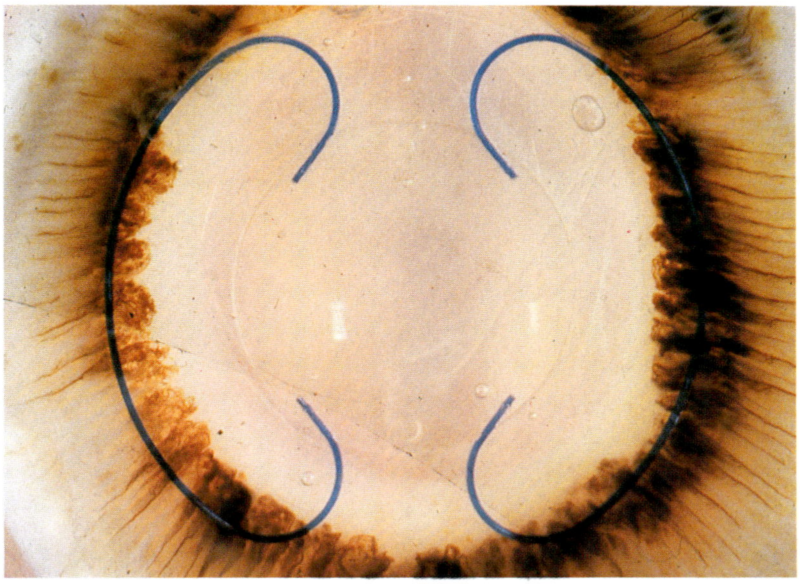

36.28 Gross photograph from behind of a rabbit eye implanted experimentally with an Anis IOL in the lens capsular sac. This lens was specifically designed in the mid-1970s for capsular fixation, and the broad C-shaped loops conform nicely to the circumference of the capsule, providing excellent centration. The cleanup of cortical material was so complete that the capsular sac is barely visible.

36.29

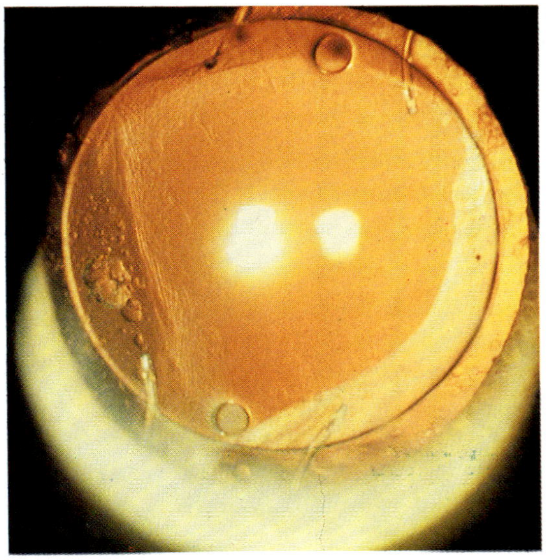

36.29 Clinical photograph of an eye implanted with an Anis lens, which has a posterior convex optic. There was no evidence of posterior capsular opacification six years after implantation. The only pearl formation and opacification is at the periphery. The radial stretch exerted by the IOL on the posterior capsule has apparently prevented central migration of proliferating epithelial cells (courtesy of Dr Aziz Anis, USA).

36.30

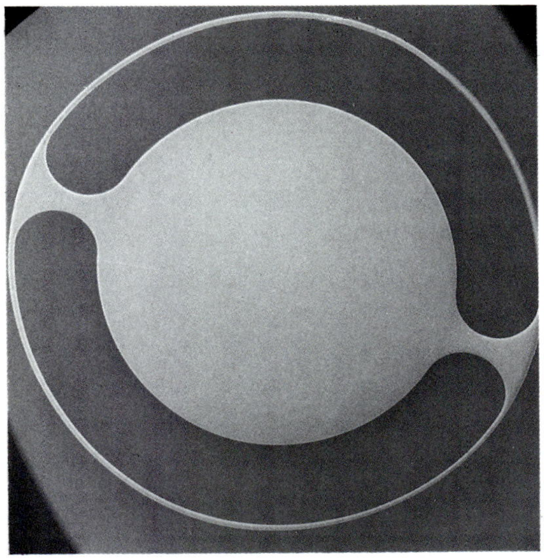

36.30 Scanning electron micrograph of a prototype one-piece all-PMMA biconvex posterior chamber lens design with an outer, supporting, 10 mm fixation ring, manufactured by Pharmacia Ophthalmics, Inc. The ring makes a 360° contact with the equator of the lens capsular sac and stretches the posterior capsule to assure contact between the posterior capsule and the biconvex optic (magnification x10).

36.31

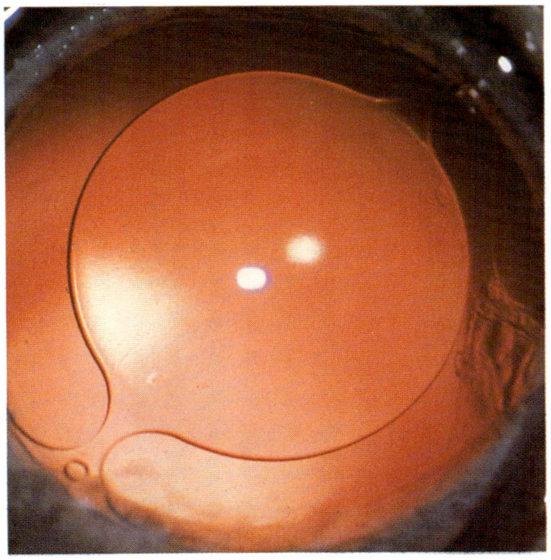

36.31 Clinical photograph of a rabbit eye implanted via the intercapsular technique, with the prototype lens illustrated in **36.30.** The photograph was taken 8 weeks postoperatively, and the excellent clarity of the media is demonstrated. The edge of the remaining anterior capsular flap is barely visible at 12 o'clock and is more prominent near 6 o'clock. The posterior capsule is stretched firmly against the posterior surface of the biconvex lens optic.

In conclusion, it is emphasized that, although ciliary fixation may achieve good clinical results over a long period of time, the precise and symmetrical placement of haptics within the capsular sac should achieve results that are even better (**36.32**).

36.32

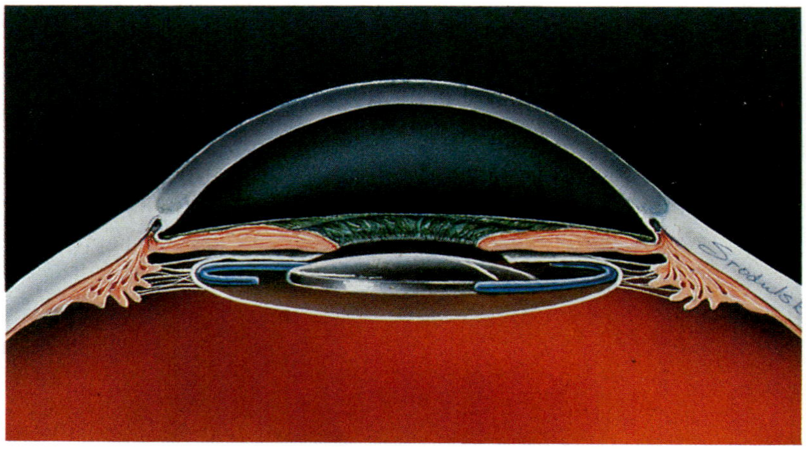

36.32 Schematic illustration of a sagittal section showing the anterior segment of the eye with a capsule-fixated posterior chamber lens (artist: Krystna Srodulski).

Further reading

Apple D.J., Reidy J.J., Googe J.M., Mamalis N., Novak L.C., Loftfield K. and Olson R.J. A comparison of ciliary sulcus and capsular bag fixation of posterior chamber intraocular lenses. *J. Am. Intraocul. Implant Soc.* **11,** 44–63, 1985.

Apple D.J., Lichtenstein S.B., Heerlein K., Letchinger S.L., Park R.B., Brems R.N. and Piest K.L. Visual aberrations caused by optic components of posterior chamber intraocular lenses. *J. Cataract Refract. Surg.,* **13,** 431–435, 1987.

Apple D.J., Kincaid M.C., Mamalis N. and Olson R.J. *Intraocular Lenses. Evolution, Designs, Complications and Pathology,* Baltimore, Williams and Wilkins, 1989.

Gwin T.D. and Apple D.J. A study of posterior chamber intraocular lens fixation and loop configuration: An analysis of 425 eyes obtained postmortem. Presented at the American Society of Cataract and Refractive Surgery Meeting, Los Angeles, CA, March 27, 1988.

Hansen S.O., Tetz M.R., Solomon K.D., Borup M.D., Brems R.N., O'Morchoe D.J.C., Bouhaddou O. and Apple D.J. Decentration of flexible loop posterior chamber intraocular lenses in a series of 222 postmortem eyes. *Ophthalmology,* **95,** 344–349, 1988.

Hansen S.O., Solomon K.D., McKnight G.T., Wilbrandt T.H., Gwin T.D., O'Morchoe D.J.C., Tetz M.R. and Apple D.J. Posterior capsular opacification and intraocular lens decentration. Part I: Comparison of various posterior chamber lens designs implanted in the rabbit model. *J. Cataract Refract. Surg.,* **14,** 605–614, 1988.

Tetz M.R., O'Morchoe D.J.C., Gwin T.D., Wilbrandt T.H., Solomon K.D., Hansen S.O. and Apple D.J. Posterior capsular opacification and intraocular lens decentration. Part II: Experimental findings on a prototype circular IOL design. *J. Cataract Refract. Surg.,* **14,** 614–623, 1988.

Section 6: MANAGEMENT OF COMPLICATIONS

37: Complications of anterior chamber lenses and management

John Alpar and Peter Choyce

Definitions

An anterior chamber lens (ACL) is an intraocular lens (IOL) that is completely in front of the iris and is supported by the chamber angle.

An IOL lens is *subluxated* when it has partially moved from its proper place but is still attached at some point to the surrounding tissues; it is *luxated* when it lies completely free without tissue support. If the lens moves to a new place suddenly, it is *expelled*. If it moves slowly, it is *extruded*. The word *dislocation* may cover any of the above conditions.

A lens is *decentered* if its optical center is partially or totally removed from the visual axis.

Considering construction, the lens is 'one piece' if both the optic and the haptic are cut out of the same material. A two piece lens has an optical part into which the haptic is inserted, even if the haptic is made of the same material. Sometimes the term 'two piece' refers to the fact that two different materials have been used in construction. Technically, it should refer to the number of separate pieces whether or not the same material was used in construction. Thus the Shepard Lens, with its four extruded PMMA haptics and a different PMMA optic, is a five piece lens.

The *haptic* is that part of an IOL that has no optical function: *Closed loop* implies a configuration where the haptic material originates from and returns to the optic. An *open loop* haptic has one end attached to the optic and the other free.

Some ACLs are vaulted. A flat nonvaulted lens is termed *uniplanar*.

For optical and manufacturing purposes, the optic of an ACL is almost always rigid. The haptic, however, may be *rigid* (Choyce lens, 37.1), *semiflexible* (Kelman, Anis, Leiske, or Azar lenses) or *flexible* (Shepard, Dubroff, Stableflex^{TM}, Pannu, Simcoe, Hessburg, or Momose lenses) (**37.2**).

37.1

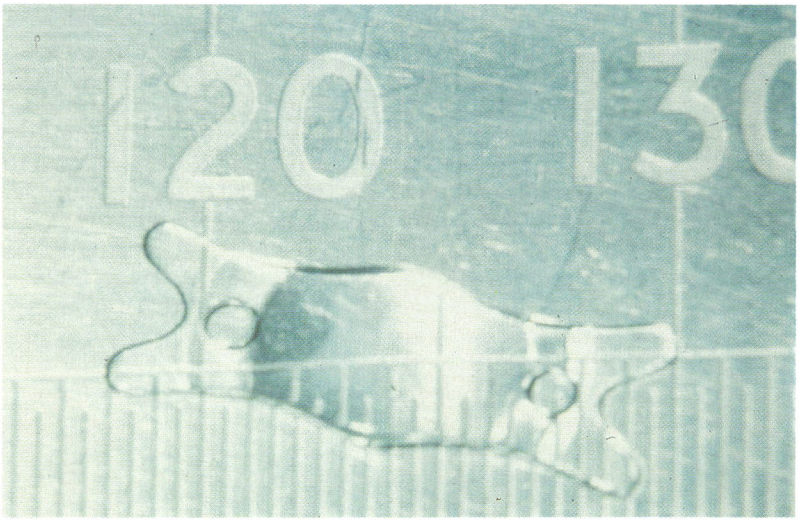

37.1 Measuring the length of the rigid Choyce IX ACL before insertion. Note the diagonal position of the lens on the ruler.

37.2(a)

37.2(b)

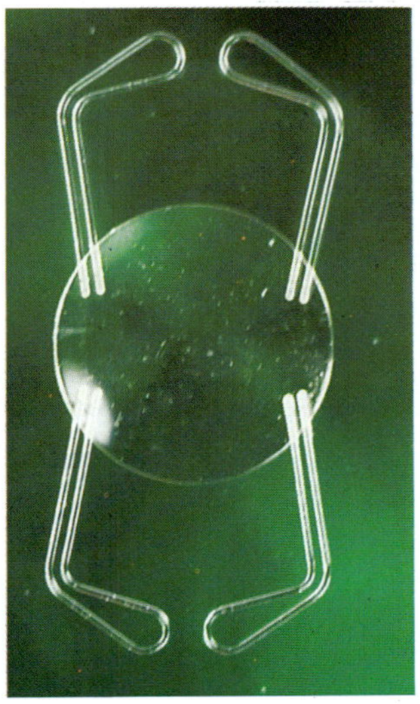

37.2(c)

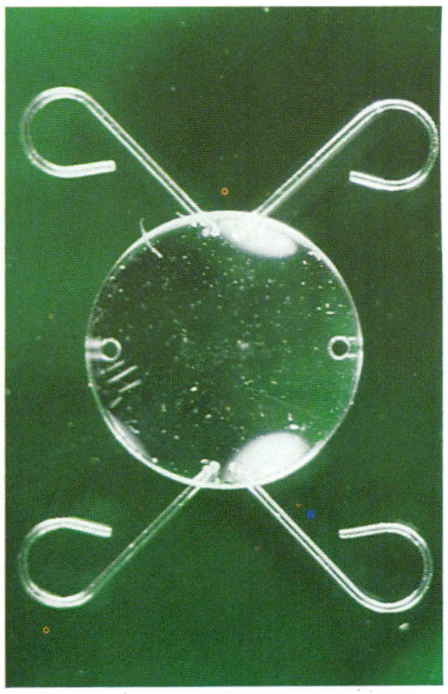

37.2(d)

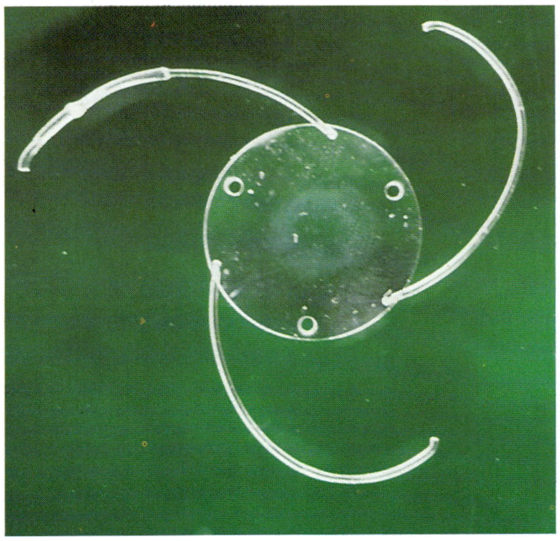

37.2 Examples of open loop ACLs of varying flexibility, all of which may be associated with unacceptable micromovement on eye rubbing, which can lead to late glaucoma and corneal dystrophy (a) Anis, (b) Stableflex^{TM}, (c) Shepard, (d) Dubroff.

General considerations

An IOL should restore maximum vision and keep it restored for the duration of the patient's life without the patient being aware of having a foreign body in the eye. Two fundamentals postulated by Harold Ridley at the dawn of IOL implantation were that the IOL will cause no harm:

'If the IOL does not move in the eye, and
If the eye does not move over the IOL.'

ACL complications are related to improper sizing, movement of the intraocular lens in the eye, movement of the tissues over the implant, change of shape of the implant (or its components) that alters the relative position of plastic and the ocular tissues, pressure of the implant on ocular tissues, optical changes, manufacturing flaws or the combination of several of the above factors.

Rigid ACL problems

One of the drawbacks of the rigid ACL is the need for very accurate *sizing* (**37.1**). Apart from the economic problems of stock, there is a need to have available, at the time of surgery, IOLs that are 0.5 mm smaller and 0.5 mm larger than the actually measured white to white + 1 mm diameter in the horizontal meridian. Serious problems can develop from improper sizing: if the lens is too small, it could *rotate* (propeller) in the eye causing corneal damage leading to endothelial corneal decompensation (ECD). This rotation is especially dangerous when the lens is implanted vertically as a primary implant. (If the lens is implanted obliquely in the near horizontal position, it will sink by gravity and may be prevented from rotating as soon as the lower two feet reach an anterior chamber diameter of the proper size). If the lens is longer than needed, increased tenderness to touch or even to blinking (especially if the lens is placed vertically) occurs, which may last for the duration of the life of the patient. This *tenderness* is the result of the lens pressing on the ciliary body, even eroding into it. If the lens is more than 0.5 mm too long, or is forced in a lengthwise direction, this erosion may occur during surgery, leading to severe intraoperative hemorrhage.

The rigid lens may *decenter* when it rotates or shifts in any other way. This is especially true of the Choyce lens (**37.3, 37.4**). Decentration often leads to optical problems: diminished vision, prism effect, glare and diplopia. In such a situation the lens must be replaced. Fortunately, the replacement of rigid lenses is not difficult nor dangerous if a viscoelastic substance is used.

Even with a vaulted ACL, adequate iridectomies are important to prevent pupillary block. If the lens is implanted as a secondary procedure, additional iridectomies may be necessary and the lens is placed in such a way that the feet do not lie near openings in the iris or near anterior synechias of the iris. If the lens is implanted as a primary procedure, adequate iridectomies must be made, but distant to the feet of the lens, and are best performed midstromal *after* implantation of the IOL. If the iridectomy is basal or nearly so, and the lens rotates postoperatively, some part of the haptic will end up in the coloboma. Although this will stop further rotation, the pressure will now be on the ciliary processes (**37.5**). This increases tenderness and may lead to low grade cyclitis, hemorrhage or cystoid macular edema (CME).

37.3

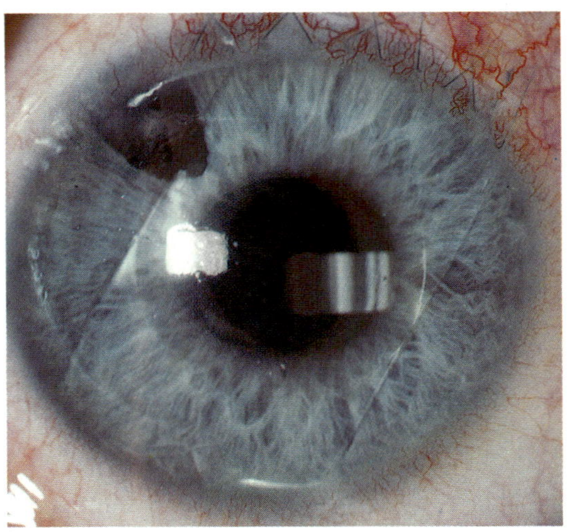

37.3 A 33-year-old white male one day after surgery, using an obliquely placed Choyce Mark VIII with a round pupil.

37.4

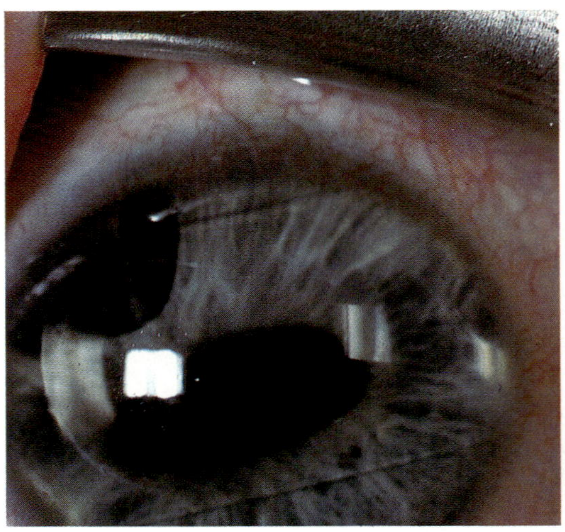

37.4 Same eye as in **37.3** 3.5 years later. Note the lens has rotated and decentered upwards, and the commencement of ovalling.

37.5

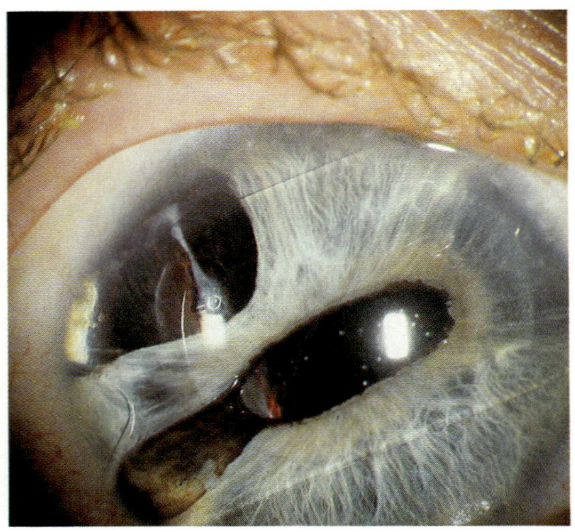

37.5 Same eye as in **37.3**, seven years after surgery. Note the callus formation with uveal ectropion inferiorly. The iridectomy has been stretched and one footplate has slipped through the iridectomy and is eroding the ciliary body.

Movement of the foot towards the vitreous will also cause the opposite foot (or feet) to rise and hit the cornea, leading to corneal endothelial decompensation. The coloboma stretches and the lens may slip through the iridectomy into the vitreous cavity (**37.6**).

The problem of vitreous

Presently many ACLs are used in complicated cases after vitreous loss, or as a secondary lens implant when there is no capsule left to support a posterior chamber lens.

One must clearly realize that vitreous entering the anterior chamber during the primary procedure is greatly different from vitreous that has been in the anterior chamber for some time, or vitreous that is present in the vitreous cavity weeks or months after an intracapsular cataract extraction. Whereas the freshly damaged vitreous must be carefully removed from the wound, from the anterior chamber, from the surface of the iris, and from the pupillary plane, the vitreous found during secondary implantation can be 'plowed back' into the retropupillary space by using viscoelastics in conjunction with a Sheets' glide or with the intraocular lens. Adherent strands of vitreous in the anterior chamber should always be cut with scissors rather than freed with a spatula, as great care should be taken not to put stress on the vitreous base and predispose the eye to later retinal detachment. Occasionally, it may be necessary to abscise vitreous at the level of the wound. In either primary or secondary implantation, formed vitreous or vitreous strands can make the implantation of a flexible ACL difficult: correct feet placement, proper centering of the lens, and avoidance of corneal/intraocular lens touch are major problems. Unrecognized vitreous presence in the anterior chamber may lead to late decentration of such a lens. The complications from vitreous are least apt to occur with rigid lenses.

37.6

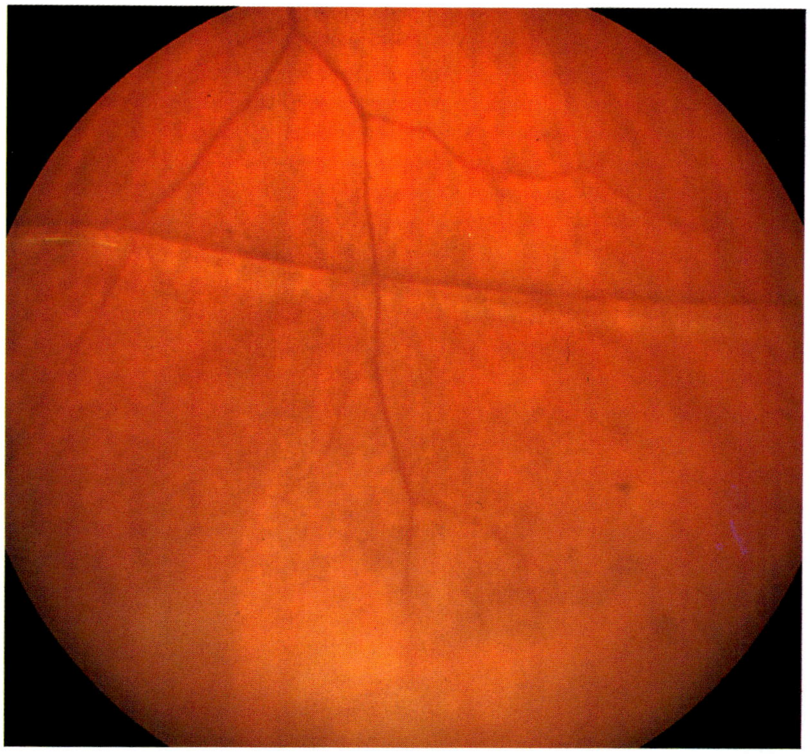

37.6 Dislocated Choyce VIII lens on the retina (courtesy of Dr Henry Hirschman, USA).

Pupil block

Pupillary block in the presence of inadequate iridectomy is common with all lenses, but especially so with the rigid lenses, even when they are vaulted anteriorly. The main clinical sign of such block is 'internal iris prolapse'. It can be solved easily with the creation of an extrapupillary iris opening by midstromal surgical or YAG laser iridotomy (see **44.11, 44.12**).

Incomplete iridectomies with the pigment epithelial layer left intact can easily be made complete with either neodymium YAG or Argon lasers. If such lasers are not available, it is enough to enter the eye between two sutures and touch the pigment epithelial layer with a spatula. Immediately the coloboma will open and the chamber deepen, and the pupillary block be solved.

The oval pupil

One of the main problems of the ACL is that the correct placement of the feet is often difficult. Certainly, viscoelastic maintenance of the anterior chamber, or the use of a Sheets' glide (or even two, introducing the lens between the two glides) makes the placement of the distal feet more accurate. However, even lenses that appear to have been well inserted and the position of the feet checked with laryngeal or dental mirrors, or a Koeppe Lens on the table, may show feet displacement on gonioscopy a week or so later.

There are generally four feet that need to be in the chamber angle. To place the upper haptic in the angle and keep it there during a primary implantation, the surgical entry wound has to have a ledge under which the feet can be tucked *under direct visualization*. However, even such a direct check does not exclude the possibility of superior iris incarceration or iris tuck (**37.7**). This is the case even in secondary implantation, when the incision can be made on the temporal side of the cornea and the lens introduced obliquely or horizontally.

37.7

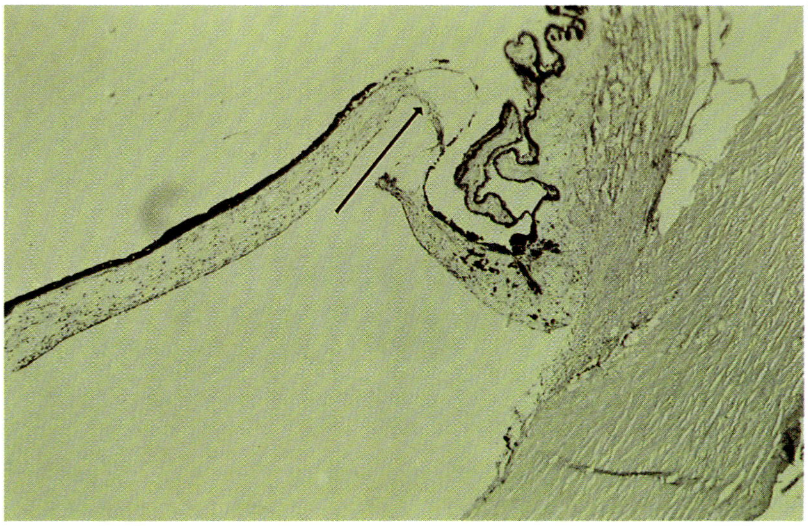

37.7 Histology showing the iris tuck of a Choyce VIII lens (arrow shows the position of the footplate).

If possible, the iris tuck should be corrected during the initial surgery (see Chapter 12). If a tuck is not corrected, ovalling will occur, which may be stationary. More often it progresses along the longitudinal axis of the IOL (**37.8**). (If ovalling is perpendicular to the axis, it is usually the result of retraction from organized vitreous.) Gradually, the lens-induced ovalling can become so extreme as to cause a slit-like pupil. Usually this is only a cosmetic problem, but sometimes optical problems, low grade uveitis or increased tenderness and dislocations (**37.9**) may be observed.

Whereas acute ovalling is the result of 'on-the-table' iris tuck, late ovalling of originally round pupils (**37.3–37.5, 37.10, 37.11**) is caused by a different mechanism. The foremost reason for late ovalling is callus formation on the iris: where the PMMA is in contact with the iris tissue, a callus forms (**37.12**). The callus, which is a protective reaction of the iris tissue, everts the pupillary pigment epithelium and pulls the pigment surface of the iris outwards (ectropion pupillae). A callus can also form around the feet of the lens and in the chamber angle (**37.11–37.13**). It can be an aid to fixation. The contraction of the callus, especially that on the iris surface near the pupil, can lead to gradual progressive pupillary distortion (**37.12**).

Rigid ACLs also have a tendency to 'sink back' into the eye (*posterior settlement*). If eyes having such lenses are checked with a gonioscope yearly, a deepening of the anterior chamber and of the chamber angle (**37.11, 37.13**) is found, with the iris crawling up around the feet. The

37.8

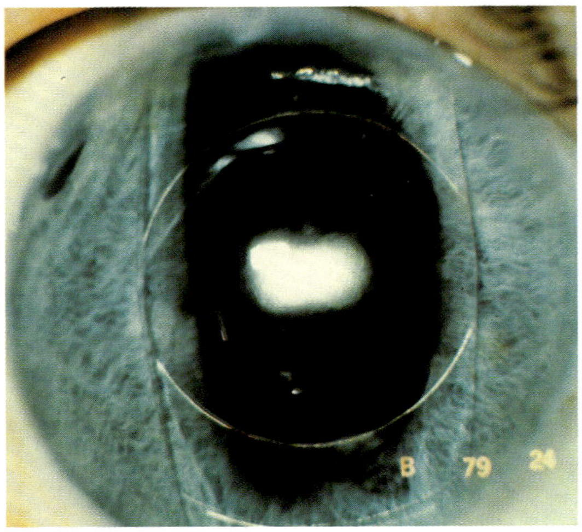

37.8 Ovalling of the pupil after vertical placement of the Choyce VIII lens with iris tuck.

37.9

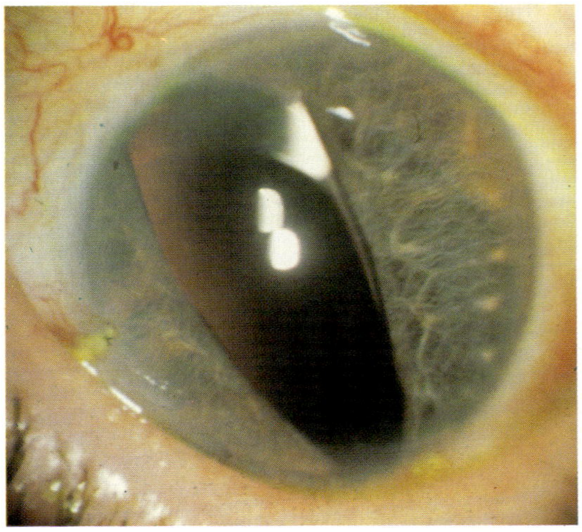

37.9 Choyce VIII lens: extreme ovalling has led to dislocation of the lens into the posterior chamber. Urgent explantation was required (courtesy of Dr Maurice John, USA).

37.10

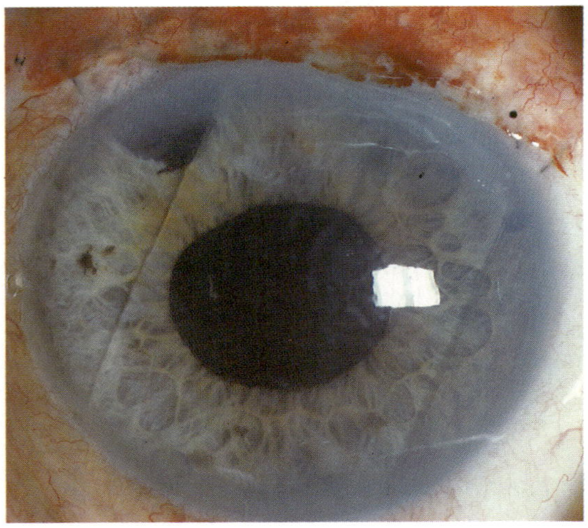

37.10 Choyce VIII lens after surgery with a round pupil.

37.11

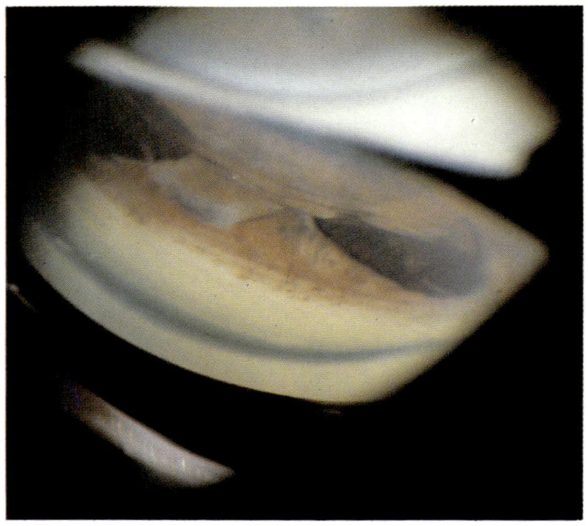

37.11 Gonioscopy of same eye as in **37.10** four years later, showing callus and erosion of feet through the iris into the ciliary body.

37.12

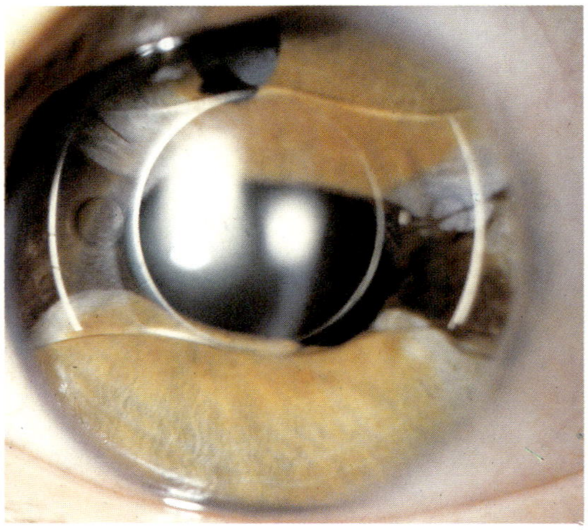

37.12 Callus formation with ectropion pupillae five years after the horizontal placement of a Choyce IX lens in a child.

37.13

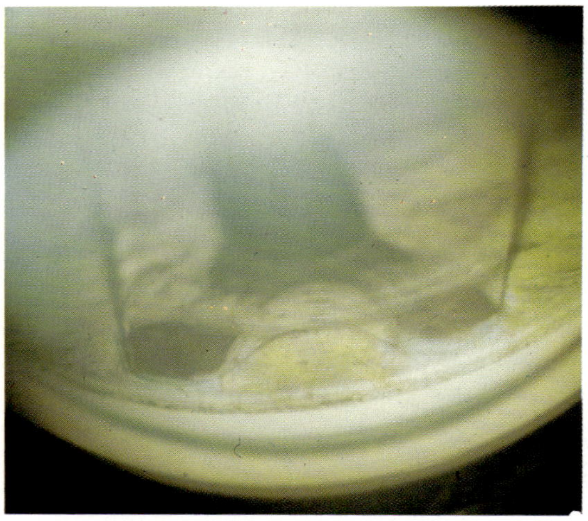

37.13 Gonioscopy showing callus formation and iris fibrosis around the lower feet of a Choyce VIII lens. Note the posterior settlement and increased pigmentation of the trabecular meshwork.

iris is actually not 'tucked', as in the acute cases, but a flat sliding is observed. Gradually, pupillary distortion develops from iris stretch. This process takes many years to develop and does not necessarily cause tenderness.

Whether the implantatión is primary or secondary, pupillary constriction greatly facilitates the guiding of the lens into the chamber angle and the avoidance of tuck. If a marked degree of tucking is discovered during the immediate postoperative period, it should be corrected through a reoperation. Using a stab incision, an iris hook can be passed without losing the chamber and the footplate lifted towards the cornea, so freeing the trapped iris. Viscoelastic material or balanced salt solution may be injected parallel with the lens axis under the feet to help iron out the tucked iris.

Late ovalling must be followed carefully. If it progresses and is accompanied by clinical signs of inflammation, even of low grade (**37.14–37.16**), or tilting (**37.17–37.19**), the intraocular lens should be replaced. Likewise, if callus formation is extensive, leading to pupillary disfiguration, lens exchange is recommended. However, if there are no symptoms indicating corneal, uveal, or retinal problems the lens can be left *in situ*, provided the patient can be observed very closely and is cooperative.

37.14

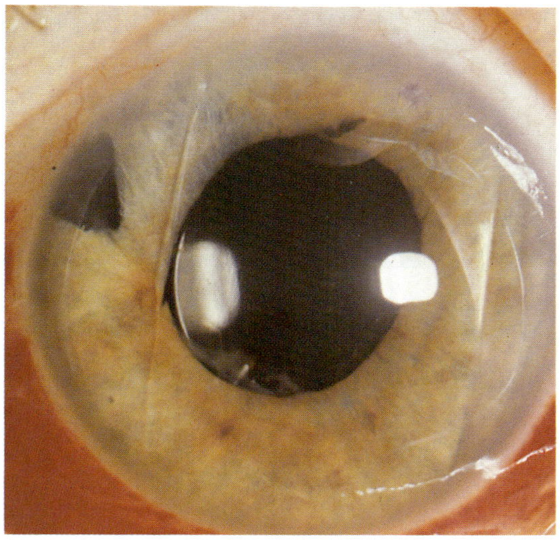

37.14 Choyce VIII lens with a round pupil after surgery.

37.15

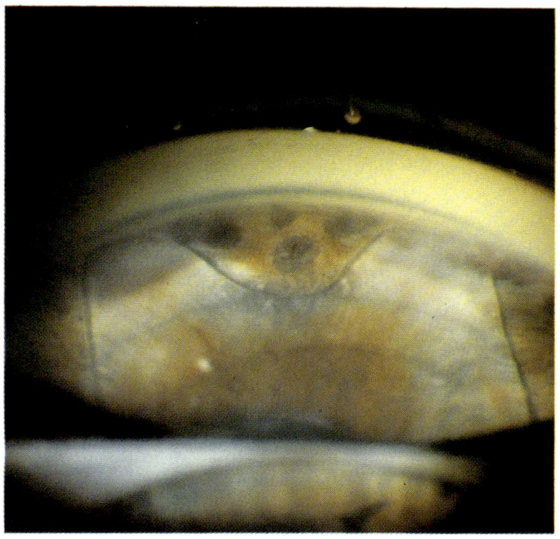

37.15 Same eye as in **37.14**. Six years later gonioscopy shows that although the feet are correctly placed, there are signs of chronic inflammation. Note the callus, fibrosis and pigmentation.

37.16

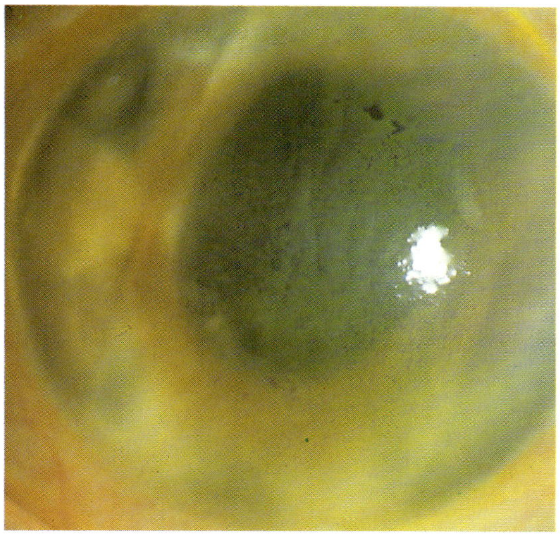

37.16 Same eye as in **37.14**, with corneal decompensation seven years after surgery.

37.17

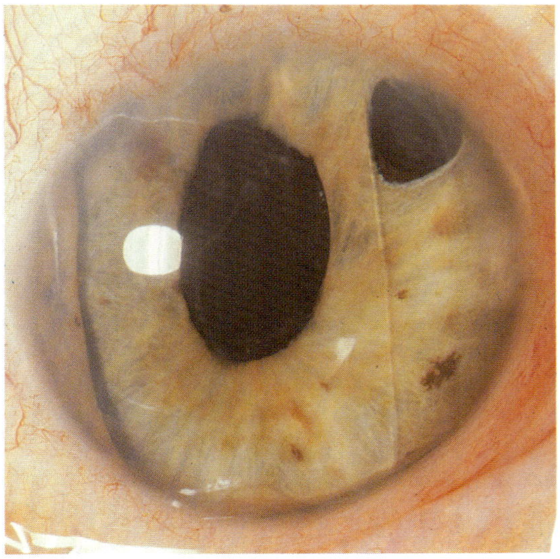

37.17 Late ovalling four years after surgery.

37.18

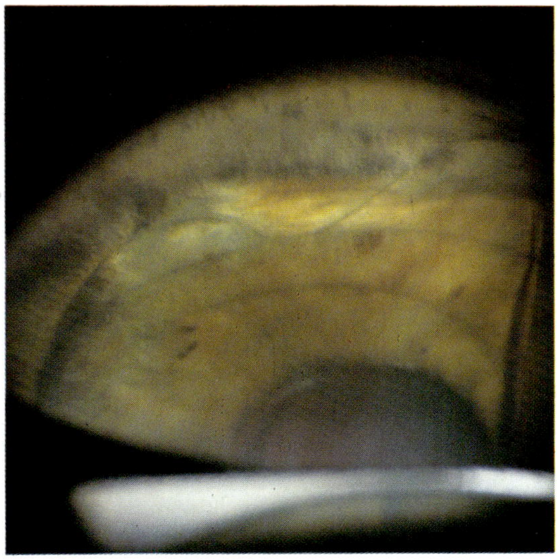

37.18 Same eye as in **37.17** seven years after surgery with a tilted lens: gonioscopy shows one foot in the iris, the other against the cornea.

37.19

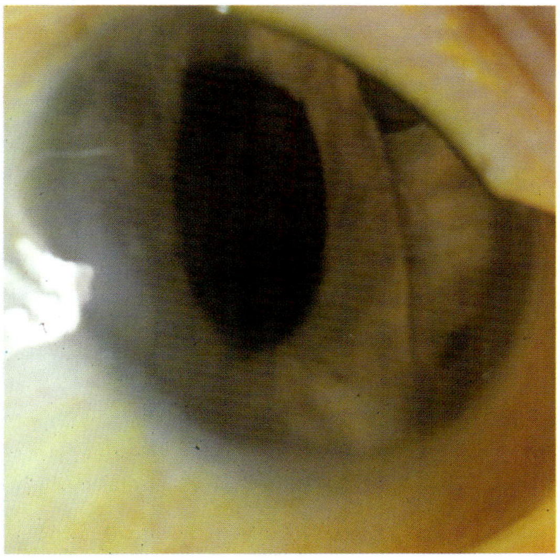

37.19 Same eye as in **37.17**, eight years after surgery showing corneal decompensation.

Haptic incarceration

It should be emphasized that the proximal feet of any lens must be placed under a corneoscleral ledge by direct observation, and reinspected during suturing. If one foot is discovered in the wound within three days, it must be replaced surgically. A stab incision at the limbus at 90° to the lens, near the superior limbus, will allow the passing of a spatula that can dislodge the incarcerated haptic.

If discovered late, severe hemorrhage may occur from the already vascularized wound. Soft haptics of flexible lenses are especially easily entrapped in the vascularized sclera (**37.20**). If gonioscopy shows no reaction around the foot, the above maneuver may be tried. However, the surgeon must be prepared to convert immediately to the opening of the wound if he experiences any resistance to the mobilization of the plastic.

If the haptic is protruding through the wound, immediate corrective surgery is mandatory because of the danger of endophthalmitis, wound leak, endothelial touch and endothelial corneal dystrophy. Amputation of the offending haptic without removing the IOL is not a solution: it destabilizes the intraocular lens leading to subluxation. If the haptic cannot be replaced and the wound sutured, the intraocular lens has to be removed.

Incarcerated haptic usually means tilted intraocular lens. Apart from the somewhat diminished optical performance, the danger of endothelial damage is considerable (*see* **39.11**) and only in exceptional circumstances should the surgeon temporize. Some flexible haptics can snap out of the chamber angle through rubbing or squeezing the eyes, and end up in the wound. The vast majority of incarcerations, however, are displaced during surgery and the problem is not recognized.

37.20

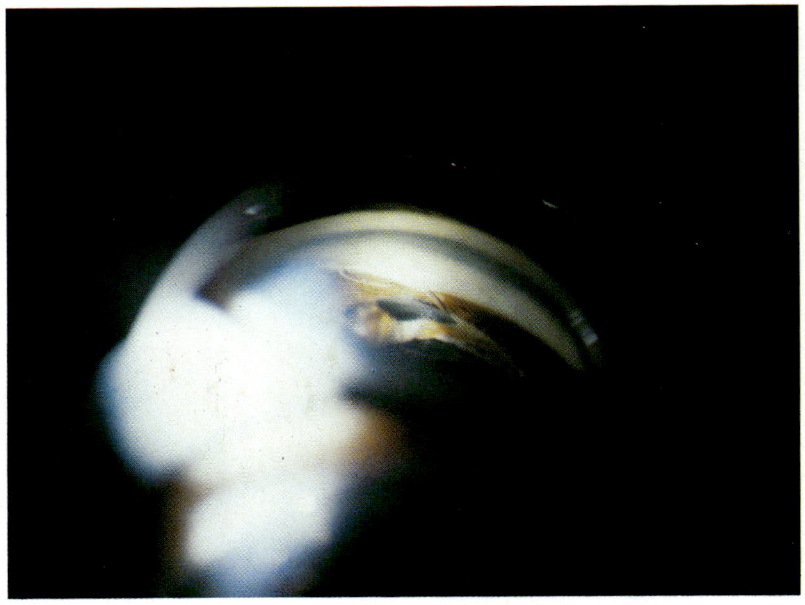

37.20 Gonioscopy showing a flexible open loop (Shepard) ACL with one foot in the wound several weeks after surgery, although it was noted to be in the correct position on the operating table.

Flexible ACL problems

The more flexible the ACL, the less is the likelihood of the problems found with rigid lenses, such as rotation, tenderness, decentration, pupil block, posterior settlement, and ovalling. However, other and more severe problems may arise from *micromovement*. Semiflexible ACLs may be associated with all the aforementioned problems, but to a lesser degree.

Open loops have fewer complications than closed loops and the best compromise is generally considered to be a one piece semiflexible open loop (Kelman) design with four point fixating haptic and an anterior vaulted optic (see **12.3**).

The movement of *closed loop lenses* (e.g., Leiske, Azar, Hessburg,) creates constant rubbing against the iris, leading to iris overgrowth around the loops (**37.21**). The iris, in self-protection, encapsulates the loops. Such adhesions do stop the rotation of the intraocular lens, but the micromovement continues. A low grade iritis is present, leading to CME and also to ECD. Since most of these lenses are in eyes that do not have posterior capsular protection and do not have the protective intact anterior hyaloid membrane, the barrier deprivation syndrome develops with all its devastating consequences. In severe cases the peripheral iris synechiae around the feet expand. The subsequent 'zipping-up of the angle' can lead to glaucoma. Furthermore, the closed loop lenses, usually already vaulted (two plane) to minimize pupillary block, will vault more on blinking if placed vertically, or upon rubbing the eye. While vaulting from compression of the loop, the lens can rise and hit the cornea, while the loop continues to irritate the iris. Such lenses should never be used and must be removed as soon as possible. Owing to the incarceration of the loops in the iris, the lens cannot 'slip out' of the eye. If force is applied, the iris might be torn (even iridodialysis can develop) and severe hemorrhage will be encountered. The technique of removing such lenses requires a separate side incision through which the invaginated loop can be amputated and rotated out of the eye (see p. 255).

37.21

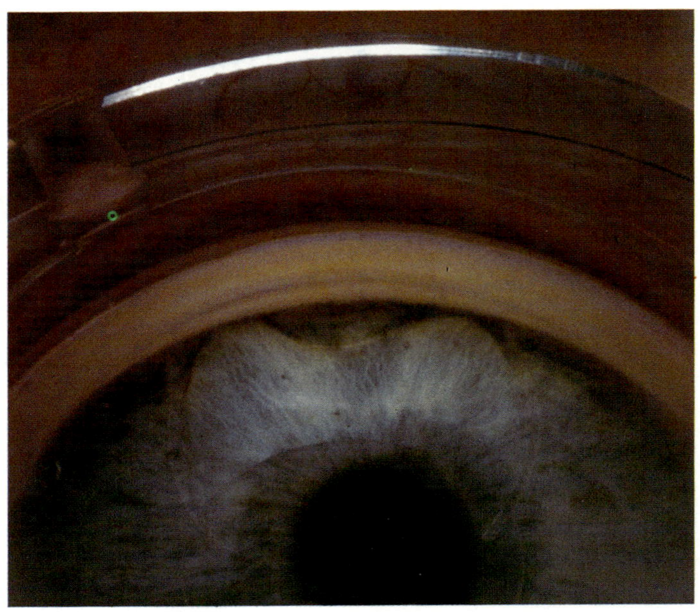

37.21 Gonioscopy showing iris overgrowth around a closed loop (Azar) ACL (zipping-up of the angle) (courtesy of Dr Jan Worst, The Netherlands).

Flexible lenses with *open loops* (e.g., Simcoe C-Loop – double or triple, Dubroff, Stableflex, Pannu, Shepard and Momose Lenses), can have the loop/angle contact on a large surface (**37.22**), especially if they are crammed into a small diameter anterior chamber. Vaulting and corneal touch is a reality, although theoretically the very flexible loops are supposed to slide along the iris surface in the iris plane and not to vault. Unfortunately, the sliding also leads to iris–lens synechias (**37.23**), zipping-up of the angle (**37.24**), neovascularization (**37.25**), uveitis, CME, and eventually ECD. These complications are worsened by any degree of eye rubbing. If a lens leads to no problems and the patient can be followed closely, the IOL does not need to be removed.

37.22

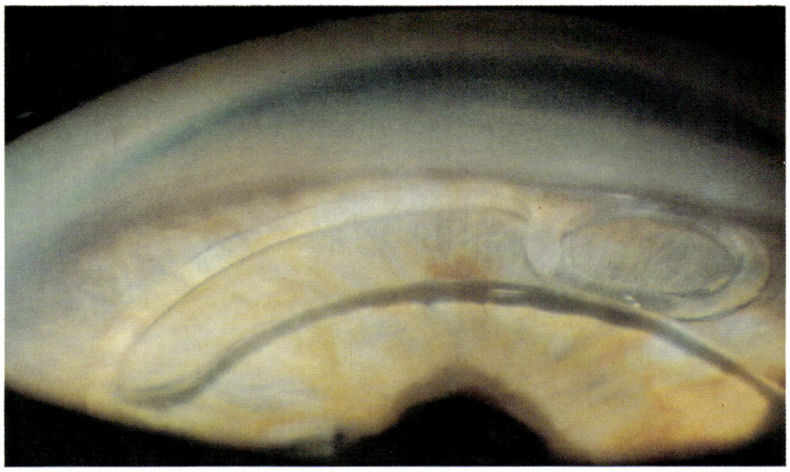

37.22 Gonioscopy showing the extensive loop–angle contact of a flexible (Pannu) ACL due to cramming of haptics against the optic.

37.23

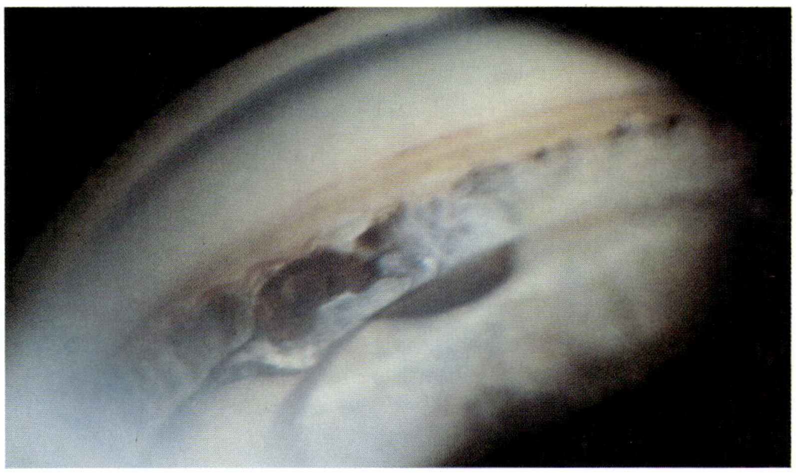

37.23 Gonioscopy of a Pannu lens with one foot embedded in the iris associated with neovascularization and iris–lens synechias.

37.24

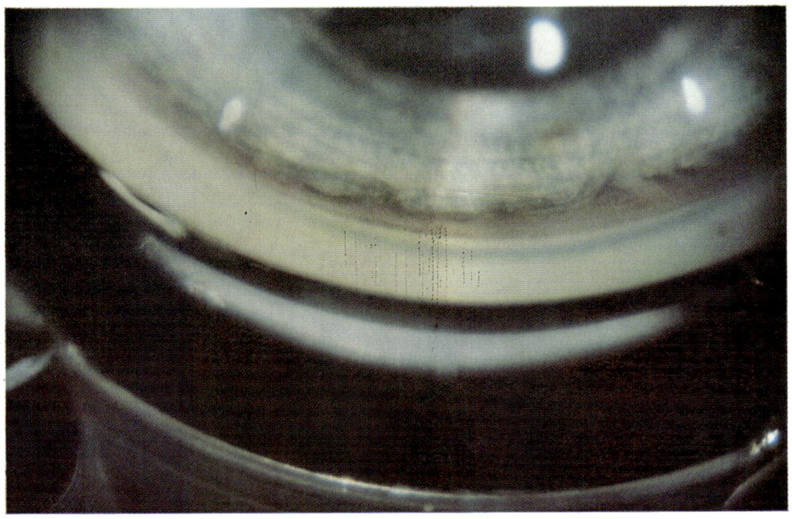

37.24 Gonioscopy showing the zipping up of angle with an open loop (Stableflex^{TM}) ACL.

37.25

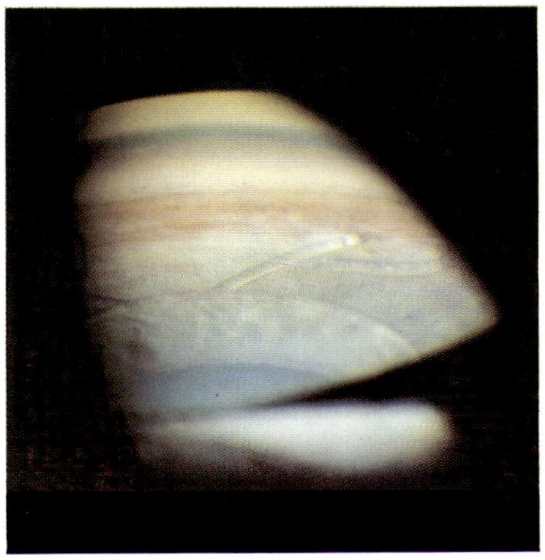

37.25 Gonioscopy showing that micromovement of the flexible open loop (Shepard) ACL induces neovascularization.

Displacement

Decentration of flexible lenses is usually caused by formed vitreous in the anterior chamber, generally just above the pupillary plane. If the presence of vitreous is recognized, then vitrectomy through the original incision has to be performed even in secondary implants. One of the signs is the difficulty of placing the intraocular lens: the flexible lens keeps coming out of the eye or is always being pushed towards one side, usually that nearer to the incision (vitreous kick syndrome). Also, the pupil cannot be constricted to a very small central opening with intracameral miotics.

Sometimes, however, the vitreous cannot be identified on the table and the centration of the intraocular lens seems to be satisfactory. Only at a later visit will the condition present itself clearly. If the decentration is small and stable, the vision good, the position of the feet such that the cornea is not threatened, and the patient can be followed regularly, a conservative approach is called for. Otherwise, a pars plana vitrectomy needs to be performed. Limbal vitrectomy would be less helpful and more dangerous to the cornea. The vitrectomy entrance is usually 180° from where the vitreous is located in the chamber. The aim is complete control of both the retroirideal and the anterior chamber vitreous.

In the case of a *blunt trauma* to the eye, a rigid or semiflexible intraocular lens can become an intraocular missile, cutting through the intraocular tissues or extruding through the ruptured surgical wound. Such intraocular lenses must be removed. The damage has to be repaired and the eye allowed to quieten down. If the condition permits, and if true need demands it, a lens of different design could be implanted later or epikeratophakia surgery performed.

Uveitis glaucoma hyphema syndrome

Micromovement in the eye may lead to *chafing* of the iris and *hemorrhage*. *Glaucoma* may develop from angle changes of all the ACL designs, from extensive peripheral anterior synechiae formation, from debris (pigment, blood cells, other material), from blocking the trabecular meshwork, or from bleached-out erythrocytes (ghost cells). The triad of uveitis, glaucoma and hyphema is termed the *UGH syndrome* (**37.26, 37.27**). If the vitreous is involved, the term is *UGH plus syndrome*. Ghost cell glaucoma is mostly present if the hemorrhage involves the vitreous cavity (UGH plus syndrome).

UGH or UGH plus syndromes can be relieved only through the removal of the intraocular lens, irrigation of the anterior chamber and, in the case of vitreous hemorrhage and ghost cell glaucoma, through a pars plana vitrectomy. The eye must then be allowed to rest and recover. Anti-inflammatory and anti-glaucomatous therapy is given as needed.

37.26

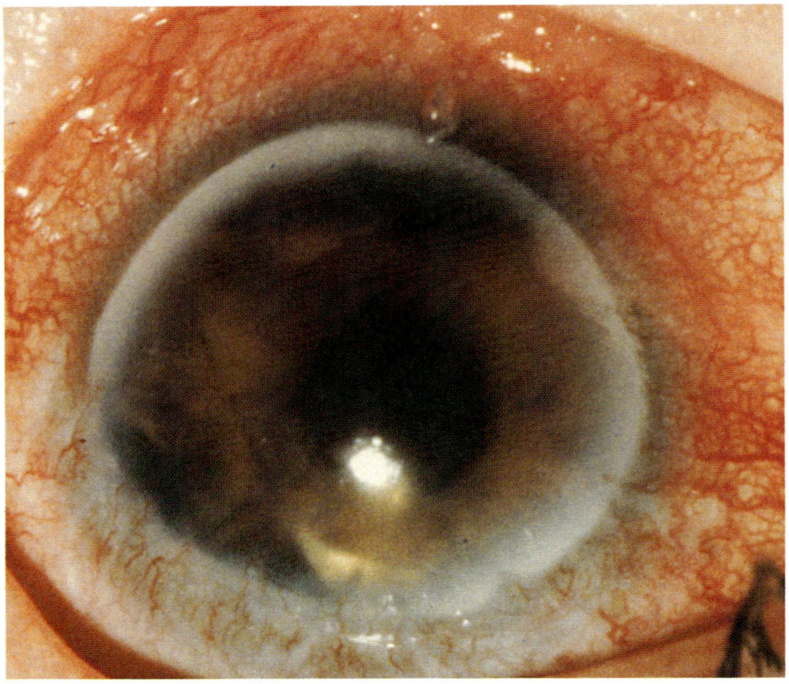

37.26 UGH syndrome from a rigid (Choyce) ACL.

37.27

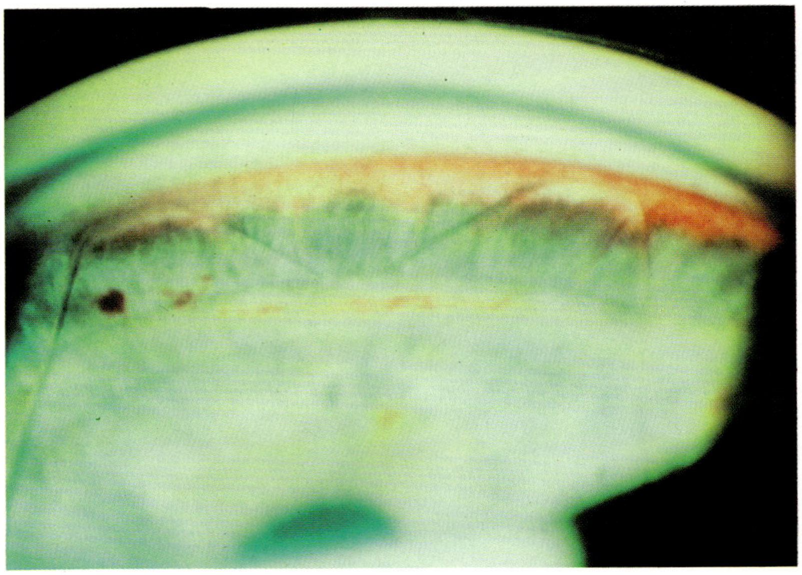

37.27 Gonioscopy of an eye with glaucoma and hyphema showing angle neovascularization and hemorrhage from a poorly finished rigid ACL.

Corneal melting syndrome

Several cases have been reported with rigid ACLs where corneal melting and perforation occurred in the absence of infection, at about half the distance between the limbus and the apex of the cornea (**37.28**). Histological examinations have not shown inflammatory changes. The keratitis is similar but more centrally placed than that associated with rheumatoid arthritis. Evidence that the syndrome is ACL related is circumstantial only, as corneal melting has also been recognized after cataract surgery without implantation in predisposed individuals.

The treatment of corneal melting syndrome is penetrating keratoplasty and the removal of the offending intraocular lens. A posterior chamber lens can be implanted and sutured, either to the iris or to the sclera through the pars plana.

37.28

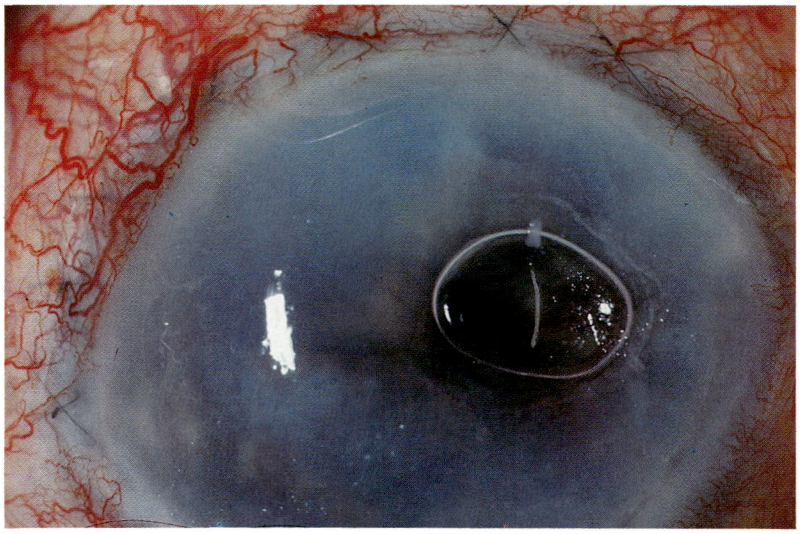

37.28 Corneal melting syndrome with a perforation 3 months after insertion of a rigid ACL.

Improper placement of lenses in the eye

With the drive to invent and manufacture a universal lens that can be used under any circumstances, recommendations have been made for the placement of posterior chamber lenses into the anterior chamber angle in the case of vitreous loss. Some of these lenses were single plane; some angled. The majority of such placements have led to corneal decompensation. If any such patient comes to the attention of a practitioner (**37.29**), the lens should be removed unless there is absolutely no sign of inflammation, peripheral synechias, neovascularization of the iris around the feet of the lens, and unless the patient can be observed at regular intervals for both gonioscopy and estimations of endothelial cell density.

Some ACLs have been implanted back to front (**37.30**). These placements generally lead to late corneal decompensation and such lenses should be removed as soon as the condition is recognized.

37.29

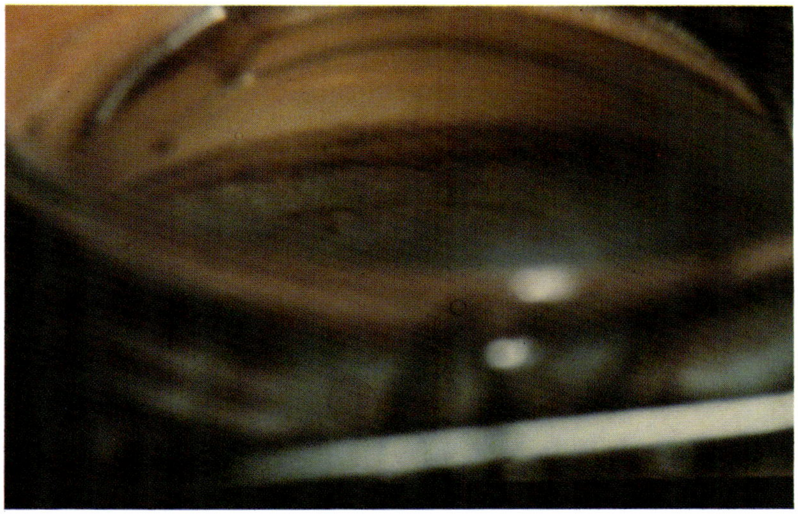

37.29 C-looped posterior chamber lens placed in an anterior chamber angle. Note the position of the polypropylene haptic against the corneal endothelium.

37.30

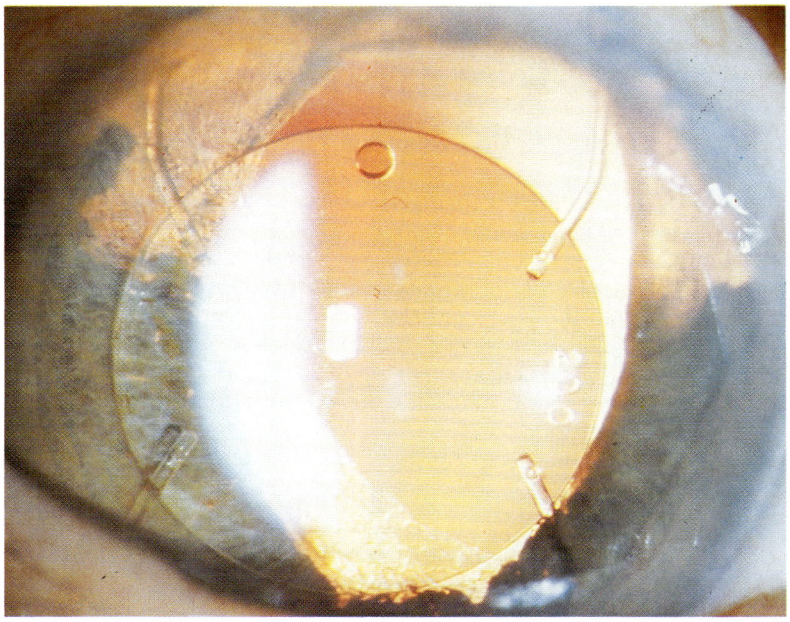

37.30 Placement of flexible (Azar) ACL back to front. Note the peripheral synechias and gross iris atrophy (courtesy of Dr Ralph Anderson, USA).

Cystoid macular edema

Cystoid macular edema can develop without noticeable endophthalmodonesis. The majority of such patients have low grade, subclinical uveitis.

It is difficult to evaluate the efficacy of therapy in CME since a large percentage resolve spontaneously. It has been shown that *systemic*, nonsteroidal anti-inflammatory agents have very little effect on CME, mainly because of insufficient ocular drug level. Systemic steroid therapy should be avoided because of the risk of side effects when given in high dosage.

The recommended treatment is intensive *topical* therapy with corticosteroids and nonsteroidal anti-inflammatory agents. Steroid eye drops should be given two hourly and reduced to six hourly after three days. Indomethacin eye drops should be given six hourly. The intraocular pressure must be monitored. If uveitis persists despite treatment, lens explantation may be considered.

Manufacturing quality

In spite of improved quality control, on occasions one still finds rough edges of both the optic and haptic components, especially at the rims of the holes drilled for insertion of the haptics (*see* **17.6, 17.8**) and at the injection gates of injection-molded intraocular lenses. These can lead to iris erosion and severe hemorrhage.

Sometimes the feet of one piece rigid intraocular lenses are not placed evenly and do not touch a flat surface simultaneously. If one depresses one foot of such a lens with forceps, the foot opposite and diagonal to the depressed foot will rise (**37.31**). If such a lens is implanted, UGH syndrome is inevitable.

To prevent such problems:

- Ignore sales talks and advertisements, especially those that employ superlatives.
- Check the companies for their safety record and use only those with an established reputation.
- Examine every intraocular lens carefully under magnification before opening the sterile package and reexamine it after the lens has been taken out from the package before implanting it into the eye.
- Rigid and semirigid, anterior chamber, angle-fixated lenses should be placed on a flat surface. All the feet should touch the surface equally. If on tapping one foot, an opposite foot is seen to rise, warpage is indicated.
- Verify the diagonal length before implantation.

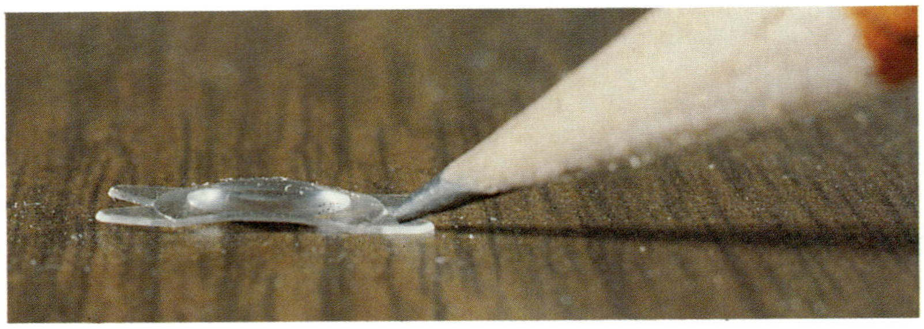 37.31

37.31 Warped rigid ACL. Note the position of the feet when one side is pushed with a pencil (courtesy of Dr Tom Ellingson, USA).

In summary, the long-term complications and morbidity from ACLs lead to caution in their recommendation. Closed loop ACLs should never be used. Only if an iris claw lens is unavailable and there is insufficient capsular support for a posterior chamber lens should an ACL be considered. The choice would then be an obliquely implanted Choyce Mark VIII or IX lens or a one piece Kelman lens with semiflexible loops.

38: Complications of posterior chamber lenses

John Pearce

Pupil trap or capture

Pupil trap (capture) means that part or all of the posterior chamber lens is anterior to the iris plane. It generally occurs later rather than earlier after surgery. Usually, early pupil capture can be corrected (**38.1**), but late capture is associated with synechias to the capsule, which are extremely difficult to break (**38.2**). The incidence reported in the literature after posterior chamber lens (PCL) implantation is approximately 1% for eyes without other pathology. In glaucoma eyes the incidence has been recorded as high as 28%.

Prevention is achieved by avoiding asymmetric fixation of loops in the bag and sulcus, unless the lens is specifically designed for capsular bag/sulcus fixation, and electing for capsular fixation, so that the optic is then deeper in the eye and more posterior to the iris. Angulated loop haptics are preferred to uniplanar, and single piece, profile cut PMMA lenses may resist anterior dislocation better than three piece lenses with polypropylene haptics. If the lens is sulcus fixated or uniplanar, the pupil should be constricted at the end of surgery. Mydriasis in the early postoperative period should be avoided, except in the presence of developing synechias.

Complications of pupil capture include a low grade *uveitis* leading to pupil block glaucoma, uveitis associated with *cystoid macular edema* (CME) and pigment deposits on the lens. Pupil block glaucoma may require Yag laser or surgical iridectomy.

Treatment of early pupillary capture is possible provided firm synechias have not developed. Dilation of the pupil and then constriction may help (**38.1**), as may pressure over the haptics with two glass rods. Late pupil capture may occur months after surgery and is usually due to progressive fibrosis between the anterior and posterior capsule or between the capsule and iris in association with sulcus placement. At this stage it is extremely difficult and often impossible to reposition the lens, which can be safely left provided there is no persistent iritis, CME or visual problems from lens edge glare (**38.2**). There may be refractive consequences with an increase in myopia (**38.3**).

38.1

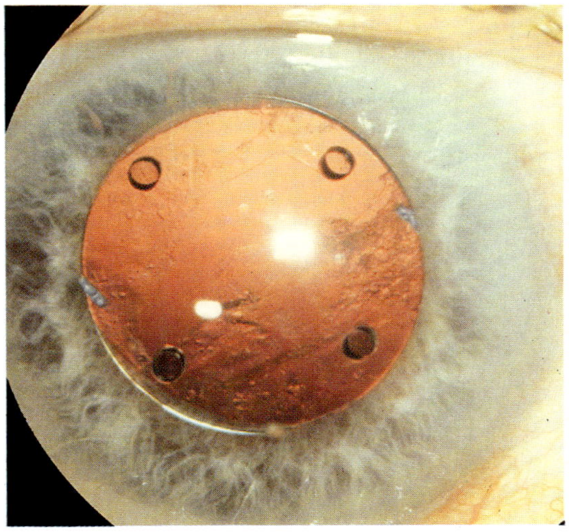

38.1 A sulcus-fixated Simcoe lens with polypropylene loops associated with anterior dislocation of the optic on pupillary dilation. Recurrences were prevented by topical miotics.

38.2

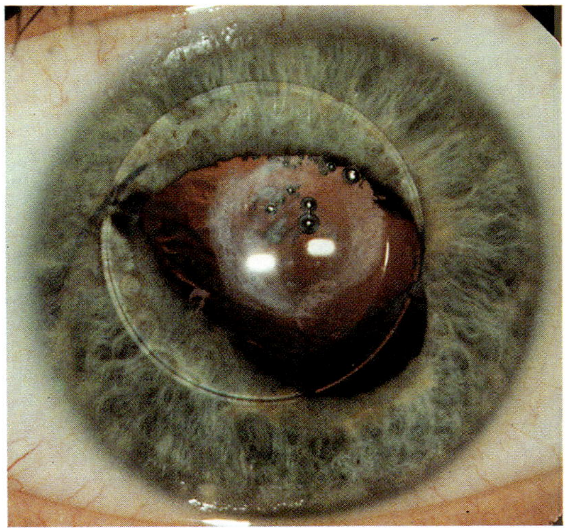

38.2 Total pupillary capture in a case of congenital cataract one year after surgery. Note that one polypropylene haptic has cut through the iris (which has healed behind). In the absence of symptoms no treatment was required (courtesy of Prof Karl Jacobi, FRG).

38.3

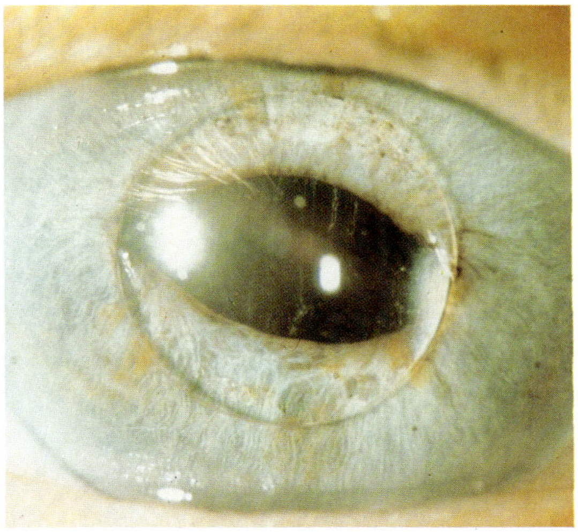

38.3 Total pupillary capture associated with an increase of myopia.

Loop malposition

Malpositioning of a loop occurs whenever either loop is not located either in the capsular fornix or in the ciliary sulcus. The cause is usually poor visibility of the loop during insertion, or late rotation or migration.

If the patient is asymptomatic, no treatment is required (**38.2, 38.4, 38.5**). Associated iritis should be treated with topical steroids. Recurrent hyphema may require loop amputation and explantation.

38.4

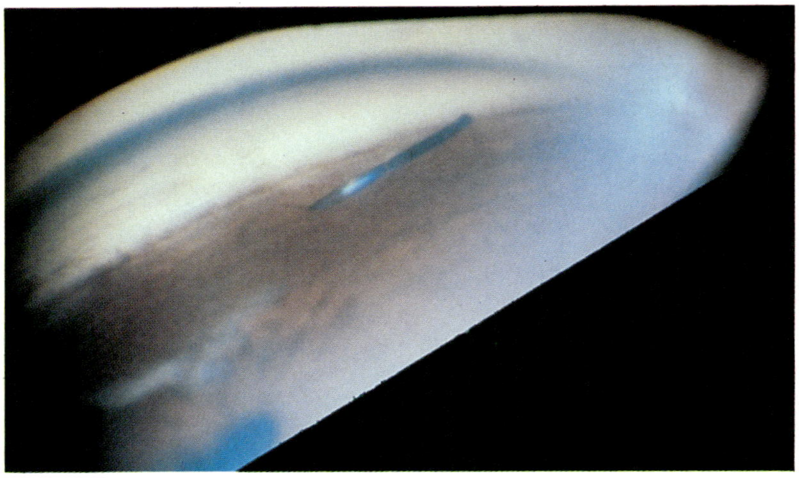

38.4 Gonioscopy showing erosion of the loop of a sulcus-placed Sinskey lens into the anterior chamber (courtesy of Dr John Alpar, USA).

38.5

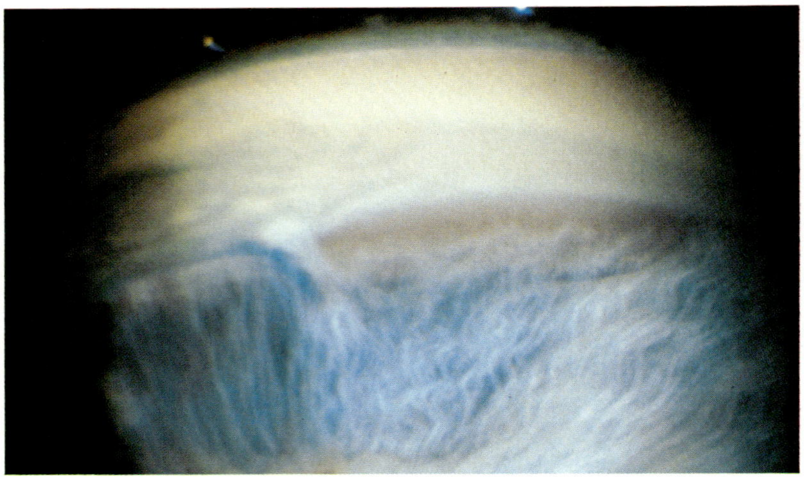

38.5 Gonioscopy showing closed loop of an Anis lens eroding through the iris (courtesy of Dr John Alpar, USA).

Decentration of the optic

With the advent of multifocal lenses, there is now a location point to allow the surgeon to detect small amounts of decentration. These are of no clinical significance. Apple found that 71% of 75 posterior chamber lens autopsy eyes had an optic edge or dialling hole within the pupillary aperture or within 0.5 mm of the pupil margin. This was seen in 92% of cases with asymmetric placement of the haptics and in 50% of cases with symmetric placement. Decentration may be minimized by avoiding asymmetric placement, by avoiding polypropylene loops and by ensuring complete clearance of the peripheral lens cortex. The chance of symptoms, especially glare during night driving, may be minimized by choosing 6.5 or 7.0 mm optics without dialling holes. The effects of optic decentration will be made worse by surgical decentration of the pupil (**38.6**).

Treatment of decentration depends on the presence of visual symptoms (**38.6**). Topical miotics may be helpful (**38.7**), but the presence of severe symptoms requires surgical interference. For discussion of the techniques for repositioning or explantation see Chapter 39.

38.6

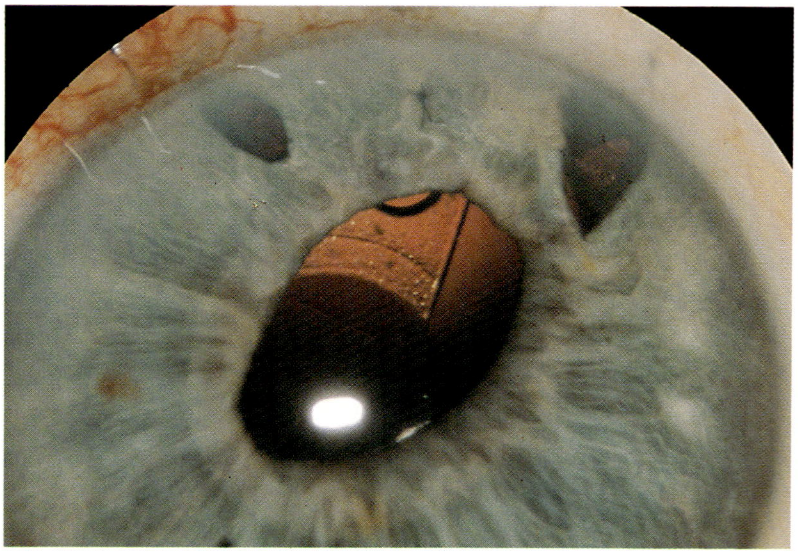

38.6 Decentration of a 4.0 mm optic of a Pearce tripod lens associated with a decentered pupil caused by a malplaced iris suture. The patient was asymptomatic and no treatment was required.

38.7

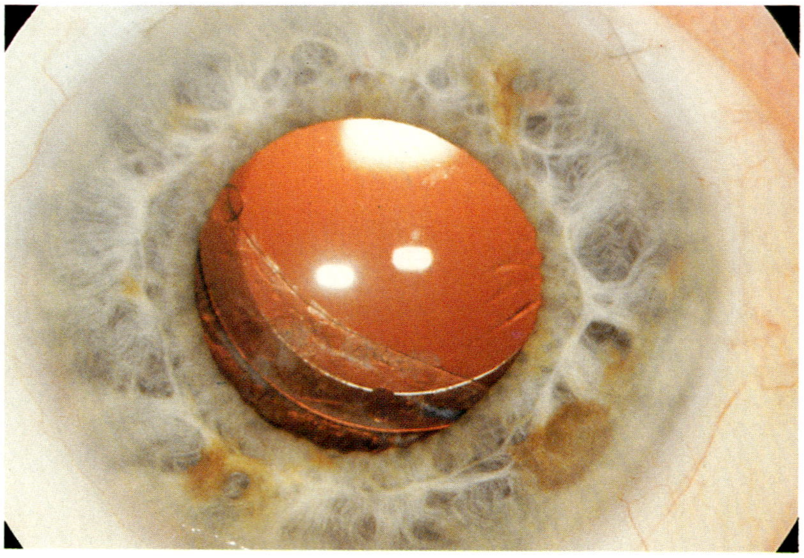

38.7 Three piece PCL with superior decentration due to capsular fibrosis. Symptoms were relieved with topical pilocarpine.

Windscreen wiper syndrome is when the optic moves in the vertical meridian causing blurring with head movements. It is due to a vertically placed lens without capsular fixation and a short or deformed haptic. It is avoided by capsular fixation or, if sulcus fixation is necessary, by placing haptics of adequate length (14 mm) in the horizontal position. Treatment may be accomplished by fixation of a loop with an iris suture, or by rotation of the lens into the horizontal position with a Sinskey hook, or by explantation and exchange (p. 256).

Sunrise syndrome (**38.8**) indicates vertical displacement of the optic superiorly. It may be caused by eccentric capsular bag fibrosis, especially when a three piece lens has been placed in the bag horizontally or when a solid disc lens has been used. The latter, if the effects are severe, necessitates lens exchange as it is impossible to recenter permanently a disc lens by rotation. Another cause is inferior zonular rupture with a horizontally placed lens in the bag. Careful inspection is therefore necessary at surgery before treatment can be planned.

38.8

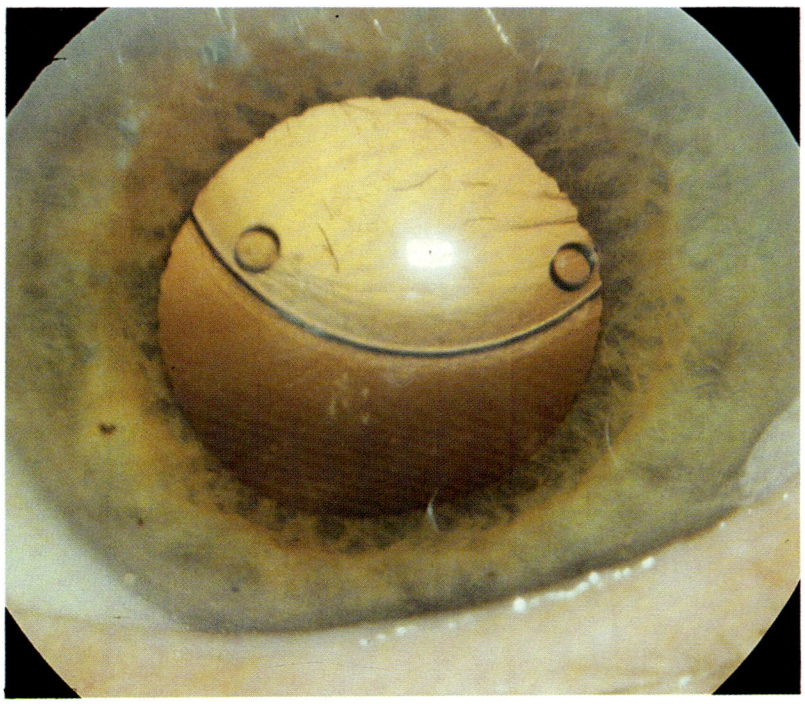

38.8 Sunrise syndrome requiring surgical intervention.

Sunset syndrome is when the lens gradually sinks down towards 6 o'clock. It is caused by movement of the lens through an inferior zonular rupture or a large tear in the posterior capsule. Symptoms are due to lens edge glare or aphakia in the visual axis. It is important to treat the lens before the 'sun has set' since, once in the vitreous, surgery becomes more complex, and if allowed to remain in the posterior segment, the lens may induce iritis, CME or retinal detachment. First, after full mydriasis, it is necessary to establish the position of the capsule and/or zonular rupture and then note if there is adequate posterior capsule in another meridian to support the lens (**38.10**). If there is insufficient intact posterior capsule the lens can be exchanged for a single piece anterior chamber lens. A McCannel suture (p. 251) to the iris can also be valuable to a loop of the lens and should be performed after trapping the optic in front of the pupil. However, in the long term this may prove more traumatic than a simple lens exchange.

Horizontal displacement may be associated with zonular dehiscence, but is more usually induced by capsular fibrosis in association with asymmetric placement (**38.9**).

38.9

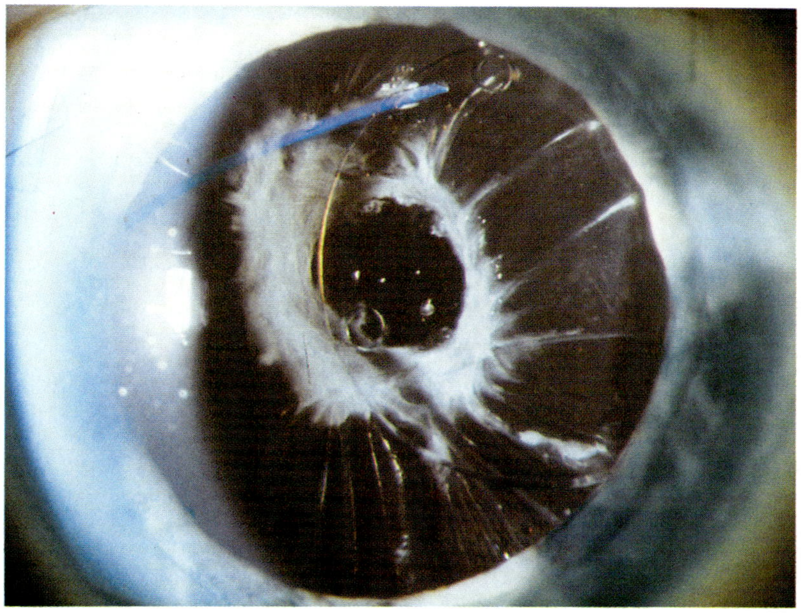

38.9 Horizontal decentration associated with capsular fibrosis. The left-hand loop is encapsulated and the force from the contracting leaves of the capsule has squeezed the edge of the optic towards the right. The right-hand loop and optic lie in front of the leaf of the anterior capsule, which does not exert any opposing force. This loop then either becomes deformed or migrates through the zonules onto the pars plana (courtesy of Prof. Karl Jacobi, FRG).

38.10

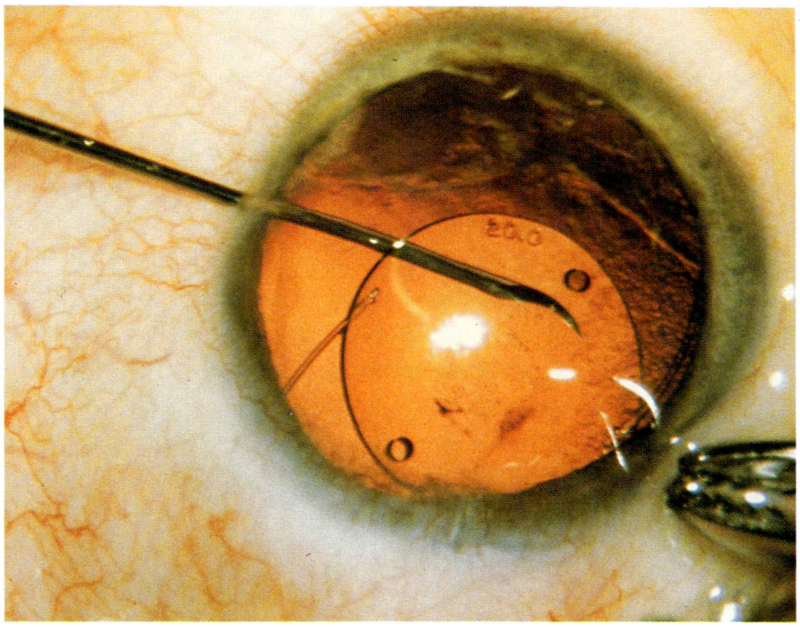

38.10 Sunset syndrome showing the use of a hooked needle under full mydriasis to rotate the lens into a meridian of adequate capsular support (courtesy of Prof. Karl Jacobi, FRG).

Pigment dispersion glaucoma

Raised intraocular pressure is associated with transillumination defects of the iris pigment epithelium, and gonioscopy shows a densely pigmented trabecular meshwork. There may be recurrent attacks of blurred vision associated with glaucoma, iritis and microhyphemata. The condition (**38.11**) should not be confused with transillumination defects caused by the original surgery (**38.12**), which emphasizes the importance of noting transillumination defects on slit-lamp microscopy in the early postoperative period.

Pigment dispersion may be avoided by capsule fixation using angulated haptics. Mild cases may be treated with topical steroids, anti-glaucoma therapy and cycloplegics. However, if the intraocular pressure cannot be controlled medically, trabeculectomy is required with a simultaneous exchange for an anterior chamber lens.

38.11

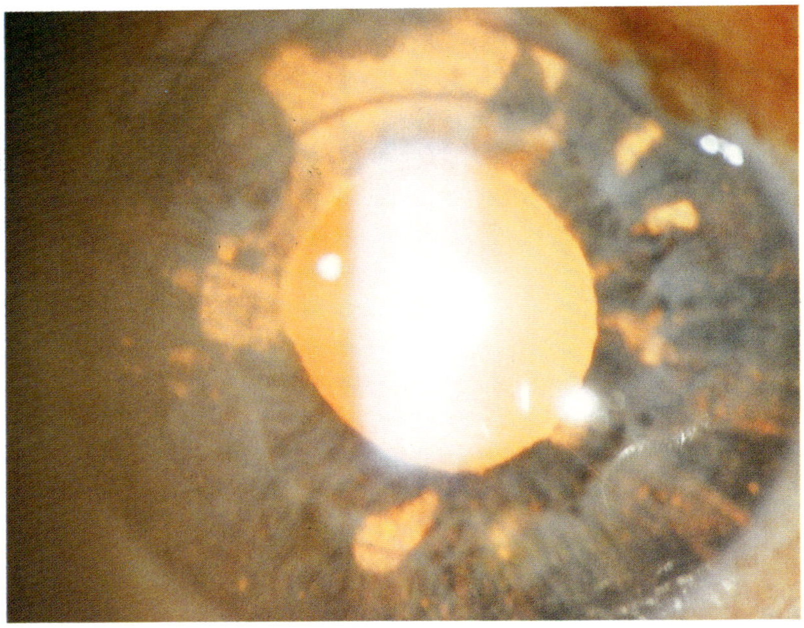

38.11 Pigment dispersion glaucoma with transillumination defects and iritis, necessitating exchange for an anterior chamber lens.

38.12

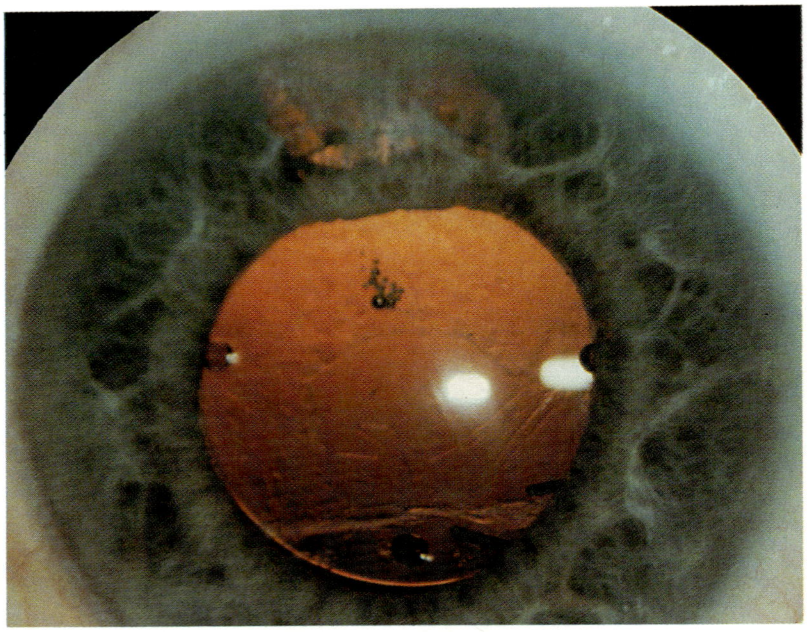

38.12 A surgically induced, symptom free, transillumination defect seen at 12 o'clock.

Fibrinoid reaction

A transient deposit of fibrin-like material is sometimes seen in the pupillary aperture following extracapsular cataract extraction and posterior chamber lens implantation. Characteristically, there is little or no cellular uveitis. A network of fibrin spreads from the margins of the iris across the pupil (**38.13**), usually between the second and fifth postoperative days. When the reaction is severe, the fibrin coalesces and becomes adherent to the anterior surface of the lens (**38.14**).

Treatment is with steroid drops one hourly and intensive mydriasis using topical phenylephrine and atropine. If the reaction does not subside within 24 hours, 4 mg betamethasone may be injected onto the floor of the orbit. Prophylaxis with preoperative and postoperative topical indomethacin is recommended in high risk cases. The condition usually resolves within two weeks of treatment, the fibrin net disappearing peripherally at first and centrally more slowly. Rarely, a film of fibrin does not clear from the anterior lens surface and will require YAG laser membranotomy.

Known associations are exfoliation syndrome, the oriental eye, diabetes mellitus and the glaucoma eye. Fibrinoid reaction has been noted by the author on two occasions in the second eye of a patient with an allergic diathesis (eczema and asthma). The possibility of phacoanaphylaxis contributing to the etiology exists, and close follow up is recommended for all such cases. Walinder *et al.* described an incidence of 28% among eyes with exfoliation syndrome, rising to 40% among those with glaucoma capsulare. Miyake *et al.* noted an incidence of 18% among eyes in Japan *not* treated with topical indomethacin against a 4% overall incidence. There has been no link between style or type of implant, viscoelastic agent or irrigating solution. Fibrinoid reaction is not prevented by surface modification of the lens with heparin. The condition may occur without lens implantation, but is extremely rare unless there is other ocular pathology.

Pathogenesis is not clearly understood, but is related to the breakdown of the blood–aqueous barrier, to release of a humoral substance and possibly to metaplasia of the epithelial cells at the edge of the anterior lens capsule into fibroblasts. This pseudometaplasia of the lens epithelium as a causative factor has been carefully investigated by Nishi and is enhanced by contact with PMMA. In addition he has found that the fibrin reaction does not occur in eyes where the epithelial cells have been purposely removed.

38.13

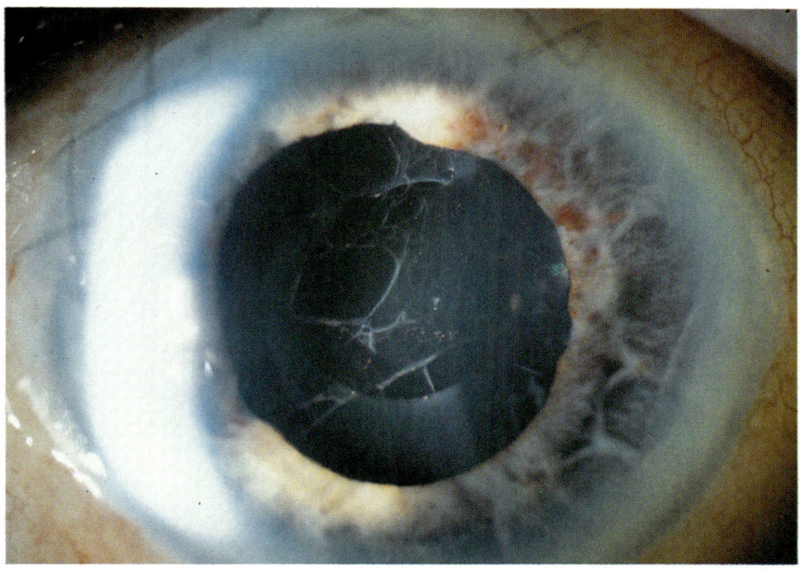

38.13 Early appearance of fibrin three days after insertion of a hydrogel lens into the capsular sac. Note the smooth curved edge of the anterior capsule inferiorly. The fibrin net extended across the pupil with a space between it and the anterior lens capsule. Note also the petechial hemorrhages on the iris surface and the small sphincter erosions.

38.14

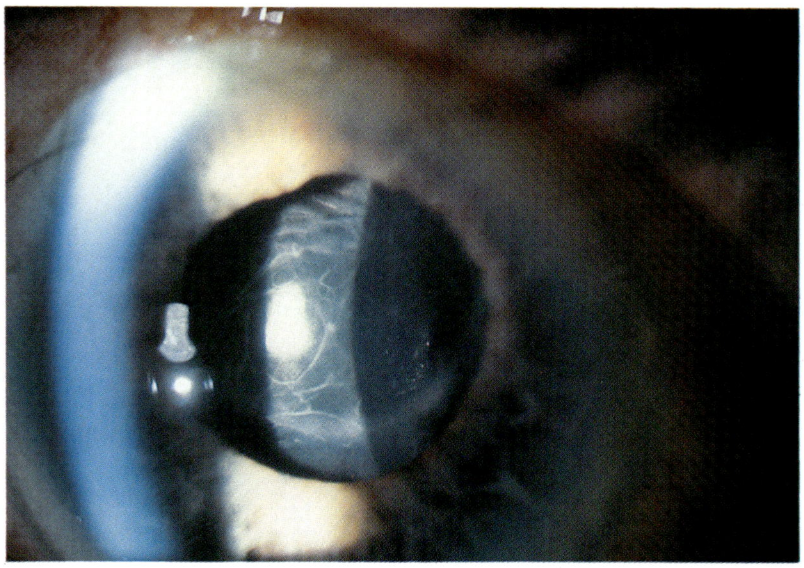

38.14 Same eye as in **38.13** eight days after surgery. The fibrinous exudate has become adherent to the surface of the lens and lens capsule.

Further reading

Apple D.J., Reidy J.J., *et al.* A comparison of ciliary sulcus and capsular bag fixation of posterior chamber intraocular lenses. *Amer. IOI Soc. J.* **2,** 44, 1985.

Brems R.N., Apple D.J., Pfeffer B.R., Park S.B., Piest K.L. and Isenberg R.A., Posterior chamber intraocular lenses in a series of 75 autopsy eyes. *J. Cat. Refract. Surg.*, **12,** 367, 1986.

Masket S. Pseudophakic posterior iris chafing syndrome. *J. Cat. Refract. Surg.*, **12,** 252, 1986.

Miyake K., Maekubo K., Miyake Y. and Nishsi O. Pupillary fibrin membrane. *Ophthalmology,* **96,** 1228–1233, 1989.

Nishi O. Fibrinous membrane formation on the posterior chamber lens during the early postoperative period. *J. Cat. Refract. Surg.*, **14,** 73–77, 1988.

Smith P.J. Pigmentary open-angle glaucoma secondary to posterior chamber intraocular lens implantation and erosion of the iris pigment epithelium. *Amer. IOI Soc. J.*, **2,** 174, 1985.

Smith S.G. and Lindstrom R.L. Intraocular lens complications and their management. *Slack Thorofare NJ.*, 1988.

Walinder P.K., Olivius E.O.P., Nordell S.I. and Thorburn W.E. Fibrin reaction after extracapsular cataract extraction and relationship to exfoliation syndrome. *J. Cat. Refract. Surg.*, **15,** 526–530, 1989.

39: IOL repositioning, removal and exchange

Robert Osher and Piers Percival

When a surgeon considers secondary surgery for implant-induced complications, care must be taken to fully weigh the benefits of the procedure against the risk, and determine the likely outcome against the probable result if no surgery takes place. The patient must be informed accordingly. In some instances, surgical removal (explantation) may cause more damage in the short term than would conservative treatment. There is little point in advising explantation if this will lead to the need for keratoplasty a few months later, when the alternative may delay such a need for several years. In such cases it is better to inform the patient and wait. Explantation may be performed more easily at the time of simultaneous keratoplasty. In other cases, such as recurrent anterior subluxation of a pupil supported lens, a simple iris suture may be all that is necessary to extend the life of the cornea and possibly obviate keratoplasty. In the case of posterior chamber lens decentration causing symptoms, repositioning of both haptics into the ciliary sulcus may suffice. Whatever surgery is contemplated, the decision will depend on the patient's symptoms, the likely prognosis from conservative treatment, the surgeon's ability and the availability of appropriate equipment, which for explantation should include a machine for anterior vitrectomy.

Implant repositioning

Spontaneous anterior or posterior subluxation of a *pupil supported (iris clip) lens* may be corrected by mydriasis, gravitational positioning of the head, and then miosis. If recurrent, however, topical miotic therapy or a McCannell suture (**39.1–39.6**) will be required. The latter will stabilize the implant, protect the cornea from further intermittent touch, and allow safe mydriasis for fundoscopy. Posterior subluxation, if fixed by posterior synechias and asymptomatic, should be treated conservatively. Total dislocation into the anterior chamber will require implant removal.

39.1

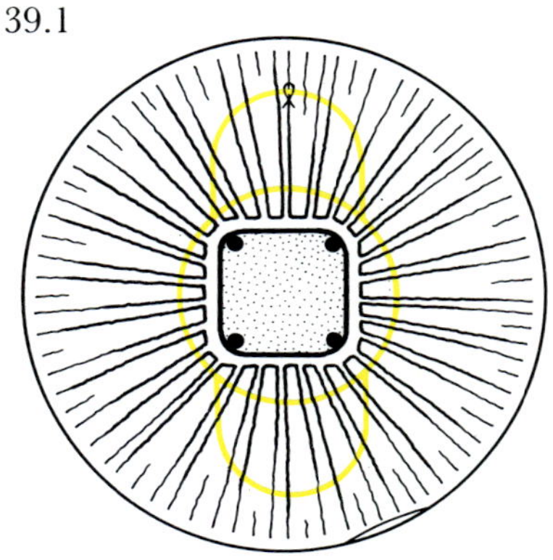

39.2

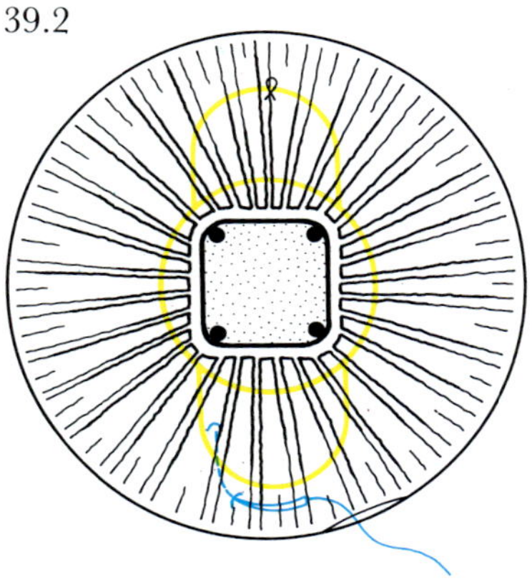

39.3

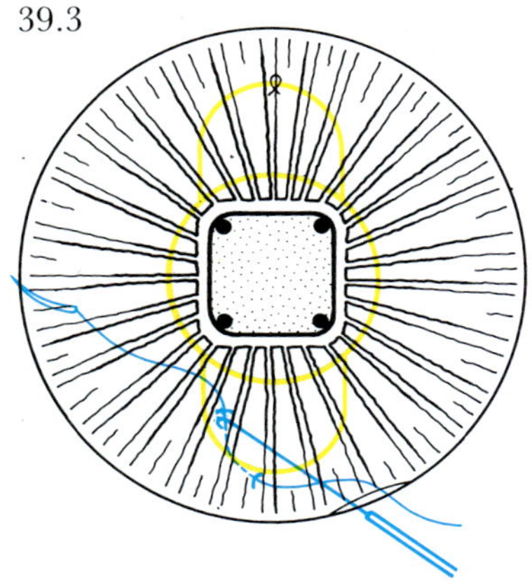

39 4

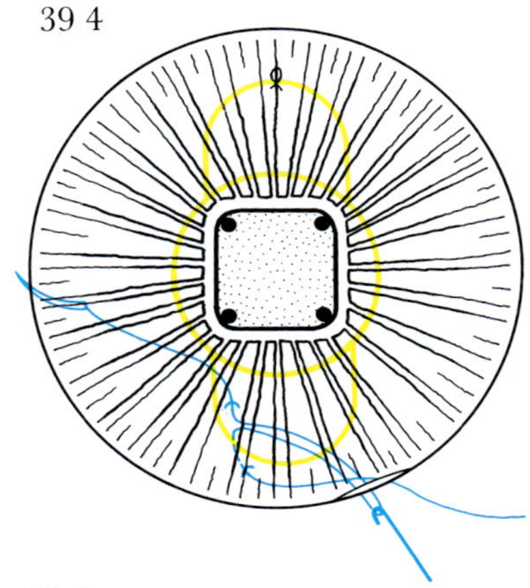

39.1 The McCannell suture for recurrent subluxation of an iris-supported lens: a 2 mm section is made at the limbus adjacent to the loop that is unstable and the anterior chamber is filled with sodium hyaluronate. The IOL is repositioned with a spatula, hook or Rycroft cannula and the pupil constricted with intracameral acetylcholine.

39.2 A 10/0 polypropylene suture mounted on a sharp-pointed 5 mm needle is inserted through the section, taking a deep bite of iris and haptic loop, and is made to exit through the cornea above the bite through the iris.

39.3 The needle is allowed to rest on the surface of the eye. The polypropylene stretching between the iris and cornea is caught with a hook.

39.4 The polypropylene is looped out of the eye with the hook and the loop cut with scissors. The needle carrying one half of the loop can then be removed.

39.5 The knot is tied at the section, care being taken to allow the loop of polypropylene running through the iris to remain loose.

39.5

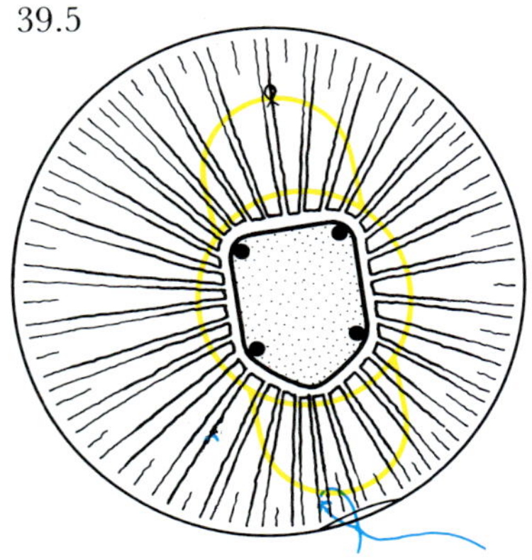

39.6

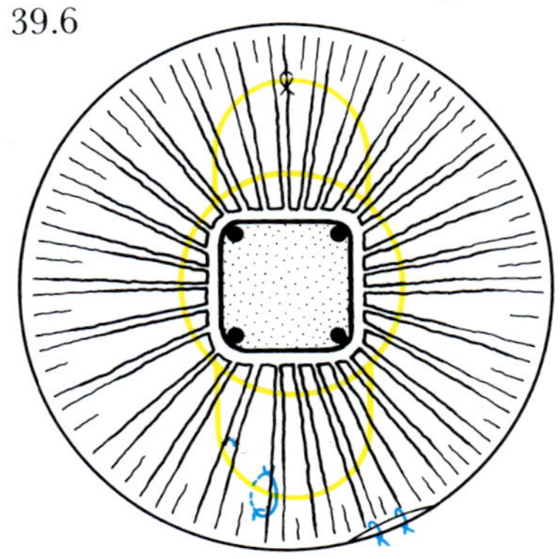

39.6 The knot is placed into the eye and carefully rotated downwards, away from the section. A small mark remains in the cornea from the midperipheral perforation.

A *posterior chamber lens* (PCL) with looped haptics may require repositioning if it is sufficiently decentered to cause symptoms. Inspection with a Goldmann three-mirror lens at the slit lamp under mydriasis should be made to assess the position of the haptics and the state of the zonule. If the position is asymmetric, a lens may be dialled with two hooks clockwise, so that both haptics come to lie in the ciliary sulcus. If loops are found to be deformed, removal and exchange may be required. If a PCL is descending through an area of zonular disinsertion (sunset syndrome), it may be possible to reposition the lens into the sulcus horizontally, 90° to the area of disinsertion. More usually, these lenses require removal or scleral fixation sutures. An unstable PCL that rocks with head movements (windscreen wiper syndrome) may be stabilized with an iris or scleral fixation suture.

An *anterior chamber lens* (ACL) rarely requires repositioning alone. However, this may be required in the early postoperative period on the diagnosis of a massive iris tuck, or the inadvertent placement of a haptic into an iridectomy or the identification of a haptic lying in the wound.

Implant removal

The most important reason for removing a lens is continuing intraocular damage to the cornea, iris, drainage angle or macula. Additional reasons can include patient discomfort or refractive surprise (**Table 39.1**). Surgical techniques are demanding as further ocular damage can readily occur, resulting in more lasting effects on the potential for vision. The surgeon should have access to a vitrectomy machine, intraocular scissors or a haptic amputator, and a series of microhooks. The use of viscoelastic material is invaluable, will lessen damage to the corneal endothelium and may help in the dissection of tissues adherent to the lens.

Table 39.1 Reasons for implant removal

Corneal decompensation
Implant induced glaucoma
UGH syndrome
Unstable or mobile IOL
Chronic macular edema
Patient symptomatology
Refractive surprise

Reasons for removal

Corneal decompensation: Early peripheral corneal edema associated with a well-positioned ACL or iris-supported lens, should be carefully watched as many years may elapse before vision fails. Yet focal corneal edema may be reversed if an offending haptic is promptly eliminated. Once the patient develops symptoms of failing vision (**39.7, 39.8**), penetrating keratoplasty may be considered. Elderly patients may be treated conservatively with topical sodium chloride or a bandage contact lens. Younger patients may require implant removal or exchange at the time of penetrating keratoplasty (see Chapter 41). A stable ACL with a deep anterior chamber may be left, but an iris clip lens should always be removed.

39.7

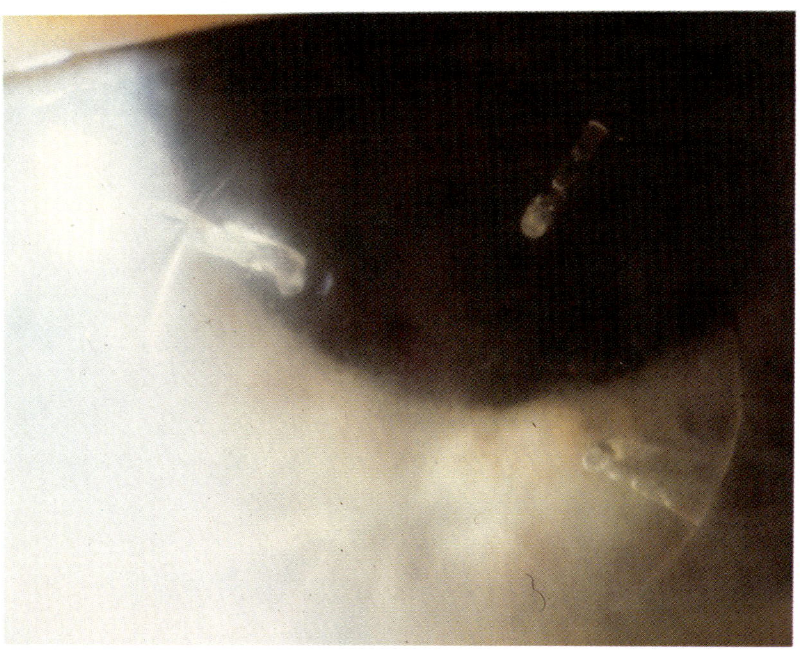

39.7 Bullous keratopathy resulting from a mobile iris clip lens (courtesy of Mr Bruce Noble, UK).

39.8

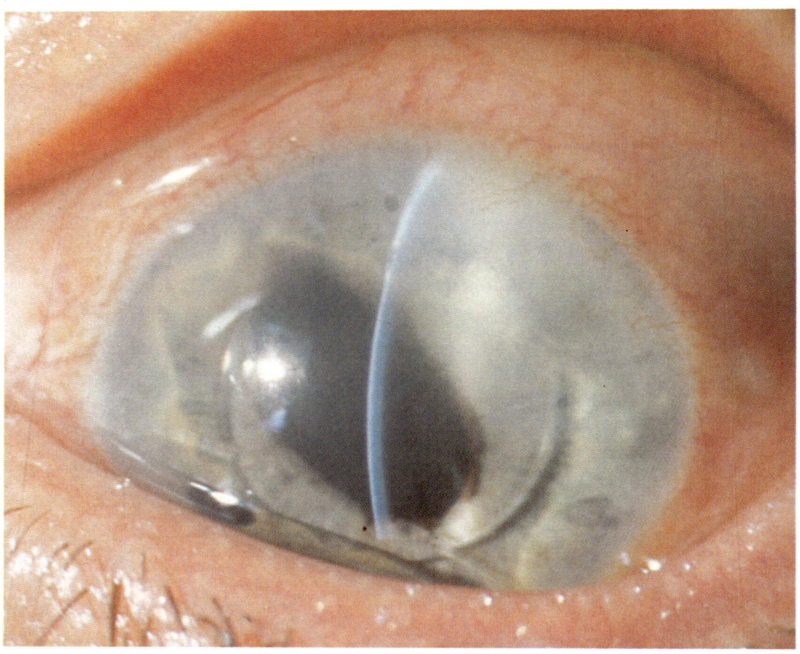

39.8 Closed loop ACL complicated by ovalling of the pupil, angle 'zip-up' from the anterior synechias and corneal edema. This was exchanged for a sutured PCL during simultaneous keratoplasty (courtesy of Mr Roger Gillie, UK).

Implant-induced glaucoma when uncontrolled by medical means. Examples include pigment dispersion from iris chafing by a pupil-supported or sulcus-fixated IOL (**39.9**), or 'angle zip-up' caused by micromovement of an ACL.

Uveitis glaucoma hyphema (UGH) syndrome: Any persistent uveitis, if uncontrolled, merits implant removal when complicated by secondary glaucoma (**39.10**), or recurrent hyphema. Exchange is not usually recommended in the presence of chronic uveitis.

39.9

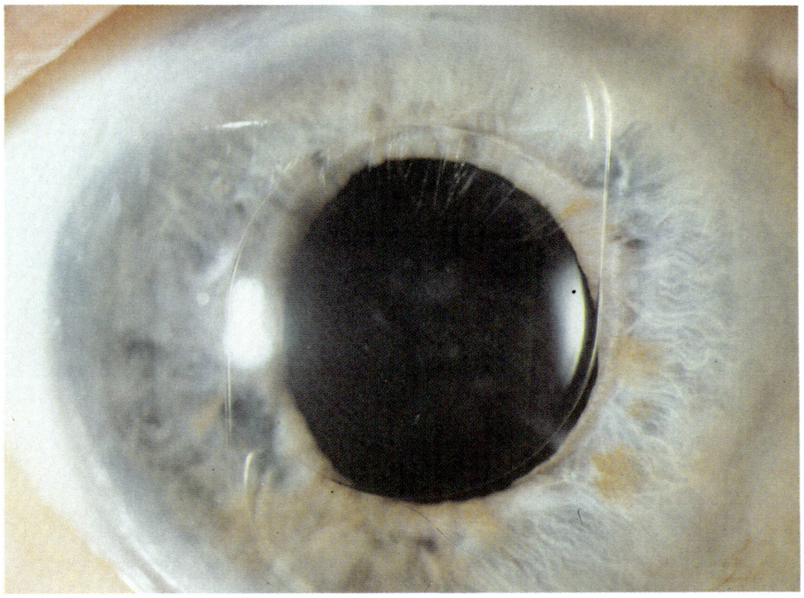

39.9 Pigment dispersion glaucoma resulted four years after a sulcus placement of a PCL. Conservative treatment failed to control the intraocular pressure. Trabeculectomy was performed with exchange for a semiflexible ACL. The glaucoma has since remained controlled without medication. Photographed three years after the lens exchange.

39.10

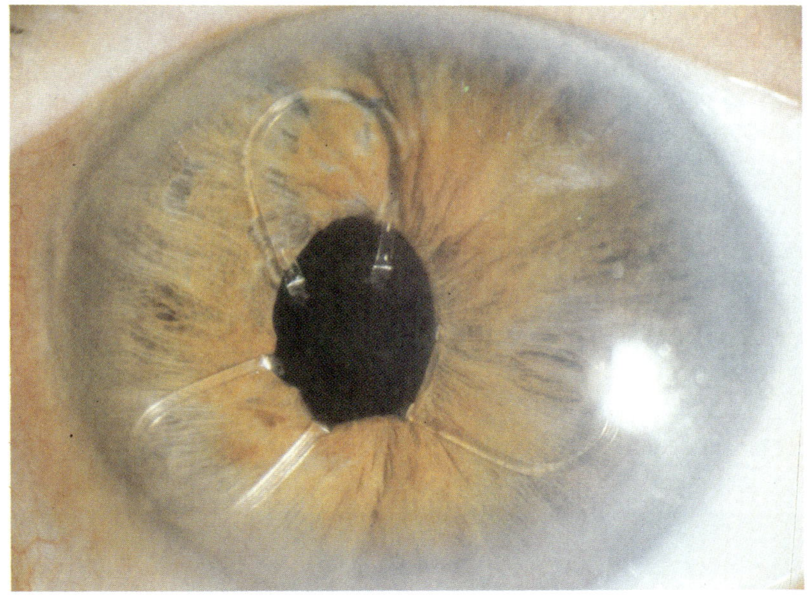

39.10 Well placed iris-supported posterior chamber Severin-style lens. One year after surgery there were recurrent episodes of ciliary injection, with iridocyclitis and secondary glaucoma. Acuity was reduced to 20/80. Failed medical treatment led to trabeculectomy with explantation.

An unstable or mobile IOL should be removed if associated with macular edema or uveitis or potential corneal decompensation. Evidence for instability may be shown by intermittent corneal touch, rocking, or rotational movements in the anterior chamber seen with the slit lamp. Total dislocation into the vitreous of any style of implant creates a risk of macular edema and retinal detachment. Such a lens should ideally be repositioned or removed using advanced vitreoretinal techniques. However, if these techniques are not available, the risks of complications from further surgery may outweigh the risks from conservative treatment. Occasionally, removal is necessary because of extrusion (**39.11**).

Chronic cystoid macular edema, when associated with implant-induced uveitis, warrants removal. This may be suggested by implant malposition, by iris synechias to any part of the implant optic or haptic, or by vitreous adherence to the implant. In cases of vitreous adherence to the cataract section (vitreous wick syndrome), vitrectomy without lens explantation will often result in a reversal of the macular edema.

39.11

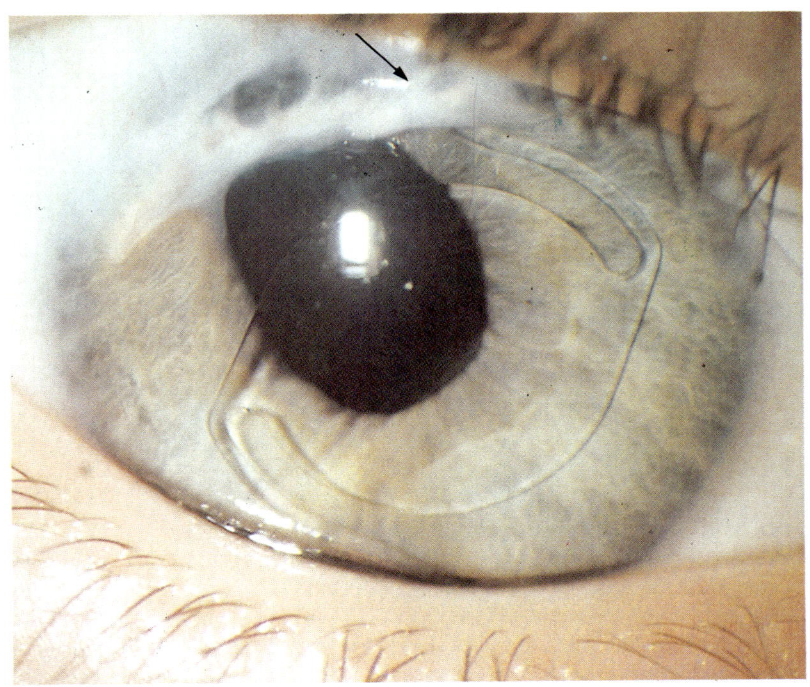

39.11 Extrusion of the knuckle of a semiflexible one piece ACL through the peripheral cornea (arrow). This was an oversized lens that had been implanted in a child's eye in the mistaken belief that the eye would grow to accommodate the lens. The section is scarred with incarcerated iris and vitreous (courtesy of Mr Bruce Noble, UK).

Patient symptomatology: Intolerable symptoms may include diplopia caused by decentration of an anterior (**39.12**) or posterior chamber lens (**39.13**), lens edge or dialling hole glare if not controlled with topical miotics (see **39.23**), persistent tenderness from an anterior chamber lens, or dissatisfaction with the IOL performance. Prolonged postoperative pain is usually only a problem following implantation of a rigid ACL. There is no specific treatment and if the pain persists the implant may have to be removed. Simply instructing the patient not to rub the eye may have beneficial effects. Performance may be impaired by iatrogenic damage (**39.14**), implantation of an erroneous lens power, or occasionally by optical aberrations (**39.15**).

39.12

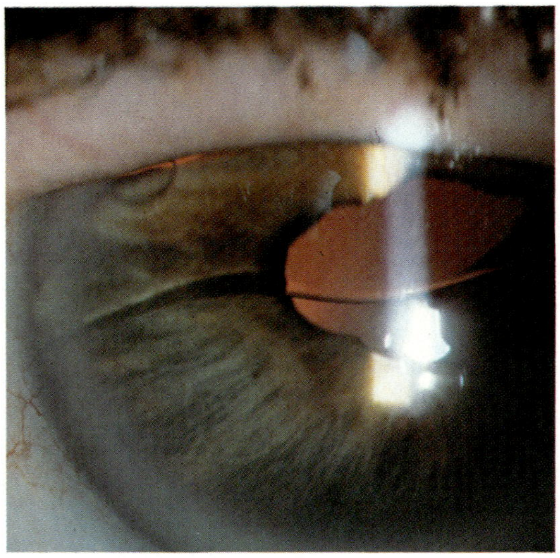

39.12 Upwards slippage of a rigid ACL, which produced intolerable diplopia and lens edge glare.

39.13

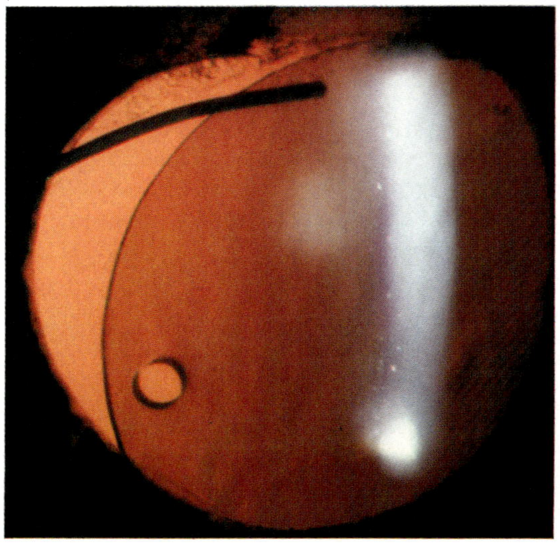

39.13 Decentration of a sulcus-placed Sinskey-style lens, with lens edge and dialling hole glare requiring lens exchange.

39.14

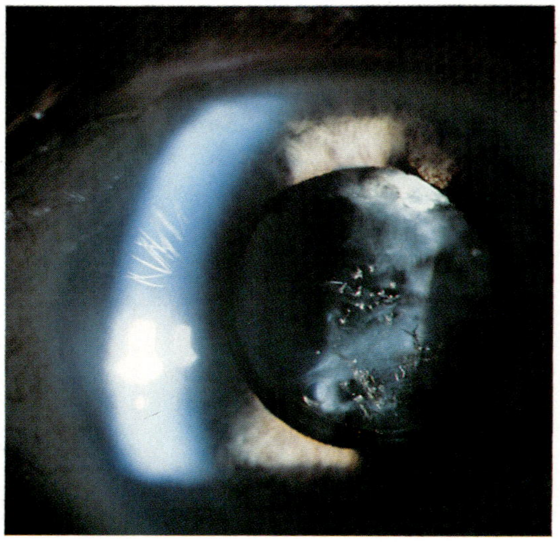

39.14 Iatrogenic damage to a PCL following inadequate clearance of the lens cortex, showing multiple Yag laser explosions within the substance of the implant, which produced glare and loss of image quality.

39.15

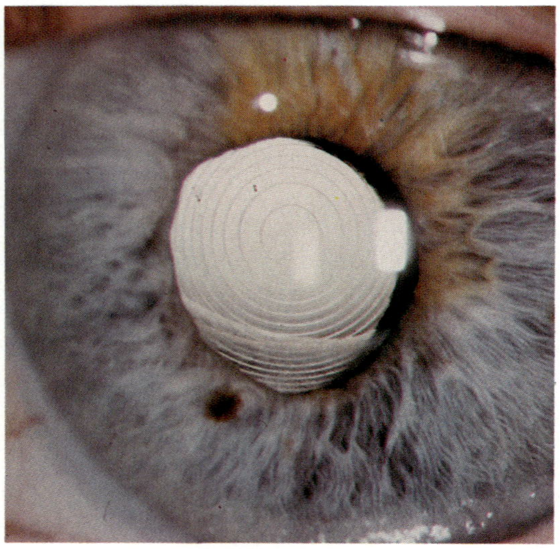

39.15 Well-centered diffractive type of bifocal IOL. The patient was intolerant to the resulting quality of vision, but symptoms resolved following lens exchange (courtesy of Mr Bruce Noble, UK).

Methods of removal

An IOL may be removed either through a limbal section or, if simultaneous keratoplasty is performed, with an open sky technique. Care must be taken not to pull on the iris or its surrounding structures during loop amputation or implant removal, as severe iris root, ciliary body or zonule damage can lead to iridodialysis, cyclodialysis or zonulocapsular damage, respectively, as well as to hemorrhage and glaucoma. All removals or exchanges should be performed under the protection of a viscoelastic agent. An automated vitrectomy unit should be at hand. Techniques will vary according to the lens type to be removed, but it may be helpful to commence with a bevelled stab incision at the limbus to allow injection of viscoelastic and subsequent access to the anterior chamber at a site distal to the main incision.

Rigid ACLs, once grasped by sturdy intraocular or lens-introducing forceps, will slide easily out of the chamber. Care must be taken to assess the presence of iris synechiae prior to surgery and, if present, these must be lysed by a jet of sodium hyaluronate or cut with Sutherland scissors. A scleral incision should be angled towards the iris root so that the lens may be prolapsed up over the posterior scleral lip. If the pupil is peaked, the surgeon should not expect a return to normal since chronic histopathological changes will have occurred.

Closed loop ACLs and flexible open loop ACLs will usually be found to have their loops buried in a tunnel of iris synechias and care must be taken to avoid intraocular hemorrhage and iridodialysis. For continuous curve closed loops, the distal loop should be cut with a loop amputator that can be locked onto the loop before cutting towards its right-hand end (**39.16**). The proximal loop is cut near to the optic on the right (**39.17**) and near to the wound on the left and is removed from its tunnel with forceps (**39.18**). The optic is rotated anticlockwise with Kelman–McPherson forceps to release the distal loop from the tunnel of synechias (**39.19**), and removed using a spatula (held in the other hand) as a ramp under the optic to avoid catching the optic or rough-cut edges of loops in the posterior lip of the wound. Sometimes it is impossible to remove all the loop remnants without damaging the root of the iris (**39.20**); it is better in such cases to amputate all that can be removed and leave the rest behind. When a loop has a bend (e.g., the distal loop of an Azar lens) or a bulb or eyelet, multiple cuts may be necessary before the loop remnants can be threaded out of their synechial tunnels. After ICCE with damage to the chamber angle, the options for rehabilitation are either a contact lens or scleral fixation of a PCL (see **39.28–39.36**) or an iris-supported lobster claw lens (Chapter 13).

39.16

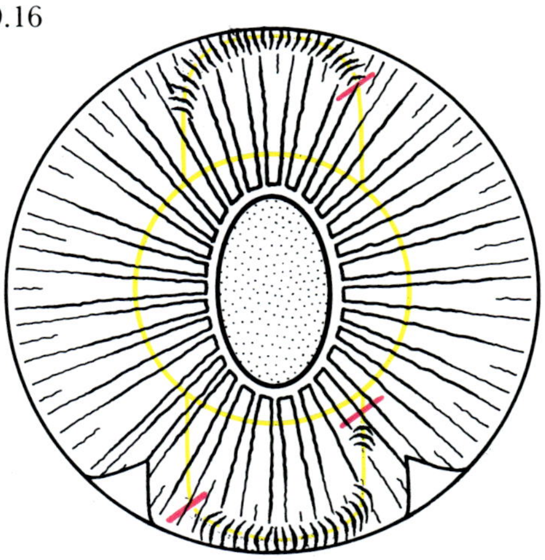

39.16 Diagram of closed loop ACL with haptics buried in the tunnels of synechias. Red bars represent the position of cuts to be made on the closed loops. The pupil should be constricted.

39.17

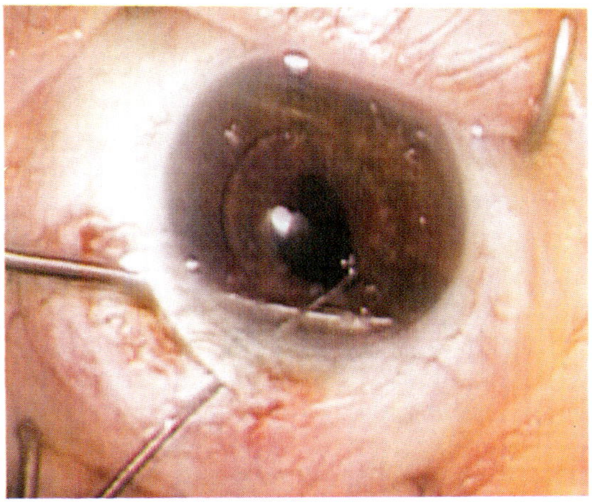

39.17 The proximal loop is cut near to the optic with a loop amputator, while the optic is steadied with a spatula or hook.

39.18

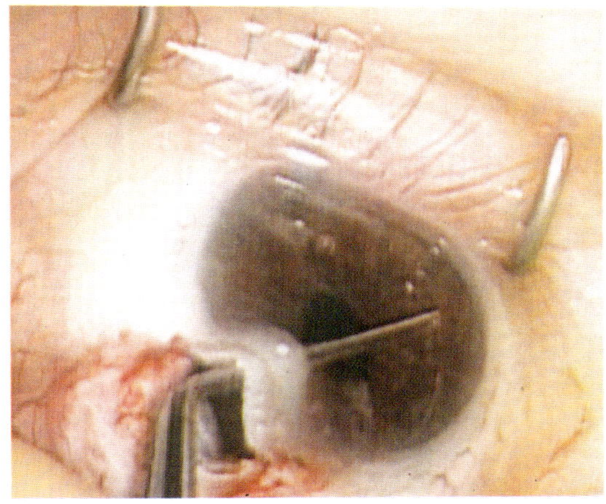

39.18 Same eye as in **39.17** showing the proximal loop being threaded out of its synechial tunnel. It is usually convenient to remove this haptic *after* removal of the main bodies of the lens.

39.19

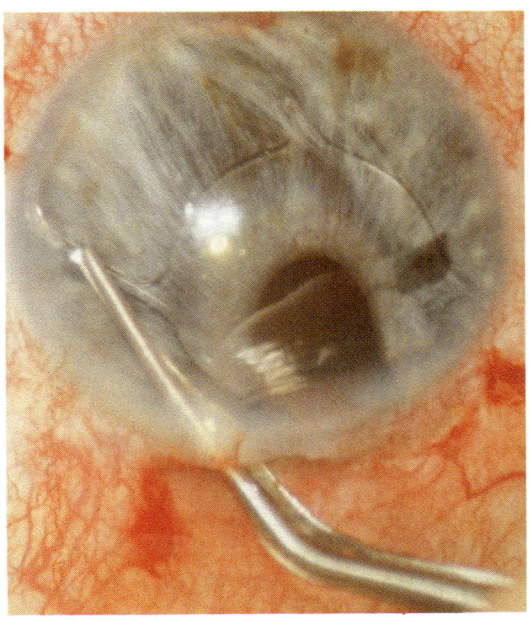

39.19 Attempted rotation of a distal loop of a Leiske lens through a tunnel of synechias with Kelman–McPherson forceps. Note the up-drawn pupil proximally because of the peripheral anterior synechias. Explantation was advised because of chronic inflammation and macular edema with secondary glaucoma.

39.20

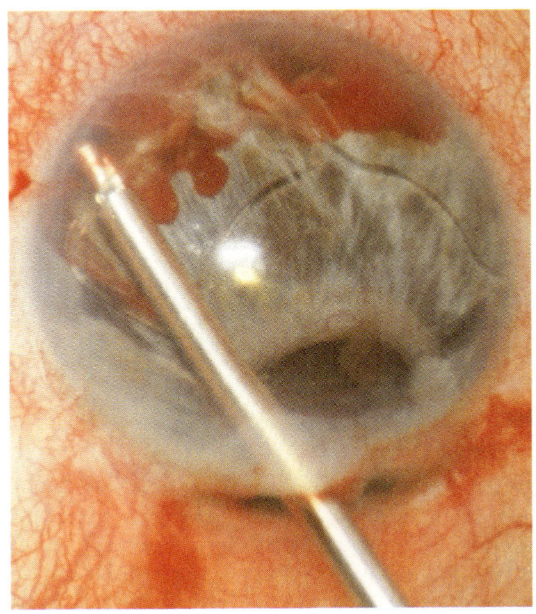

39.20 Same eye as in **39.19**. The distal loop failed to move and rotation caused a small iridodialysis and hemorrhage. The photograph shows a further cut being made with the distal loop held in the amputator.

Iris-supported lenses are removed after the cutting of any iris suture and division of synechias. If vitreous is posterior to the pupil, the anterior chamber should be maintained with either air or viscoelastic; intraocular fluid should be avoided since it may hydrate the vitreous and create positive pressure. If vitreous is drawn to the wound, or vitreous loss occurs, or vitreous synechias are present, a formal anterior vitrectomy must be performed before closure. Retrieval of a lens from the vitreous is more challenging. An anterior approach may be used, but the chamber should remain closed until the lens is in front of the iris. Two stab incisions are made and hooks introduced through each. A visible loop is caught with one (C-shaped) hook (**39.21**) and the other hook is placed underneath the lens to lift it forwards (**39.22**). The lens is trapped in the anterior chamber with intracameral miotic and it is then safe to open the eye for explantation and vitrectomy.

39.21

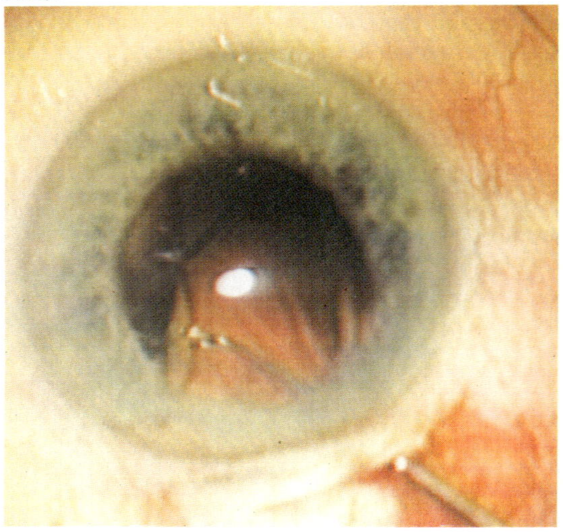

39.21 Posterior dislocation of an iris clip lens: a visible loop is caught with a C-shaped hook or intravitreal forceps.

39.22

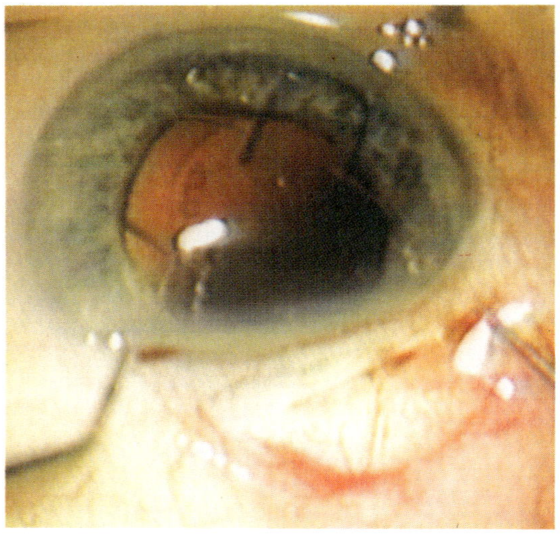

39.22 Same eye as in **39.21**. A second hook is placed underneath the lens to lift it forwards.

Posterior chamber lenses must be assessed for the shape of the haptic and style of the optic prior to surgery. If the loops are pure without bulbs or eyelets, the IOL may be rotated clockwise into the anterior chamber using two hooks (**39.23–39.25**).

Sometimes a malpositioned PCL may be managed by surgical repositioning, but the decision as to the most effective treatment cannot be taken until the position of the haptics has been properly assessed. If the haptics cannot be seen with maximal mydriasis, a limbal stab incision is made and the iris retracted or pushed for better visibility. If asymmetric placement is found to be the cause of decentration, the lens may be dialled with a one- or two-hook technique into the central position, with each haptic resting within the ciliary sulcus. It should then be deliberately decentered slightly towards each haptic and watched for spontaneous recentration. If the lens fails to recenter, a problem exists, such as loop deformation, and the treatment plan may be switched either to explantation/exchange or to stabilization with an iris suture. If the lens fails to rotate on attempted dialling, it is likely that the haptic is either in the zonules, or through a tear in the zonule or lens capsule, or possesses an eyelet or bulbous tip. Reverse rotation, further decentration towards the ensnared haptic, then rerotation may be successful in freeing the haptic. Continued failure of rotation requires amputation of the haptic and, if inaccessible, retention within

39.23

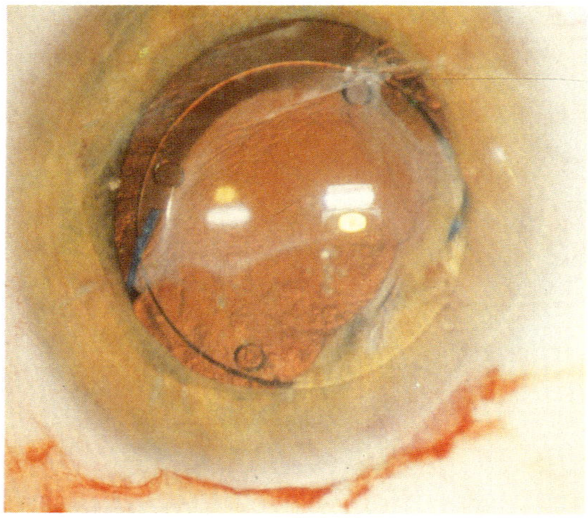

39.23 Atonic pupil and sulcus placement of a polypropylene looped lens. The lens edge and dialling hole produced intolerable symptoms of glare. Note the pupillary capture caused by adherence of the iris to the lens capsule.

39.24

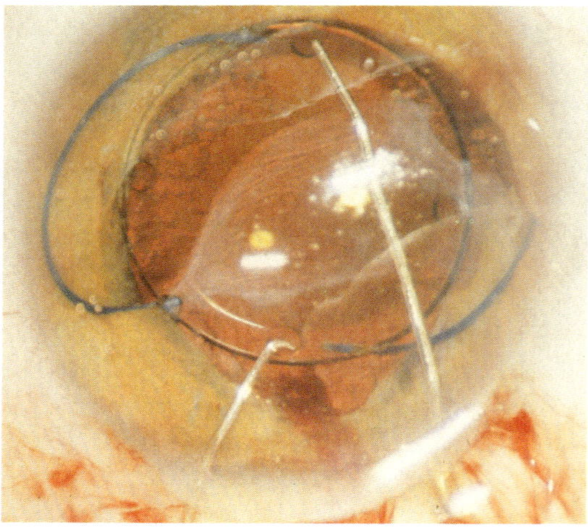

39.24 Same eye as in **39.23**. Clockwise rotation of lens and haptics into the anterior chamber using two hooks. Note the deformity of the open polypropylene loop (left-hand side).

39.25

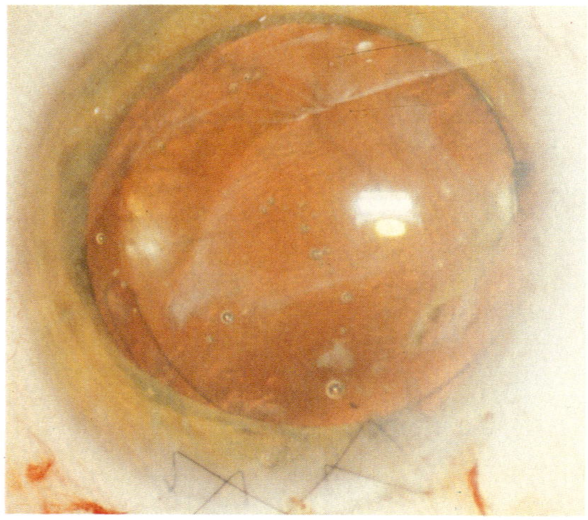

39.25 Same eye as in **39.24**. The synechias have been separated. Exchange was for a well centered, PMMA-looped sulcus-placed lens with a 7 mm optic. The symptoms were, to a large extent, resolved.

the eye. Closed-loop lenses require cutting at the apex of each loop before the rotation maneuver (**39.26**). Sometimes the entire lens and capsule will require explantation after lysis of the zonules with α-chymotrypsin.

Occasionally, it may be necessary to retrieve a PCL from the vitreous. The two-hook method should be used as for the retrieval of iris-supported lenses, and the availability of a vitreoretinal surgeon for assistance is advisable.

Regardless of the situation requiring explantation, once the lens is in the anterior chamber a spatula should be used as a ramp to prevent snaring of the optic or haptic on the posterior lip of the wound. The trailing haptic should be carefully observed to avoid damage to the iris and cornea and to prevent vitreous drag. If the lens is entangled with vitreous, a formal vitrectomy will be required.

39.26

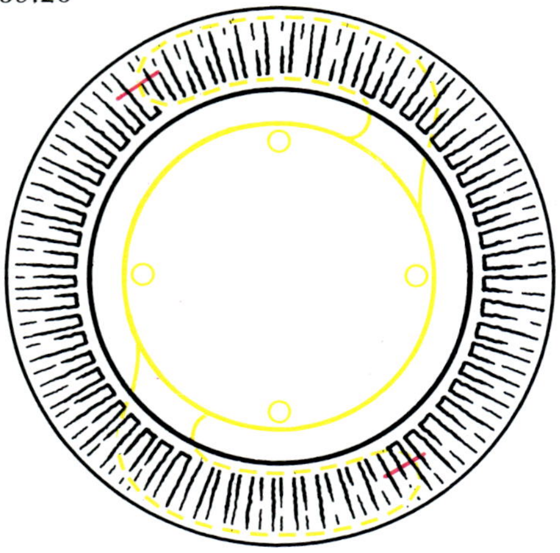

39.26 Diagram of a closed loop PCL requiring removal. Red bars represent the position of the cuts to be made on closed loops before rotation clockwise. The pupil should be dilated maximally.

Implant exchange

Implant exchange will depend on the ocular state. If idiopathic chronic uveitis or macular edema is present, exchange may be postponed and considered as a second procedure six months after implant removal. However, if a specific cause of the uveitis or macular edema can be identified, such as a malpositioned haptic, a lens exchange that solves the problem may be indicated. Wide optic, sulcus fixated PCLs may be exchanged for malpositioned PCLs (**39.25**) if the posterior capsule is intact. The peripheral anatomy of the capsule and zonule should be inspected carefully to determine the best axis of implantation and fixation. Semiflexible one piece ACLs (**39.9**) may be exchanged for PCLs in cases of pigment dispersion glaucoma or where the posterior capsule or zonule is deficient (sunset syndromes). They may also be exchanged for pupil-supported lenses or other ACLs in the absence of angle anomalies. In the presence of angle disorganization or anomaly, the implant may be exchanged for a PCL sutured to the iris through its dialling holes (**39.27**) or sutured to the sclera through the ciliary sulcus (**39.28, 39.29**).

39.27

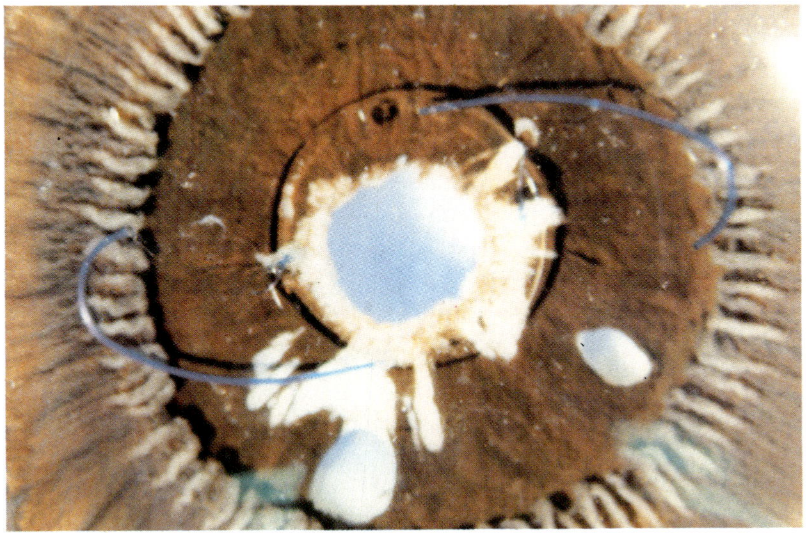

39.27 Sutured PCL following a lens exchange, photographed from behind at autopsy. Note the haptics float free on the surface of the ciliary body (courtesy of Prof. David Apple, USA).

39.28

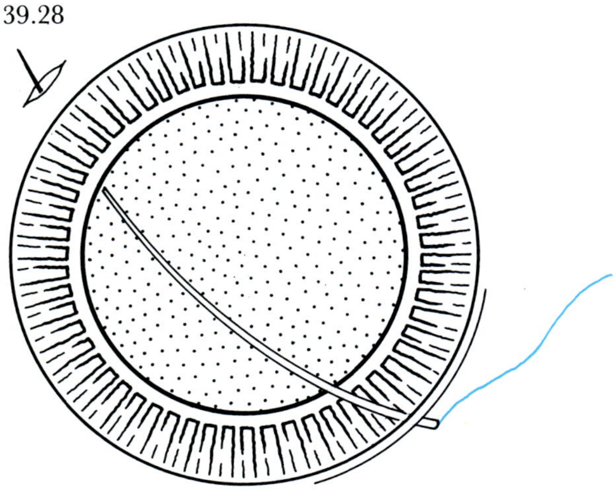

39.28 Double-armed polypropylene on a 13 mm needle is taken under the distal iris, through the ciliary body to exit through the preformed scleral incision 1 mm from the distal limbus. A 16 mm straight needle can also be used.

39.29

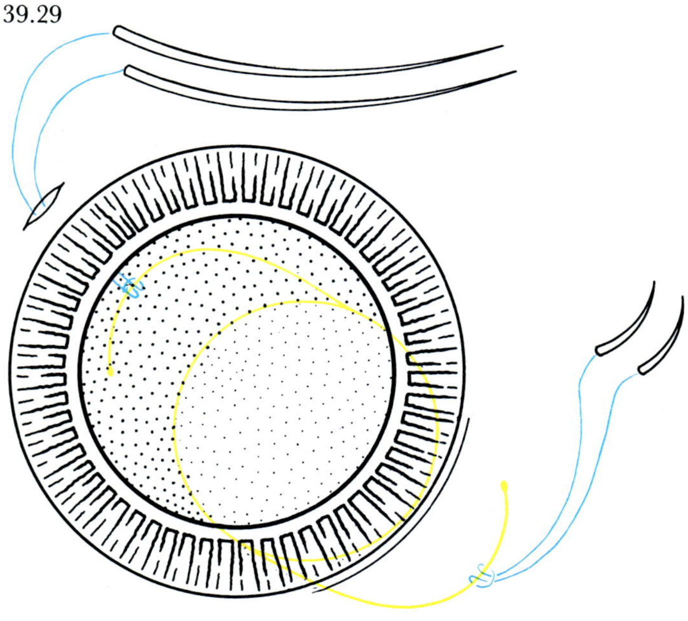

39.29 A second needle is passed parallel to the first, the polypropylene having been sutured to the implant loops. Bulbous tips to the loops are recommended to prevent the suture from slipping off the haptic.

For secondary *iris fixation*, polypropylene may be sutured through two dialling holes to the iris just peripheral to the sphincter muscle. This may be relatively easy during keratoplasty, but it is not recommended in the presence of uveitis. It should be recognized that the loops of a 14 mm lens are likely to lie on the surface of the ciliary body (**39.27**) and that for a fit into the ciliary sulcus, a lens of reduced loop span should be chosen.

Scleral fixation is generally preferred to iris fixation: for a simple technique using double-armed sutures, a proximal limbal incision is made and opposite this a small scleral incision 1 mm beyond the limbus, so that the fixating suture can be buried later. Double-armed polypropylene is sutured to the distal loop of the lens. The needle length is 13 or 16 mm. One needle is passed under the iris to exit through the preformed incision (**39.28**). The second needle is passed parallel to the first and the distal loop of the lens passed to the ciliary sulcus (**39.29**). It remains relatively easy to pass a similar suture under the iris to fix the proximal loop through the ciliary body to the sclera posterior to the section. The polypropylene knots should be tied under partial thickness flaps of sclera.

An alternative method of scleral fixation has been recommended by James Lewis, whereby single-armed sutures are inserted *ab externo,* so avoiding a blind pass through the ciliary body. Conjunctival peritomies are made to expose the sclera at the 2 and 8 o'clock meridians in order to avoid the ciliary nerves and posterior ciliary arteries. Triangular partial thickness scleral flaps are raised at least 3 mm in length from the base to the apex. A 25-gauge needle on a 1 ml syringe is inserted with the left hand parallel to the plane of the iris, through the scleral bed, commencing 1.5 mm posterior to the posterior surgical limbus. The needle tip passes through the sulcus and into the pupil (**39.30**). With the right hand, a straight 0.15 mm diameter needle attached to 10-0 polypropylene is similarly passed parallel to the plane of the iris through the sulcus in the opposite meridian and threaded through the lumen of the 25-gauge needle. The 25-gauge needle is then gently withdrawn from the eye, carrying with it the 10-0 polypropylene. A superior limbal wound is made, sufficient for entry of the PCL, and a loop of polypropylene is retrieved with a microhook (**39.31**). The loop is then cut and the ends tied to the haptics of a single piece PCL at the widest extent of the loop span (**39.32**). After injection of viscoelastic, the lens is inserted behind the iris, making sure that the inferior loop is attached to the right-hand polypropylene suture (**39.33**). Gentle tension on the polypropylene will then dial the lens horizontally into the stable sulcus position (**39.34**).

39.30

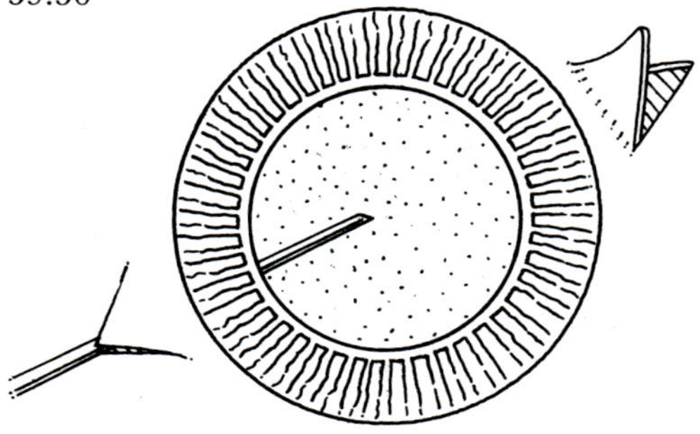

39.31

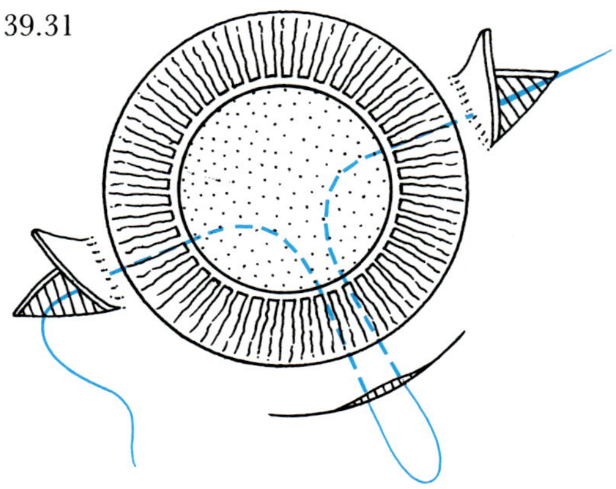

39.32

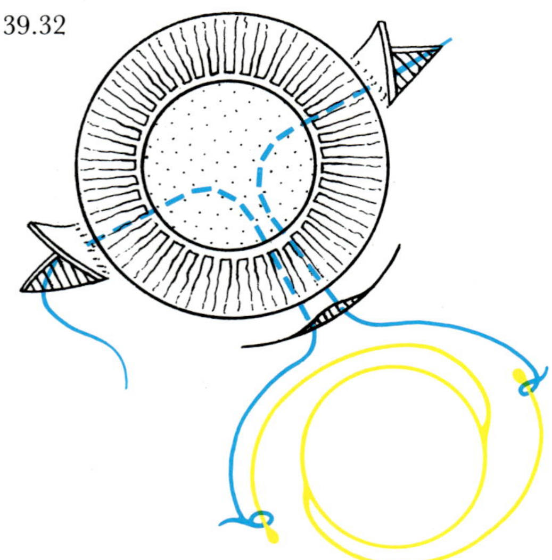

39.33

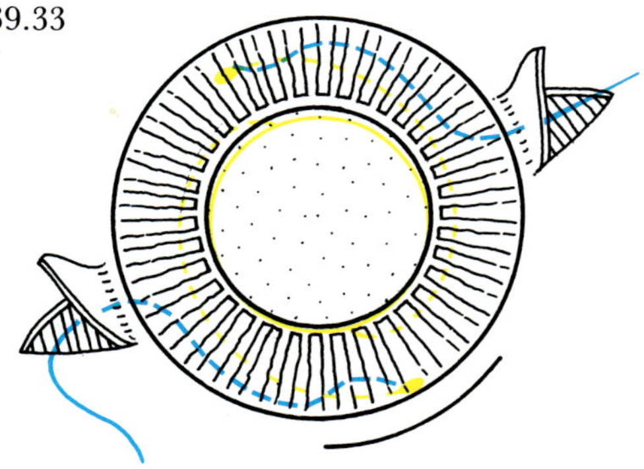

39.34

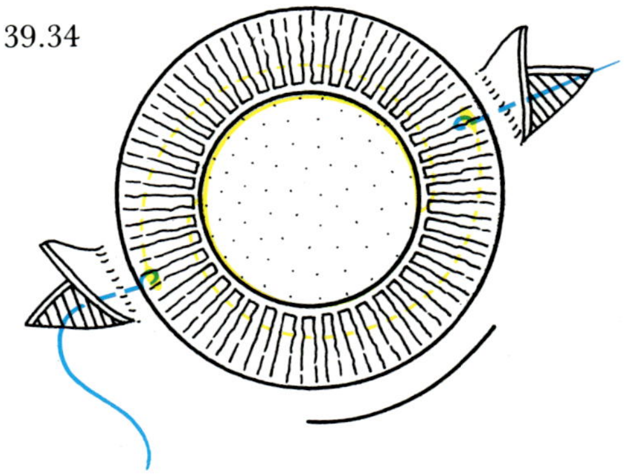

39.30 A 25-gauge needle is passed through the sclera behind the iris, where it can be seen in the posterior chamber.

39.31 The intersulcus polypropylene has been looped out of the eye.

39.32 The cut ends of polypropylene are tied to the haptics of a PCL at the maximum loop span.

39.33 Vertical placement of the PCL.

39.34 The PCL has been dialled into position by gentle tension on the polypropylene.

Next, a suture of 10-0 polypropylene on a spatulated needle is used to make a short bite in the scleral bed next to the exit site of the intersulcus polypropylene. A square knot is tied with four throws incorporating the cut end of the intersulcus polypropylene (**39.35**). The scleral flap is then closed with 10-0 nylon to bury the polypropylene knot (**39.36**). Finally, the conjunctiva over each scleral flap is closed (see also **41.17** and **41.19**).

Further reading

Apple D.J., Price F.W., Gwin T. *et al.* Sutured retropupillary posterior chamber intraocular lenses for exchange or secondary implantation. *Ophthalmology,* **96,** 1241–1247, 1989.

Duffey R.J., Holland E.J., Agapitos P.J. and Lindstrom R.L. Anatomic study of transclerally sutured intraocular lens implantation. *Amer. J. Ophthalmol.,* **108,** 300–309, 1989.

Koch D., Price F.W., Whitson W.E. and Carlson A. Techniques of suturing posterior chamber lenses. *Audiovisual J. of Cataract and Implant Surgery,* **6,** No. 1, 1990.

Koenig S.B., McDermott M.L. and Hyndink R.A. Penetrating keratoplasty and intraocular lens exchange for pseudophakic bullous keratopathy associated with a closed loop anterior chamber lens. *Amer. J. Ophthalmol.,* **108,** 43–48, 1989.

Price F.W. and Whitson W.E. Visual results of suture fixated posterior chamber lenses during penetrating keratoplasty. *Ophthalmology,* **96,** 1234–1240, 1989.

39.35

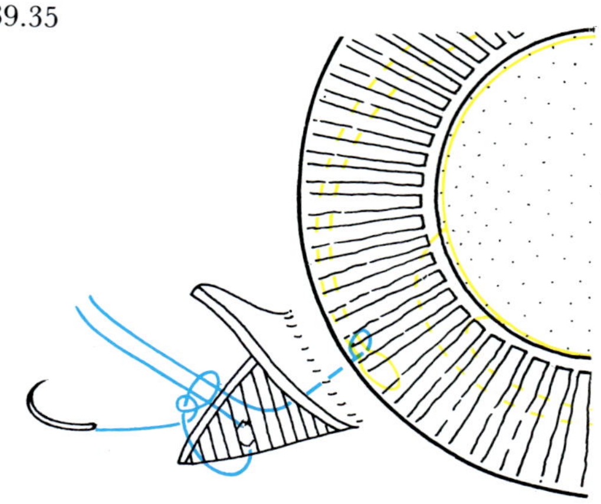

39.35 A second polypropylene needle is inserted into the scleral bed to secure the cut end of the intersulcus polypropylene.

39.36

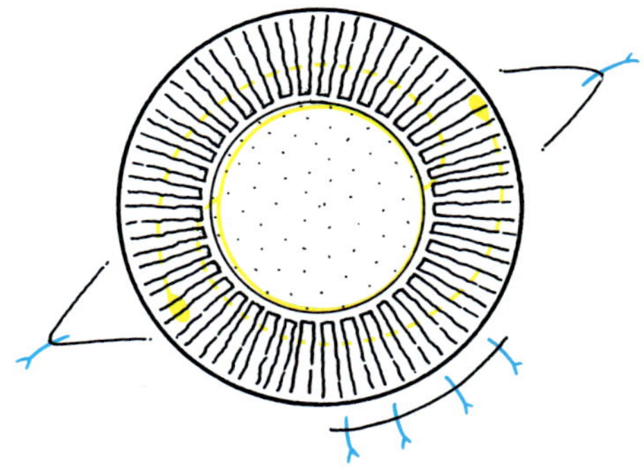

39.36 Final closure of the limbal wound and scleral flaps with 10-0 nylon.

40: Pseudophakic glaucoma and uveitis

Marvin Kwitko

Predisposing factors

Physiological and anatomical characteristics of the patient's eye may predetermine the onset of pseudophakic glaucoma:

- Small eye with a shallow anterior chamber.
- Abnormal pupillary anatomy and pharmacological responses.
- A 'difficult' eye, as in patients with diabetes, obesity, immunological sensitivity, deep set eye, or narrow palpebral fissure, is more likely to lead to surgical complications.
- Undiagnosed subluxation of the cataract.
- Outflow block from the lens material when there is a permeable capsule in a mature cataract.
- Predisposition to sustained postoperative hemorrhage, as in diabetes (**40.1**), bleeding diatheses, or long term anticoagulation.

40.1

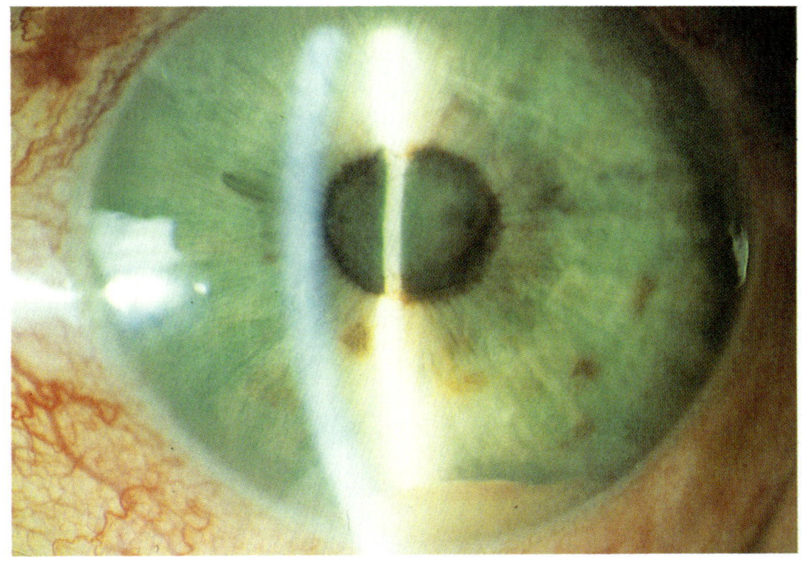

40.1 Pseudophakic glaucoma in a diabetic patient associated with postoperative hyphema and uveitis.

Two primary factors that contribute to the pathogenesis of pseudophakic glaucoma are mechanical and inflammatory. The mechanical factors consist of recurrent microhemorrhages, inflammatory cells and debris, pigment release, residual lens cortex and imperfect implant edges; these are induced by apposition of the implant to delicate intraocular uveal structures, or by the residual lens cortex blocking aqueous outflow. The inflammatory factors consist of the formation of peripheral anterior and posterior synechias, progressive pigment loss, polishing compound residue on the implant, pseudophakodonesis, neovascularization and cortex admixture with vitreous or sensitivity reactions.

Surgical factors

Sustained ocular hypertension with or without uveitis may be induced by surgical factors or complications of surgery:

- Displacement of nuclear fragments into vitreous during phacoemulsification.
- Incomplete evacuation of cortex leading to uveitis and outflow block (**40.2**).
- α-chymotrypsin leading to outflow block from fractured particles of the zonular apparatus.
- Insufficient elimination of viscoelastic agents.
- Faulty quality control of the IOL leading to uveitis and hyphema from rough edges (**40.3**), or toxic lens syndrome due to the presence of residual polishing compounds (**40.4**).

40.2

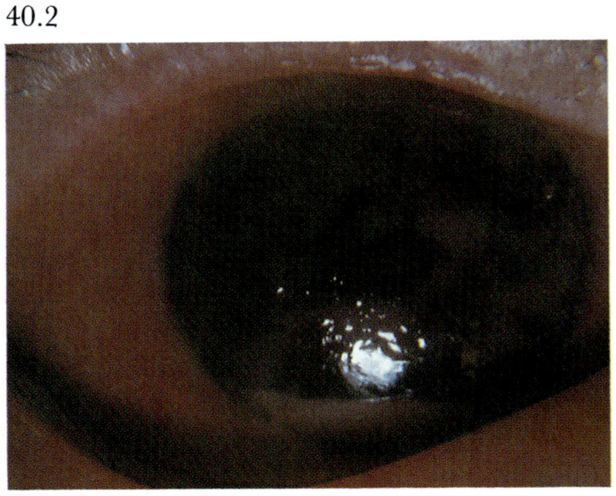

40.2 Uveitis following phacoemulsification with incomplete evacuation of the cortex: Nøte the hypopyon.

40.3

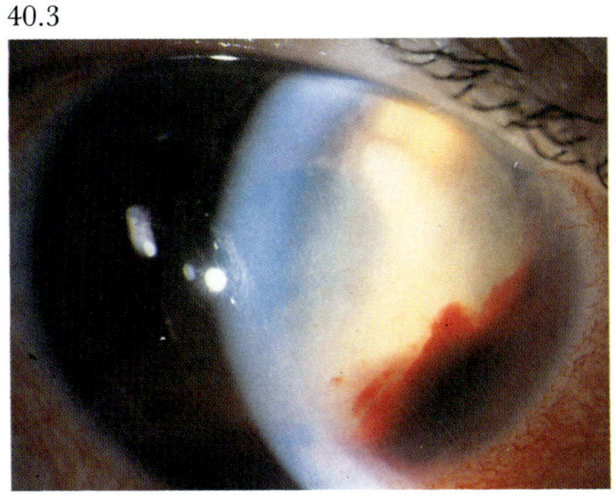

40.3 Uveitis glaucoma hyphema (UGH) syndrome with corneal edema.

40.4

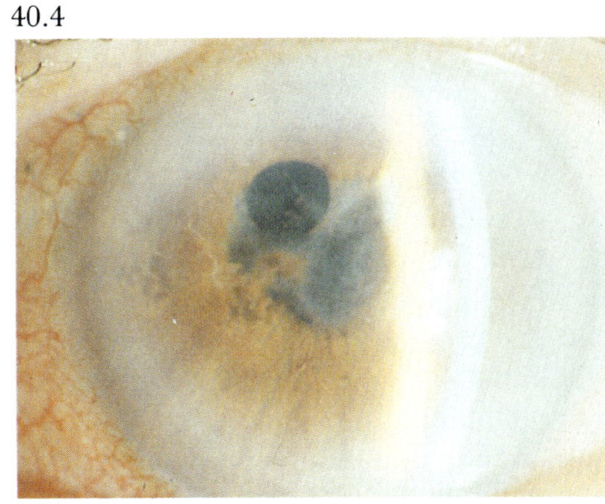

40.4 Cyclitic membrane and posterior synechias resulting from toxic lens syndrome.

- Biodegradation of implant material in contact with the vascular uveal tissue leading to inflammation and hemorrhage.
- Other lens impurities: The plastic should contain little or no monomer or additives, such as curing agents, mold release agents or hardeners. The lens may be improperly heated or stored during molding, lathing and drilling, making it susceptible to degradation. Electrostatic properties of plastic, which are exaggerated when the plastic is dry, create a force that attracts impurities, such as lint, talc and dust, to the implant. Freon, which is used in ethylene oxide sterilization, can also alter the plastic.
- Response to topical steroids in susceptible patients.
- Pupil block glaucoma caused by forwards movement of the iris–implant diaphragm when aqueous cannot circulate into the anterior chamber (**40.5**). The condition may result from inadequate removal of the lens cortex, persistent hyphema and postoperative uveitis associated with capsule contracture causing forwards movement of the implant leading to ring posterior synechias. Treatment is with intensive mydriasis and laser or surgical iridectomy.
- Phacoanaphylactic endophthalmitis: the residual cortex in the second eye of a patient who has undergone extracapsular surgery for the first, may create an immune response that can cause a severe glaucoma (**40.6**). The condition is currently quite rare.
- Progressive anterior synechias caused by micromovement of the anterior chamber lens haptics. Associated low grade uveitis leads to cocooning of the haptic by overgrowth of iris tissue and embarrassment to the filtration angle (**40.7**).
- Implant location: contact with uveal tissue, as with angle- or pupil-supported lenses (**40.8**) or with placement in the ciliary sulcus (**40.9**), may jeopardize the blood–aqueous barrier or lead to iris chafing with pigment dispersion. The consequent glaucoma may not commence until many years after surgery.

40.5

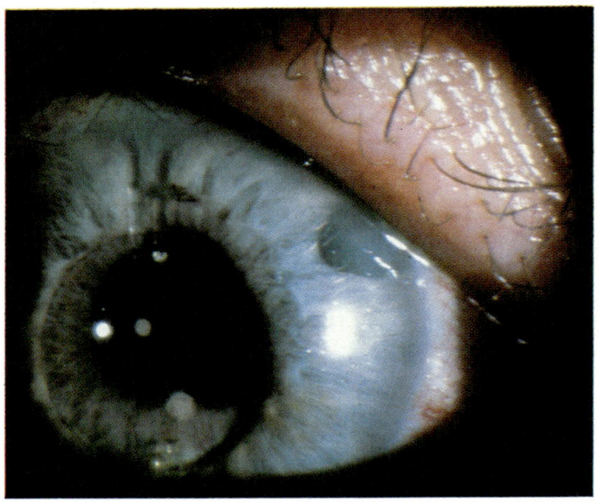

40.5 Pupil block glaucoma with internal iris prolapse. The condition was cured with Argon laser iridectomy.

40.6

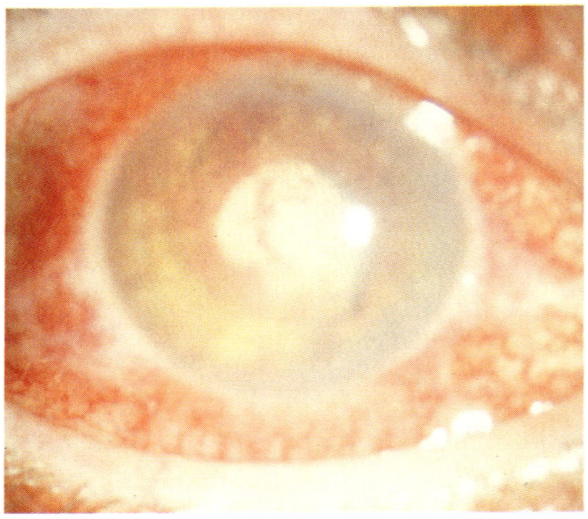

40.6 Phakoanaphylactic endophthalmitis.

40.7

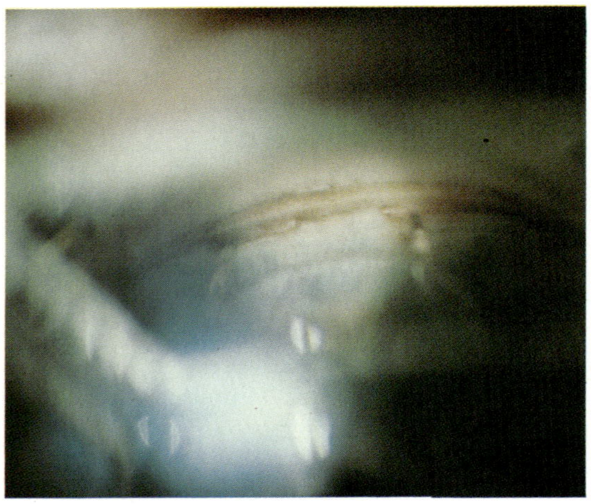

40.7 Gonioscopy showing peripheral anterior synechias enveloping a closed loop haptic of an anterior chamber lens implant.

40.8

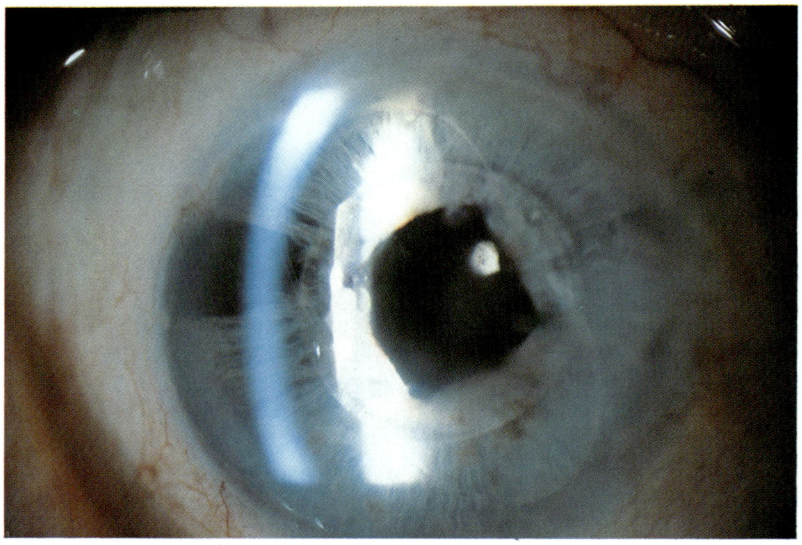

40.8 Late uveitis/glaucoma with a well placed, four loop, pupil-supported lens seen 16 years after surgery. Recurrent recent episodes of pigment dispersion with uveitis and glaucoma for 18 months were controlled medically. Note that early corneal edema is present nasally over the inferior loop. VA is still 20/40 unaided.

40.9

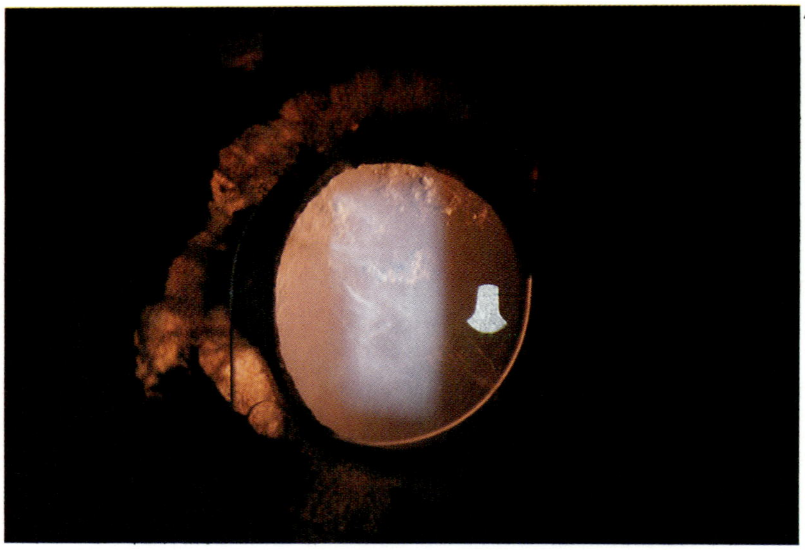

40.9 Pigment dispersion glaucoma, four years after sulcus placement of a PCL, caused by iris chafing (note the transillumination defects). Medical treatment failed. Trabeculectomy was performed with an implant exchange for a semiflexible ACL. The intraocular pressure has since remained under control (3 year follow up) without medication.

Management

Prevention, to a large extent, is obtained by meticulous cleaning of the lens cortex, removal of viscoelastic material at the end of surgery and locating the implant within the lens capsule. Postoperatively, the pupil should be kept mobile. A watch should be kept for posterior synechias and if the pupil appears small and rigid, weak mydriatics should be used.

Treatment is initially with mydriatic drops, both anticholinergic and adrenergic, beta-blockers, systemic acetazolamide and intensive steroid drops (unless the patient is a steroid responder). For severe inflammatory reactions, subtenon and orbital floor injections of betamethasone are recommended.

Topical beta-blockers should be used with extreme caution in patients with bradycardia, cardiac arrhythmias, asthma and cardiac failure, and only after consultation with a physician. Systemic acetazolamide should also be used with extreme caution in patients with bone marrow depression, hypokalemia, weight loss, confusional states, renal colic and uric acid retention. Serum electrolyte levels should be taken regularly to avoid potassium depletion.

Pupil block glaucoma or glaucoma caused by the *swelling of soft lens matter* in the posterior chamber, should be treated surgically if not alleviated by mydriatics. Sometimes argon laser iridotomy is all that is necessary (**40.10**). If not, an iridectomy is recommended (with aspiration of the soft lens matter through the iridectomy in cases with posterior chamber lenses) along with reformation of the anterior chamber with balanced salt solution. In the case of pupil block with a pupil-supported lens, it may be sufficient to create photomydriasis in one quadrant with the Argon laser in order to assist aqueous flow (**40.11**). In cases of pupil block from anterior chamber lenses after intracapsular extraction, a posterior sclerotomy should be performed to tap aqueous that has pooled in the posterior chamber, as well as an additional iridectomy with reformation of the anterior chamber. If the above measures fail, the implant should be removed in combination with an anterior vitrectomy. In order to do this after an extracapsular case, α-chymotrypsin should be injected under the iris in a circular pattern and the implant and lens capsule removed in one piece (**40.12**).

For implant-induced glaucoma, such as *pigment dispersion* from sulcus placement (**40.9**), *anterior synechias* associated with anterior chamber lenses (**40.7**) or *late uveitis/pigment dispersion* associated with pupil-supported lenses (**40.8**), if the glaucoma cannot be controlled by acetazolamide systemically and beta-blockers topically, a trabeculectomy should be performed associated with removal of the offending implant under sodium hyaluronate.

40.10

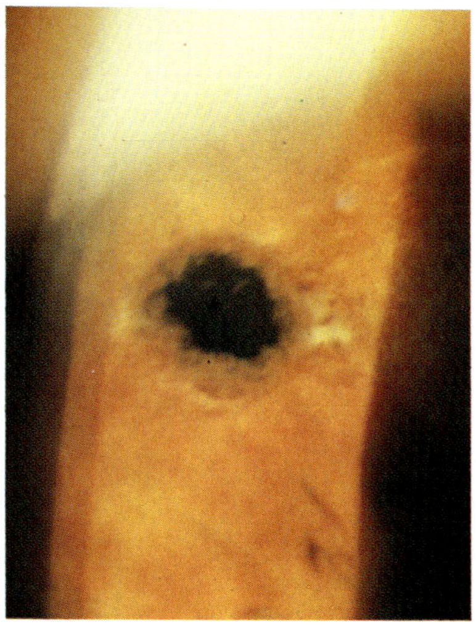

40.10 Iridotomy performed with an Argon laser.

40.11

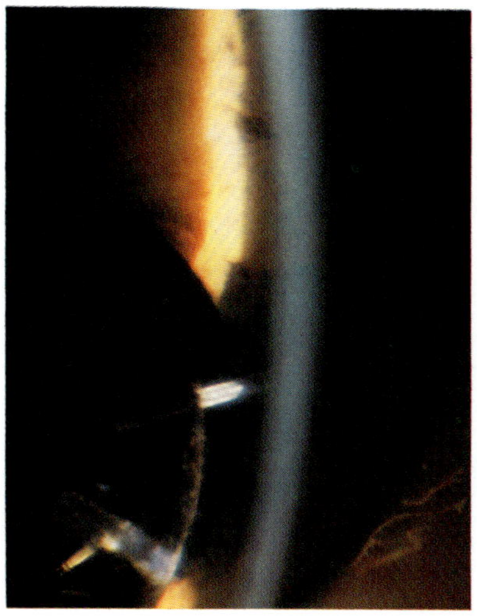

40.11 Photomydriasis with an Argon laser to create an outflow channel around an iris-supported lens implant.

40.12

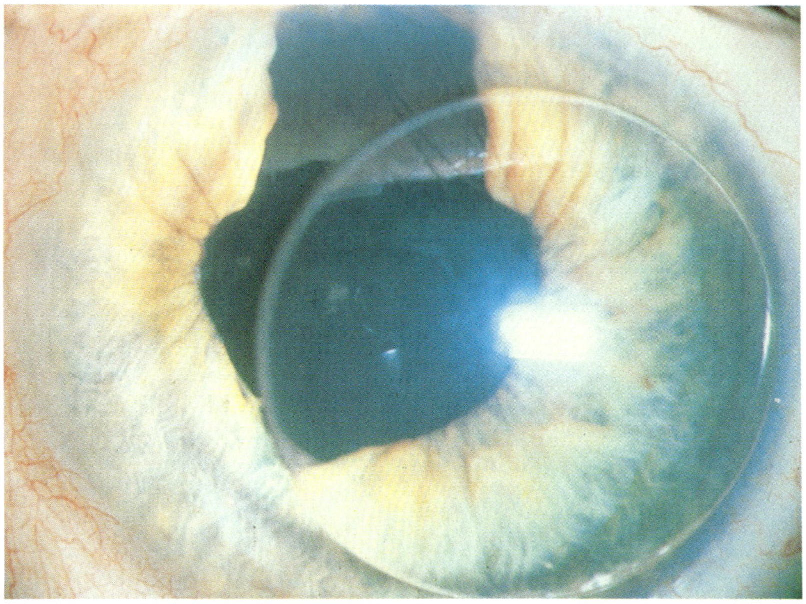

40.12 Pseudophakic glaucoma that failed to respond to medical management. The implant was removed with the associated lens capsule. A sector iridectomy was performed with vitrectomy. The patient was later fitted with a contact lens.

Further reading

Drews R.C. Prevention of blinding complications in intraocular lens implantation. *Implants in Ophthalmology*, **3**, 2–5, 1989.

Kwitko M.L. *Pseudophakic Glaucoma*. Exerpta Medical, New York, pp 301–304, 1984.

41: Pseudophakic bullous keratopathy

Peter Agapitos, Richard Duffey and Richard Lindstrom

Pseudophakic bullous keratopathy (PBK) has now become the most common reason for performing penetrating keratoplasty (PK) in North America. The mechanisms that can contribute to corneal decompensation include surgical trauma, intraocular inflammation with subsequent loss of endothelial cells, pseudophakodenesis and subsequent turbulence in the anterior chamber leading to endothelial cell loss, and inflammation from lens design, such as closed loop anterior chamber lens implants as well as lens material such as polypropylene. With age there is a slow, continuous loss of endothelial cells of 0.1–1% per year. The threshold for corneal edema from endothelial cell loss varies between 400 and 1000 cells/mm^2.

Iris-fixated implants and closed-loop anterior chamber implants are the most common types of implants that cause PBK (**41.1, 41.2**). It is much less frequent with modern posterior chamber implants and is then more likely to be related to surgical trauma than to the IOL.

Symptoms associated with early endothelial cell failure consist of variable vision, which is worse in the morning, with subsequent improvement as the day progresses and the cornea deturgesces from surface evaporation. Clinical examination of the cornea may reveal guttata, and examination of the stroma should be performed as well as examination for Waight–Beetham lines. These lines are indicative of previous stromal edema and are characteristic of Fuchs' dystrophy.

41.1

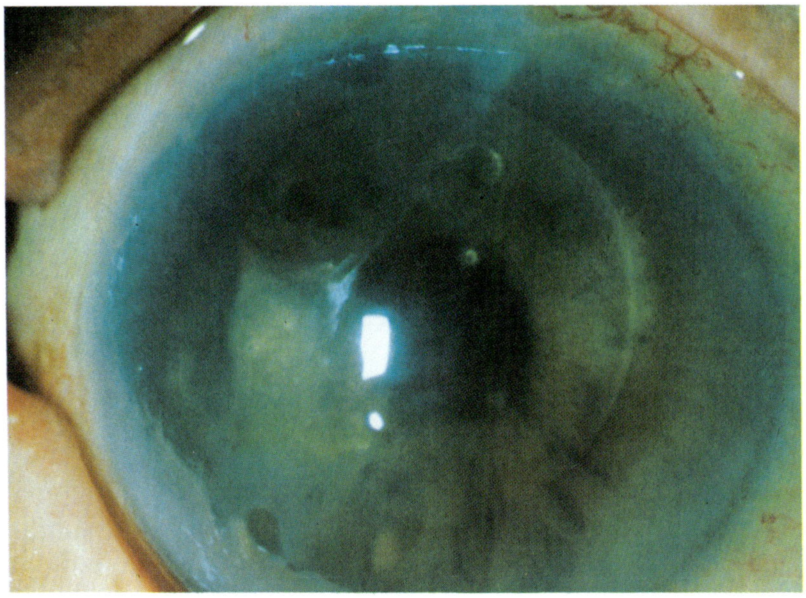

41.1 PBK caused by subluxation of a Medallion Lens (courtesy of Dr Aiko Yamanada, Japan).

41.2

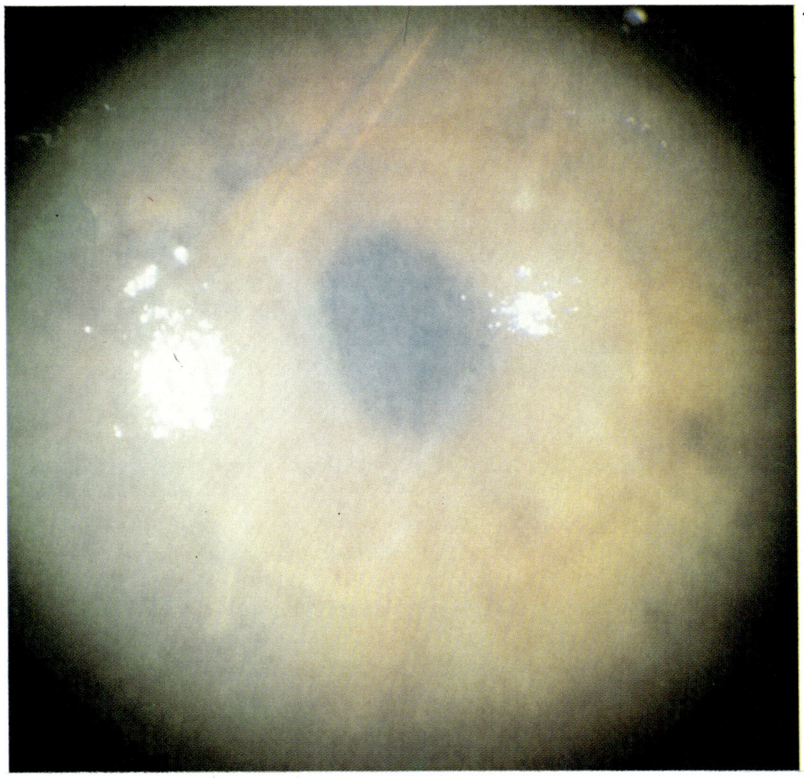

41.2 Bullous keratopathy caused by a closed-loop anterior chamber intraocular lens implant (courtesy of Dr Edward Holland, USA).

Medical treatment of PBK

Patients with PBK present with decreased vision or variable vision and pain. The pain is due to the irregular ocular surface, the development of bullae and the subsequent rupture of bullae to expose nerve endings.

Medical treatment may consist of hypertonic saline and lubricating eye drops in mild cases with reasonable vision. A reduction of intraocular pressure may help to decrease corneal swelling. Patients with PBK can become intensely inflamed and can develop a hypopyon uveitis, secondary to a persistent epithelial defect. It should be noted that they are susceptible to infections because of the instability of the ocular surface and should not be placed on long-term topical steroids. Although there is some experimental evidence to suggest that steroid drops may improve endothelial cell function, this has not been confirmed clinically. If the discomfort is not manageable by the above measures, a bandage contact lens may be considered, although careful follow-up is required because of the increased risk of infection.

Surgical treatment of PBK

The surgical treatment of PBK consists primarily of PK. This may be undertaken for visual reasons or simply for comfort. In patients with pain and no visual potential, a conjunctival flap will also produce an excellent result without the potential complications of PK. If the central endothelial cell density is greater than 1000 cells/mm^2, simple lens exchange may be performed. However, corneal edema or significant fluctuations in vision from morning edema or an endothelial cell density of less than 1000/mm^2 generally necessitates PK.

Preoperative evaluation and surgical planning

Major concurrent conditions that may cause problems postoperatively include ocular surface problems and glaucoma. Obvious rosacea blepharitis should be treated prior to surgery. If severe ocular surface problems are present, tarsorrhaphy may be performed at the time of PK. Glaucoma should also be controlled prior to surgery. Assessment of the potential visual acuity may be performed with an interferometer in the presence of limited corneal disease, or *via* entoptic phenomena when dealing with completely opaque media.

The timing of surgery is important. Once patients develop PBK they frequently go on to develop uveitis and cystoid macular edema (CME) so that it may be appropriate to avoid any delay.

Intraocular lens powers need to be calculated prior to exchange. If keratometry (K) readings are too irregular, then the opposite eye may be used, or a mean K value assumed, based on previous surgical results. In practice we have found that the mean K after 0.5 mm oversized grafts is roughly 45 D. There is some individual variation and each surgeon should develop a personal data base. Axial length measurements are performed and compared to the fellow eye and then the SRK formula is used to compute intraocular lens power. Preoperative examination of the anterior segment should also note the style of implant and fixation, formation of synechias, other distortion of anterior segment anatomy, including peaking of the pupil, and the presence of vitreous.

Principles of anterior segment reconstruction

Anterior segment reconstruction during PK should include the removal of as much of the preexisting pseudophakos as is safely possible when the position of this has contributed to the endothelial decompensation. Lysis of synechias is important and we have found that this can generally improve aqueous outflow, even if synechias have been present for a long time. Synechialysis is performed in conjunction with vitrectomy and all the vitreous should be removed from the anterior chamber as well as from iridectomy sites. An attempt should be made to remove vitreous that is attached to the posterior iris since this has been shown to contribute to cystoid maculopathy. In some cases, pupilloplasty may be performed with a 10-0 polypropylene suture to pull the iris plane taut and reduce the tendency for synechias to the corneal wound.

All closed-loop anterior chamber lens implants, all intraocular lens implants containing metallic components and most iris-fixated intraocular lenses should be removed. Well positioned PCLs may be left in place. Occasionally, a complication-free rigid anterior chamber lens can be left in place, although our current trend is to discard any kind of anterior chamber implant.

We have performed a retrospective study, comparing our intraocular lens removals in PBK *vs* intraocular lens removal and exchange and we have found that the results are virtually similar in the two series. For this reason, we advocate exchange, unless the person is aphakic in the other eye and would prefer to be aphakic in both eyes.

The next principle in reconstruction relates to which type of implant will be used and how it will be fixated. Excellent results can be obtained with the anterior chamber open-loop, four-point fixation type of semiflexible implants as recommended by Koenig *et al.* Another alternative is to suture a posterior chamber lens (PCL) to the iris, either through positioning holes or through the haptics. PCL fixation trans-sclerally, through the ciliary sulcus, is our procedure of choice, using a single piece PCL of PMMA with short C-loops. This is preferred to suturing techniques to the iris that would leave the loops free floating on the surface of the ciliary body, with the risk of pseudophakodonesis and all the known complications of a pupil-supported lens (see **39.27**).

Penetrating keratoplasty

For PK the use of oversized grafts is recommended. This has the advantages of less crowding of the anterior segment, a deeper anterior chamber, possibly formation of fewer synechias and less glaucoma. Standard storage media are utilized and either a hand-held Weck trephine or a Hessberg–Barron suction trephine (**41.3–41.5**) can be used. The host button is excised with vertical cutting scissors (**41.6**). The donor cornea is punched, endothelial side up (**41.7**).

41.3

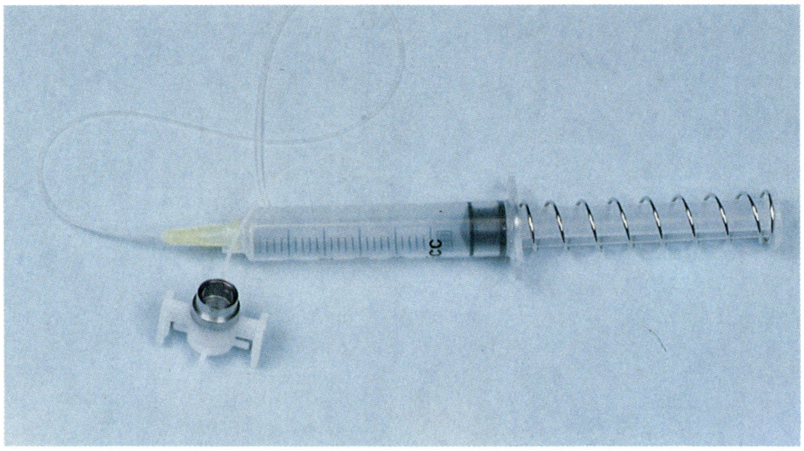

41.3 A Hessburg–Barron vacuum trephine with spring syringe to apply suction.

41.4

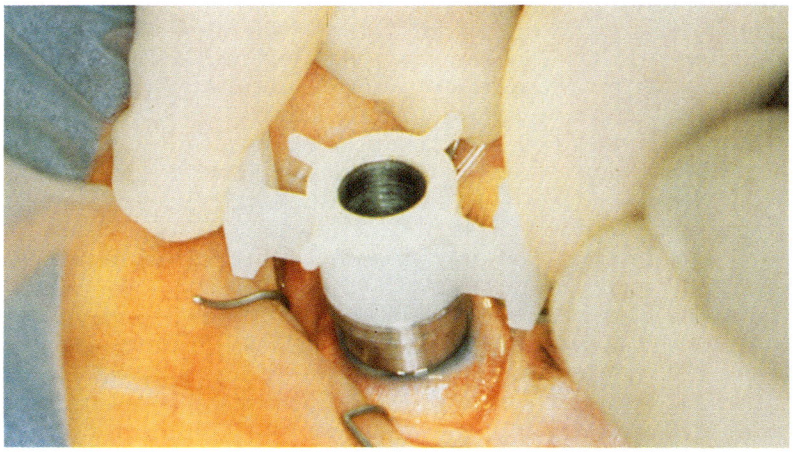

41.4 Trephination of the host cornea.

41.5

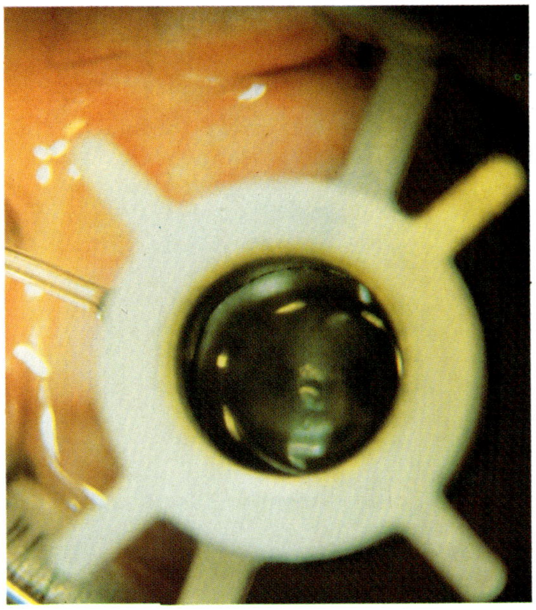

41.5 After the trephine has been suctioned into place, the cutting of the corneal wound can be observed through the center of the barrel.

41.6

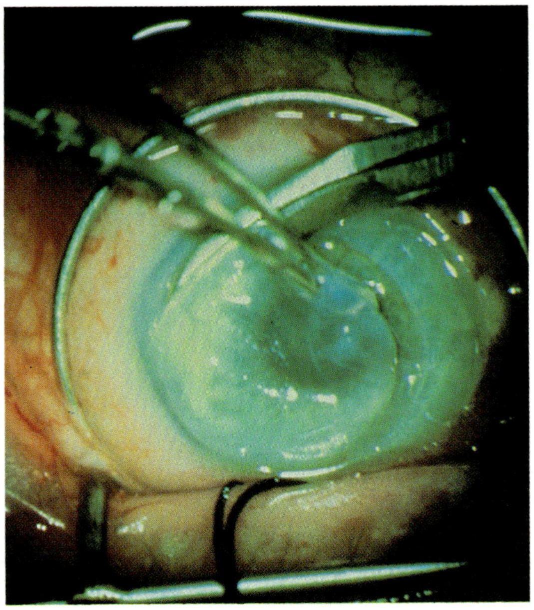

41.6 The corneal host button is excised using vertical corneal scissors. A Flieringa ring is used for all cases of aphakic and pseudophakic keratoplasty.

41.7

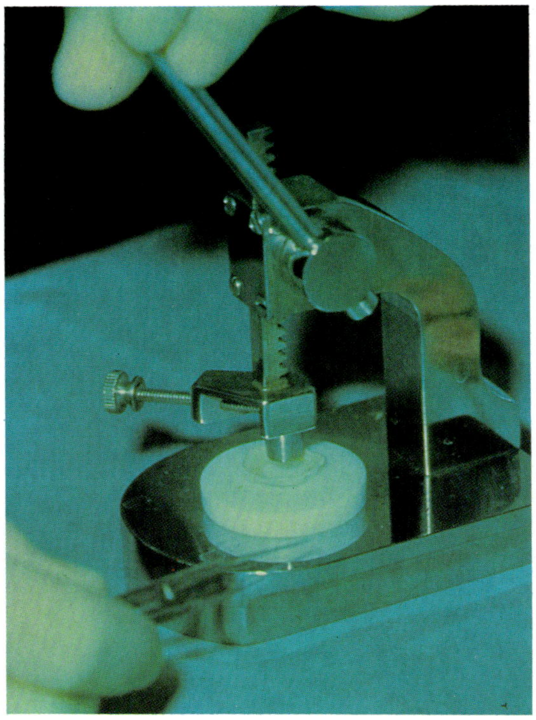

41.7 The donor cornea is punched, endothelial side first, using an Iowa press. The donor cornea is usually oversized by 0.2–0.5 mm compared with the recipient trephination.

Intraocular lens removal

When removing intraocular lenses, one must take care not to cause any damage to delicate intraocular structures. Rigid anterior chamber lenses should be cut horizontally, otherwise stretching of the ciliary body could cause bleeding. They can be easily removed in two pieces since they are not prone to encapsulation. Closed-loop anterior chamber lenses present the most difficult problem in removal. The haptics should be severed by cutting with baby Wescott scissors or a Rappazzo-style lens loop amputator (see **39.20**). After removing the optic, the haptics need to be removed, usually from a tunnel of synechias. This can be difficult when the haptic is firmly encapsulated, making it best to cut out as much as can be safely cut and leaving the remaining material *in situ*. In a Stableflex implant the double looped haptics can sometimes be hooked out of the angle and removed after the haptic has been severed from the optic (**41.8**). Severe bleeding can occur from the ciliary body when haptics have eroded into this delicate structure.

Sulcus-fixated PCLs can also be difficult to remove with possible complications of bleeding, although their removal is rarely necessary during PK.

Iris-fixated lenses are usually removed, but iridocapsular lenses may be left if the chamber is deep and the lens is well fixated without any evidence of prior uveitis or macular edema. Usually, if a suture is in place, this is cut first and removed. Platinum clips have to be bent open away from the haptic. Posterior synechias are divided and a new pupil may have to be fashioned (see also Chapter 39).

41.8

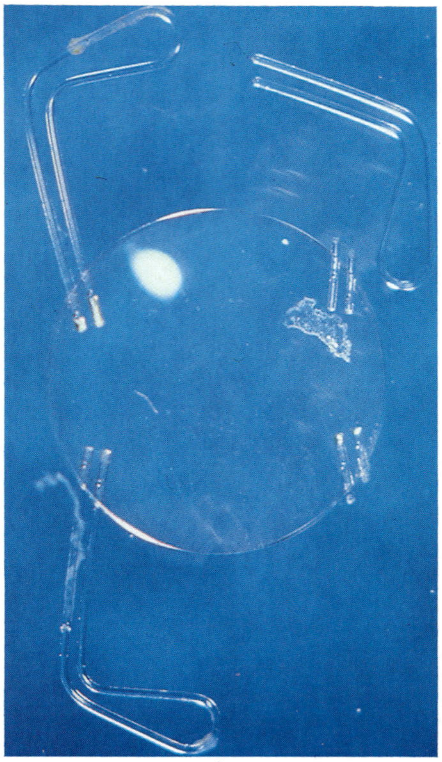

41.8 Explanted Stableflex implant. Note that on the superior haptic a membrane can be seen.

Vitrectomy and pupilloplasty

A thorough anterior vitrectomy is important. We prefer an automated vitrector with infusion, such as the Avit™. The vitrector is used to clear any iridectomies and is passed under the iris to remove vitreous adherent to the posterior iris. The two-handed technique may be necessary for this, turning out the room lights and using a light pipe in the left hand for better visibility of the vitreous strands. The iris is then swept with a Weck cell sponge to make sure there is no residual vitreous on the iris or around the angle. After it is certain that all vitreous has been removed, an effort is made to lyse any synechias. These may be evaluated using Waring's technique with a dental mirror for inspection. Often an updrawn pupil can be turned into a round pupil. An iridoplasty is performed when necessary, using an interrupted 10-0 prolene suture.

Secondary intraocular lens insertion

If using an anterior chamber implant, proper sizing is most important. Care must be taken on inserting the implant to avoid bleeding from the angle. If severe bleeding does occur, thrombin (100 units/ml) may be applied if topical adrenaline and viscoelastic tamponade are not sufficient.

If a PCL is to be inserted and if the posterior capsule is still intact, the implant may be placed in the sulcus without fixation, but only if the posterior capsule peripherally is visible for 360°. If there is uncertainty as to the zonular integrity, a trans-scleral suture is recommended.

Clinical experience combined with laboratory studies have demonstrated that trans-scleral suture fixated PCLs through the ciliary sulcus are stable and that, with care, the ciliary body vasculature can be avoided. Cadaver eye data (**41.9, 41.10**) indicate that for true ciliary sulcus fixation of the haptics, the perpendicularly passed suture should exit the scleral surface less than 1 mm posterior to the surgical limbus in the vertical meridian and approximately 0.5 mm from the limbus in the horizontal meridian, and between 0.5 and 1.0 mm in the oblique meridians (**41.11**).

Following vitrectomy, the anterior segment should be filled with an air bubble in order to draw the iris forwards and open the ciliary space (**41.12**).

41.9

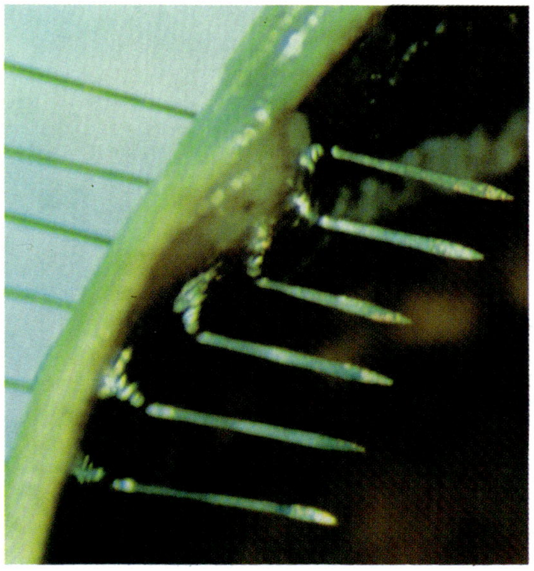

41.9 Sagittal section of a cadaver eye with straight needles passed perpendicularly through the sclera in the vertical meridian, beginning at the posterior surgical limbus and at points 1, 2, 3, 4 and 5 mm posterior to the posterior surgical limbus. This shows that the second needle from the top corresponds most closely to the location of the ciliary sulcus (published with permission from the *American Journal of Ophthalmology* and from the authors of the article 'Anatomic study of trans-sclerally sutured intraocular lens implantation', **108,** 300–309, 1989; copyright, the Ophthalmic Publishing Company).

41.10

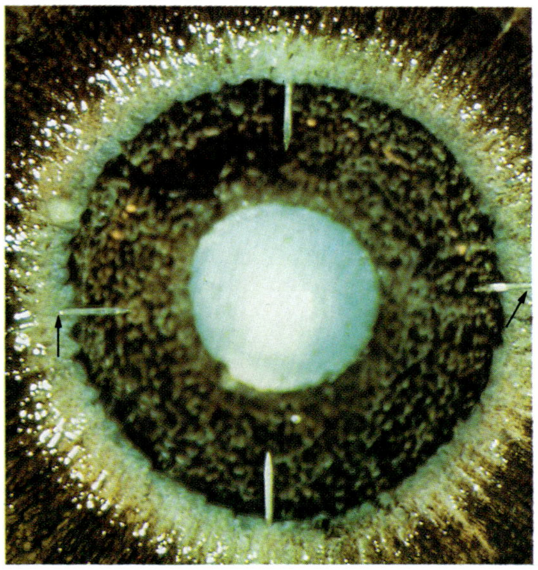

41.10 Cadaver eye sectioned at the equator showing that needles pass 1 mm posterior to the posterior surgical limbus, directly through the ciliary sulcus in the vertical meridians and 0.5 and 1 mm posterior to the ciliary sulcus in the horizontal meridians at 9 o'clock and 3 o'clock (arrows) (published with permission from the *American Journal of Ophthalmology* and from the authors of the article 'Anatomic study of trans-sclerally sutured intraocular lens implantation, **108,** 300–309, 1989; copyright, the Ophthalmic Publishing Company).

41.11

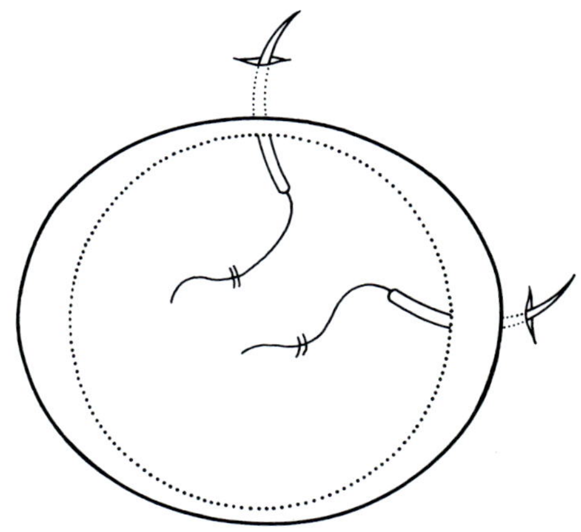

41.11 Diagram of an eye showing the relationship of the posterior surgical limbus (oval ring) to the underlying ciliary sulcus (dotted ring). Needles passed through the ciliary sulcus in the vertical meridians will exit the sclera 1 mm posterior to the limbus, and those in the horizontal meridians will exit the sclera 0.5 mm posterior to the limbus.

41.12

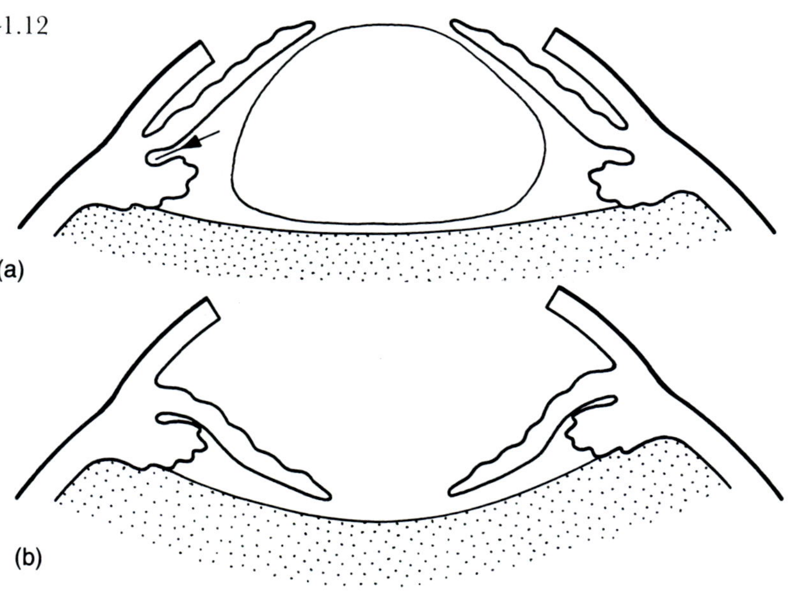

41.12 Scleral fixation of a PCL following vitrectomy during keratoplasty: (a) Cross-section of an air-filled eye with the peripheral iris pulled up against the peripheral cornea by capillary action, allowing the ciliary sulcus space (arrow) to open up for easier suture access; (b) Cross-section of a fluid-filled eye with the iris allowed to sag, thus closing the potential ciliary sulcus space and making suture placement more difficult.

A 10-0 prolene suture is tied to the haptics at their greatest spread diameter (**41.13**); for example, 13.5 mm apart on a one-piece all-PMMA, 10° vaulted 7 mm optic posterior chamber intraocular lens (such as the Iolab 6840B). The implant haptics should have bulbous tips. Care should be taken to avoid a more proximal haptic location for the suture (**41.14**). Conjunctival peritomies are performed at the 1–2 o'clock and 7–8 o'clock meridians, the sites planned for suture placement. The single-armed needle for each haptic is passed through the pupil, hugging the posterior iris surface, and into the ciliary sulcus space (**41.15**). The needle is then passed perpendicularly through the sclera between 0.5 and 1 mm posterior to the posterior surgical limbus, depending on the meridian of scleral fixation. We recommend that the vertical and horizontal meridians be avoided in favor of an oblique axis suture orientation, in order to avoid potential vascular complications relating to the perforating branches of the anterior ciliary arteries in the 3, 6, 9 and 12 o'clock meridians and the long posterior ciliary arteries and nerves in the 3 and 9 o'clock meridians.

After both sutures are passed, the implant is placed through the corneal trephination wound and the inferior haptic is directed beneath the iris as the trans-scleral suture is gently pulled up to guide and fixate the haptic into the ciliary sulcus (**41.16**). An assistant holds the inferior haptic suture taut, keeping the haptic secured in the ciliary sulcus, and the superior haptic is similarly placed.

We have demonstrated that, in many eyes, when haptic sutures are passed as above, the sutures actually pass into the ciliary sulcus through the peripheral iris root and anterior chamber angle and exit the angle through the scleral spur (**41.17**). This has not led to pupillary distortion or formation of peripheral anterior synechias in any of the eyes studied thus far, and provides the advantage of avoiding the ciliary body and its abundant vasculature, including the major circle of the

41.13

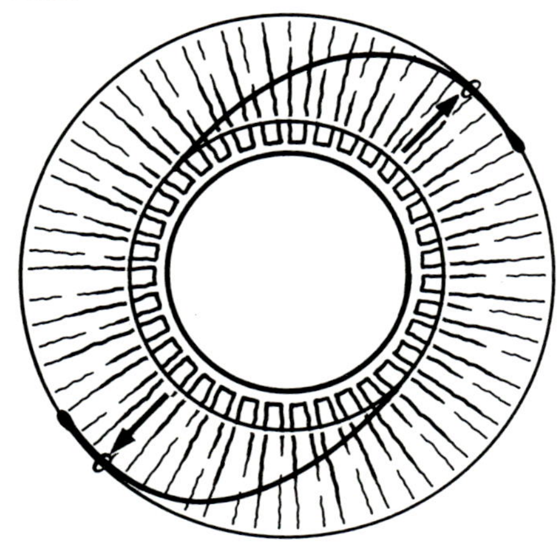

41.13 Posterior aspect of the iris showing the correct suture locations on the implant haptics (arrows), which correspond to the greatest haptic spread within the ciliary sulcus.

41.14

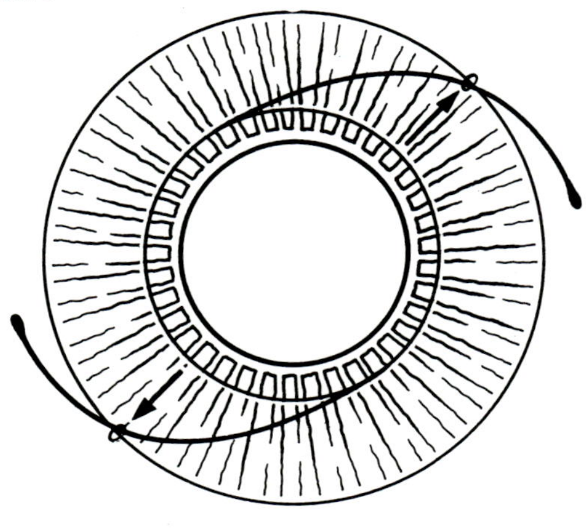

41.14 Posterior aspect of the iris showing incorrect suture locations on the implant haptics (arrows). A suture tied too proximally on the haptic causes the distal portion of the haptic to overlie the pars plana, even though the suture is placed correctly in the ciliary sulcus.

41.15

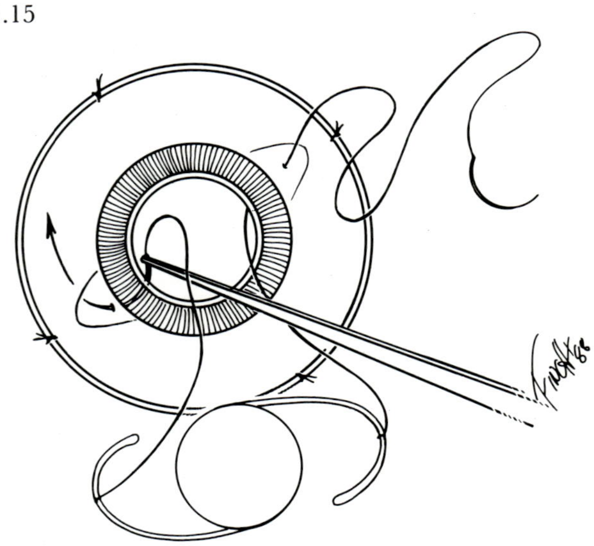

41.15 The suture is passed under the iris and through the ciliary sulcus, exiting 0.5–1 mm posterior to the surgical limbus.

41.16

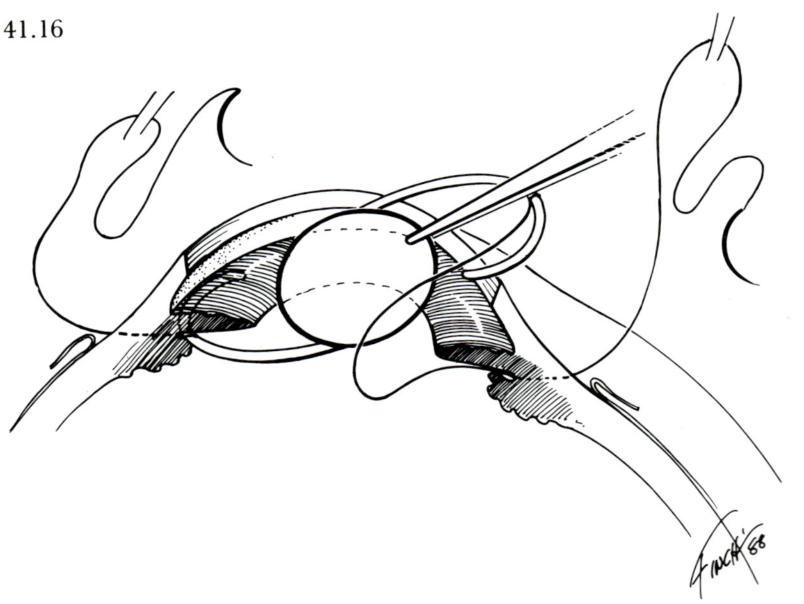

41.16 The implant is inserted through the trephination wound into the ciliary sulcus.

41.17

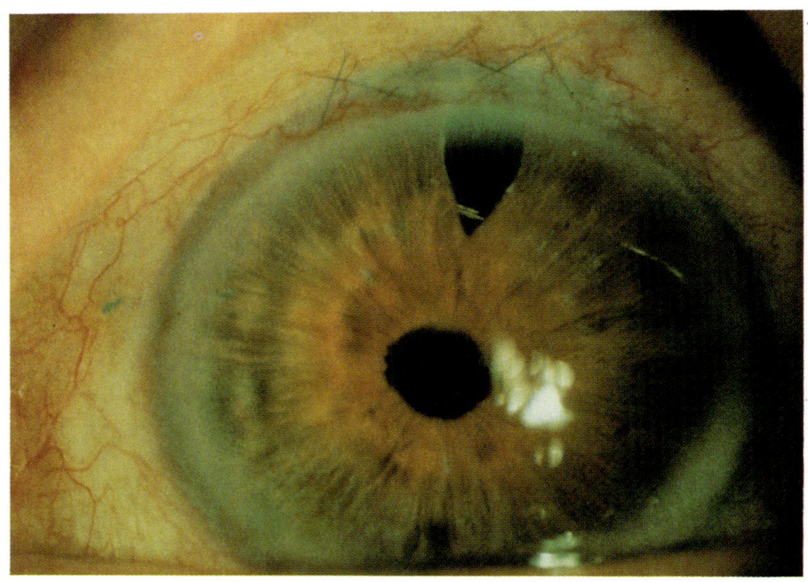

41.17 Patient with a secondary trans-sclerally sutured posterior chamber lens. The haptics are fixated at the 3 and 9 o'clock meridians with the suture visible at 9 o'clock. Note the round pupil.

iris. After trans-scleral suture passage, a second superficial bite is taken posterior to the scleral suture exit site and the suture is tied to itself, avoiding excessive tension and scleral buckling. The excess suture is then cut short and the knot flattened with a low temperature ophthalmic cautery. Alternatively, the free needle arm is tied to the top of the loop and then passed posteriorly as a long superficial scleral bite dragging the loop and single suture arm into a scleral tunnel (**41.18**). The suture is then cut flush with the conjunctival surface and allowed to retract beneath the conjunctiva and into the scleral needle track. The conjunctiva is then reapproximated at the limbus with buried 10-0 nylon sutures, making sure that the scleral knot is covered completely. Another approach is to dissect scleral flaps and pass the sutures such that they can be covered by them (see **39.35**).

We consider the above technique of posterior chamber lens fixation to be safe and compatible with the normal anatomy of the anterior segment (**41.19, 41.20**). There have been no major complications. The most frequent problem has been transconjunctival erosion of the prolene suture raising concern over the possibility of endophthalmitis. The use of a scleral flap could lessen this potential risk.

41.18

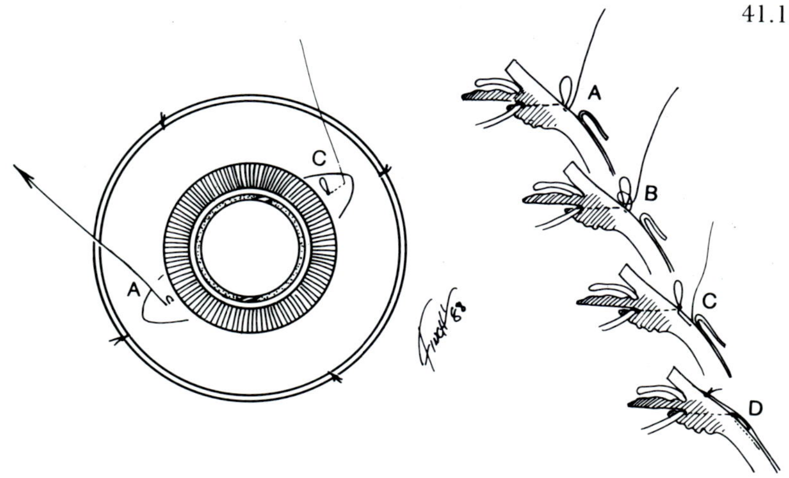

41.18 After the implant has been inserted, a second bite is taken on the sclera (A) and the suture is tied to itself (B). The suture may then be passed through the sclera, posteriorly (C), and cut flush leaving the loop long. The conjunctiva is then drawn up to cover the scleral knot and sutured at the limbus (D).

41.19

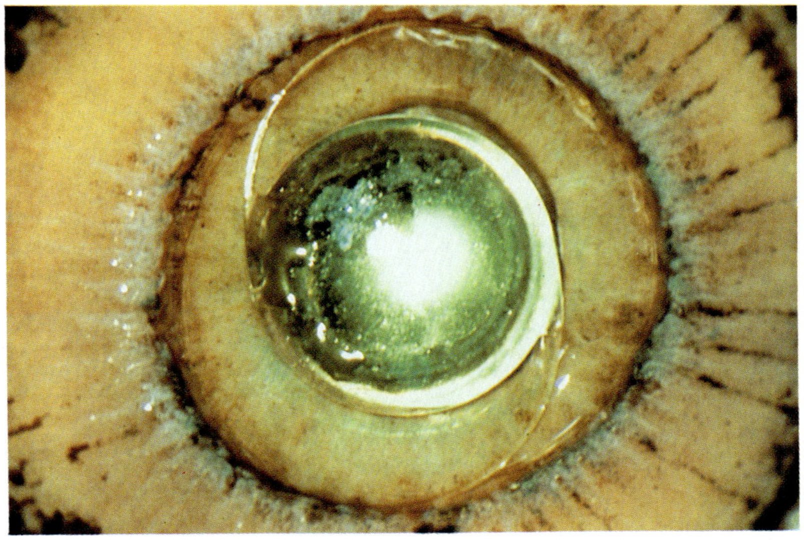

41.19 Cadaver eye showing a well-centered posterior chamber implant viewed from behind, with the haptics secured in the sulcus (published with permission from the *American Journal of Ophthalmology* and from the authors of the article 'Anatomic study of the trans-sclerally sutured intraocular lens implantation, **108,** 300–309, 1989; copyright, the Ophthalmic Publishing Company).

41.20

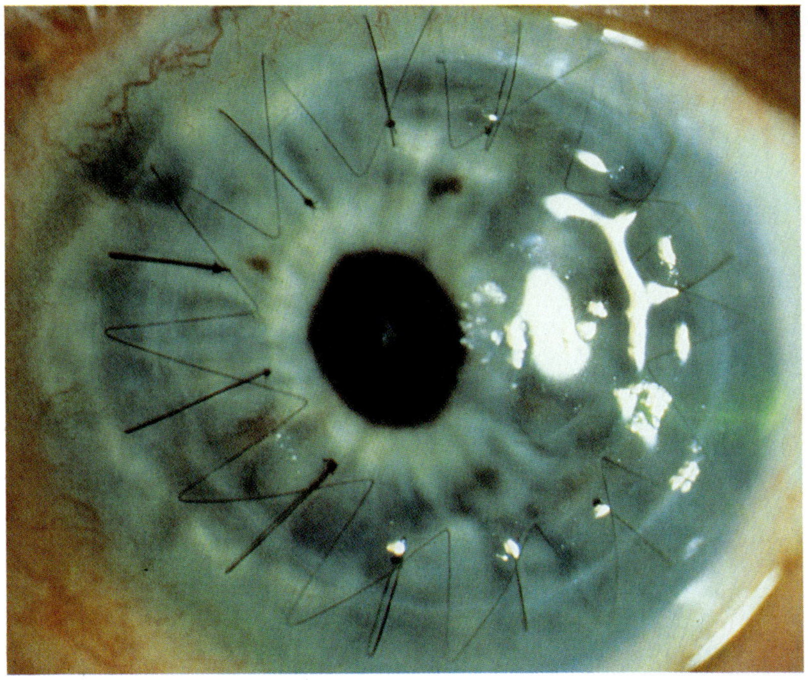

41.20 Patient with a sutured posterior chamber intraocular lens implant. Note the normal appearance of the anterior segment.

Further reading

Duffey R.J., Holland E.J., Agapitos P.J. and Lindstrom R.L., Anatomic study of trans-sclerally sutured intraocular lens implantation, *Amer. J. Ophthalmol.*, **108,** 300–309, 1989.

Koenig S.B., McDermott M.L. and Hyndiuk R.A. Penetrating keratoplasty and intraocular lens exchange for pseudophakic bullous keratopathy associated with a closed loop anterior chamber lens. *Amer. J. Ophthalmol.*, **108,** 43–48, 1989.

Speaker M.G., Lugo M., Laibson P.R., *et al.* Penetrating keratoplasty for pseudophakic bullous keratopathy. Management of the intraocular lens. *Ophthalmology,* **95,** 1260–1268, 1988.

42: Pseudophakic endophthalmitis

William Smiddy, Terry O'Brien and Walter Stark

Endophthalmitis is a potentially catastrophic complication of any intraocular surgery. Although quite rare, its possibly devastating course can irreversibly limit vision. Prompt diagnosis and effective treatment may determine the visual outcome in a high proportion of cases. Thus, the successful management of suppurative postoperative endophthalmitis requires the following five steps:

- Make the clinical diagnosis.
- Obtain proper laboratory studies.
- Initiate appropriate antimicrobial therapy.
- Modify initial therapy.
- Terminate therapy.

Now that the use of preoperative and perioperative prophylactic antibiotic is widespread, the incidence of infective endophthalmitis following cataract extraction is about 0.02–0.1%, compared with an incidence of 0.5% or higher when preoperative and perioperative (including conjunctival) antibiotics were not used. The local flora is probably the source of causative organisms in postoperative endophthalmitis, although intraocular cultures do not always correlate with preoperative external cultures.

The standard procedure is to administer prophylactic subconjunctival antibiotics (gentamicin and possibly a cephalosporin) routinely at the conclusion of surgery.

Etiologic associations

Infective postoperative endophthalmitis usually appears sporadically, but there are several circumstances under which its incidence is increased. Such increased incidence has been described following vitreous loss, with a vitreous wick syndrome, in association with filtering blebs (although with a delayed presentation), with wound dehiscence following suture removal, and in the presence of exposed nylon sutures. Localized epidemics of endophthalmitis have been described, with contamination of the intraocular lens (IOL) and irrigating solutions, and from the respiratory tracts of the operating team. The increased incidence with vitreous loss and other surgical complications may be due to the increased operating time and instrumentation, or to the enhanced access of the posterior chamber to the anterior chamber. The most effective treatment for endophthalmitis is prevention through attention to these issues.

Clinical presentation and differential diagnosis

The classic presentation of postoperative endophthalmitis is painful, decreased vision accompanied by mild to severe inflammation with hypopyon (**42.1**). Pain is the clinical hallmark of the presentation of endophthalmitis, but it may present painlessly with a degree of inflammation that is indistinguishable from the usual postoperative course.

Since there may be no clinical signs that allow the specific differentiation of endophthalmitis from other causes of postoperative inflammation, its diagnosis can be difficult. The principal differential diagnoses of postoperative endophthalmitis include increased inflammation due to retained cortex or nuclear material, coexisting iritis, coexisting proliferative diabetic retinopathy, reaction to other toxic components such as the IOL polishing compounds, IOL sterilizing agents, direct IOL toxicity, or spontaneous rupture of the hyaloid face. Noninfective, implant-related inflammation may present more acutely, with the hypopyon forming at an earlier stage and slow or no progression from the first to second postoperative day. The hypopyon may be small and visible only with a slit-lamp, emphasizing the need for proper postoperative slit-lamp examination (**42.1**) rather than just using a hand light. Inflammation associated with proliferative diabetic retinopathy usually has a more fibrinous nature and is typically painless.

Chronic vitreous hemorrhage may have escaped diagnosis preoperatively because of dense cataract, and this may mimic the

42.1

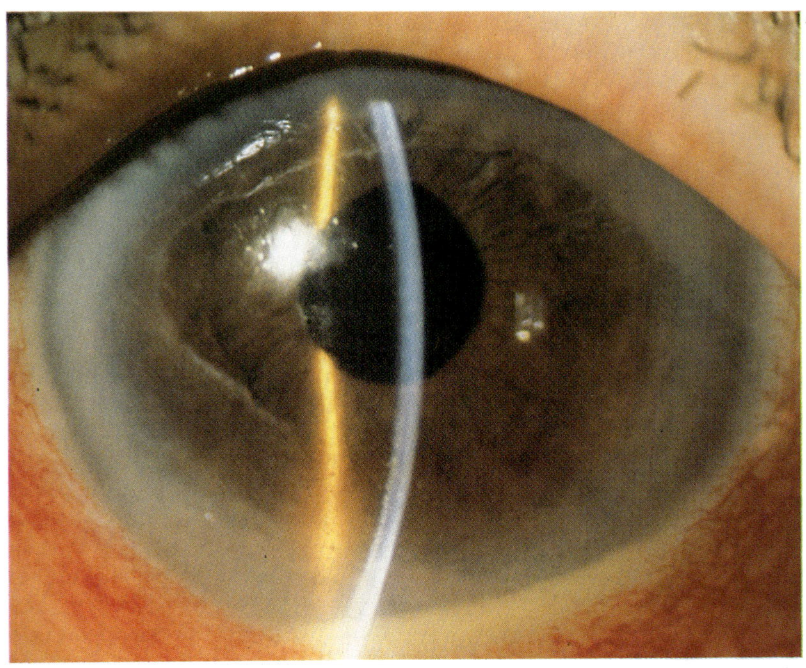

42.1 Slit-lamp photograph of the typical appearance of a patient presenting with pseudophakic endophthalmitis. It is important to retract the lower lid inferiorly when examining postoperative patients to inspect for hypopyon that otherwise may escape detection.

inflammation characteristic of endophthalmitis. However, in these cases the apparent posterior segment inflammation is increased out of proportion to that found in the anterior segment, and signs are usually painless and nonprogressive. Retinal periphlebitis has been described as an early presenting sign of endophthalmitis. Indirect evidence useful to distinguish infective endophthalmitis may include the presence of factors associated with an increased incidence of endophthalmitis, such as inadvertent filtering bleb or vitreous loss.

Visual acuity usually decreases in patients with endophthalmitis, although the specificity of this sign is poor since visual acuity decreases in postoperative inflammation from any cause. Nevertheless, profound decreased vision (light perception without projection), absence of red reflex from the fundus, and the presence of an afferent pupillary defect are among the most ominous signs.

Clinical classifications of endophthalmitis

It is clinically useful to distinguish between early acute inflammation (within 72 hours postoperatively), late acute inflammation (onset of inflammation beyond 72 hours), and delayed subacute or chronic inflammation (weeks to months following surgery). Infective endophthalmitis may present during any of these periods, but the class of organism, its virulence, and the clinical approach will be determined largely according to which of these three groups it falls.

Postoperative endophthalmitis that occurs within the first 72 hours is most frequently caused by gram-positive organisms, but may also be due to gram-negative organisms. With the most virulent organisms, the signs and symptoms may occur on the first postoperative day, but are usually more distinct by two to four days following surgery. Most cases of bacterial endophthalmitis show progressive symptoms and thus can be distinguished from noninfective causes of postoperative inflammation. Signs most specific for early acute inflammation include corneal stromal edema, fibrinous iritis, and severe vitritis. Hypopyon is diagnostic.

Late acute postoperative endophthalmitis classically occurs in patients with a filtering bleb. This association may be important to keep in mind when differentiation of sterile inflammation from infection is difficult.

Delayed subacute or chronic infection is usually caused by less virulent organisms, such as *Staphylococcus epidermidis*, the anaerobic bacterium *Propionibacterium acnes*, Nocardia, Mycobacteria, and yeasts. This group can be difficult to distinguish from noninfective causes of postoperative inflammation. Clinical signs may be masked by concurrent steroid treatment. Although *S. epidermidis* endophthalmitis is well known to present in this fashion, a more recently recognized cause is *P. acnes*. Clinical signs usually include chronic, persistent, low-grade inflammation, or an increase in low-grade inflammation several months postoperatively. Cultures should be maintained for longer than the usual time as this organism may be quite fastidious. White plaque-like opacities on the posterior capsule are characteristic, but only present in about half of reported cases. Although endophthalmitis due to gram-negative organisms rarely presents as a delayed subacute infection, *Pseudomonas cepacia* endophthalmitis has been reported to present in this fashion following IOL implantation. Fungal endophthalmitis usually exhibits fluffy aggregates in the anterior vitreous cavity.

Proper management of postoperative endophthalmitis depends upon a prompt and accurate diagnosis. The clinical signs and symptoms direct the physician to the possibility of endophthalmitis, and identification of the organism by proper specimen collection, staining, and laboratory culturing techniques follows from this suspicion.

Initial treatment

The initiation of antibiotic therapy should never precede the prompt, judicious collection of intraocular fluids for appropriate laboratory investigations. Retrobulbar anesthesia or general anesthesia is recommended, ideally in the operating room. However, under suboptimal circumstances in cases of acute infection, it is more important to obtain a prompt sample than to delay because an operating room is unavailable. Cases of delayed subacute infection are less urgent, so an operating room setting is worth waiting for.

Fluid specimens should be obtained both from the anterior chamber and the vitreous cavity. The highest yield for a positive culture is from the vitreous cavity. Of cases with a positive culture from the vitreous, one half may not show growth from the aqueous.

A small (25- or 27-gauge) needle can be inserted directly into the anterior chamber or through a preplaced deep, but not penetrating, bevelled limbal or corneal incision to collect an aqueous sample (0.1–0.2 ml). The vitreous sample usually requires a larger gauge needle because the fluid is more viscous. To avoid the difficulty of working on a soft eye, sclerotomy for the vitreous sample may be made before removing the anterior chamber sample. The sample can be obtained through the anterior incision by placing the needle posterior to the lens and lens capsule. A pars plana incision may be better, since it allows for a pure vitreous cavity sample and avoids the theoretical disadvantage of creating a communication between the anterior and posterior chambers. A vitreous suction and cutting instrument may be preferred (**42.2**), since aspirating nonfluid vitreous with a needle may

42.2

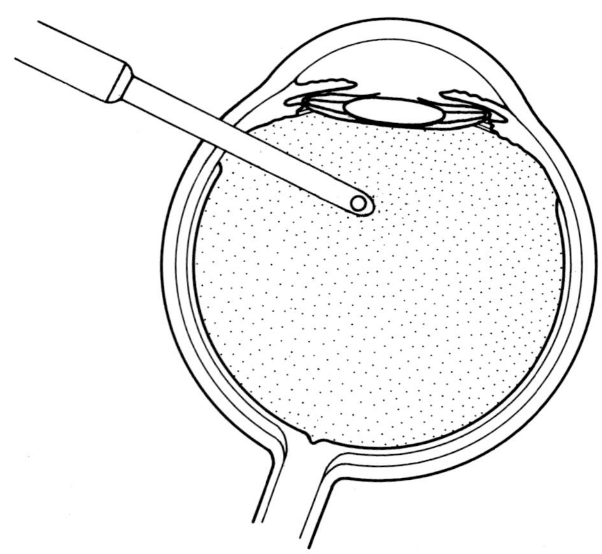

42.2 To obtain a vitreous sample for culture a vitrectomy instrument is preferred to needle aspiration in order to minimize vitreous traction on the retina.

result in undue vitreous traction, which may be the cause of later retinal detachment. Sometimes, however, a fluid sample is readily obtainable with the needle only. Regardless of the type of probe used, its tip should be visualized directly before beginning aspiration. If a vitrectomy is being performed, a 0.3–0.6 ml sample can be obtained during the initial stages of the vitrectomy by splicing a syringe into the aspiration line using a three-way stopcock (**42.3**), and collecting an undiluted sample by manual suction before beginning the infusion. The three-way stopcock can then be adjusted to allow conventional vitrectomy aspiration when the intraocular infusion is started. The infusion-diluted sample from a more complete vitrectomy can be filtered through a disposable filter system, and the filter may be removed under sterile conditions and cut into pieces for placement in appropriate culture dishes.

The aqueous and vitreous samples should be plated for microbiological evaluation as soon as possible, and taken immediately to the laboratory for incubation and staining. A proper selection of culture plates should be collated in advance, including blood agar, chocolate agar, and thioglycollate broth specimens, as well as a Sabouraud agar plate for fungus growth. If prior laboratory studies or other clinical signs indicate atypical organisms, other special media such as Lowenstein–Jensen or Middlebrook–Cohn agar for Mycobacterium or Nocardia should be used. If antibiotics have already been instituted, devices can be used for antibiotic neutralization to improve the rate of bacterial recovery. Anterior chamber and vitreous cavity samples should be plated separately. A system and media for anaerobic culture and transport (such as Brucella agar with 5% horse serum) should also be available. Immediate Gram- and Giemsa-stained slide smears, as well as unstained specimens, should be prepared.

42.3

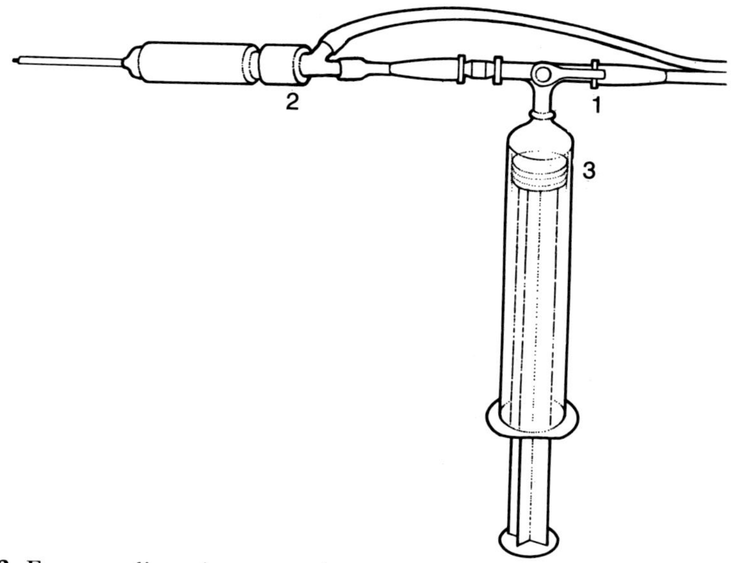

42.3 For sampling vitreous a three-way stopcock (1) is inserted into the aspiration tubing near the vitrector handpiece (2) so as to minimize dead space in the tubing. The sample is collected into the syringe (3), before commencing infusion, so that is is undiluted.

Etiologic organisms

Cultures collected in a standard way from patients suspected of having postoperative endophthalmitis have been found to yield positive results in about 75% of cases (**Table 42.1**). The vitreous specimen is more likely (but not always) to yield a positive culture than is the anterior chamber specimen, especially when vitrectomy is performed.

Table 42.1 Culture results in infective endophthalmitis

			Percentage of culture-positive cases					
Series	*Number*	*%*	*Gram-positive staining*	*S. epidermis*	*S. aureus*	*Streptococcus*	*Gram-negative staining*	*Fungal*
Forster (1974)	23	43	60	20	10	20	40	10
Forster (1980)	140	56	58	18	9	21	29	13
Diamond (1981)	26	100	77	38	12	23	15	8
Puliafito (1982)	17	100	82	59	12	0	18	0
Rowsey (1982)	7	77	79	30	15	0	15	8
Olsen (1983)	40	75	90	38	24	28	7	3
Bohigian (1986)	82	62	76	29	18	25	18	6
Driebe (1986)	83	75	76	38	21	12	16	8
Stern (1989)	26	73	89	52	5	16	11	0

Forster R.K. Endophthalmitis: Diagnostic cultures and visual results. *Arch. Ophthalmol.*, **92,** 387–392, 1974; Forster R.K., Abbott R.L. and Gelender H. Management of infectious endophthalamitis. *Ophthalmology*, **87,** 313–319, 1980; Diamond J.G. Intraocular management of endophthalmitis. A systematic approach. *Arch. Ophthalmol.*, **99,** 96–99, 1981; Puliafito C.A., Baker A.F., Haaf J. and Foster C.S. Infectious endophthalmitis; review of 36 cases. *Ophthalmology*, **89,** 921–928, 1982; Rowsey J.J., Newsome K.L., Sexton D.J. and Harms W.K. Endophthalmitis; current approaches. *Ophthalmology*, **89,** 1055–1065, 1982; Olsen J.C., Flynn H.W. Jr, Forster R.K. and Culbertson W.W. Results in the treatment of postoperative endophthalamitis. *Ophthalmology*, **90,** 692–699, 1983; Bohigian G.M. and Olk R.J. Factors associated with a poor visual result in endophthalmitis. *Am. J. Ophthalmol.*, **101,** 332–341, 1986; Driebe W.T., Mandelbaum S. and Forster R.K. Pseudophakic endophthalmitis. Diagnosis and management. *Ophthalmology*, **93,** 442–448, 1986; Stern G.A.. Engel H.M. and Driebe W.T. The treatment of postoperative endophthalmitis. Results of differing approaches of treatment. *Ophthalmology*, **96,** 62–67, 1989.

A positive culture result has been defined as growth on two or more media, or confluent growth on at least one solid medium plate at the inoculation site. Contamination must be suspected when there is scanty growth or growth only on a transfer specimen.

The most common class of bacteria comprises the gram-positive organisms, present in 58–90% of the culture-positive cases (**Table 42.1**) and of which *S. epidermidis* is the most common. At least half of infections are due to coagulase-negative staphylococci. Twelve different species have been identified and it is wrong to dismiss these as skin contaminants or nonpathogens.

The incidence of resistant staphylococci is increasing. Virtually all staphylococci isolates are resistant to penicillin, many are resistant to methicillin, though by a different mechanism, and there is frequent cross-resistance to cephalosporins.

Other common gram-positive isolates in cases of acute postoperative endophthalmitis include *Staphylococcus aureus* and streptococcal species.

Gram-negative bacteria are reported to cause 7–40% of culture proven endophthalmitis cases (**Table 42.1**). Most common are Proteus and pseudomonas species. Others include *Hemophilus influenzae*, and Bacillus species (especially after trauma).

Fungi are responsible for up to 13% of cases (**Table 42.1**), but may cluster in an epidemic fashion. The principal causes of postsurgical fungal endophthalmitis are Aspergillus, Candida, and Paecilomyces species.

Antibiotic therapy

The preferred initial intravenous agent should include an aminoglycoside in combination with a broad spectrum antibiotic that will be effective against staphylococci (**Table 42.2**). Intravenous methicillin is preferred over cefazolin or other cephalosporin antibiotics, because there is less nephrotoxicity when combined with an aminoglycoside; however, the increasing incidence of methicillin-resistant strains limits its use. Vancomycin therapy in combination with an aminoglycoside may be precluded because of ototoxicity and nephrotoxicity. However, if subsequent culture reports demonstrate a methicillin-resistant strain, consideration should be given to substituting intravenous vancomycin, or sodium fusidate (which is less toxic) may be given parenterally and topically. This is active against resistant staphylococci. Recent studies have suggested suboptimal intraocular penetration with parenteral vancomycin; hence third-generation cephalosporins are increasingly recommended. Peak and trough serum levels of aminoglycosides should be monitored after the initial four to five dosages and the dose altered accordingly. Renal function tests, such as serum creatinine levels, should also be monitored to detect nephrotoxicity at its earliest stages so that the therapy can be modified.

Cefazolin and an aminoglycoside are preferred for subconjunctival or topical antibiotics (**Table 42.2**).

The selection of these medications for the treatment of early acute postoperative infection is based on their ability to combat the most likely etiologic organisms. If there is a known cephalosporin allergy, or past anaphylaxis has been noted with penicillin, vancomycin may be substituted.

If there is reason to suspect a specific organism, the initial choice of antibiotics can be altered. For example, when a fulminating course of postoperative inflammation with proptosis, ophthalmoplegia, and ring corneal abscess suggests *Bacillus cereus* infection, intravenous (and intravitreal) clindamycin should be substituted for cefazolin because of its synergistic effect with gentamicin against Bacillus species. Specific etiologic entities may be suspected on the basis of epidemiologic information about other current outbreaks, and the initial antibiotics chosen accordingly. Subconjunctival injections of ceftazidime have been found to be effective in preventing experimental endophthalmitis due to *Pseudomonas aeruginosa* and may therefore be more effective than cefazolin when this is suspected.

Table 42.2 Therapy of suspected acute postsurgical bacterial endophthalmitis

Route	*Agents*
Intravitreal injection	Cefazolin (2.5 mg) and gentamicin (0.1 mg) (Vancomycin 1.0 mg)
Subconjunctival injection	Cefazolin (100 mg) and tobramycin (20 mg)
Intravenous infusion	Methicillin (200 mg/kg/day) and tobramycin (3–7 mg/kg/day in three divided doses)
Topical application	Cefazolin (50 mg/ml) and tobramycin (14 mg/ml), one drop alternately every 30 min.

The general consensus is to use topical, intravenous, periocular and intravitreal antibiotics (**Table 42.2**).

Broad spectrum intravitreal antibiotics (for example, gentamycin with cefazolin or vancomycin) should be administered at the time the cultures are taken, despite the risk of retinal toxicity. The volume of injection fluid should be minimized, if possible to 0.1 ml, and directed away from the posterior retina (**42.4, 42.5**).

If a fungal infection is confirmed, periocular miconazole and intravenous amphotericin B should be initiated. Intravenous miconazole or oral ketoconazole can be substituted if amphotericin B is contraindicated. Intravitreal antifungal agents should be reserved for the most refractory cases, since their efficacy has not been fully established.

Corticosteroid therapy in bacterial endophthalmitis is controversial and should be delayed for at least 24 hours after initiation of antibiotics. Steroids are given subconjunctivally, peribulbarly or systemically in order to reduce damage to intraocular tissues by minimizing the host inflammatory response. They are contraindicated in fungal endophthalmitis.

42.4

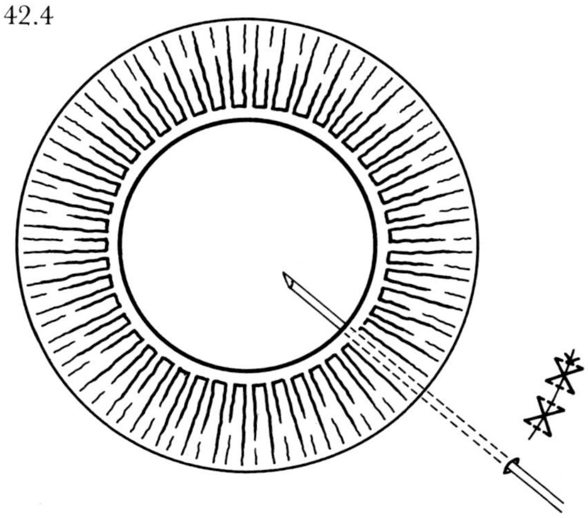

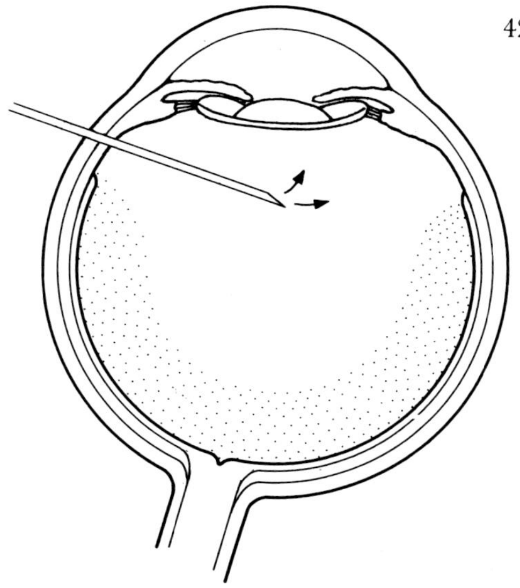

42.5

42.4 Antibiotic injection after vitrectomy. The 25 gauge needle, mounted on a 1 ml syringe, is inserted bevel up, 3 mm posterior to the limbus, adjacent to the sutured sclerotomy.

42.5 Antibiotic is injected into the midvitreous space slowly, so as to minimize intravitreal currents and avoid directing the antibiotic towards the retina.

Vitrectomy

The role of vitrectomy in the treatment of endophthalmitis has not been completely defined. Visual results in patients undergoing vitrectomy are worse than in those not undergoing vitrectomy, but this may be owing to a selection bias towards cases of poor prognosis. The rationale for at least a core vitrectomy is to decrease the infectious and inflammatory load and allow for a larger sample collection. However, subsequent retinal detachment has been described in up to 21% of cases, although this may be due to the selection bias. The consensus is to perform vitrectomy only on patients with more severe inflammation or if there has been an unsatisfactory response to initial medical therapy.

The technique for performing a vitrectomy should involve removal of as much inflammatory and infectious debris as possible while maintaining visibility of the posterior pole. Visualization of the vitrectomy instruments should be maintained at all times during the surgery, and if visualization is too poor, it may be necessary to conclude after performing only a central core vitrectomy in order to avoid complications from further surgery. A long (6 mm) infusion cannula is recommended in these cases, since it may not be possible to visualize the cannula tip. If the anterior chamber is full of clotted or inflammatory debris, and the IOL or posterior cavity cannot be visualized, the anterior chamber can be washed out with the vitrectomy instrument through a small limbal incision. Alternatively, the debris may be cleared using a 23-gauge butterfly needle for infusion and a Ziegler blade or blunt cannula to create an outflow path at a separate site (**42.6**).

The central portion of the posterior capsule is usually excised to maximize visibility of the posterior segment, but because the IOL has usually been placed only a few days previously, care must be taken to avoid dislodging the lens. There may be layers of thick inflammatory debris and tissue on the retina which may be carefully removed using the fluted extrusion needle. The retina may be very friable and susceptible to bleeding or retinal break formation. After completing the vitrectomy and closing the sclerotomies, intravitreal antibiotics are injected (**42.4**).

42.6

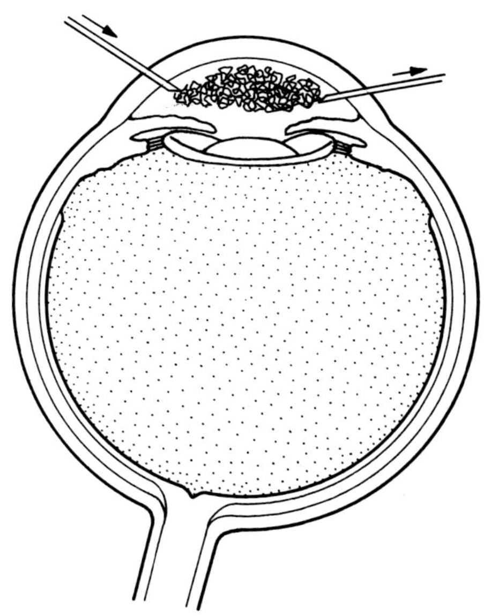

42.6 Removal of anterior chamber debris: While infusing with a 25 gauge butterfly needle at the limbus from one side, a Ziegler blade or blunt cannula is used to evacuate the contents from another side.

Retention of implant

Removal of the IOL is not usually necessary or recommended, except with culture-proven fungal endophthalmitis or when conventional therapy has failed. Removal of prosthetic materials from other parts of the body is usually indicated in cases of infection and generally results in improvement or cure. However, this does not seem to be necessary in the eye, as indicated by both clinical and experimental results, even in cases of pseudomonas endophthalmitis.

Modification of initial therapy

The isolate is checked for sensitivity to the antibiotics being used, but remember the possibility of contaminants on the culture plates. A very light growth or isolation of a certain organism in only one medium may make the pathogenicity of that organism suspect.

Once an organism is specifically identified the antibiotics can be adjusted. For example, once *S. epidermidis* has been identified the aminoglycoside may be discontinued. Conversely, medications with poorer coverage of gram-positive organisms, such as cefazolin and methicillin, can be discontinued once a gram-negative organism has been identified.

Serum gentamicin levels should be monitored for their peak and trough level to maximize their efficacy. In addition, because of the potential for renal toxicity, creatinine levels should be monitored, particularly in high-risk patients. Oral probenecid may be used to potentiate penicillin and cephalosporin therapy by prolonging serum and, hence, the intraocular concentration. Additional intravitreal antibiotics can be instilled after 48–72 hours if the clinical response has been unsatisfactory.

Most infections will improve with therapy over 7–10 days, after which antibiotics can be terminated. However, prolongation of therapy is necessary if the clinical response is poor. Systemic steroids should be continued only during the 5–7 days of the most severe inflammation, whereas topical steroids may be continued for several weeks. An important principle in modifying treatment is to do so only for definitive reasons and in a logical sequence.

If a patient has been managed without vitrectomy initially and there is no clinical improvement within 72 hours, a vitrectomy is advocated. Repeat cultures are often negative but should still be collected. Persistent reculturing and repeat intravitreal antibiotics may effect a cure in some cases and in others a fungal or anaerobic infection should be suspected.

Visual results

The virulence of the organism and the promptness with which therapy is instituted are the predominant factors in determining visual outcome.

Culture-negative cases improve the prognosis, possibly owing to misdiagnosis, infection due to less virulent organisms or early presentation. 20/400 or better vision may be retained in 100% of culture-negative cases, but in only 50% of culture-positive cases. Gram-positive organisms are more common than gram-negative organisms and carry a better prognosis.

Future improvements may be made with the new third-generation cephalosporins, for example, ceftazidime for *Pseudomonas aerugionosa*. Advances are also being made among the fluorinated quinolones, which are broad spectrum antibiotics with excellent penetration of blood ocular barriers. The new cephalosporins may be helpful prophylactically, both subconjunctivally and systemically, but the main cornerstones for success will remain a sterile operating environment, a high index of suspicion when trouble arises, and then prompt diagnosis and treatment.

Further reading

Allen H.F. and Mangiaracine A.B. Bacterial endophthalmitis after cataract extraction, II: Incidence in 36,000 consecutive operations with special reference to preoperative antibiotics. *Trans. Am. Acad. Ophthalmol.*, **77**, 581, 1973. *Arch. Ophthalmol.*, **91,** 3–7, 1974.

Driebe W.T., Mandelbaum S. and Forster R.K. Pseudophakic endophthalmitis. Diagnosis and management. *Ophthalmology*, **93,** 442–448, 1986.

Jones D.B. Initial management of postoperative pseudophakic microbial endophthalmitis, in Stark W.J., Terry A.C. and Maumenee A.E. (Eds), *Anterior Segment Surgery*. Baltimore, Williams & Wilkins, pp 339–49, 1987.

Mandelbaum S. and Forster R.K. Postoperative endophthalmitis. *Int. Ophthalmol. Clin.*, **27,** 95–106, 1987.

Olsen J.C., Flynn H.W. Jr, Forster R.K. and Culbertson W.W. Results in the treatment of postoperative endophthalmitis. *Ophthalmology*, **90,** 692–699, 1983.

Meisler D.M. and Mandelbaum S. Propionibacterium-associated endophthalmitis after extracapsular cataract extraction. Review of reported cases. *Ophthalmology*, **96,** 54–61, 1989.

Section 7:
THE POSTERIOR CAPSULE

43: Factors affecting opacification

Piers Percival

There are two main mechanisms whereby the posterior capsule may opacify. One is the migration of epithelial cells onto the capsule (**43.1**) with proliferation into Elschnig's pearls (epithelium). The other involves lens epithelial metaplasia into myofibroblasts that induce fibrosis (**43.2**) and contracture of the capsule (fibrosis).

Epithelium, once within the visual axis, may reduce visual acuity (VA) to less than 20/100 within six months (**43.3**), but fibrosis reduces the vision very slowly and it may be many years before treatment is necessary (**43.4**).

43.1

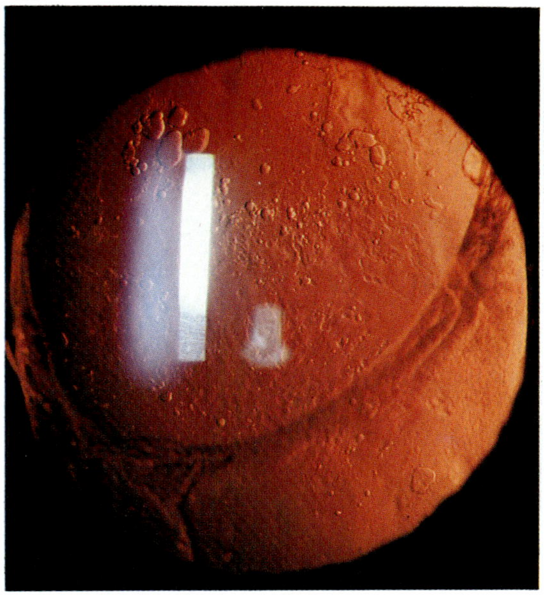

43.1 Epithelium two years after bag placement of a 12 mm hydrogel lens. Note the arcuate rim of the anterior capsule inferiorly; VA 20/80.

43.2

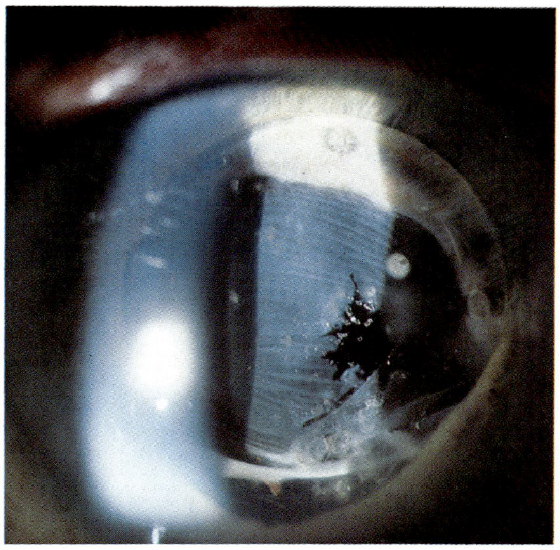

43.2 Capsular fibrosis associated with sulcus placement of the posterior vaulted lens. Note the pupil capture superiorly. The small YAG capsulotomy was performed with difficulty and was associated with lens pitting.

43.3

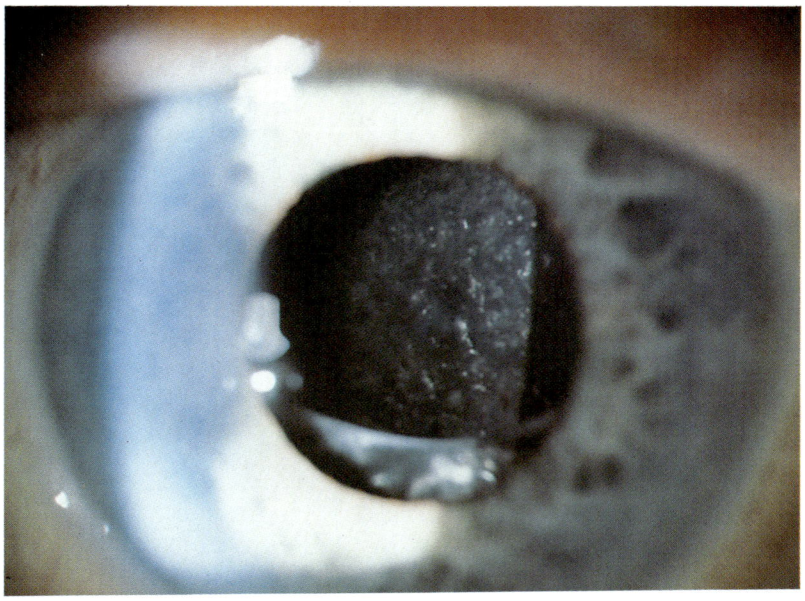

43.3 Epithelium two years after bag placement of a looped lasergap lens with a posterior encircling ridge. Note the crescent of anterior capsule inferiorly; VA 20/100.

43.4

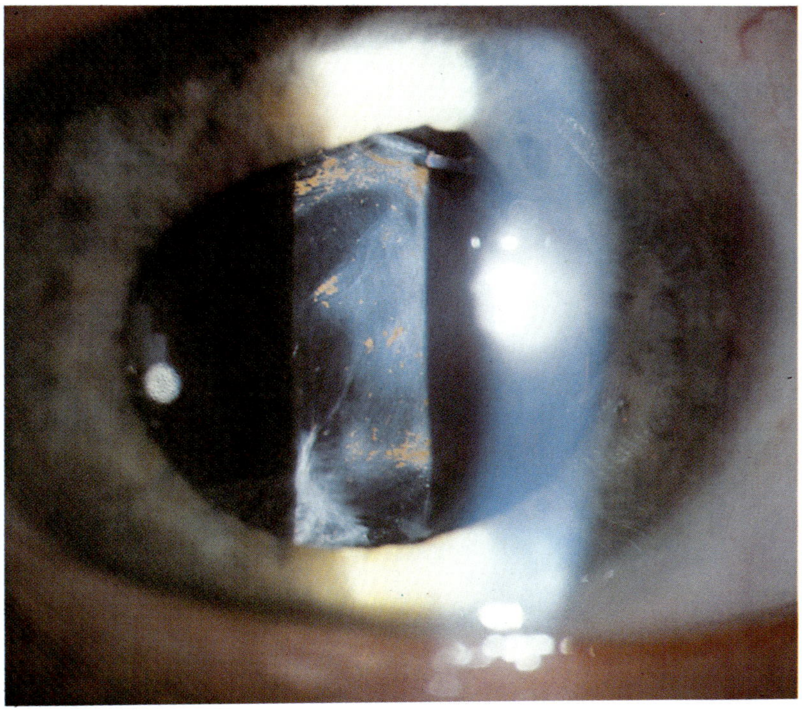

43.4 Fibrosis and pigment deposition on a posterior capsule five years after implanting a sulcus-placed posterior vaulted lens; VA 20/15; no symptoms.

Other changes in the posterior capsule include folds, which may be due to zonular weakness or dehiscence at 90° to the direction of the folds, and wrinkling (**43.5, 43.6**), which is associated with a lax capsule. Both folds and wrinkling are compatible with normal vision and usually do not require treatment. Stretch marks caused by looped haptics in the bag and seen at surgery will vanish within a few days, provided there is a tight and even stretch of the posterior capsule. If the stretch is not even, then linear wrinkling may remain. A plaque that cannot be cleared at surgery will thicken postoperatively (**43.7**) and should be treated by primary capsulotomy or a neodymium YAG laser a few weeks later.

Occasionally, an opening may appear spontaneously in the clear posterior capsule some years after surgery. This does not imply malpositioning of the lens as this may happen in eyes without implants.

43.5

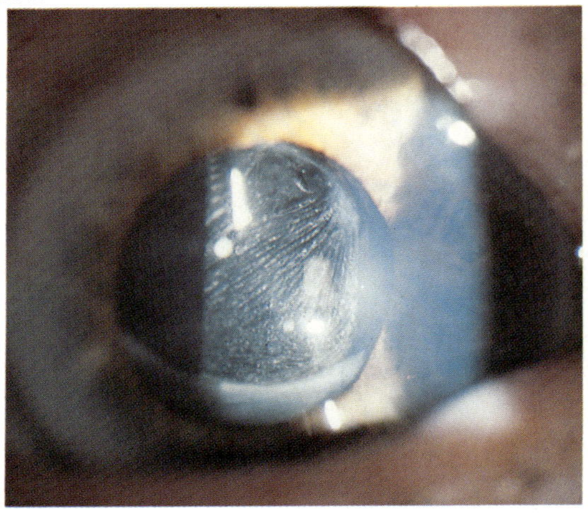

43.5 Wrinkling of a posterior capsule behind a bag-placed meniscus lens; VA 20/20 nine months after surgery.

43.6

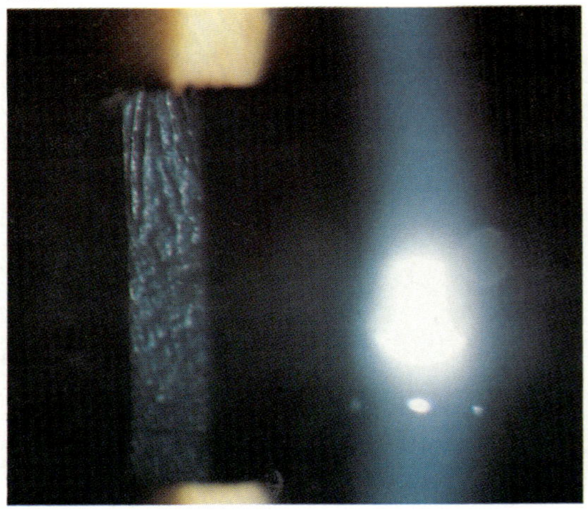

43.6 Wrinkling behind a one piece ridged lasergap lens; VA 20/15.

43.7

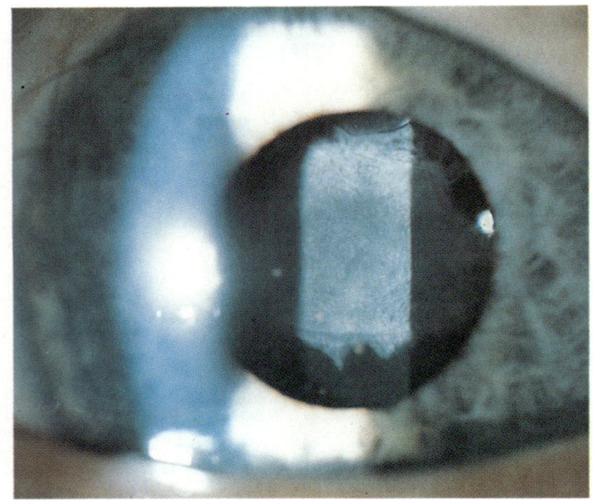

43.7 Central fibrotic plaque behind a bag-placed posterior chamber lens; VA 20/60; patient aged 59.

Epithelium and IOL design

The edge of any optic may provide a barrier to the ingrowth of unaltered epithelial cells, despite proliferation into pearl formation outside the optic edge. The tighter the stretching of the posterior capsule, the greater is the barrier effect; this is best seen with convex posterior (CP) or biconvex optics supported by angulated loops (**43.8, 43.9**).

Anis has found that if there is an encircling haptic support to CP lenses, there is also a molding effect with circular wrinkles that form a fibrous ring (**43.9**). The ring may be at the edge of the optic or inside the edge, but wherever it is, it produces an additional barrier to epithelial ingrowth. This is in contrast with those open looped CP lenses that have a two-point contact in the fornix of the lens capsule, producing a linear fold behind the center of the optic and a less even stretch of the central capsule.

43.8

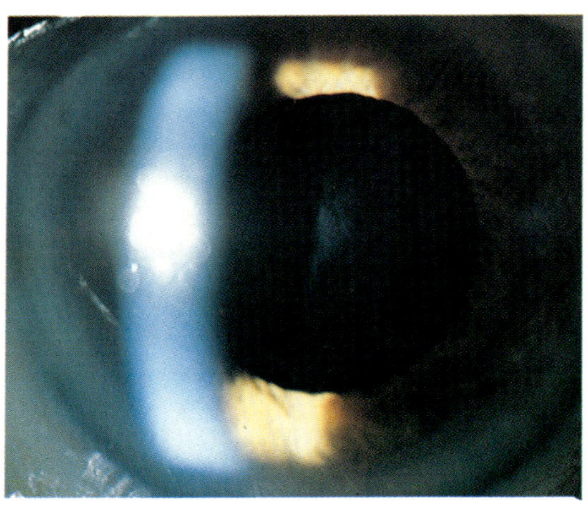

43.8 Optically clear lens and capsule seven years after convex posterior lens implantation.

43.9

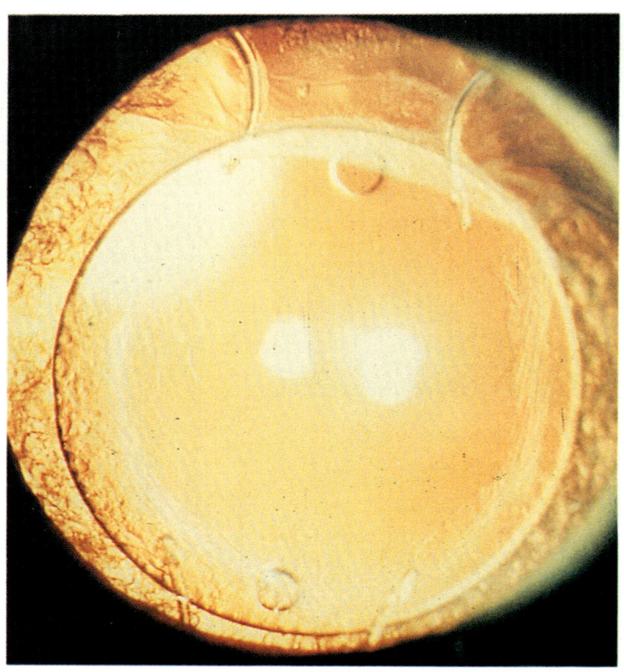

43.9 Convex posterior Anis lens with the encircling haptics in the capsular bag. Note the ingrowth of epithelium stops at the optic edge (right-hand border) and at the fibrous ring (inside left-hand border; courtesy of Dr Aziz Anis, USA).

A third barrier to ingrowth of the epithelium is the fusion of the residual rim of the anterior capsule to the posterior capsule (Soemmering's ring). However, judging by the high incidence of epithelial ingrowth after ECCE without lens implantation (approximately 45% in three years), this is an unpredictable event.

Convex anterior (CA) lenses, which are plano posterior, do not stretch the capsule in the same way as CP lenses and are associated with a higher incidence of epithelium, even when bag encapsulated and with forwards angulation of the haptics, both of which help to increase the contact with the posterior capsule.

Hydrogel lenses behave differently. Even when CP and with a forwards curvature of the haptics inducing a tight fit against the posterior capsule postoperatively, they are too soft to offer resistance to epithelial ingrowth (**43.1**).

Lasergap lenses are designed to expose a space between the back of the lens and the posterior capsule, but whether this is achieved by a complete circumferential ridge, or incomplete with bosses, or a meniscus (concave posterior) lens, they are associated with a high incidence of epithelium (**43.3, 43.10, Table 43.1**).

Epithelium may occur in all ages and degrees of cataract maturity, but has a slightly yet progressively higher incidence the younger the age of the patient.

43.10

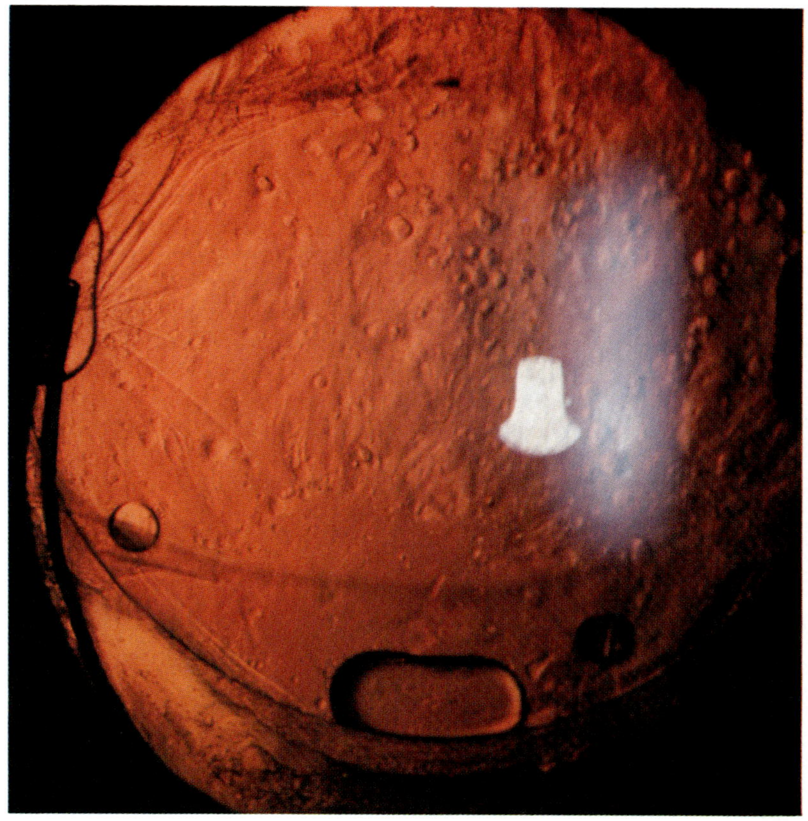

43.10 Epithelium three years after a bag placement of a lasergap lens with four bosses.

Results

Comparative capsulotomy rates for epithelium are shown in **43.11** and **Table 43.2**. Eyes were taken from 1320 consecutive posterior chamber implants with intact capsules at surgery, operated on between 1982 and 1987. Each eye was examined at the end of two, three and five years after surgery. Perforating injuries and secondary implantations were excluded. The need for capsulotomy was taken as opacification that reduced VA to less than 20/40 or opacification with patient dissatisfaction of VA 20/30 or 20/40. At two years 22 eyes (18 patients) were not traceable, 148 were lost from death and 1150 were examined. At three years 781 eyes were examined and at five years 229 were examined.

The Sinskey lenses and the majority of Pearce lenses were sulcus placed. The lasergap and hydrogel lenses were capsule placed. All had angulated haptics, yet the incidence of epithelium for lasergap and hydrogel lenses was found to be more than ten times higher than that for CP lenses.

43.11

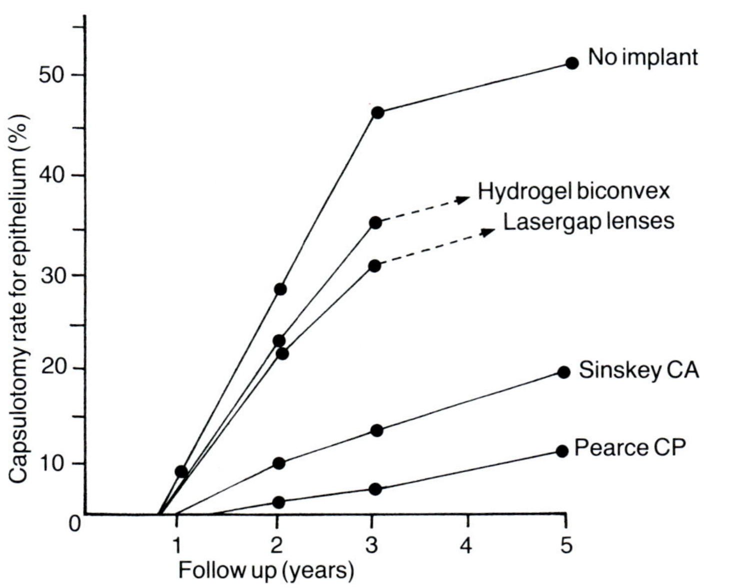

43.11 Incidence of epithelium with different lens styles.

Table 43.1 Incidence of capsulotomy for epithelium among 327 lasergap lenses seen 3 years after surgery

Lasergap style	*Eyes*	*Capsulotomy*	%
Circumferential ridge	250	73	29
Four posterior bosses	43	10	23
Meniscus	34	5	15

Table 43.2 Comparative need for capsulotomy (Caps.) for epithelium among eyes examined

	Examination								
	At 2 years			*At 3 years*			*At 5 years*		
	Eyes	Caps.	%	Eyes	Caps.	%	Eyes	Caps.	%
Sinskey CA	83	4	4.8	73	6	8.2	68	9	13.2
Pearce CP	431	4	0.9	296	7	2.4	161	9	5.6
Lasergap	434	77	17.7	327	89	27.2	0		
Hydrogel CP	202	33	16.3	85	26	30.5	0		
No implant*	88	20	22.7	80	34	42.5	67	31	46.2

* These cases were taken from an earlier series

Factors contributing to fibrosis

Contact with PMMA enhances the myofibroblastic differentiation of epithelial cells in some eyes, so that although proliferation of unaltered cells is inhibited, there may develop a slowly progressive smooth fibrotic sheet over the posterior capsule.

The opacification sometimes follows the configuration of wrinkling seen in an early postoperative period (**43.2**). Fibrosis is more common in CP than other lens types, whether of looped or disc configuration, but Anis, Arnott and Galand agree that if the CP optic has an encircling haptic in the fornix of the lens capsule, there is a greater evenness in the stretching of the capsule and this results in a clearer capsule centrally (**43.9**) than that produced by J-looped or by disc lenses. Fibrosis is enhanced by chronic inflammatory syndromes; for example, asymmetric or sulcus-placed polypropylene loops associated with decentration or pupil capture (**43.2, 43.12**); implantation associated with past glaucoma surgery or the glaucoma triple procedure (**43.13**); eyes with a tendency for uveitis, as in diabetes, a past history of iridocyclitis or surgery in children. Uveitis, by leading to posterior synechias to the lens capsule, also predisposes to pupil capture, which can perpetuate a low grade inflammatory syndrome. The predisposition to fibrosis may be lessened by ensuring bag encapsulation (**43.14**).

We found hydrogel lenses in uncomplicated eyes to be virtually free from the development of fibrosis.

Of the 781 implanted eyes examined at three years (**Table 43.2**), 49 were associated with the glaucoma triple procedure or past filtration surgery. The incidence of capsulotomy for fibrosis in these eyes was 20.4%. With these eyes excluded, the incidence of fibrosis was 3.7% among CP sulcus-placed looped lenses and 1.7% among other lens types. Fibrosis associated with CP sulcus-fixated lenses increased with time to 6.8%, so that at five years their combined incidence for capsulotomy was 12.9%.

43.12

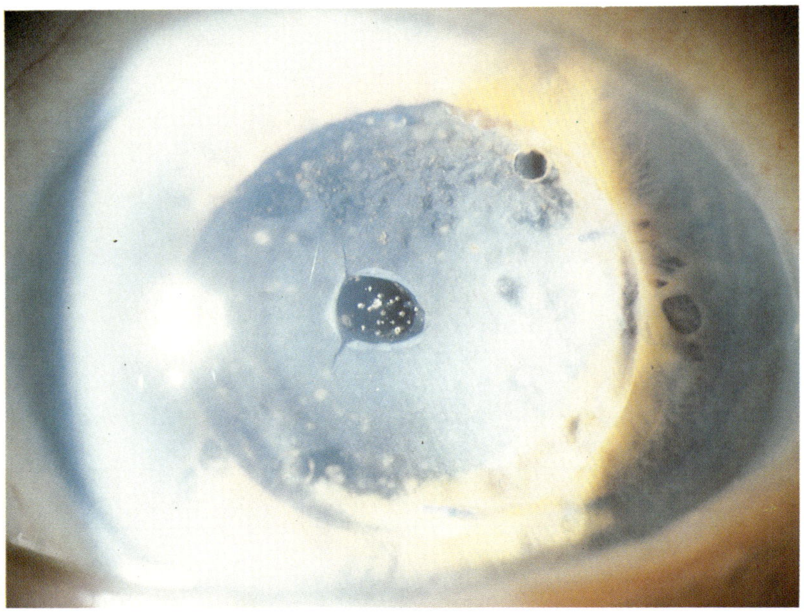

43.13

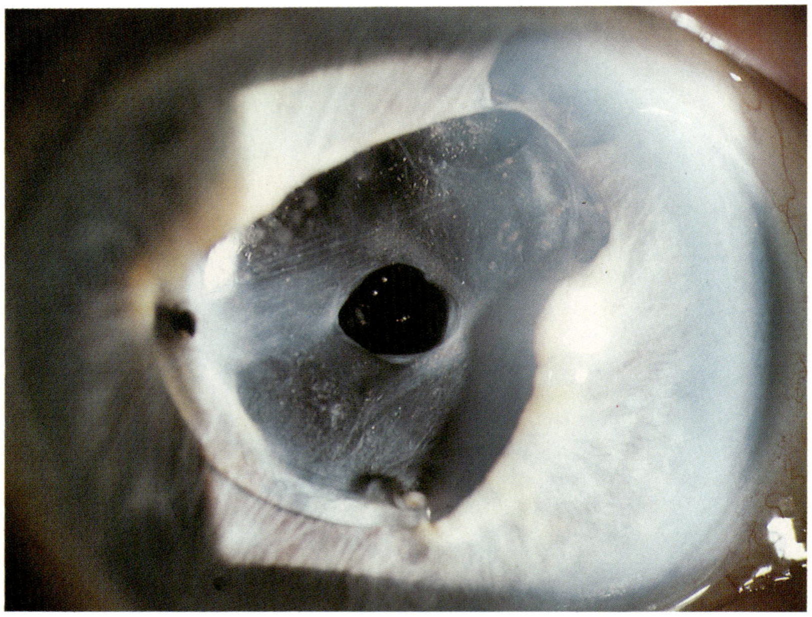

43.14

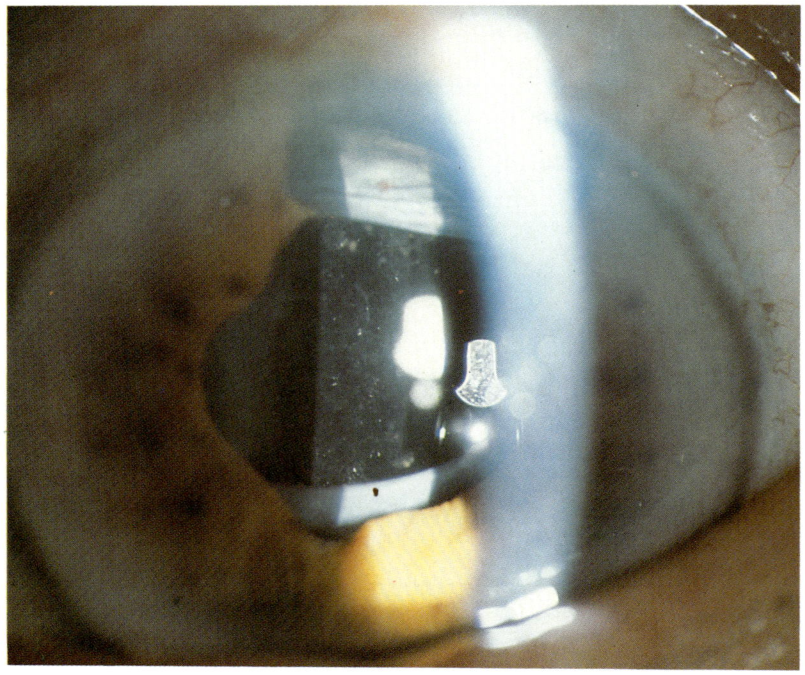

43.12 Capsular fibrosis associated with posterior synechias and pupil capture of a sulcus-placed posterior vaulted lens. Note the difficult small YAG laser capsulotomy associated with pitting of the posterior lens surface. Precipitates are present on the anterior lens surface.

43.13 Glaucoma triple procedure with a sector iridectomy, inferior sphincterotomy and sulcus placement associated with capsular fibrosis and pupil capture. Note that the YAG capsulotomies for fibrosis are smaller and more difficult to perform than those for epithelium.

43.14 Glaucoma triple procedure with a sector iridectomy, inferior sphincterotomy and bag placement. Note the iris lens clearance and the masking of pupil defects by the anterior flaps of the capsule. Visual acuity 20/30 three years after surgery.

Which lens?

The recommended design for minimizing the need for secondary capsulotomy should be an all PMMA lens with encircling haptics or haptics of a soft C configuration with a loop span of no more than 12.5 mm. The haptics should be angulated forwards and the optics should be convex posterior or biconvex. Satisfactory iris lens clearance should be seen postoperatively and, if so, pupil capture will be avoided.

It should be anticipated that when these CP lenses are properly encapsulated, the capsulotomy rate at five years will be less than 10%. The preferred optic diameter is 6.5 mm.

For eyes that are predisposed to uveitis or associated with glaucoma surgery, consideration should be given to the new surface-modified lenses (see p. 115), which show a marked inhibition of cellular reaction.

Further reading

Cobo L.M., Oshsawa E., Chandler D., Arguello R. and George G. Pathogenesis of capsular opacification after extracapsular cataract extraction. *Ophthalmology*, **91,** 857–863, 1984.

Santos B.A., Pastora R., Del Monte M.A. and O'Donnell F.E. Comparative study of the effects of optic design on lens epithelium in vitro. *J. Cataract Refract. Surg.,* **13,** 127–130, 1987.

Sterling S. and Wood T.O. Effect of intraocular lens convexity on posterior capsule opacification. *J. Cataract Refract. Surg.,* **12,** 655–657, 1986.

44: YAG laser technique and complications

Robert Drews

The simultaneous development of the YAG laser for use as a wound-free surgical tool by Danièle Aron Rosa (**44.1**) and Franz Fankhauser represents one of the major contributions to eye surgery of this decade. With it many procedures that were hazardous and inexact can now be performed safely, with optical precision.

The neodymium YAG laser utilizes an yttrium–aluminum–garnet crystal, artificially contaminated with neodymium to produce an extremely bright coherent monochromatic light in the infrared of wavelength 1060 nm. While this output is fortuitous in many respects, it has two disadvantages: (a) the light is invisible, so a second HeNe laser beam must be added to the apparatus for focusing; (b) the infrared YAG laser output cannot be conducted by fiber optics and requires a much more complex system of lenses, mirrors, and prisms to conduct it to the patient's eye (**44.2**). The high cost of early YAG lasers has been reduced in many devices, but these optical restraints and the need for high reliability of operation and precise, reproducible output has kept the price of the better YAG laser devices quite high (**44.3**). Considering the thousands of cases that can be performed with such a device however, the cost per case becomes acceptably low if the initial investment can be met.

44.1

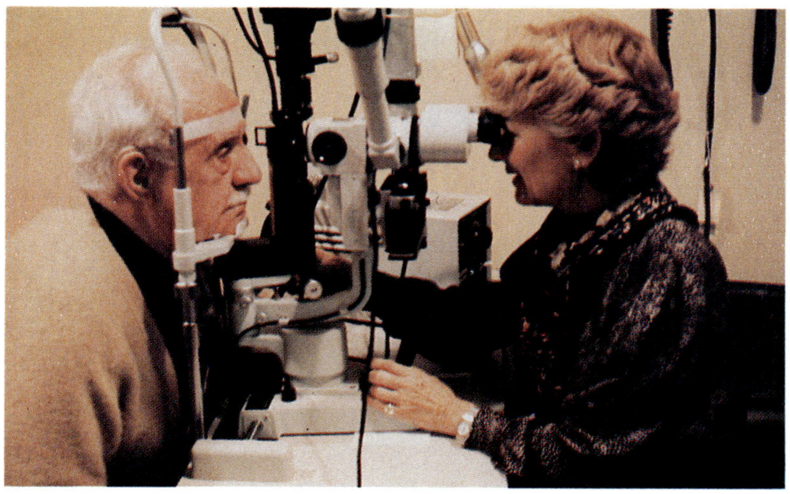

44.1 Danièle Aron Rosa teaching YAG laser posterior capsulotomy.

44.2

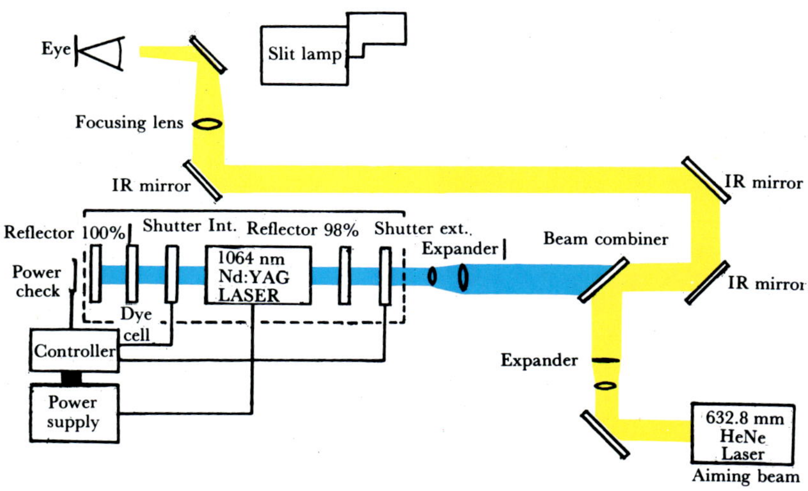

44.2 The mechanical, physical, and optical requirements of a reliable YAG laser are significant (courtesy of Rodenstock).

44.3

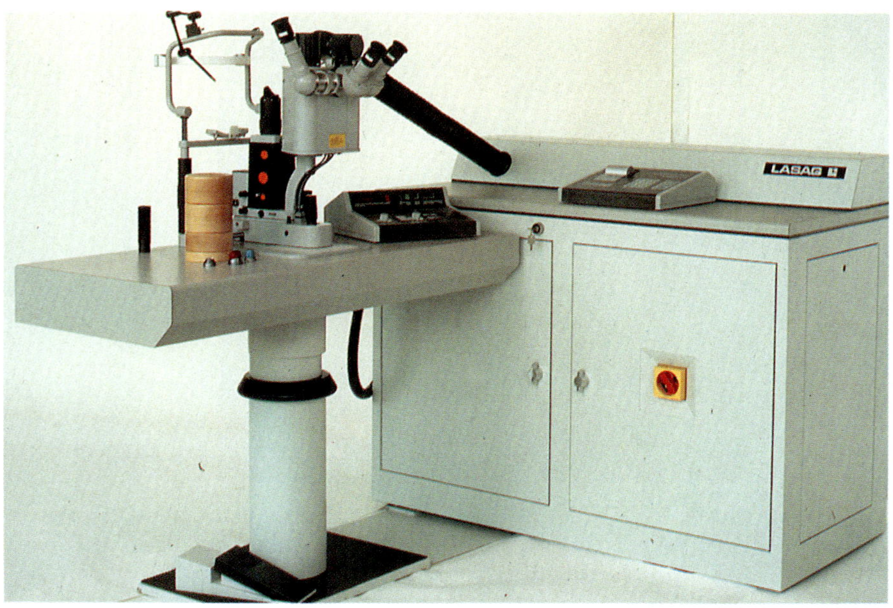

44.3 The Rolls-Royce of YAG lasers: the Lasag® unit developed in cooperation with Franz Fankhauser (courtesy of Sigmacon).

The power input requirements for a YAG laser are much less than those for an Argon laser, and no special wiring or cooling is needed. The output is quite different. In contrast to the Argon beam, the YAG laser beam is focused (**44.4**). This has two effects: firstly, structures far enough in front of and behind the focal point do not receive enough energy to be damaged, even when no plasma is formed. Hence the YAG laser's great safety. Secondly, the focal point itself is about 50μm in diameter and receives more than a million watts of energy in less than a billionth of a second. Whereas the beam from an Argon laser must strike something opaque, be absorbed and turned into heat, the energy from a YAG laser is so enormous per unit area per unit time that the molecules receiving it are unable to respond. Instead, the electrons are stripped away from the nuclei. Since it is electrons that bind atoms together into molecules, wherever the YAG laser beam strikes, the material is vaporized. A hole is produced.

A very high energy, local shock wave is also produced, which may tear a taut lens capsule, for example, and create a defect much larger than the 50μm hole that the direct hit produced. On the other hand, this shock wave dissipates extremely rapidly with distance and usually forms no threat to surrounding structures in the eye. To compare the precision of such a hole (**44.5**) to the risk of a perforating wound, trauma, and the imprecision of a needling procedure (Chapter 45) is ridiculous. Millions of procedures have now been performed with YAG lasers. The safety record is, predictably, unprecedented.

However, the YAG laser remains an optical knife. It requires surgical judgment, skill, and conservative application to avoid problems. Safety with the YAG laser requires an appropriate case selection, and the delivery of the minimum amount of energy necessary. Most papers that report YAG laser complications, particularly of high elevations of intraocular pressure, record excessive energy levels released within the eye: this has lead the Food and Drug Administration, USA, to warn that if more than 150 bursts are needed, the probability of complications increases substantially. Effective use of the YAG laser requires that the media must be clear (**44.6**). Even such an overlooked problem as drying of the cornea secondary to the use of anesthetic can degrade the YAG beam image (remember that the YAG is effective because it is focused) and make it necessary to use higher energy levels. The presence of lens precipitates or pigment on an intraocular lens can significantly impede a capsulotomy. YAG laser pits will themselves absorb further YAG laser energy that is applied to the same area and so grow enormously, thus blocking effective action on the posterior capsule.

If the patient's eye is moving or there is difficulty focusing the laser beam peripherally, a contact lens such as an Abrams, Goldmann (nonmirrored), or a specially constructed YAG laser lens (**44.7**), will help. If there is difficulty in focusing, first be sure that the media are clear, and then try a higher magnification. This will reduce the depth of focus and make focusing more critical. If there still seems to be difficulty in focusing, the unit should be recalibrated and the oculars adjusted while firing at some black paper.

44.4

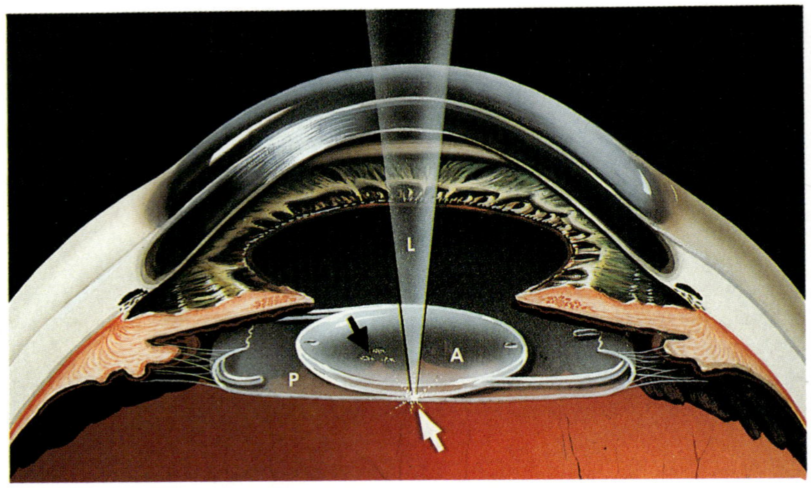

44.4 Both the safety and efficacy of the YAG laser are due to the focused nature of its beam (courtesy of the Highlights of Ophthalmology).

44.5

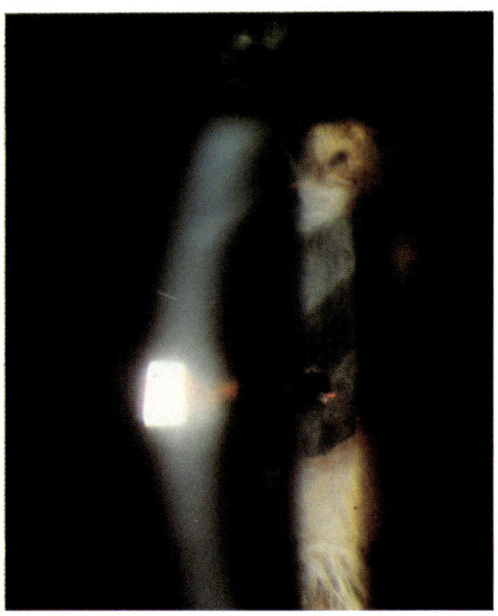

44.5 A single YAG laser pulse produces a very small discrete hole, which may be enlarged by the shockwave that the laser burst produces.

44.6

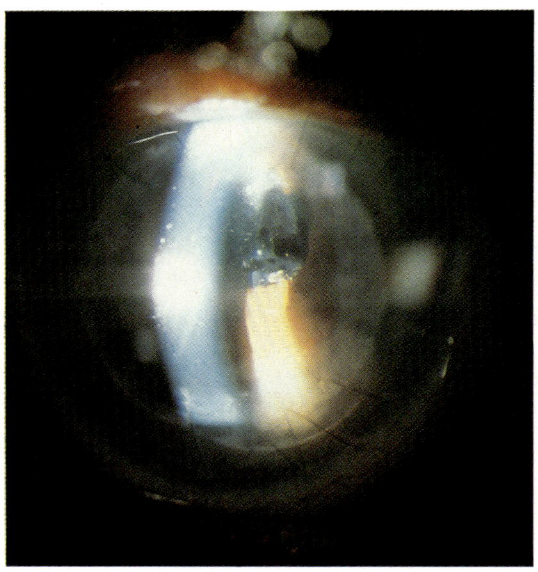

44.6 A capsulotomy through a cloudy graft may be extremely difficult. Even the taking of an intraocular pressure before capsulotomy may produce enough drying and roughening of the corneal surface to interfere.

44.7

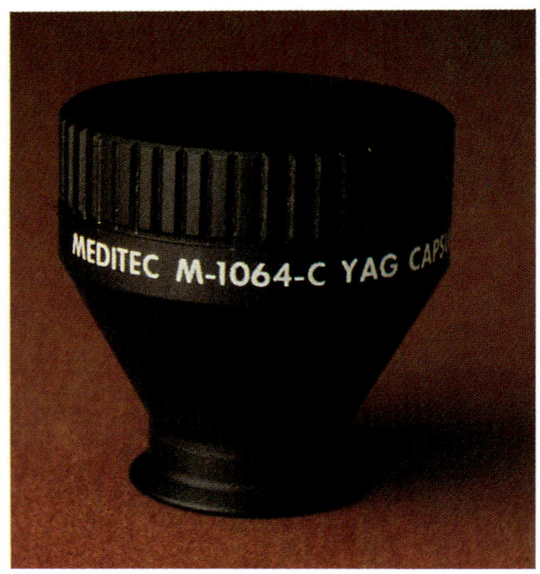

44.7 The use of a contact lens can be of particular help where stabilization of the eye, magnification, and a better view of the peripheral structures are desired.

Accidental damage to the cornea may occur if the patient moves, or while the surgeon attempts a peripheral iridectomy in an extremely shallow chamber peripherally. Fortunately, such damage is in such a very small area (**44.8**) that it heals rapidly with no consequence. Pitting of an intraocular lens (**44.9**) can be harder to avoid, especially if the lens is of low molecular weight (molded) PMMA. Fortunately, such pits are rarely of significance to the patient, but they will grow enormously if fired at repeatedly. The YAG laser should not be used through glass IOLs, which may shatter.

44.8

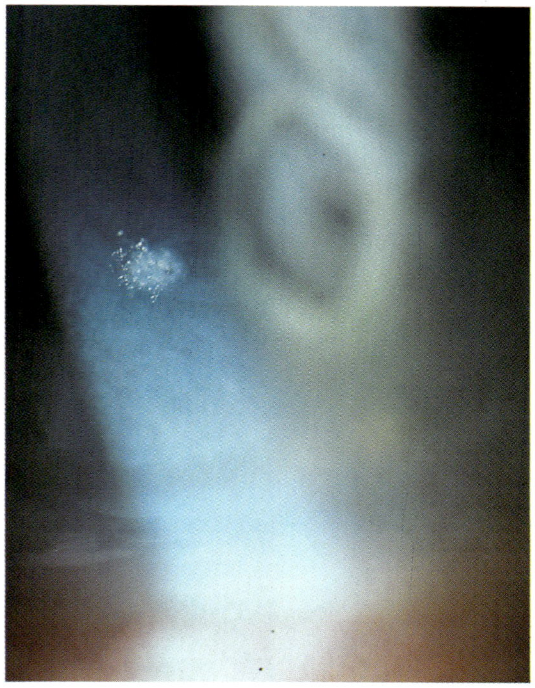

44.8 YAG laser damage to the cornea is dramatic but minor, and disappears in one to two days. Even the endothelial defect is usually undetectable after 48 hours.

44.9

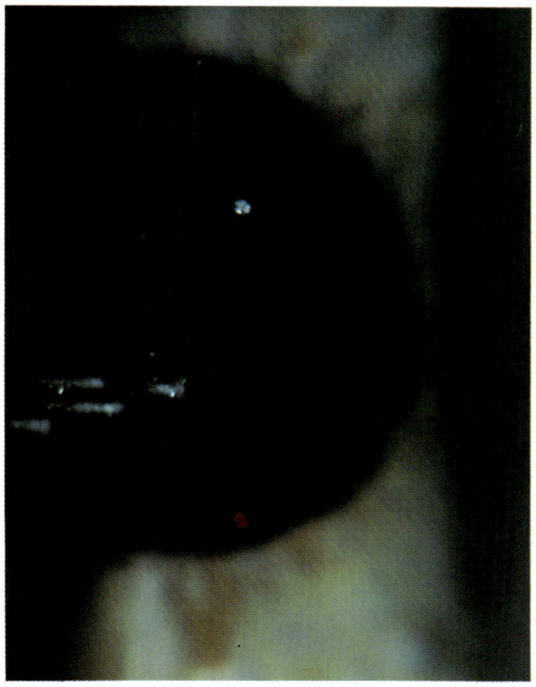

44.9 YAG laser marks in an intraocular lens are permanent, but usually do not affect vision. Additional laser bursts should not be applied in the same area, since the marks can enlarge rapidly.

Iris abnormalities

In most cases, YAG laser iridotomy is easier and superior to Argon laser iridotomy. The hole is smaller, there is less tissue damage and no charring. YAG laser holes tend to become larger with time and seldom heal over, as may occasionally occur in an Argon iridotomy. Rarely, in a gray iris a combination of both instruments is needed (**44.10**).

YAG laser iridotomy is especially useful in the early postoperative period when an anterior chamber lens produces pupil block with iris bombé (**44.11**). Laser iridotomy should be done near the intraocular lens where the chamber is deepest; it can afford an immediate cure (**44.12**).

44.10

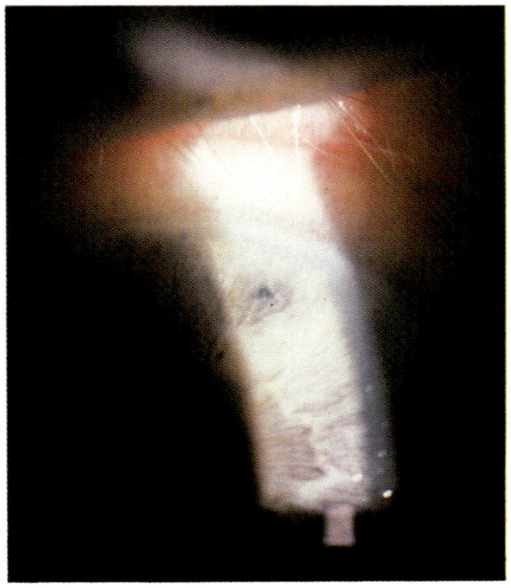

44.10 Iridotomies in this gray iris were impossible with either the Argon or YAG lasers; a combination succeeded nicely.

44.11

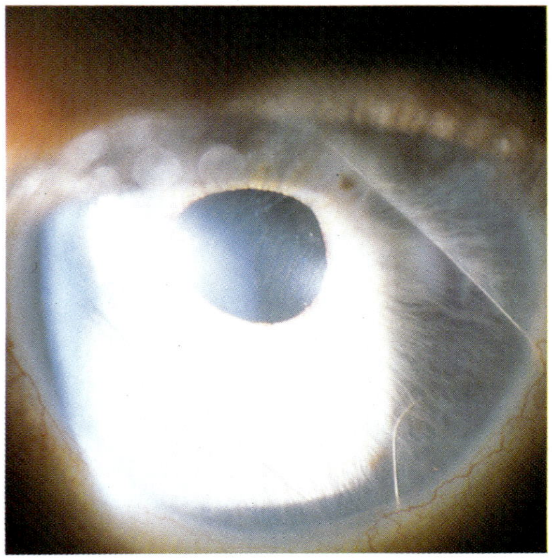

44.11 Pupil block produced by an anterior chamber lens, with bombé of the iris over the edges of the IOL.

44.12

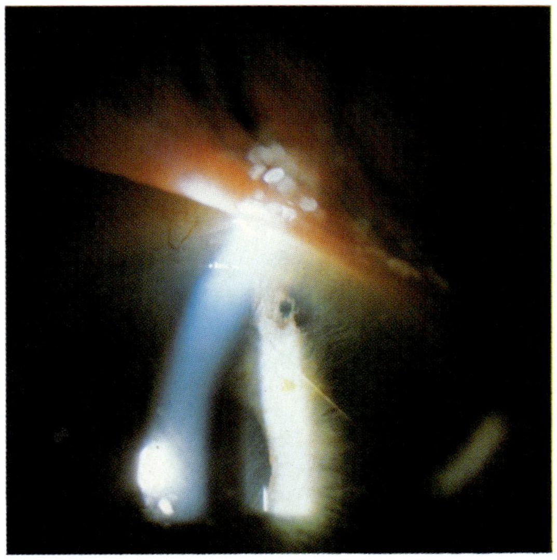

44.12 Application of the YAG laser to the case shown in **44.11** is most safely done near the edge of the intraocular lens, where the anterior chamber is deepest.

It may be tempting to improve mydriasis in patients with chronic glaucoma who are about to have cataract surgery (**44.13, 44.14**), but such cases often bleed, the dilatation obtained is still inadequate, and there is a chance of high elevations of intraocular pressure, especially in patients with compromised facilities of outflow. This procedure is not recommended. Major iris bleeding (**44.15**) is most likely in patients on anticoagulants, but otherwise is usually easily controlled simply by pressing on the eye to raise the intraocular pressure.

Accidental notching of the normal pupil (**44.16**) is more dramatic than that in eyes that have been on chronic miotics, but is of no significance to the patient.

44.13

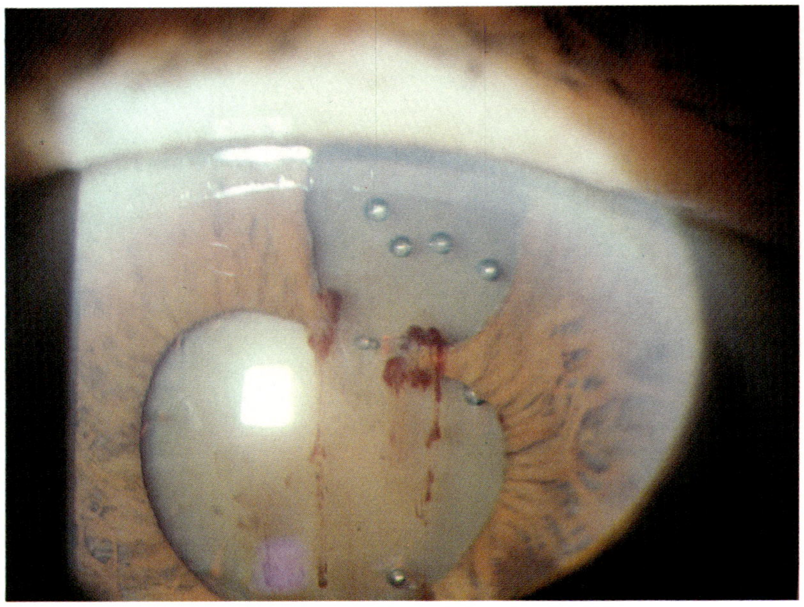

44.13 YAG laser sphincterotomy in a glaucoma eye prior to cataract surgery, which produced bleeding, a rise in intraocular pressure, and a ragged cut.

44.14

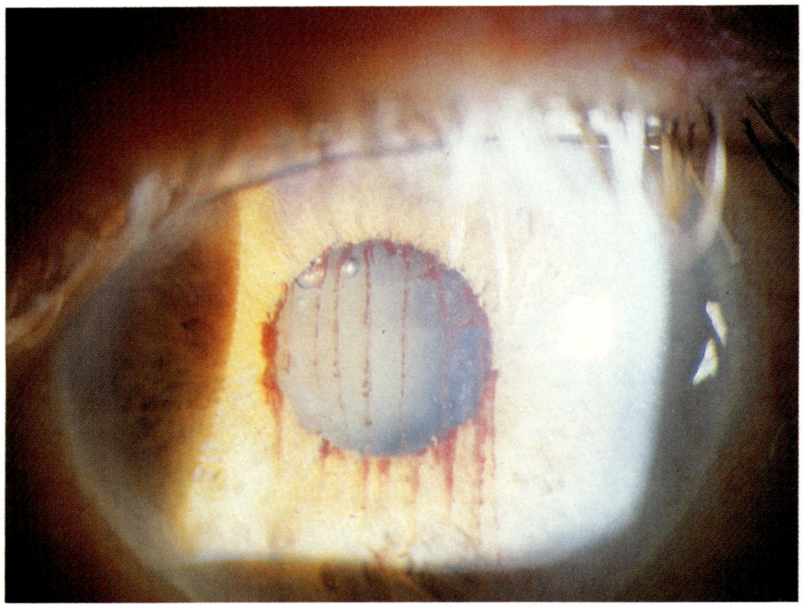

44.14 An attempt to improve mydriasis in a glaucoma eye with multiple notches at the pupil margin. Note the cascading hemorrhages.

44.15

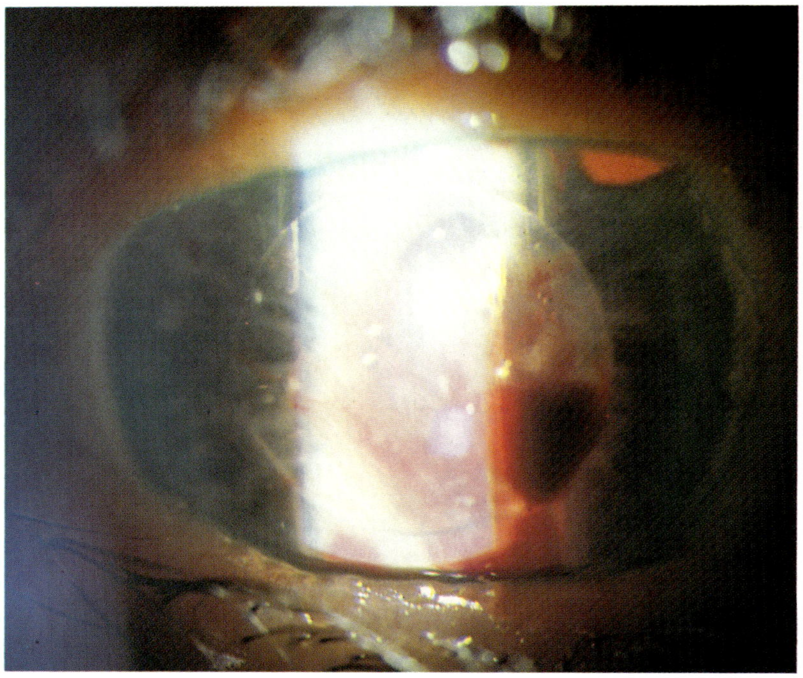

44.15 Major hemorrhage is usually easily controlled by pressing gently on the eye to raise intraocular pressure.

44.16

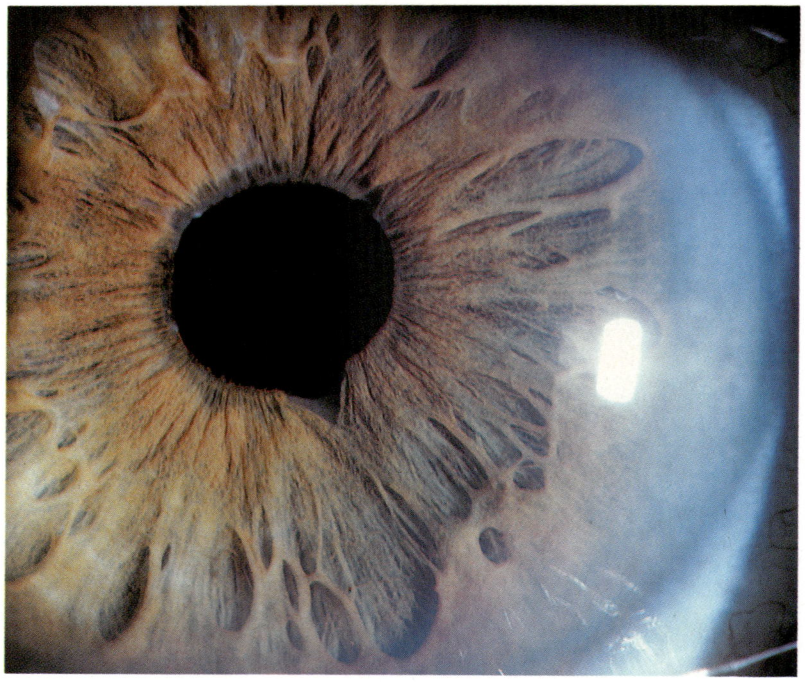

44.16 An inadvertent sphincterotomy in a normal iris is inconsequential.

While a discrete strand of vitreous or capsule to a wound with peaking of the pupil may be lysed with excellent results (**44.17, 44.18**), often the relief is incomplete (**44.19, 44.20**), and most commonly no effect at all is obtained, unless an inordinate number of bursts are used. Still, in the appropriate case with a discrete strand, this is an excellent way to relieve an early cystoid macular edema secondary to vitreous and iris traction.

The dissection of posterior synechias and other material off the anterior surface of an intraocular lens (including the anterior lens capsule) is relatively safe and easy (**44.21, 44.22**). Since optical breakdown occurs at and anterior to the focus of the YAG, it is easy to avoid damaging structures beyond the focal point by being careful not to focus too deeply.

44.17

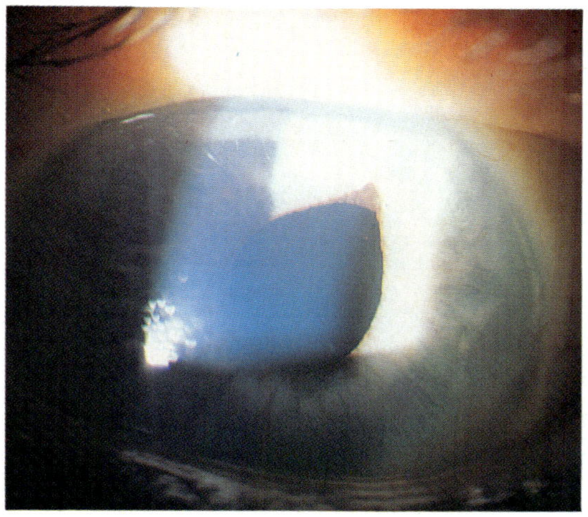

44.17 A discrete band of vitreous tenting the iris and producing chronic iris chafing and cystoid macular edema.

44.18

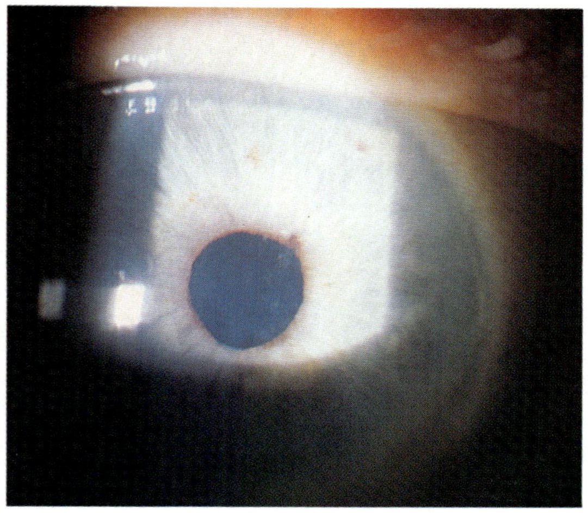

44.18 Treatment of the eye in **44.17** with a YAG laser.

44.19

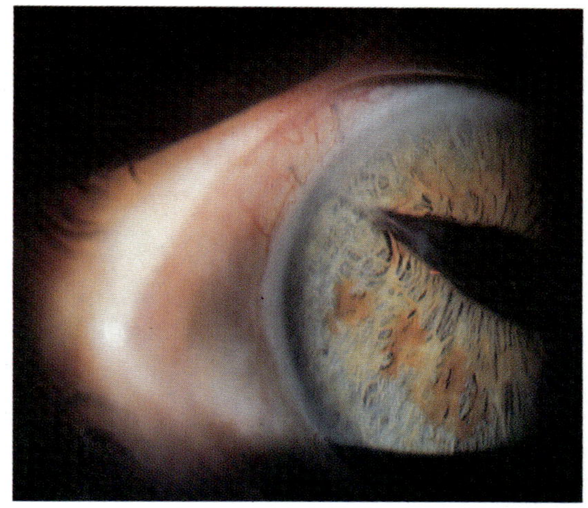

44.19 Vitreous adherence to the wound causing pupillary peaking.

44.20

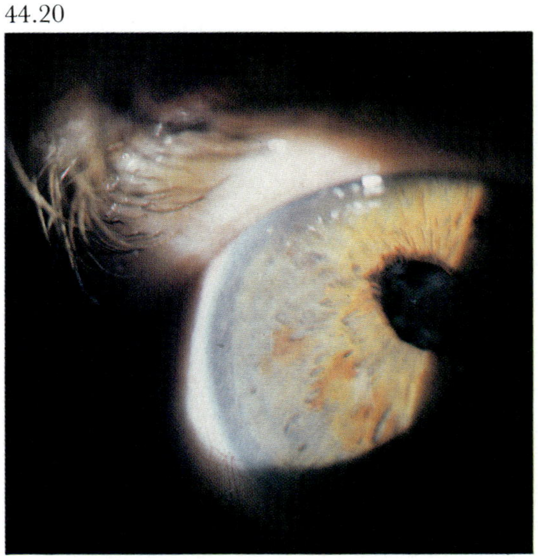

44.20 Treatment of the eye in **44.19** achieved an improvement, but not a round pupil. It is almost impossible to lyse broad bands or sheets of vitreous with a YAG laser.

44.21

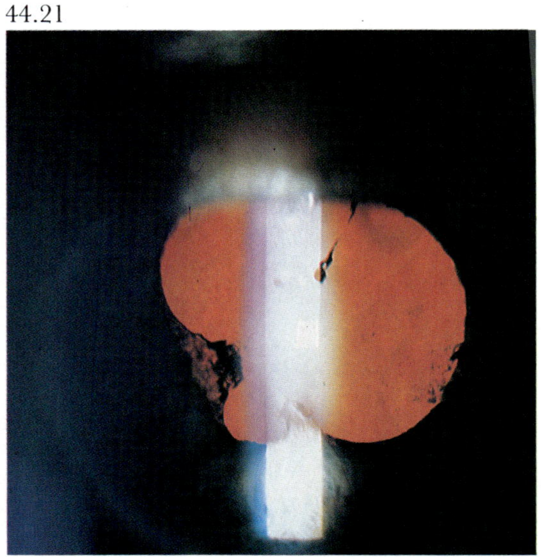

44.21 Posterior synechias and debris on the anterior surface of an intraocular lens.

44.22

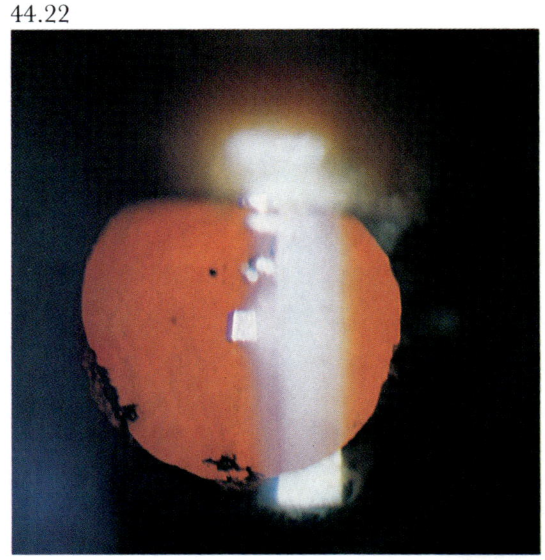

44.22 Lysis of posterior synechias seen in **44.21**.

Anterior capsule and nucleus

The use of the YAG laser for anterior capsulotomy is controversial. Unless surgery is to be performed at once, however, it is important that the capsulotomy be made with discrete openings (**44.23**). If the YAG marks are placed too close together, the capsule will gape, allowing excessive aqueous access to the lens (**44.24**). Complete anterior capsulectomy (250 bursts or more) will invite acute congestive glaucoma if surgery is delayed.

A different pattern may be necessary if an 'envelope' incision is contemplated (**44.25**). Avoid vertical incisions, as these may tear with delivery of the nucleus. Anterior capsulotomy is particularly useful in the mature cataract (**44.26**) where conventional capsulotomy can be frustrating, incomplete, and lead to later surgical difficulties.

Anterior capsulotomy openings, when discrete, will heal so that delay of surgery is safe (**44.27**), as long as rapid maturation of the lens does not occur.

The use of the YAG laser on the nucleus (**44.28**) can give some fascinating insight into nuclear anatomy, and is being used by some to soften a nucleus in preparation for phacoemulsification. Unfortunately, an enormous amount of energy is required and the crumbling of such a nucleus may make delivery by expression difficult.

44.23

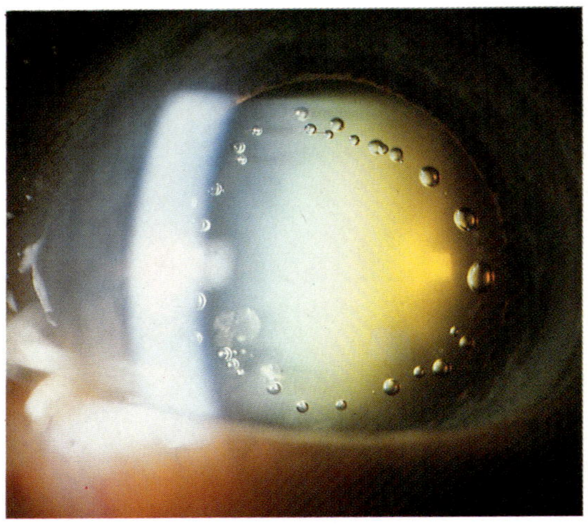

44.23 Unless surgery is to be performed immediately, an anterior capsulotomy should be done with discrete openings.

44.24

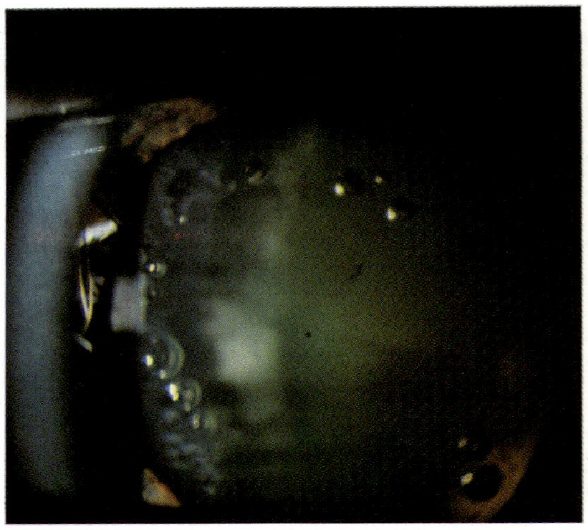

44.24 An unwanted large defect in the anterior capsule at 10.30 o'clock, produced by laser openings being made too close together.

44.25

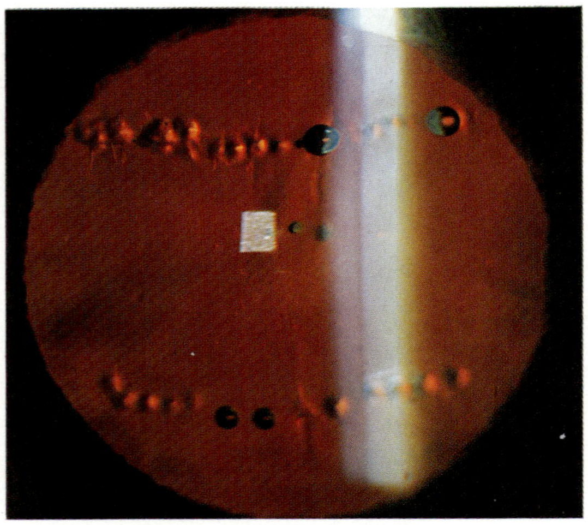

44.25 For an envelope incision, the vertical parts of the capsulotomy should be performed at surgery.

44.26

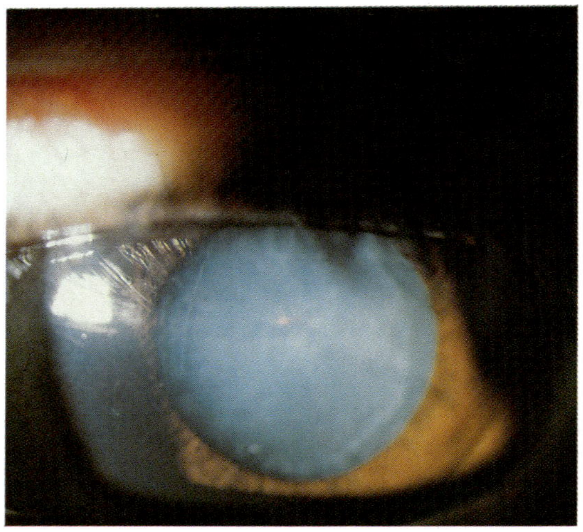

44.26 Laser capsulotomy in a mature cataract. Begin at 6 o'clock and work upwards on both sides, since the liquid cortex tends to cascade through the holes and obscure the capsular area below the openings.

44.27

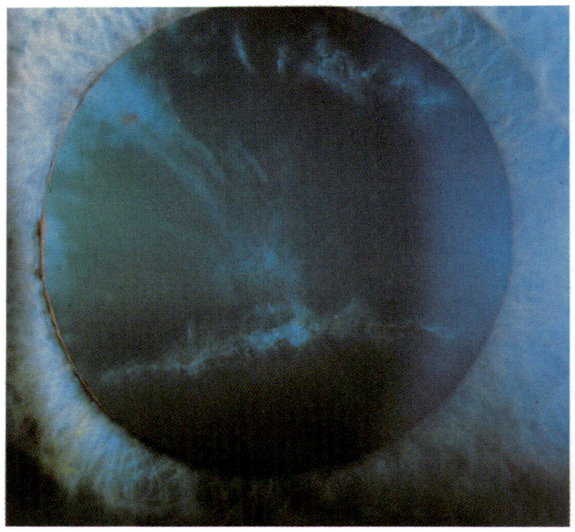

44.27 An eye 4.5 months after a YAG laser capsulotomy, showing that the perforations have healed without complication.

44.28

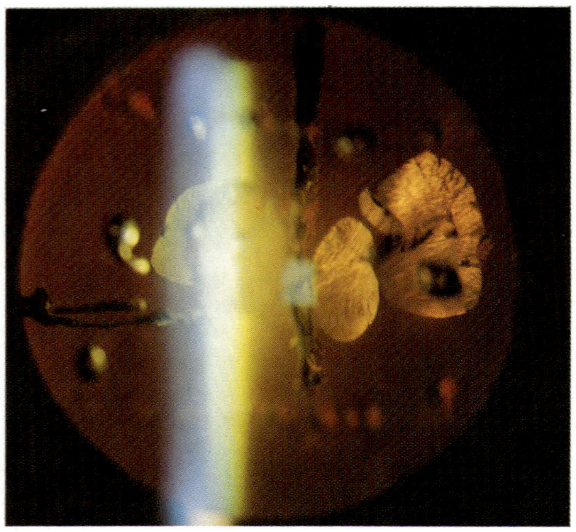

44.28 Application of YAG laser energy to the nucleus showing fans of opacity in front and behind the nucleus, and radial clefts.

Posterior capsulotomy

The YAG laser was invented for posterior capsulotomy. The temptation to make a circle of multiple YAG laser marks (**44.29, 44.30**) should be resisted as this requires an unnecessary amount of energy. Instead, two or three YAG laser applications may be all that is needed (**44.31**), especially if the posterior capsule is under tension and the laser is focused onto the lines of stress. The recommended power should be less than 1.5 mJ for each application, unless the membrane is thickened by fibrosis. Miraculous restoration of vision is possible in apparently complex cases (**44.32, 44.33**). In very difficult, thick membranes it is

44.29

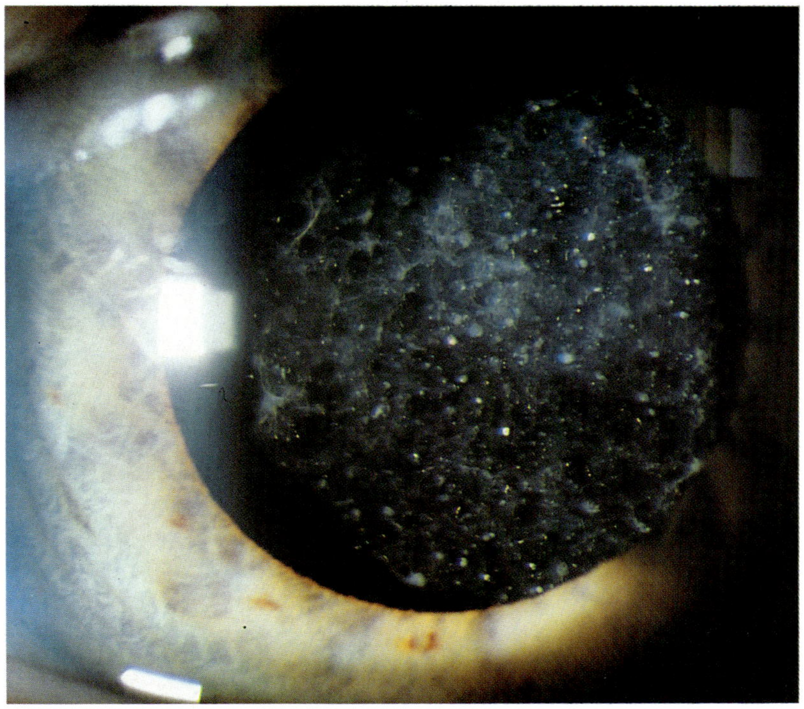

44.29 Dense posterior capsule opacification with Elschnig pearl formation.

44.30

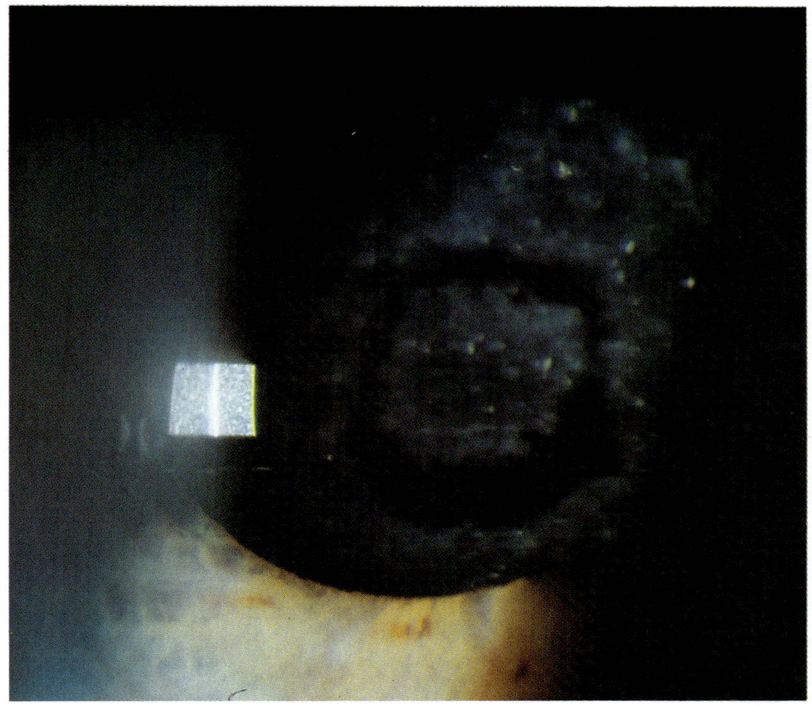

44.30 Treatment of the eye in **44.29** by a circular posterior capsulotomy that required more applications than necessary.

44.31

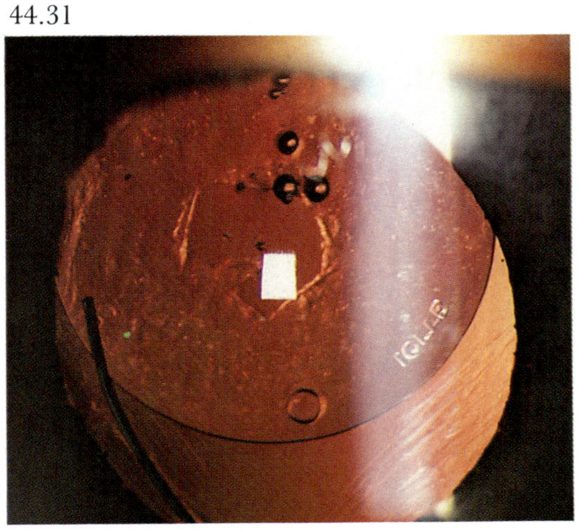

44.31 An ideal 2 mm opening produced by three YAG laser applications.

44.32

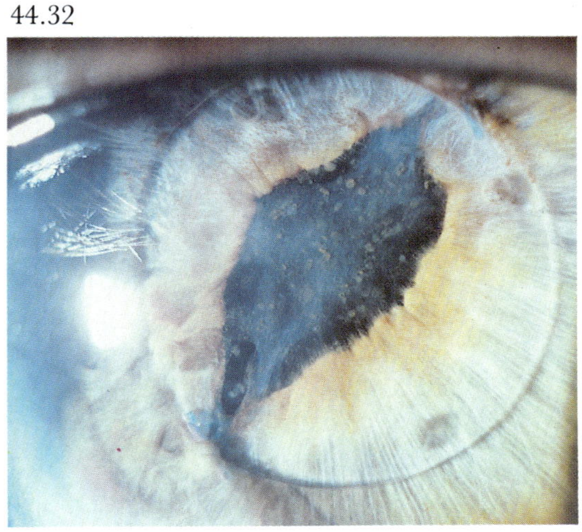

44.32 A dislocated IOL had been managed by double entrapment in the pupil. Inflammation from an iris chafing syndrome resulted in a pupillary membrane with a visual acuity of 3/200.

44.33

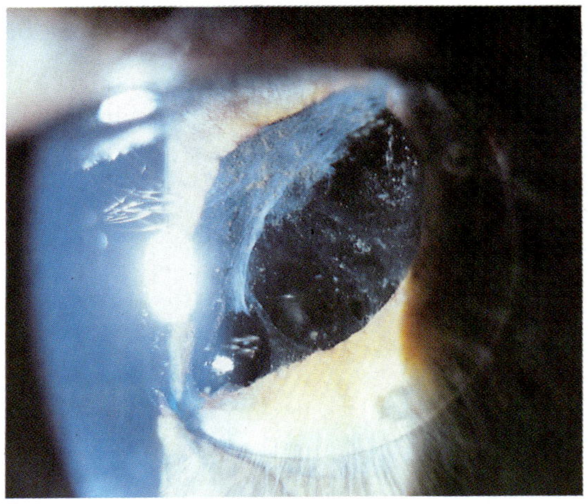

44.33 The YAG laser clearance of the pupillary membrane in **44.32** restored 20/40 vision (limited by chronic macular edema).

best to remember that a small hole in the thinnest part may suffice (**44.34, 44.35**). If vision is not improved by a 1 mm opening, it is not likely to be improved by a larger one!

Retinal detachment (**44.36**) following YAG laser capsulotomy is unusual, occurring in less than 1% of cases. However, it may be difficult to see through a small capsulotomy opening and a high index of suspicion is needed. The incidence is less than that following surgical discission.

Finally, in cases where the opening is difficult to achieve and then rapidly closes again, be aware that you may well be dealing with a neoplastic reaction: rubeosis, fibrous downgrowth, or epithelial downgrowth (**44.37**).

44.34

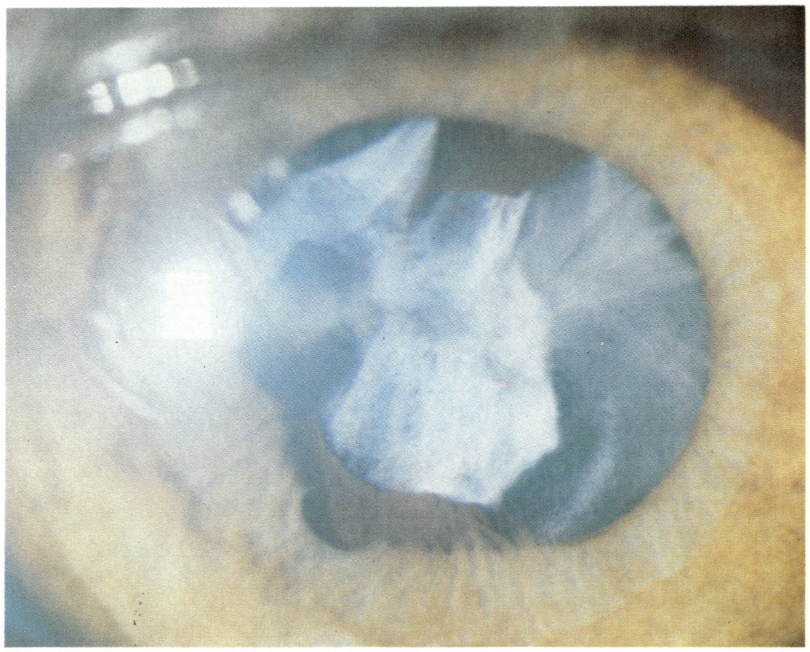

44.34 Dense fibrotic plaque.

44.35

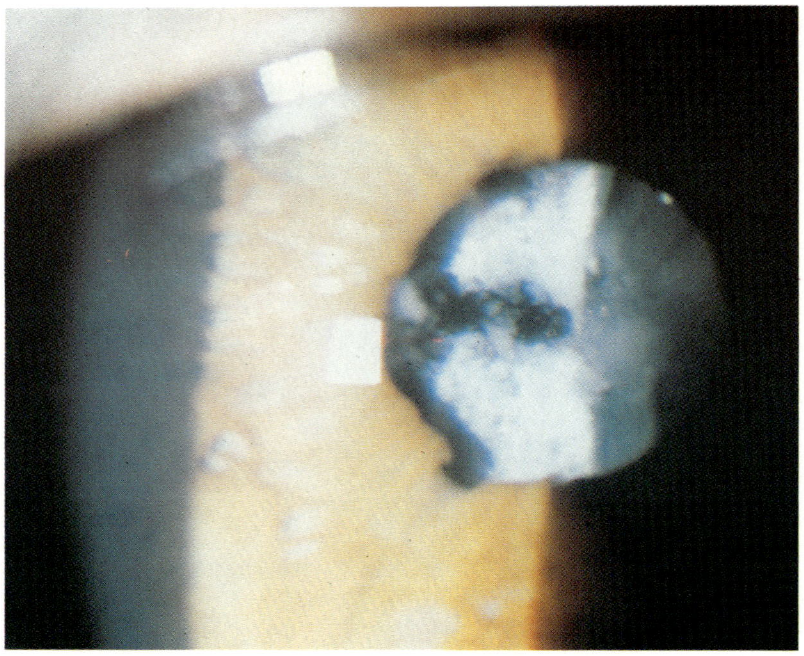

44.35 An adequate opening in the eye in **44.34** made by choosing a relatively thin part of the membrane for treatment.

44.36

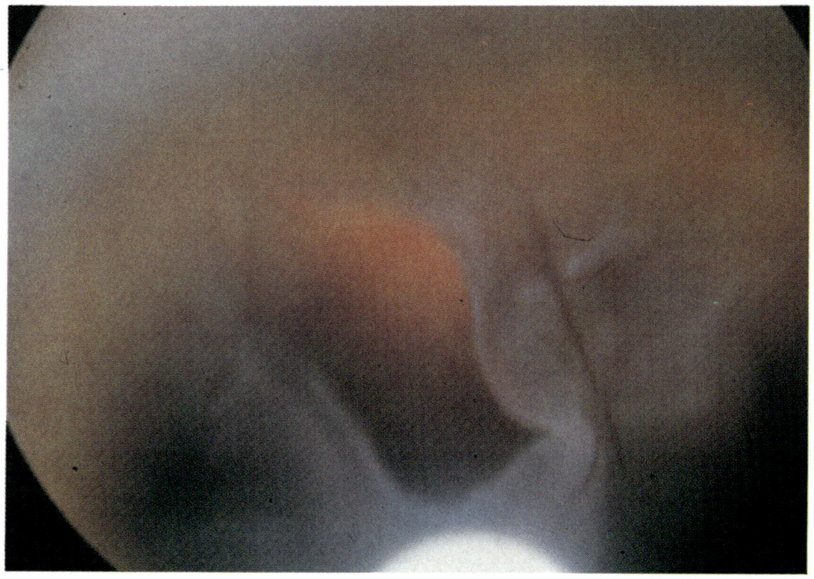

44.36 Retinal detachment occurring within three weeks of a YAG capsulotomy.

44.37

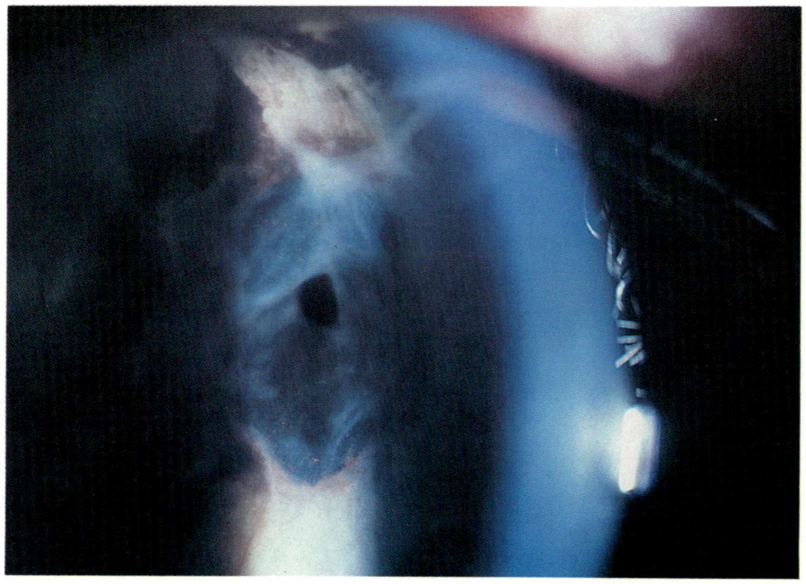

44.37 Difficult capsulotomy in a patient with epithelial downgrowth. The membrane reformed within a few weeks.

Further reading

Drews R.C. Anterior capsulotomy with the neodymium YAG laser: results and opinions. *Am. Intra-Ocular Implant. Soc. J.*, **11,** 240–244, 1985.

L'Esperance F.A. *Ophthalmic Lasers: Photocoagulation, Photoradiation, and Surgery.* St. Louis, C.V. Mosby, 1983.

Schwartz L., Spaeth G. and Brown G. *Laser Therapy of the Anterior Segment: A Practical Approach.* New Jersey, Slack, 1984.

45: Surgical capsulotomy

John Pearce and Piers Percival

The pars plana approach

Edward Epstein first proposed the posterior approach to the posterior capsule by way of the pars plana in 1957, and in 1980 Lindstrom and Harris revived interest with the explosion in the use of posterior chamber lenses with extra capsular cataract surgery.

Advantages: minimal surface and/or subconjunctival anesthesia is required, as there is no iris contact; vitreous cannot be pulled into the anterior chamber or wound (thus lessening the risk of retinal detachment, pupil block glaucoma, and IOL decentration); and as the anterior chamber cannot be lost there is no corneal endothelial damage.

Disadvantages: the possibility of vitreous hemorrhage; possible damage to the vitreous base; and possible endophthalmitis, although in the authors' experience this has not occurred in over 100 cases.

Technique

The operation can be performed in an outpatient operating room providing there is an operating microscope and sterile operating conditions.

- Informed consent should be obtained from the patient.
- Surface anesthesia and full pupillary dilatation with topical phenylephrine 10% and cyclopentolate 1%.
- Skin preparations and operating drape.
- Barraquer's wire lid speculum.
- A small bleb of subconjunctival local anesthesia, such as lignocaine 2%, is injected in the infratemporal and supranasal quadrant.
- Looking through the operating microscope the supranasal globe is gripped with toothed forceps, such as Colibri or St. Martins, and the globe is penetrated to 3.5 mm from the limbus perpendicularly in the infratemporal quadrant with a discission knife or needle (**45.1, 45.2**). The point of the knife is then seen in the pupil behind the posterior chamber lens, the capsule is engaged superiorly and cut down towards 6 o'clock (using a sawing motion if densely fibrosed (**45.3**)), and the knife withdrawn.
- Subconjunctival antibiotics and steroids are given.
- The patient is discharged on topical steroids.

This technique can also be performed with the patient sitting behind a slit-lamp microscope, but in the authors' opinion sterility of the operating field is questionable in such a situation. Surgical capsulotomy may be preferred to YAG laser capsulotomy when the posterior capsule is very densely fibrosed.

45.1

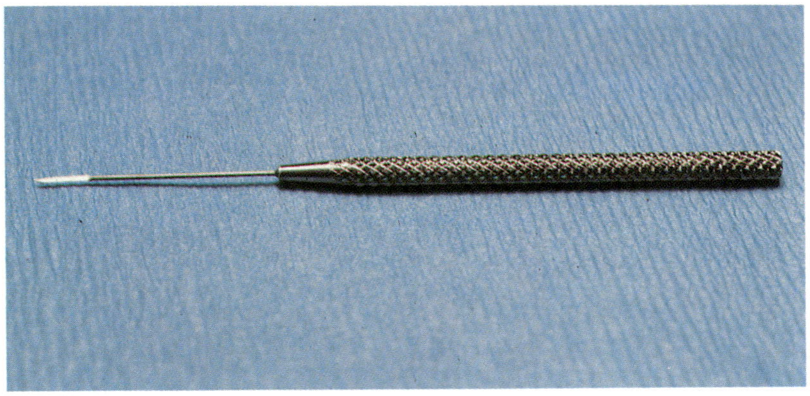

45.1 Pearce micro discission knife designed specifically for the purpose.

45.2

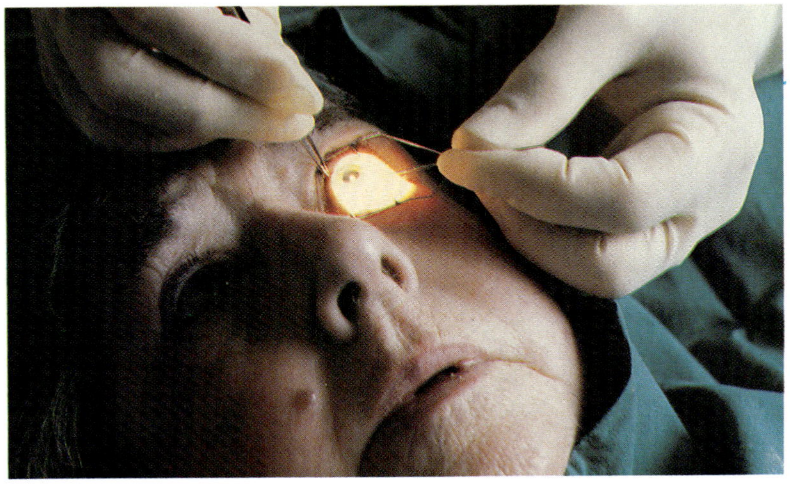

45.2 Pars plana capsulotomy performed as an outpatient operation.

45.3

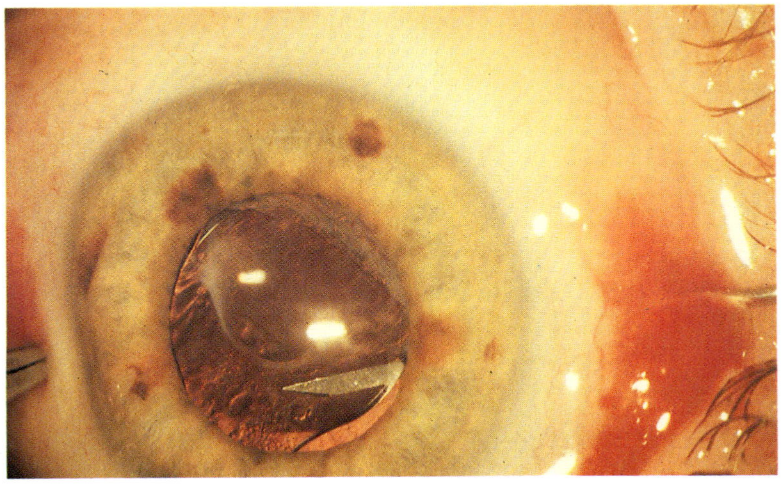

45.3 Completion of the capsulotomy before the knife is withdrawn.

Limbal approach

A stab incision is made through peripheral cornea with a blade of 1 mm width (such as the standard diamond blade) to penetrate the cornea and iris (**45.4**), angulated towards the edge of the implant. The capsulotomy needle will be introduced through this iridotomy behind the lens, which is less traumatic than introduction in front of the iris, with the necessary hooking back of the pupil margin and possible forwards displacement of the implant. This procedure also covers the difficulties of possible posterior synechias or inadequate mydriasis.

The needle is prepared by taking a standard hypodermic (or subconjunctival) needle and bending the tip *towards* the lumen so that it just projects beyond the diameter of the shaft (**45.5**). The width of this will now enter the 1 mm incision without escape of aqueous, and the very short projection of the tip will enable tearing of the capsule without penetrating the anterior hyaloid. If there is a firm contact between the posterior lens surface and the capsule (as with convex posterior lenses, especially in cases of capsular fibrosis), the needle should be attached to a syringe of sodium hyaluronate and passed behind a front of viscoelastic material, which will cause the necessary separation (**45.6**). If it is considered that the anterior chamber may shallow, or if there is pupil capture to relieve, or if there is PMMA in the anterior chamber, then sodium hyaluronate should be placed in the anterior chamber beforehand (**45.7**).

Capsulotomy is made by passing the needle *beyond* the midpoint of the pupillary area, turning the tip from a sideways position so that it faces backwards, engaging with the posterior capsule, tearing, turning the tip back to a sideways position and removing it from the eye. No suture should be necessary (**45.8**).

45.4

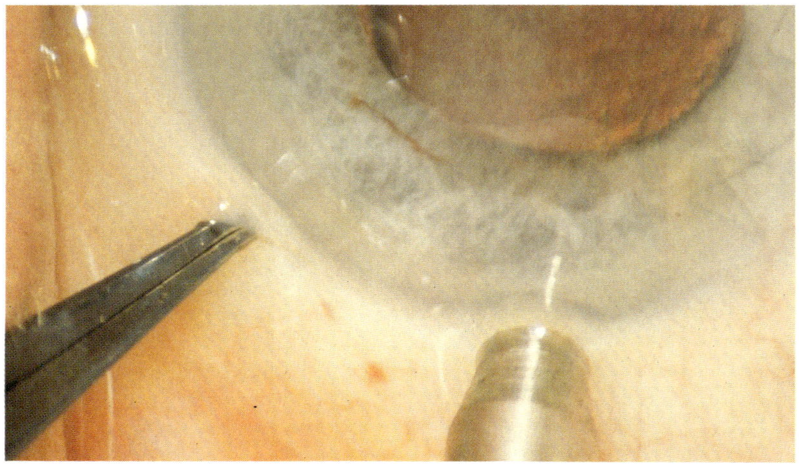

45.4 Plunge of a 1 mm diamond blade to penetrate the cornea and iris.

45.5

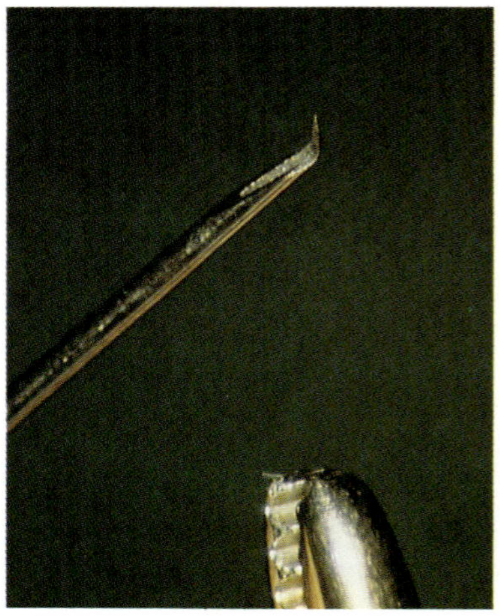

45.5 The tip of a hypodermic needle has been bent with Spencer Wells forceps so that the tip projects just beyond the diameter of the shaft.

45.6

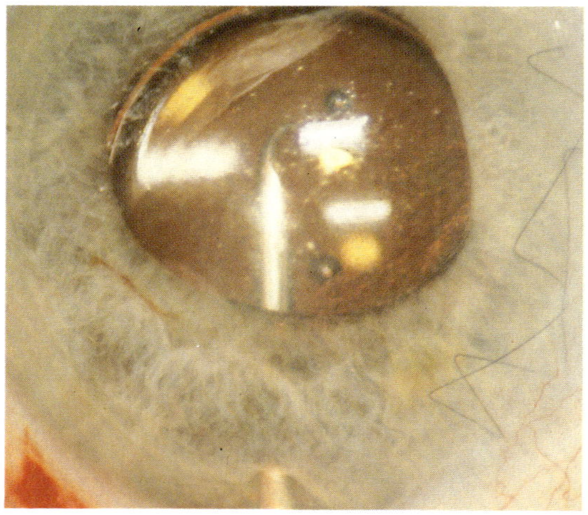

45.6 Needle enters behind a front of sodium hyaluronate underneath the implant.

45.7

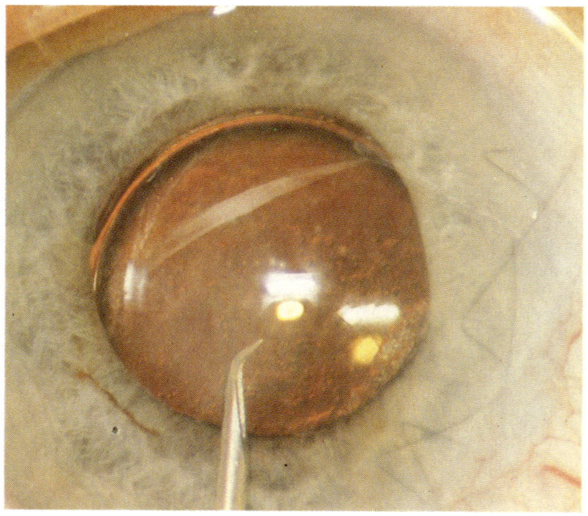

45.7 Prior to the procedure in **45.6**, sodium hyaluronate may be injected in front of the implant.

45.8

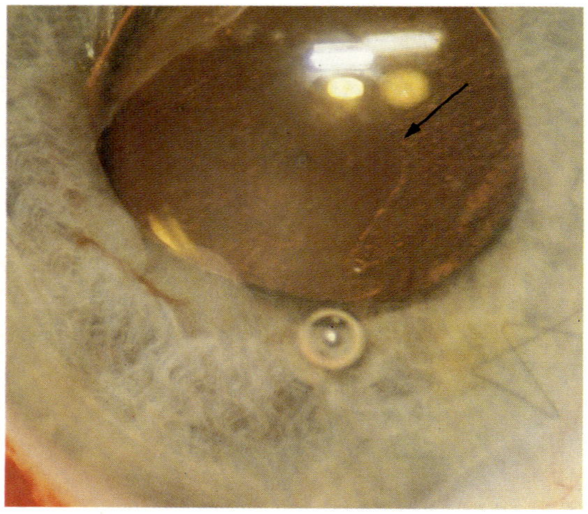

45.8 The arrow indicates the edge of the capsulotomy. Note the pupil and implant position remain undisturbed.

Further reading

Mashoudi N. and Pearce J.L. Retrospective study of 67 cases of secondary pars plana posterior capsulotomy. *Brit. J. Ophthalm.*, **69**, 364–367, 1985.

Smith G.S. and Lindstrom R.L. *Intraocular Lens Complications and their Management*. Slack. Inc. Thorofare, p.148, 1988.

Section 8:
EPILOGUE

46: The changing scene in Asia

Arthur Lim

Blindness due to cataract will double by the year 2000, in part due, as in other age-related problems, to the increased life expectancy made possible by modern science, but largely as a result of poverty and poor organization of human resources worldwide.

Cataract problem

Cataract is a massive problem, accounting for more than 50% of preventable or curable blindness in the developing countries. The main problem facing these countries is that there are just not enough surgeons to operate. The backlog in Asia of unoperated patients is estimated at well over 10 million, with consequent major social and economic problems. In India alone, the estimate is that 6 million persons are blind from cataract, which accounts for 55% of India's blind population. In some countries, such as Bangladesh, nonophthalmologists have been trained to perform cataract operations in order to resolve the massive backlog. Another alternative is to utilize ophthalmologists from countries where there is an excess, such as from Japan. Unfortunately, this practice is complex and raises many political issues. Again, unfortunately, the increased efforts of WHO and non-governmental organizations hardly cope with the number of new victims of cataract, let alone the backlog of millions.

The implant controversy

Many ophthalmologists have viewed implantation surgery as irrelevant in the developing countries. This view is wrong. The wealthier communities within the developing countries will enjoy the benefits of modern technology, as they enjoy the benefits of better housing, communications and nutrition. Patients who can afford to pay will always demand the best.

Effective communication has enabled wide dissemination of information on the latest technology, at least in the cities, and ophthalmologists throughout Asia are moving rapidly towards microsurgery and implantation. However, in contrast, so many rural communities remain neglected that some still do not even have access to the primitive technology of cataract camps. In developing countries, the major problems that confront the use of lens implantation will remain financial, including the cost of trained personnel, of operating microscopes, of implants and of viscoelastics.

Newly industrialized countries

The line that separates a developed from a developing nation is arbitrary. Newly Industrialized Countries (NICs), including South Korea, Taiwan, Hong Kong and Singapore, have the characteristics of a developed country, and are poised for further economic growth. In these countries there is an explosive demand for high technology. **Table 46.1** relates the implant experience of the Ministry of Health in Singapore.

There is great variation in the per capita income among the countries in Asia (**Table 46.2**). The NICs have improved communications, and now the population is well-informed concerning the miracles of modern technology. It has been predicted that soon the demand for implant surgery will spread to every major hospital throughout Asia, and it is only a matter of time before the wealthier countries meet the demand for implantation even in their rural communities. But what of the existing mass blindness? This will not be easily solved as the countries with poor economic development are likely to remain in a hopeless situation until they can be helped by their wealthier neighbors.

Table 46.1 Intraocular lens implants performed in Singapore*

Year	*No. of Implants*
1982	32
1983	154
1984	485
1985	1135
1986	2176
1987	4921
1988	6319

* Courtesy of the Ministry of Health, Republic of Singapore.

Table 46.2 Per capita income of Asian countries*

Country	*Per Capita Income (1985) (US$)*
Japan	8,316.00
Hongkong	6,311.00
Singapore	5,847.00
Taiwan	3,142.00
South Korea	1,954.00
Malaysia	1,574.60
Thailand	579.41
India	220.00
Nepal	139.00
Bangladesh	128.61

*Source: *Far Eastern Economic Review Asia Yearbook 1987* (the per capita incomes of Japan, South Korea and Taiwan have increased considerably more recently).

Low cost implant surgery

For those who accept the need for implant surgery, it is essential to minimize the cost yet maintain safety. With extracapsular cataract extraction (ECCE) and posterior chamber implants (PCI), the surgeon should be able to achieve 20/40 (6/12) vision or better in 95% of patients who have no other ocular pathology. The basic factors for success of ECCE and PCI are as follows:

- Trained microsurgeon.
- Good operating microscope with a coaxial light for the important red reflex to show up features not otherwise seen (**46.1–46.3**).
- Soft eye by compression for at least 10 minutes and a well-dilated pupil.
- Infusion fluid with 1:1,000,000 adrenaline to keep the pupil dilated (**46.4**).
- Can-opener method of anterior capsulectomy with the bent tip of a disposable needle (**46.5**).

46.1

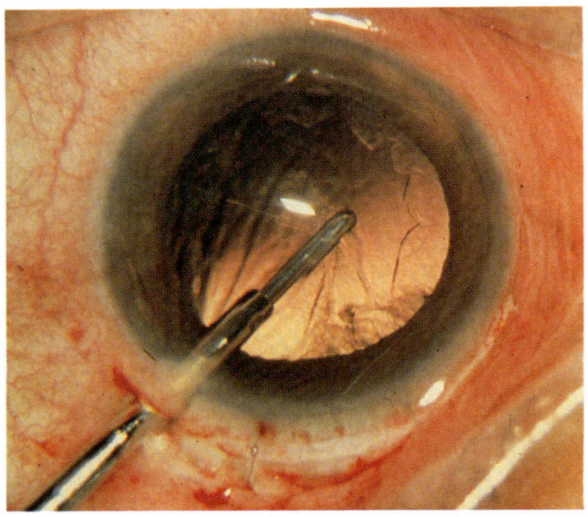

46.1 Radiating black lines converging on the aspirating port indicate that the posterior capsule is impacted into the aspirating port. The instrument must not be moved until aspiration is released, as movement may tear the posterior capsule. The edge of the anterior capsule and some cortex are also seen. Note the use of red reflex.

46.2

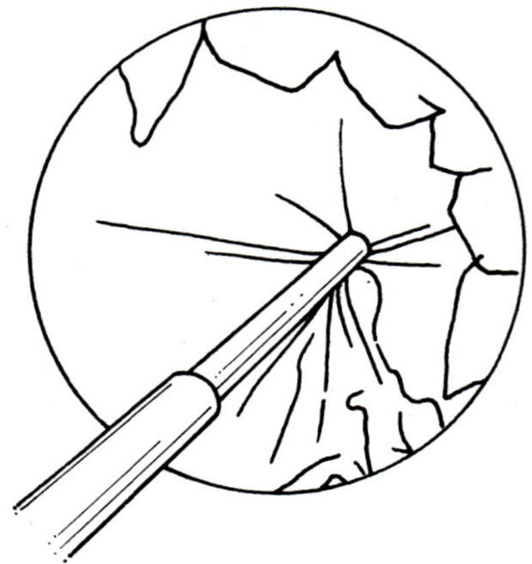

46.2 Diagram of **46.1**.

46.3

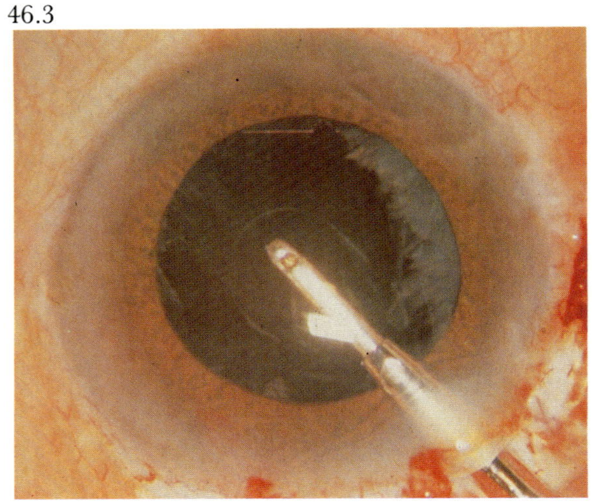

46.3 A ring reflex that surrounds the aspirating cannula is due to indentation of the posterior capsule by the aspirating cannula. It indicates that the posterior capsule is intact and bulging against the cannula.

46.4

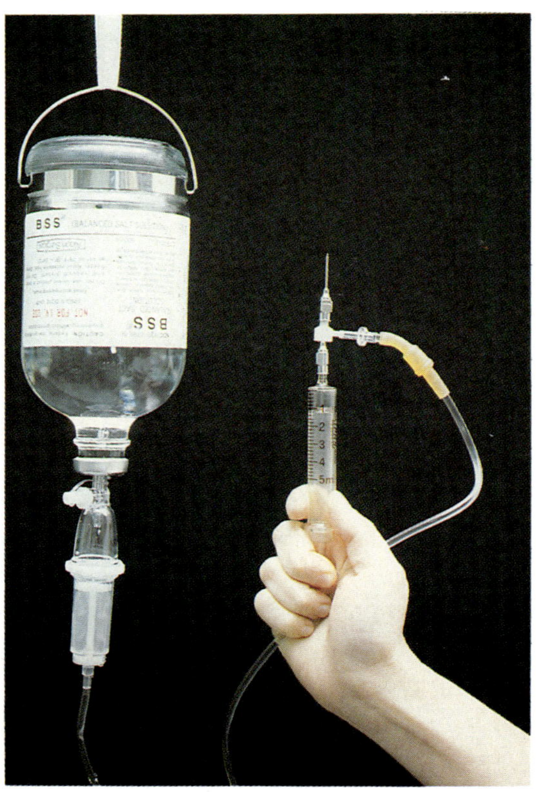

46.4 A balanced salt solution with adrenalin 1:1,000,000, suspended 600 mm above the eye. This irrigating solution flows into the infusion cannula through a nylon connector. A 5 ml syringe is connected to a McIntyre coaxial cannula. (Note the position of the hand to enable suction by moving the thumb and index fingers away from the palm.)

46.5

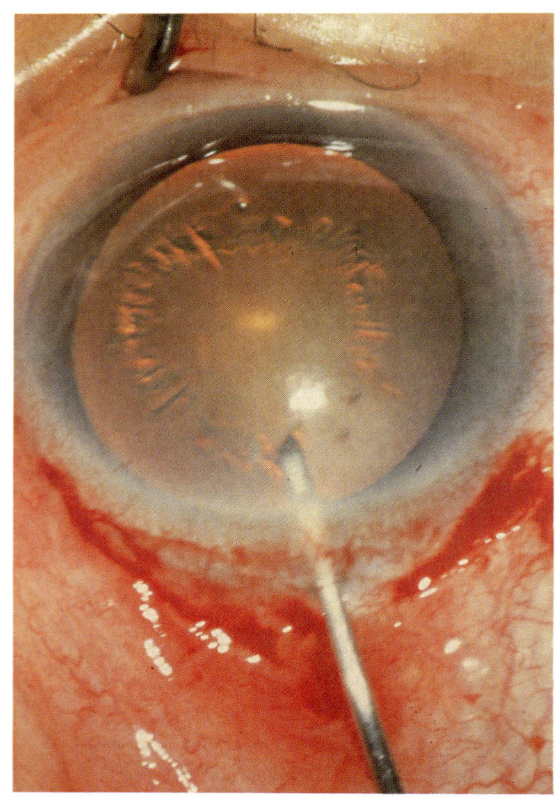

46.5 Forty small cuts on the anterior capsule made under an irrigating fluid with adrenalin 1:1,000,000, to maintain dilatation of the pupil.

- Cortex removal by nonautomated irrigation/aspiration (**46.6–46.9**).
- Sulcus placement may be favored by some surgeons beginning to learn ECCE (**46.10, 46.11**). This is useful when there is poor mydriasis, but see Chapter 14.

Some factors that contribute to expense may be considered useful but are not essential for successful surgery. These include the use of a diamond knife, viscoelastic material, BSS® or BSS PLUS®, mechanical aspiration and phacoemulsification.

46.6

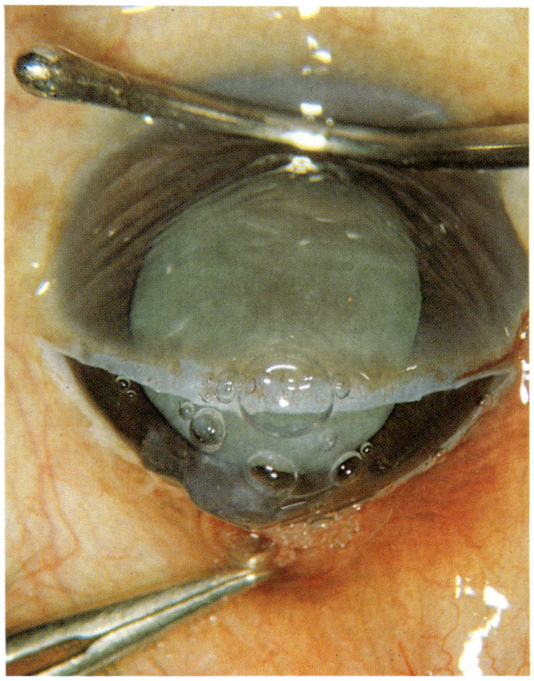

46.6 Expression of nucleus by gentle pressure inferiorly and counter pressure on the scleral lip superiorly. The instrument should not run across the center of the cornea.

46.7

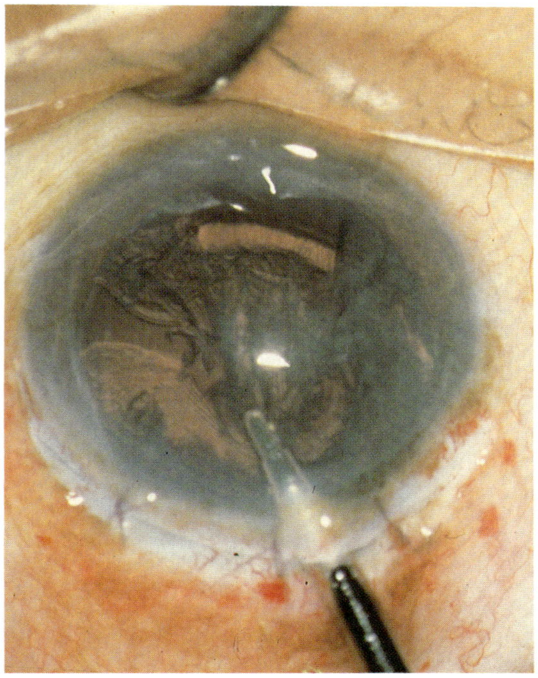

46.7 After closing the chamber with 2–4 sutures, the cortex is engaged with gentle suction using a 0.3 mm port and stripped from behind the anterior capsule and iris towards the center with a McIntyre coaxial cannula.

46.8

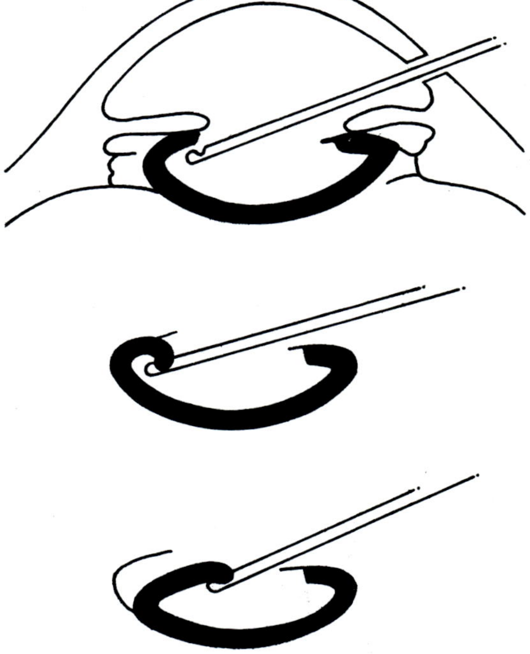

46.8 Diagram illustrating the procedure in **46.7**.

46.9

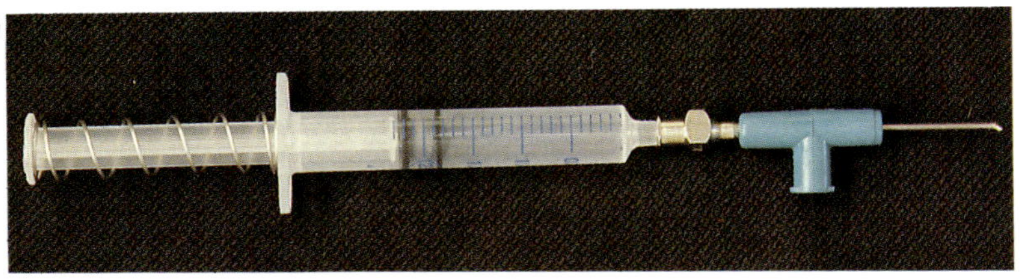

46.9 The Pearce coaxial cannula is very similar to the McIntyre coaxial cannula and may be used one-handed with a spring round the plunger to provide a controlled suction.

46.10

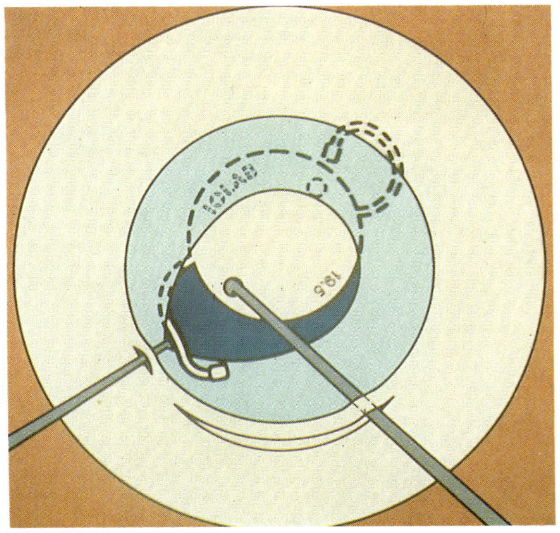

46.10 Two-handed insertion of an implant: After gliding the inferior loop behind the iris and placing the optic behind the pupil, the superior loop is placed behind the iris by dialling the optic with a Sinskey hook, while the other hand retracts the iris.

46.11

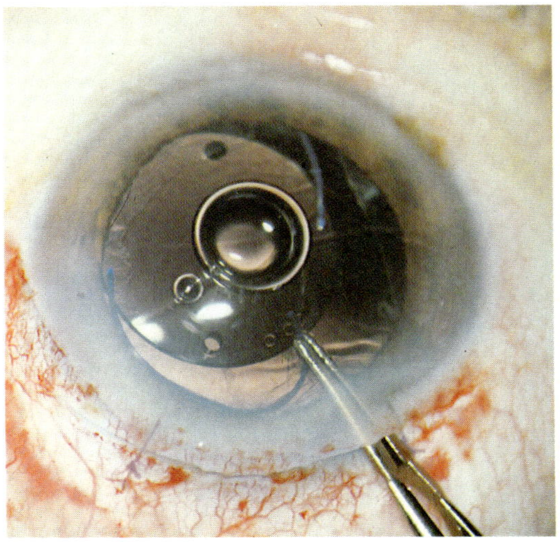

46.11 One-handed insertion of an implant by flexing the superior loop downwards with Kelman–McPherson forceps, then pronating the hand to allow the loop to slip behind the iris.

Further reading

Lim A.S.M. *A Colour Atlas of Posterior Chamber Implants,* Philadelphia: Saunders, 1985.

Lim A.S.M. Impact of technology on mass blindness in Asia. *Jpn J. Ophthalmol.,* **31,** 375–383, 1987.

Lim A.S.M. Holmes Lecture – the impact of rapid changes on management of blindness conditions. *Trans. 11th Asia–Pacific Academy of Ophthalmology,* pp 88–101, 1987.

Lim A.S.M. and Chiang C. Education – Review of low cost implant technique. *Implants in Ophthalmology,* **3,** 30–36, 1989.

Lim A.S.M. Ophthalmology in Asia in the year 2000, *Asia–Pacific J. Ophthalmology,* **1,** 18–21, 1989.

47: The problems of cataract surgery in developing countries

Mark Wood, Cosme Naval and Piers Percival

It is estimated that of 50 million cataract sufferers, there are 20 million in the world today who see less than 20/200 owing to bilateral cataract. Most of these are found among the 4000 million inhabitants of the so-called developing countries. The problems are:

- Lack of resources to meet the cost of capital equipment and the ongoing costs of disposables and implants.
- Inadeqiate infrastructure – often ophthalmology may not be covered by a country's health facilities in certain areas.
- A dearth of trained ophthalmologists prepared to help the masses of semiliterate blind in rural communities.
- Population longevity and the fact that, in tropical latitudes, cataract occurs earlier in life than in temperate zones. (In India, for the age range 50–65, the prevalence of cataract is six times that in North America).
- Dissatisfaction with aphakic spectacles. Although aphakic spectacles offer the cheapest form of optical correction following cataract surgery, the problems of accurate fitting, visual distortion and discomfort may lead to little motivation for replacement when they are scratched or broken.
- Impracticability of contact lenses because of the dry and dusty conditions, the scarcity of clean water, the inadequacy of personal hygiene and the expense of continual replacement.

Kenya

In Kenya the population is 22 million and there are approximately 30 trained ophthalmologists (but two-thirds are in private practise), yet the eye service there is considered to be better than in many other African states. Surveys performed between 1976 and 1983 revealed an incidence of acuity less than 10/200 (WHO definition of blindness) of 0.7%, and an incidence of acuity less than 20/200 (American definition of blindness) of 1.7%. This incidence is nine times that found in the USA. The incidence by cause is shown in **Table 47.1** and suggests that approximately 60,000 see less than 10/200 and 150,000 see less than 20/200 primarily because of cataract. Dr Randy Whitfield, working for the Kenya Ophthalmic Programme, in 1986 reported a total of 7,132 cataract operations in the fifteen units staffed by ophthalmologists and a further 1,223 performed by Clinical Officers outside these units. Clinical Officers usually do three years medical training, a further year in ophthalmology and, if selected for cataract surgery, another year of surgery at a recognized unit before they can work on their own. At the Kikuyu Eye Unit (**47.1**), as elsewhere in Kenya, uncomplicated cataracts are delegated to these Clinical Officers. Each year, 2000 surgical cases pass through the unit, but many are complicated eyes and these require the undivided attention of ophthalmologists. Ophthalmologists have little time for the additional burden of lens implantation and, at present, IOLs are unavailable unless donated from other countries.

47.1

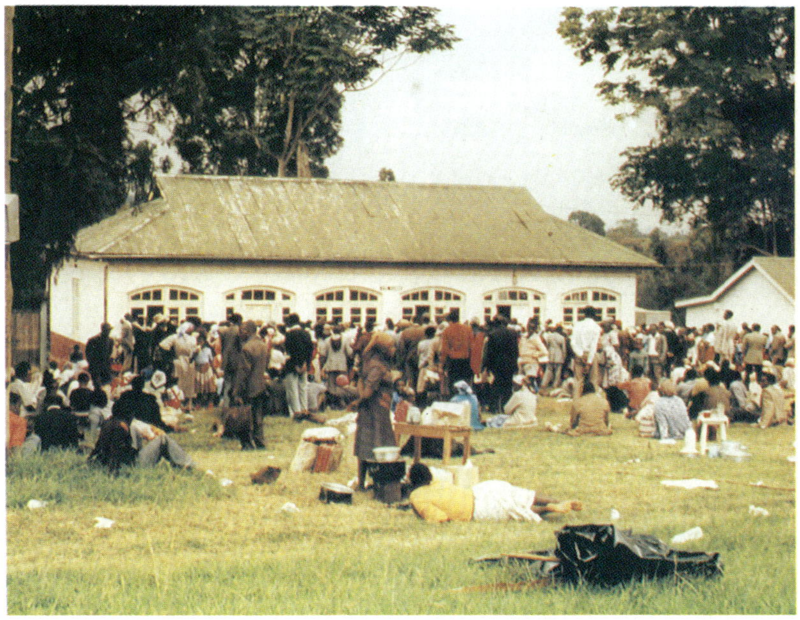

47.1 A routine clinic at the Kikuyu Eye Unit, Kenya.

Table 47.1 Causes of blindness in Kenya, 1983

Cataract	38%
Trachoma	19%
Glaucoma	9%
Senile macular degeneration	7%
Refractive error	6%
Other and unknown causes	21%

The Philippines

Salceda, Caparas and Alejo-Ramirez surveyed the cataract problem in the Philippines in 1988. Based on a nationwide survey conducted in 1987, they reported an incidence of blindness (inability to count fingers at a distance of 3 m) in 1.07% of the population. Of the blindness, 87% was due to cataract, implying that there were 502,860 Filipinos living blind from bilateral cataract; in some the cataract would be untreatable because of coexisting pathology, such as glaucoma. A questionnaire sent to the 271 practising eye surgeons revealed that only 5% of this half-a-million backlog was being tackled each year, and that 23% of surgeries were being performed without payment. Of the ophthalmologists, 80% practise only in the large cities and some practise routine lens implantation. However, 50% of the population are semiliterate and rural, often living in areas where the government health facilities do not include an ophthalmologist. Modern medicine, including lens implantation, may be brought to rural areas by nongovernmental organizations (**47.2, 47.3**), but this makes little inroad into the enormous backlog.

As a result of the survey, a national cataract program has now been proposed to encourage the contribution of existing ophthalmologists, as well as the services of third-year ophthalmic residents. The target is an additional 35,000 operations per year. Outreach to the under-privileged is possible, but requires a political will as well as serious technical, financial and administrative support.

47.2

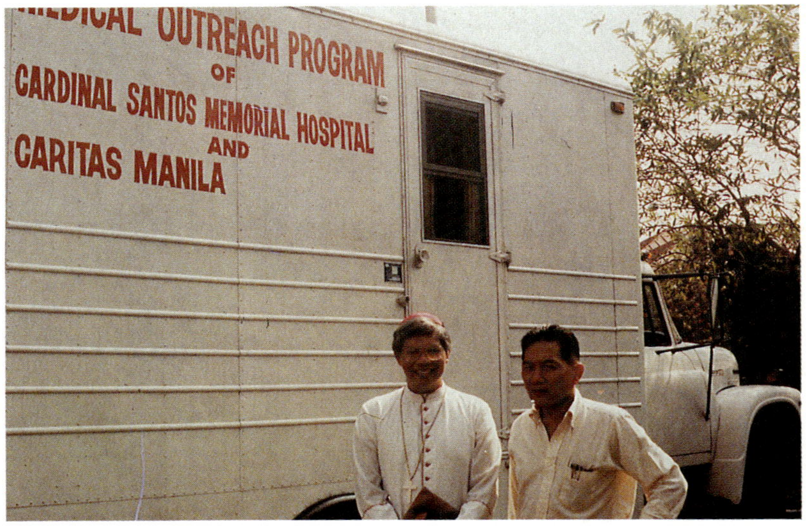

47.2 Mobile bus fully equipped for ECCE, donated by the Swiss Lenten Organisation to Caritas, Philippines, seen with Bishop Teodoro Buhain, Director of Caritas, and Dr C. Naval, in charge of the cataract mission to rural areas, where most of the funding for lens implantation comes from charity.

47.3

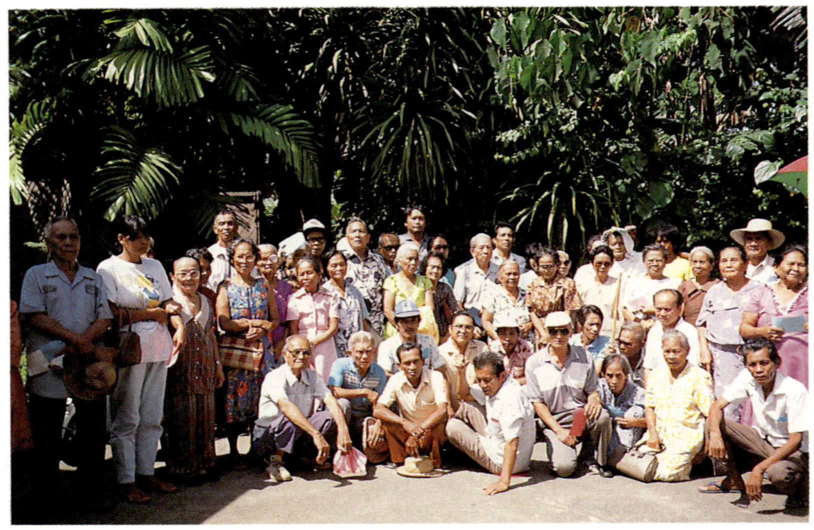

47.3 Four days work without trained assistance at a rural hospital in the Philippines.

Dilemmas and solutions

The above descriptions from two different countries give some insight into the massive problems that exist. Considering the time, training and expense, should implants even be considered? Yet is it fair to expect people contributing to the society of a country to work under the handicap of aphakia? Progress must be made and, assuming that IOLs provide the optimal method of visual rehabilitation, should they be used only by fully trained ophthalmic surgeons or should unqualified personnel be trained specifically for the purpose? Is it better to recommend intracapsular surgery with anterior chamber or iris claw lenses under loop magnification, or is it better to recommend extracapsular surgery with placement of the lens into the envelope of the lens capsule under microscopic control? The latter requires more dedicated training and more expensive equipment, but when correctly performed is safer for the patient and does not require follow-up care. Both methods will produce a proportion of patients whose vision will ultimately fail, but the relatively low incidence of capsular opacification after the safer method must be countered by the potentially serious hazards of glaucoma, uveitis and corneal decompensation more likely after the former method.

Clearly, there is a place for surgery without lens implantation by specifically trained personnel (as in Kenya) for the backlog of elderly people who may have little more to contribute to society. Implantation may be reserved for those still active in the community, and it is both feasible and practicable to train personnel specifically for this. Whether the well-tried intracapsular methods advocated by Daljet Singh of Amritsar, India, are superior to the extracapsular methods advocated by Lim (Chapter 47) and others in terms of cost effectiveness and patient tolerance, only time will tell.

Further reading

Pretorius, M. A practical guide for IOL surgery and study of anterior chamber IOL *vs* posterior chamber IOL in third world countries. *Implants in Ophthalmology*, **3,** 68–70, 1989.

Young P.W. and Schwab L. Intraocular lens implantation in developing countries. *Ophthal. Surg.*, **20,** 241–244, 1989.

48: Low cost surgery

Piers Percival

The aim of this atlas has been to provide clear guidance as to those methods that are both effective and safe for surgeons training themselves in the practise of IOL implantation. Sophisticated techniques have evolved to give a high precision routine for cataract surgery. Phacoemulsification inside the bag of the lens capsule or after continuous circular capsulorhexis is ideal when combined with small incision surgery. However, it should be appreciated that not all the methods that appear to be the most advanced are necessarily the most effective. Examples of such advanced methods and their disadvantages may be listed:

- Small incision surgery is technically more difficult because of the reduced arc of instrumentation available.
- 'Small incision lenses', or foldable IOLs, when rolled or folded may have the overall diameter reduced from 6.5 to 3 mm, but in the rolled or folded form the lens may still require a wound of 4 mm in length for insertion. There may be doubt whether the reduction from 10 mm, the incision length necessary for standard ECCE, has much influence on postoperative events. Introduction of a lens in its flat state is theoretically safer for the cornea.
- Automated lens irrigation/aspiration (I/A) requires a high volume of irrigating fluid, which can have disastrous consequences on the corneal endothelium, especially if phacoemulsification is used with a prolonged irrigation time or with hard nuclear fragments bouncing in the anterior chamber. Foot control of I/A is less sensitive and less adaptable when complications arise than is finger control.
- BSS® is 16 times more expensive than lactated Ringer's, and has little proven advantage clinically, when low volume irrigating methods are used.
- The routine use of viscoelastic agents is expensive, but this and the possible rise of intraocular pressure may be outweighed by the need. A soft eye may be consistently achieved by peribulbar anesthesia with a 20-minute oculocompression and, except in complicated cases, this will obviate that need. Low-cost viscoelastics, such as the polycarbonate Cellugel®, are included in **Table 22.1** (p. 139).
- The routine use of intracameral acetylcholine or carbachol is expensive, and is unjustified since when the lens is placed in the capsular bag there is no iris touch and there is no need for intraoperative miosis.

However, safety should not be compromised by oversimplification. There are still areas in the world where, although cataract is the most common cause of blindness (**48.1**), treated cataract may be the second most common cause. Disasters may be prevented by ensuring that the surgeon is properly equipped with basic tools (**48.2**) and does not rely on outmoded methods, which although possibly quicker or cheaper, defeat their object by producing unreliable results. The following essentials are recommended for any surgeon seriously considering IOL implantation.

48.1

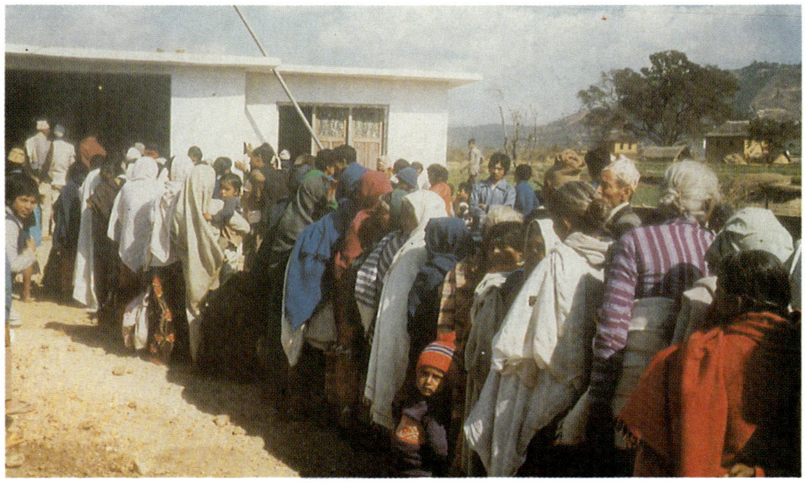

48.1 Patients waiting for treatment in Nepal (courtesy of Dr Jan Worst, The Netherlands).

48.2

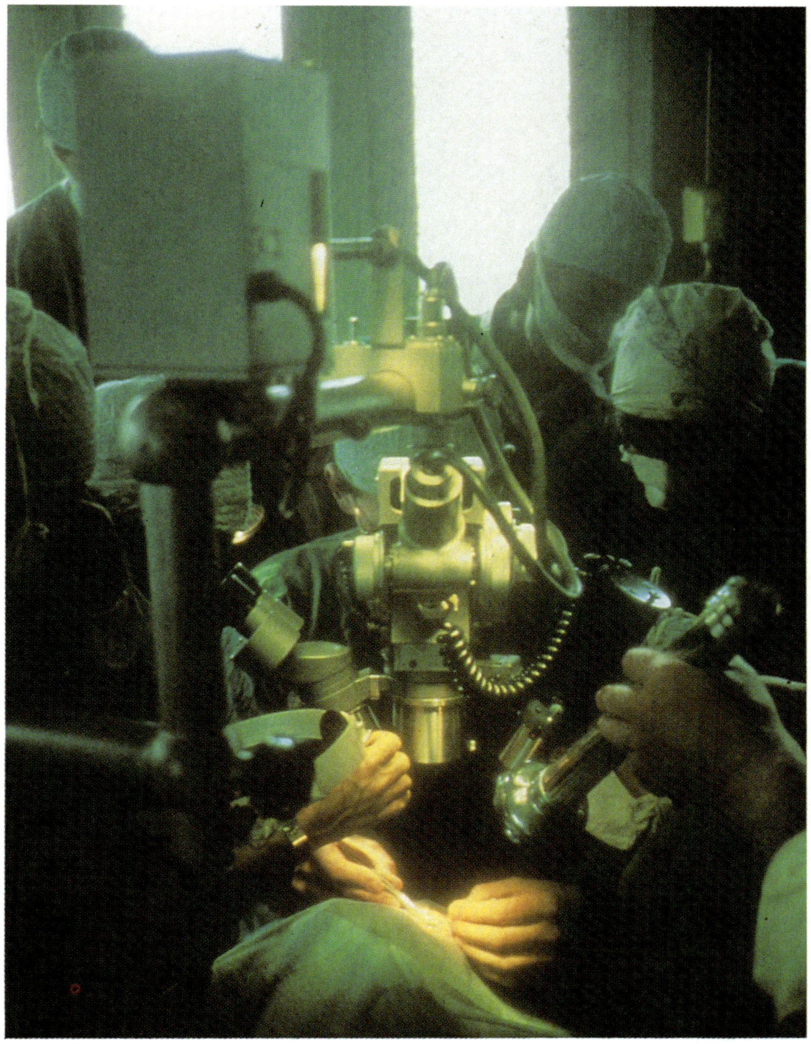

48.2 Dr Jan Worst teaching microsurgery in Nepal

Essentials for cost effective surgery

- A clean operating field. Note that a polythene drape (**48.3**) is necessary to prevent the implant from touching the lid margin during its insertion.
- A coaxial operating microscope (**48.2**). Although an expensive outlay, the advantages are incision control, easier hemostasis, accuracy of suturing, visibility and elimination of foreign particles, early diagnosis and treatment of intraoperative complications, accuracy of IOL placement and greater surgical confidence. Routine ECCE should not be attempted without a microscope.
- Peribulbar local anesthesia should be recommended for all except the mentally disturbed, uncooperative or very nervous. An oral premedication, such as temazepam 10 mg, may be given one hour before surgery. Thirty minutes before surgery take 1500 units of hyaluronidase and dissolve this in a 20 ml bottle of lignocaine 2% with adrenaline 1:200,000 (the adrenaline is optional). This will provide for 10 cases. Using a 10 ml syringe, withdraw 2 ml and add 5 ml of plain bupivacaine 0.5%. Inject 3.5 ml of this mixture above the orbital floor infratemporally (**48.4**) and 3.5 ml below the orbital roof superomedially (**48.5**) (see also pp 170–171). Cover with a pad and simple oculopressor, such as the Honan Balloon, for 20–30 min at 30–35 mmHg (**48.6**). This method obviates the need for a facial block and will guarantee a soft eye at surgery.

48.3

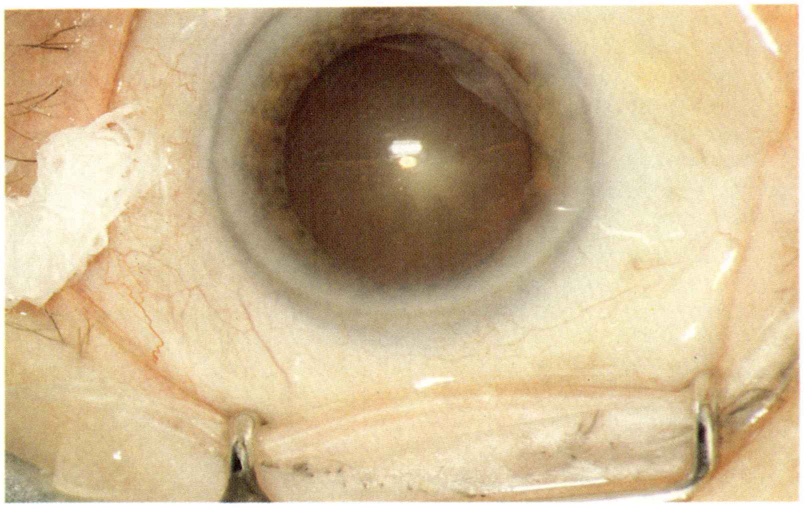

48.3 A clean field. Note that a polythene drape is reflected under the upper lid margin, that the corner of a gauze swab acts as a wick to drain any excess fluid from the conjunctival sac, and that the exposure is adequate without a superior rectus suture.

48.4

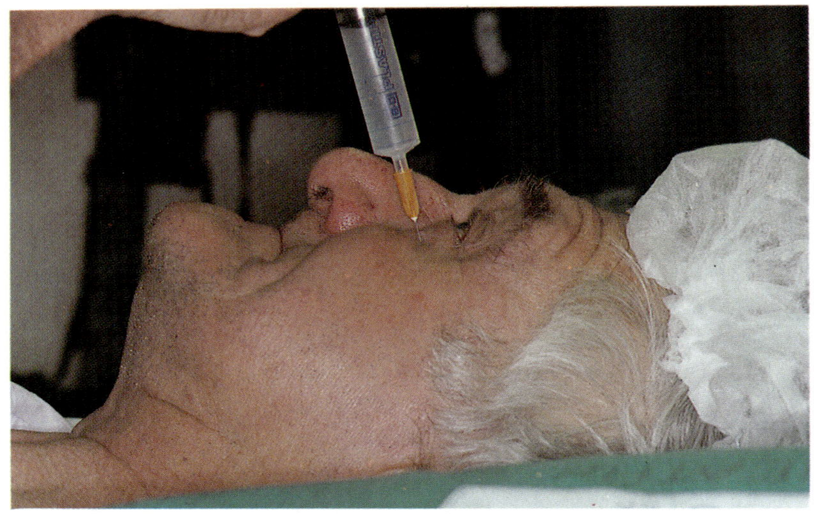

48.4 Peribulbar anesthesia: the needle is directed posteriorly.

48.5

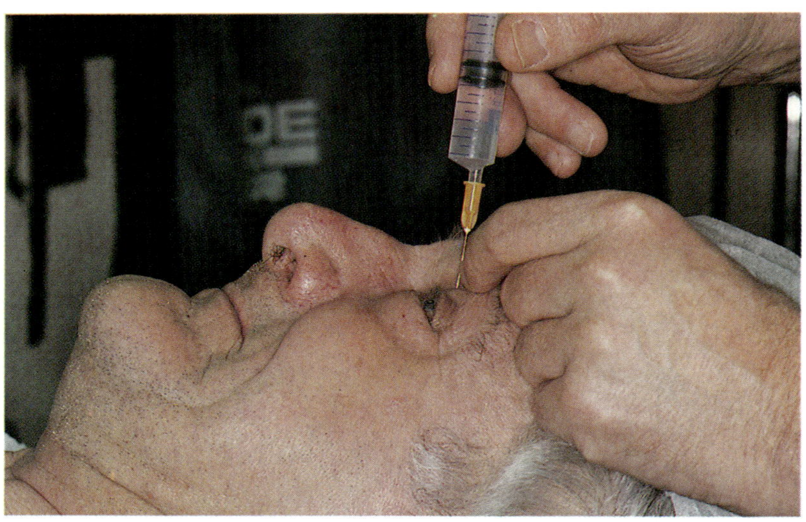

48.5 Peribulbar anesthesia: the needle is directed posteromedially.

48.6

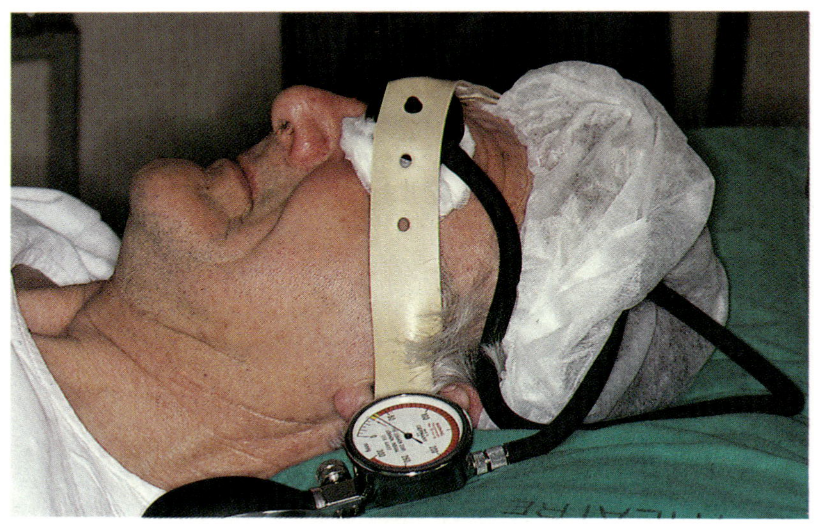

48.6 Honan Balloon applied for the duration of the preceeding operation.

- The extracapsular approach's advantages over the intracapsular's are a shorter wound, simpler instrumentation (**48.7**), fewer postoperative complications, secure compartmentalization of the eye without the worry that the vitreous face may protrude, IOL stability, physiologic positioning of the IOL and a reduced need for postoperative visits. Postoperative capsule opacification can be minimized by IOL selection (see p. 285) and the duration of surgery can be averaged at under 15 minutes.
- Hand-held instruments for nucleus and cortex extraction (**48.8**), although disposable, usually may be reautoclaved until blocked or broken. For low-volume irrigation Hartman's (lactated Ringer's) solution is safe, 1 liter lasting for more than 10 cases (**48.9**).

48.7

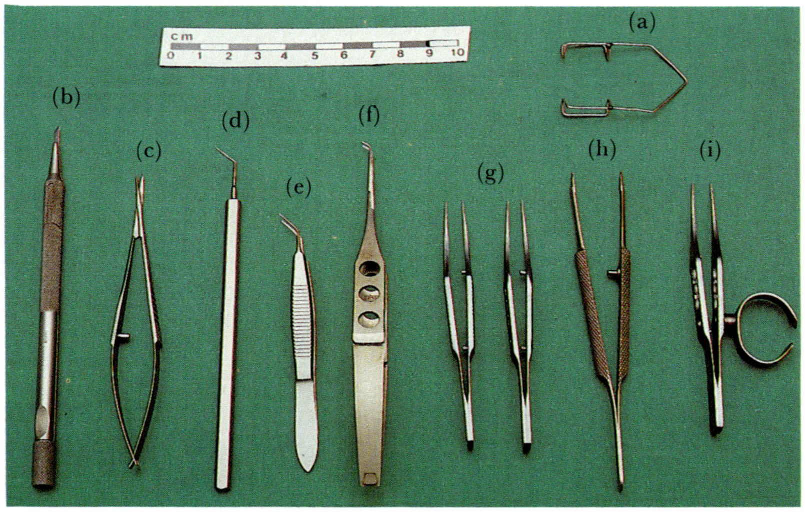

48.7 Basic setting for the envelope method of ECCE: (a) Wire speculum; (b) Disposable blade on a holder for incision (if diamond unavailable) and cutting suture material; (c) Fine curved capsulotomy scissors for cutting the capsule after lens implantation; (d) Sinskey dialling hook; (e) Kelman–McPherson forceps; (f) Clayman lens introducing forceps; (g) Pair of titanium suture tying forceps with platforms; (h) Needle holder; (i) Atraumatic notched forceps. Additional instruments that may be necessary include: artery forceps; superior rectus forceps; straight scissors; small gallipots; micropore sponges.

48.8

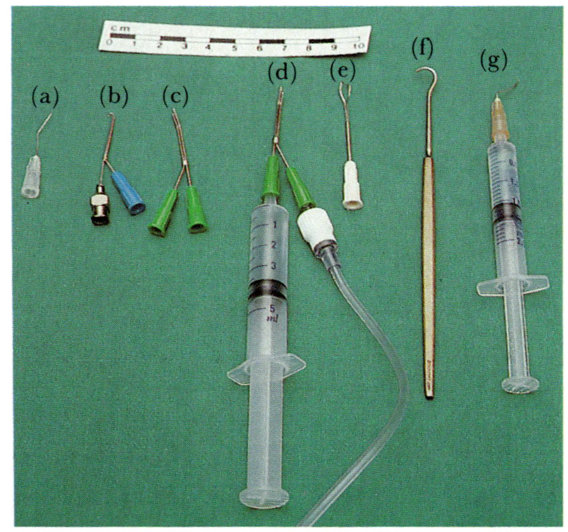

48.8 Hand-held instruments for lens extraction: (a) 30-gauge cannula for reformation of the anterior chamber; (b) J-shaped double cannula for aspiration at 12 o'clock; (c) Double cannula with the aspirating port pointing to the right – the tips have been bent with artery forceps to overcome problems of a deep set eye (the Simcoe cannulas are a useful alternative as is also the McIntyre coaxial cannula, see **46.4**); (d) Pearce double cannula: the irrigating arm is fed by a connecting tube to a drip, the aspirating cannula with a 0.3 mm port pointing to left is attached to a 5 ml syringe; (e) Anis irrigating vectis; (f) Lens expressor; (g) Capsulotomy needle on 2 ml syringe.

48.9

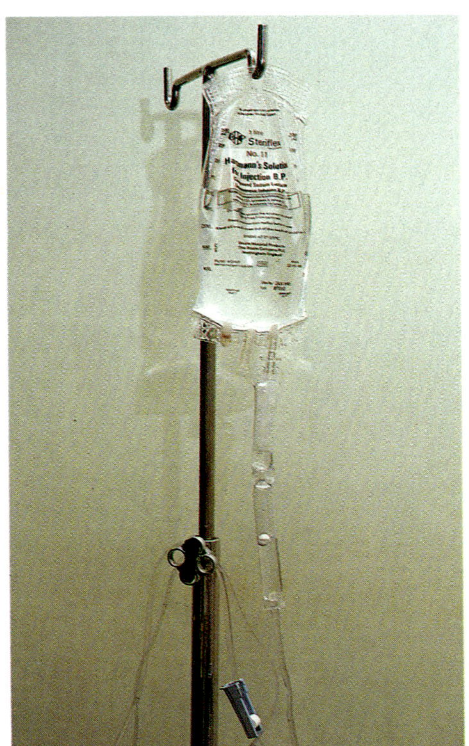

48.9 1 liter of Hartman's solution into which has been injected 1 ml of 1:1000 adrenaline, with an intravenous setting for adjusting the flow. An additional connector tubing should be changed for each case.

48.10

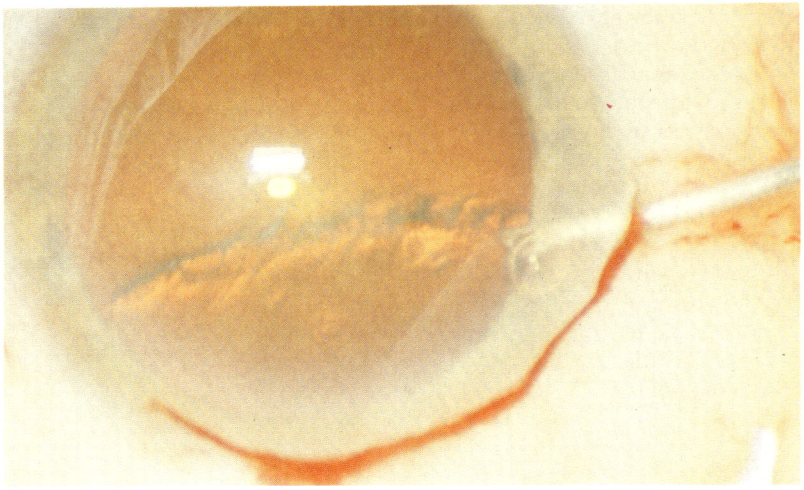

48.10 A linear capsulotomy.

48.11

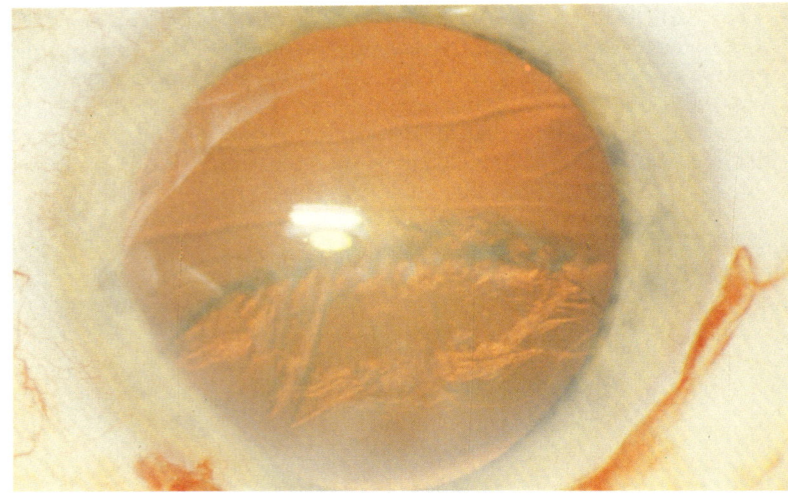

48.11 Using a lens expressor inferiorly (not shown) and counter pressure superiorly with vectis, the nucleus can be seen to prolapse through the linear opening.

48.12

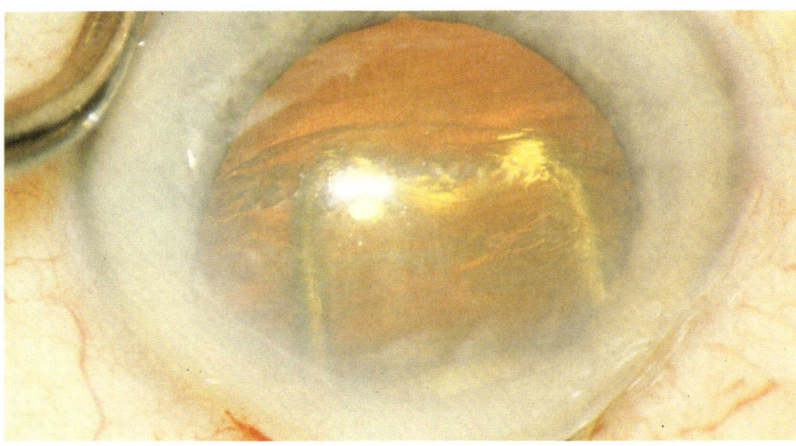

48.12 The nucleus may then be lifted out of the eye with an Anis irrigating vectis. The cornea is neither indented nor reflected.

48.13

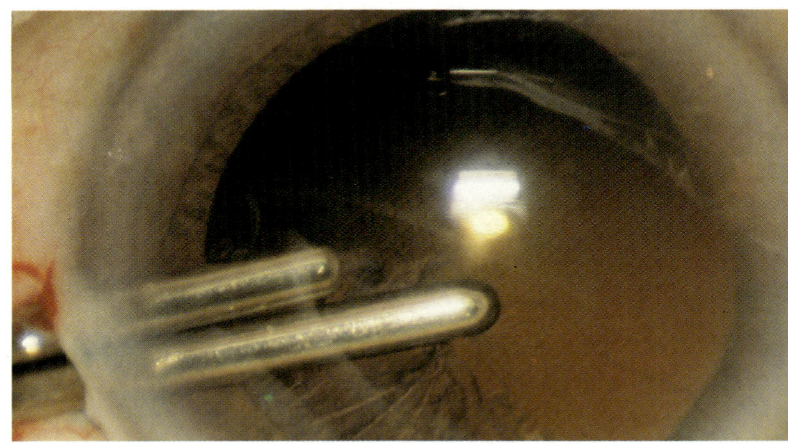

48.13 For removal of the cortex at 12 o'clock, the double cannula may be inserted temporally, with the aspirating port pointing up underneath the upper flap of capsule. Note, in this example, the radiating lines at the aspirating port that indicate posterior capsule capture and necessitate immediate reversal of aspiration (see also **46.1**).

48.14

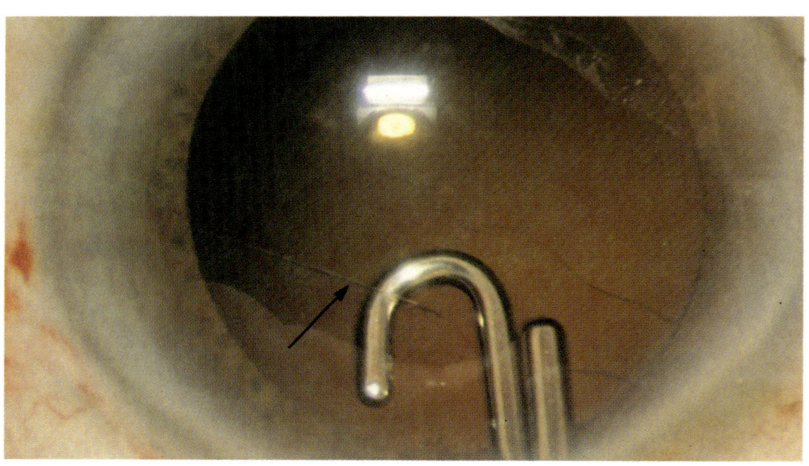

48.14 The use of a J-shaped cannula is an alternative for aspiration at 12 o'clock. The J is placed underneath the rim of of the anterior capsule (arrow).

48.15

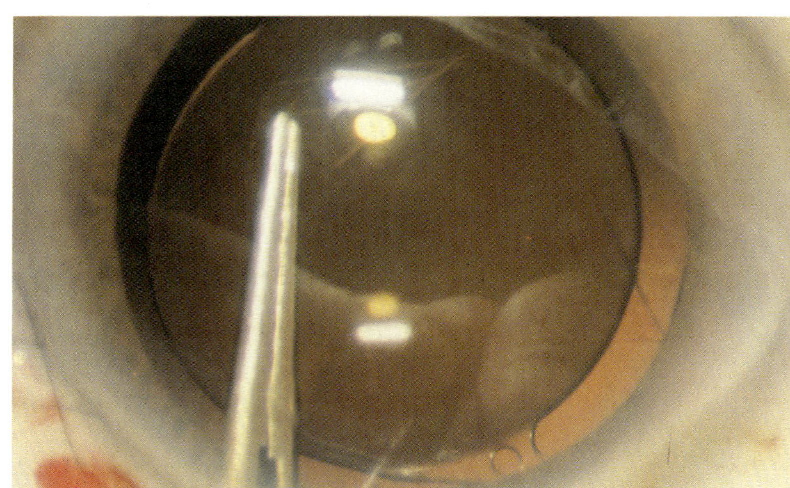

48.15 After placement of the IOL in the capsular sac and incision to one side of the anterior capsule, smooth capsulorhexis is completed with Kelman–McPherson forceps.

- Lens placement into the capsular sac rather than the ciliary sulcus will avoid erosions into the iris or ciliary body, granulomatous reactions, iris capture, and pigment dispersion glaucoma. The intercapsular (envelope) method (**48.10–48.15**) has the advantages of protection of intraocular structures during surgery, near certainty of IOL placement, and retention of the anterior capsule to support a sulcus-placed IOL in the event of posterior capsule rupture. Continuous circular capsulorhexis offers the surest method for total capsular fixation and perfect centration.
- An autoclave: Expediency cannot be compromised by the risk of infection or the intraocular introduction of toxic chemicals.
- Lens power calculation: Axial length biometry and choice of lens power have transformed cataract surgery into an art whereby large numbers of patients do not require glasses after surgery. Even high refractive errors may be fully corrected and the use of astigmatic techniques and bifocal implants heighten further the achievements that are now possible.
- A diamond knife gives a clean and well-sutured wound that is a prerequisite for trouble-free convalescence. Scissors crush and stainless steel is insufficiently sharp. A diamond, if carefully cleaned in salt-free fluid (e.g., distilled water) under the microscope by the surgeon, will repay an endless dividend of satisfaction for upwards of 500 cases.

Armed with the tools that are right and aided by a specialist nurse who will care for the instruments, the surgeon rapidly improves in confidence, temperament and enjoyment of the work that has to be done. Attention to detail and prevention of problems before they occur are essential to success and nowhere in the world should this be impossible.

Further reading

Lim A.S.M. and Chiang C. Education – Review of low cost implant techniques. *Implants in Ophthalmology*, **3,** 30–36, 1989.

Percival P. Low cost surgery on Mindanao: a Third World initiative from the UK. *Implants in Ophthalmology*, **4,** 22–26, 1990.

Appendix I

Visual Acuity Equivalents

Distance at 6 m			*Near at 35 cm*	
America	*UK*	*Europe*	*Jaeger*	*Point size*
20/20	6/6	1.0		
20/30	6/9	0.66	J1	N4.5
20/40	6/12	0.5	J3	N6
20/60	6/18	0.33	J6	N9
20/80	6/24	0.25	J8	N12
20/100		0.2		
20/200	6/60	0.1	J16	N24

Index

References are given by page number where illustrations are supplemented by information in the text or where information is solely textual. Bold figures refer to illustration numbers by chapter and refer to specific illustrative features only.